NURSING IN SOCIETY
A HISTORICAL PERSPECTIVE

FIFTEENTH EDITION

JOSEPHINE A. DOLAN, R.N., M.S., Pd.D.
Professor Emeritus and Special Lecturer, University of Connecticut

M. LOUISE FITZPATRICK, R.N., M.A., Ed.D., F.A.A.N.
Dean and Professor, College of Nursing, Villanova University

ELEANOR KROHN HERRMANN, R.N., M.S., Ed.D.
Associate Professor, School of Nursing, Yale University

W. B. SAUNDERS COMPANY
PHILADELPHIA • LONDON • TORONTO • MEXICO CITY • RIO DE JANEIRO • SYDNEY • TOKYO

W. B. Saunders Company: **W. B. SAUNDERS COMPANY**
Harcourt Brace Jovanovich, Inc.

The Curtis Center
Independence Square West
Philadelphia, PA 19106

Listed here is the latest translated edition of this book together with the language of the translation and the publisher.

Japanese (13th Edition)—Seishin Shobo Ltd., Tokyo, Japan

Library of Congress Cataloging in Publication Data

Dolan, Josephine A.
Nursing in society.

Includes bibliographies and index.
1. Nursing—History. 2. Nursing—Social aspects—History. I. Fitzpatrick, Louise. II. Herrmann, Eleanor. III. Title. [DNLM: 1. History of nursing. WY 11.1 D659n]
RT31.D64 1983 362.1'73 82-48503
ISBN 0-7216-3135-5

Cover Illustration: St. Sebastian Nursed by St. Irene

Artist: Georges de La Tour

Founders Society Purchase, Ralph Harman Booth Bequest Fund

Nursing in Society ISBN 0-7216-3135-5

Last digit is the print number: 9 8 7

PREFACE

The fifteenth edition of *Nursing in Society* continues the ongoing presentation of the proud heritage of nursing since the inception of this book by Miss Minnie Goodnow in 1916. This new edition welcomes two nurse historian contributors, Dr. M. Louise Fitzpatrick and Dr. Eleanor Herrmann.

This book is designed to meet the need for a concise yet systematic history of nursing for those who wish to orient themselves in this field of endeavor without perusing extensive and detailed documents. To meet this objective the book has been written for the student of nursing, the busy practitioner of nursing and other members of the health team as well as persons interested in the evolution of health fields.

The fascinating story of the evolution, emergence and expansion of nursing from a simple practical skill to a complex profession has been compressed into sixteen chapters. Nursing is depicted against the societal setting and the cultural and scientific background of the history of mankind. Nursing history is linked to social history, and the title of the book is a reflection of this relationship, as are the chapter titles.

The story of nursing is recounted not as the chronological reporting of events and personalities but as an interpretation of the response of nurses to the needs of people for retaining, attaining and/or regaining health as well as for care during sickness. From the farthest reaches of time, in the most primitive settings, the nurturing efforts and independent role of the nurse in response to survival needs were directed toward keeping people healthy as well as comforting the sick. The development of this wellness-illness component of nursing is woven throughout the chapter contents.

The emergence of nurses, their freedom or restraints to practice, their status, their successes or failures, their recognition of opportunities for progress or unwillingness to remove obstacles to achieve a high quality of care are described in the chapter summaries entitled *The Heritage of Nursing*. Here the image that nurses have portrayed over the years is summarized. Each opening chapter illustration focuses on the continuous strong leadership of nurses in response to human needs in the societal setting of the period.

In this edition the concept of history of nursing has been broadened to include *nursing anthropology*. Chapters 2 and 3 focus on ancient cultures and the response to cultural diversity that has resulted in transcultural nursing. These aspects of understanding those who are served as well as those who serve unite in historical and anthropological significance. There is stronger documentation of the role and status of nurses from primary source materials. Information on the significance of our long historical contribution has been enhanced.

Religious influences played an important role in emphasizing the plight of the sick and poor and the need for human dignity, in elevating the status of women, in encouraging men to select nursing as a career and in stimulating the emergence of dynamic nurse leadership. Those recruited to nursing were socially skilled, intellectually endowed and as knowledgeable scientifically as the times permitted. The sound independent and interdisciplinary approach to client care has been researched in greater depth.

The cover depicts the famous painting by Georges de La Tour, now housed in the Detroit Institute of Arts. It was selected because of its beauty and its symbolic representation. St. Irene is providing independent nursing care in an emergency situation. The light is symbolic of nursing. It has been associated with those great nurses who have brought and still bring *light* into an otherwise dark period of travail; who *lighten* many another's sorrows and fears; who *enlighten* those in need of knowledge of health and illness; and who make another's load *lighter* by assuming the task, like Simon of Cyrene, of helping to carry a person's burden. The *light* of compassion, refreshment and peace has *glowed* through time because of many a caring nurse. It is of interest that the works of art, by great artists, that depicted the importance of St. Irene caring for St. Sebastian were painted in the 17th century on the basis of early Christian documentation. When the bubonic plague of that period struck victims like arrows entering their bodies, they began pleading to St. Sebastian to intercede for their recovery. The great artists of the period researched and found that a nurse, St. Irene, was a potent force in St. Sebastian's care.

It has been recognized that many current problems have deep roots in the past and have been perpetuated by tradition. To assist in achieving an understanding of our current plight in education for practice as well as in professional collaboration for greater client accountability and satisfaction, many new data have been included. An expansion in the historical coverage of the progress and problems of nursing education has been incorporated, as have the highlights and impact of studies of nursing, recognition of the other health professions, and collaborative opportunities. Also emphasized is the ongoing struggle to retain professional autonomy to provide true professional nursing care and thus support efforts to achieve client accountability.

There has been an attempt to orient the reader to the recurring issues of the present by recounting the recognition of these problems by nurses in the past as well as their successes in wrestling with similar perplexing situations. A selective process had to be utilized in the interest of accomplishing a concise presentation of this significant field. The authors recognize the important contributions of many past and present individuals and groups whose achievements it has not been possible to include.

In a book of this size, an attempt to cover all important contributions is necessarily curtailed. Thus, only certain highlights of each period can be presented. The chapters have been rearranged to produce a more logical sequential development. There is greater emphasis on the emergence of the role and function of the nurse and the delivery of nursing services, especially in the last one hundred years.

Extensive revisions have caused deletion of some material and replacement by more significant data in focusing on present-day nursing. Many new illustrations enhance the visual presentation and serve as an elaboration of the content.

The explosive force of constantly advancing scientific knowledge and the electrifying influence of quick communication of new discoveries and developments have changed the frontiers of civilization. Recorders and interpreters of history can describe only briefly the most important aspects of human development in one small volume. In a review of the wealth of books and articles, only the most pertinent could be mentioned.

It is hoped that this book will increase understanding of the relationships of the physical, biological, psychological, social, cultural and spiritual aspects of life to nursing as a humanistic science and will enable the student to see the correlation between these and the role of the nurse.

Grateful appreciation is due to the many persons who have generously assisted in the location of new data, in granting permission to use material, and in reading, criticizing and preparing the manuscript for publication. We are deeply grateful to the Detroit Institute of Art for permission to reproduce the de La Tour for the cover of this book. Our deepest gratitude is extended to Ms. Katherine Pitcoff, Nursing Editor, W. B. Saunders, for her inspiration, support, patience and assistance in our efforts.

We sincerely hope that with all its limitations *Nursing in Society* will stimulate an appreciation and pride in the heritage of nursing.

JOSEPHINE A. DOLAN

M. LOUISE FITZPATRICK

ELEANOR K. HERRMANN

CONTENTS

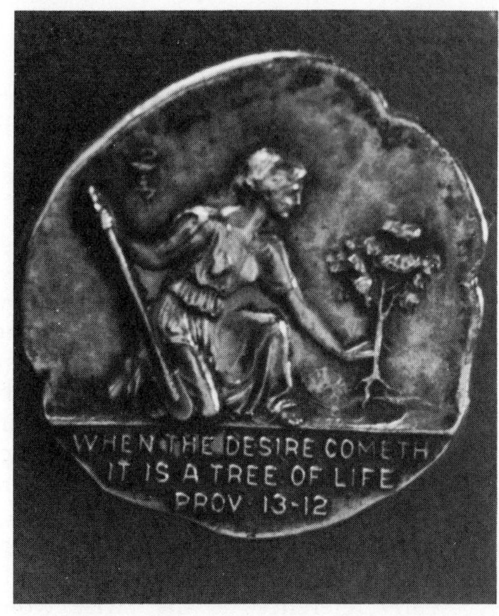
WHEN THE DESIRE COMETH
IT IS A TREE OF LIFE
PROV 13-12

A symbolic representation of the nurse's timeless nurturing skills, on the pin of the National Organization for Public Health Nursing. (Dolan collection.)

1 The Genesis of Nursing

Nursing as an art to be cultivated and a profession to be followed is modern; nursing as a practice originated in the dim past where some mother among the cave dwellers cooled the forehead of her sick child with water from the brook. . . .

Sir William Osler[1]

The task of identifying and describing the emergence of the role of nursing in the history of humanity is truly a monumental one. There is no way to document the existence of this form of nurturing during prerecorded history, except for the indisputable fact of the survival of the human race. Nursing emerged with the inception of the history of humanity and has been essential for the ongoing sustenance of the human race. From the dawn of civilization the *art of nurturing* has been *essential to the preservation of life*.

Throughout time there have been needs basic to the maintenance of life, and concern for these has formed the unique components of nursing.[2] Provision for these needs continues to challenge families, communities and deliverers of health care.

ROLE OF THE NURSE

Nursing evolved as an *intuitive* response to the desire to keep people *healthy* as well as to provide comfort, care and assurance to the sick. This response emanated from certain women who proved to be particularly adept at providing a healthy home environment, protecting children and caring for elderly and sick members of families. They shared their services with neighbors during periods of illness. One can imagine that the nurse figure in the community was a very capable, concerned and compassionate woman who assumed the nurse role as a societal assignment. Some "nurses" were much more effective than others in coping with people and their personal and family crises. Nursing was not a role expected of

[1]Osler, William: *Aequanimitas*. Philadelphia, Blakiston Co., 1932, p. 156.

[2]Henderson, Virginia: *Basic Principles of Nursing Care*. London, International Council of Nurses, 1960, pp. 9, 10.

all women; it was assumed by those who had the desire and ability to truly nurture.

INCEPTION OF A KNOWLEDGE BASE

The first nurses were independent "generalists" who had the freedom of action to be as creative as their intellectual and personal skills permitted. Although their initial response was intuitive, new information was discovered through problem solving and a body of knowledge gradually developed and expanded. The incorporation of this knowledge into the overall nurturing effort may have accounted for very early references to the "wise women" of the community.

The necessity of teaching was an important ingredient of nursing from earliest times. The early nurses taught clients as well as successors and passed on the accumulated knowledge orally and therefore by tradition.

The essence of their service was reflected in the *caring-curing* component of commitment to the person who needed the special knowledge and skills of the nurse. Assessment of these needs preceded a regimen, the ingredients of which included warmth, sincerity of manner, listening, comforting, reassuring, nourishing, cleansing and simple procedures for the care of the sick.

The positive action of nurses involved the recognition of the need for maintenance of health (attaining, retaining and/or regaining health) in addition to caring for, and consoling the ill and the uncomfortable.

Empirical Practices

Intuitively, the nurse figure found foods for as balanced a diet as possible. She even discovered that certain foods were poisonous and investigated until she was skillful at withdrawing the deleterious substances from the staple items in the diet. During this process, she ascertained that certain foods caused vomiting or diarrhea, and this knowledge then formed a part of her folk healing. She also selected such natural objects as seeds, nuts, leaves, roots, herbs and bark from trees and devised ways of extracting medicinal ingredients from these raw materials. Because of their value, these folk remedies and plant lore have been passed on through the ages. Many of these herbal remedies have been used throughout the centuries. The value of natural products continues to be recognized, and they form the basis of many modern-day medicines.

Tenderness, concern, love and hope were expressed in simple remedies, such as touching (laying on of hands), rubbing a painful area or aching body with soft motions, applying heat or cold and concocting herbal mixtures. Herbal teas and ointments were compounded from products of nature, and recipes were treasured by families through the years. Thus, *empirical practices* in nursing evolved.

In retrospect this nurse figure performed the duties not only of nurse but also of nutritionist, pharmacist, physical therapist and social welfare worker. The setting for the delivery of care was the home.

ANCIENT THEORIES OF DISEASE

Many baffling problems needed to be studied and solved; among them was the cause of sickness. External causative factors of trauma or illness, such as a fall that resulted in a noticeable bruised area, could be seen or understood (although malevolent forces were blamed for causing the fall). However, humans were baffled and bewildered by spontaneous illness. The sudden ache inside the body, the paroxysms of sharp and throbbing pain, the inability to retain the food, the loss of sight, the muscular spasms and the loss of movement of one side of the body with concomitant loss of vocal expression were incomprehensible and were considered to have supernatural causes.

Ancient disease concepts appeared to be associated with the following areas:

1. *Sorcery*. A sorcerer had the ability to use magical ritual formulas to compel the supernatural forces to produce injury, disease or even death in another person. This power over another was associated with the ability to "hex," or to cast an evil spell. As a consequence, the fear-ridden body of the victim reflected physiological disor-

ders. In many cultures children were considered to be particularly susceptible.

2. *Magic.* There were two types of magic—*homeopathic* (imitative) and *contagious.* In homeopathic magic it was assumed that things that resembled each other were the same. Therefore, one injured an image of one's enemy in the belief that consequently the victim would be injured. Contagious magic assumed that things once in contact with a person remained always in contact, and therefore what was done to one affected the other. It was believed that a person should never permit himself to become dissociated from any part of his body because of the danger of someone's gaining control of him and working his occult powers. In many cultures the shaman or root doctor was believed to possess countermagic.

3. *Breaking a Taboo.* A person was believed to be automatically punished if he broke a taboo. The cultural acceptance of this fate was so strong that the person often wasted away for no apparent reason.

4. *Intrusion of a Disease Object.* Illness was believed to be induced by the entrance into the body of some small object. Its removal was accomplished by the medicine man's sucking it out and then removing it from his own mouth. When the power of suggestion seemed to have motivated the illness, the sight of an object's being removed had a healing effect on the victim.

5. *Bodily Invasion by a Spirit.* The demonic theory of disease emphasized the possession of the body by the devil or other evil spirits that caused physical and mental distress, disease and even death.

6. *Loss of the Soul.* The soul could be enticed to leave the body by an evil spirit or a sorcerer. During the soul's wanderings, an injury could befall it and prevent its return. A soul-catching ceremony would then be required to effect its return.

7. *Dreams.* Dreams seemed to cause sickness. The elements of the dream acted as a suggestive mode of behavior. It was and is still believed that the soul leaves the body during periods of dreaming.

Empirical practices were thus combined and supplemented with *occult* practices. The causes of illness were believed to be beyond nature as humans observed it; they were supernatural, visible signs of *malevolent gods.* Indeed these gods *struck* a person with such force and suddenness that he frequently became paralyzed and unable to speak. This condition was referred to as a *stroke.* Fear of the unknown has been terrifying to people throughout time. In a desperate search for an explanation, primitive people developed the *theory of animism,* which holds that everything in nature is alive with invisible forces and is endowed with supernatural powers: good spirits bring blessings; evil spirits (demons) bring trials, tribulations, sickness and death.

It was imperative that a solution be found by which the body could be freed from the influences of evil spirits. The solution seemed to revolve around *submission, sacrifice* and *supplication.* Submission resulted in the attitude that "what cannot be cured must be endured." Sacrifices were made of animal and sometimes human victims. The very young, the physically and mentally handicapped and the aged were the unfortunate ones selected to placate irate evil spirits. Supplication was expressed through prayer.

Preventive Measures

Ancient peoples searched for a means of protection from these malevolent forces. When worn or carried, *amulets* were believed to protect the wearer from evil influences, black magic and disease. *Talismans* were objects that were supposed to bring good luck.

ROLE OF THE MEDICINE MAN

When illness reached such proportions that input was needed from someone with skills different from those of the nurse figure, the "physician figure" emerged. He was called a *shaman, medicine man* or *witch doctor.* This person was a male with *disease-oriented skills* who assumed a solemn supervisory relation to illness and its cure.

The shaman treated disease almost entirely through psychotherapeutic maneuvers, conducting religious rituals to eject the evil spirits from the body of the patient. A man of mystery, a man, apart from the group, who practiced precise details of ritualistic treatment, the shaman derived power from the "medical mystique." Primitive medicine stood midway between magic and religion.

The shaman's function evolved as an extension of the role played by the nurse. His therapy was a fear or shock technique to rid the body of evil spirits. The technique, which appealed to all the senses, might be to refuse the sick person rest and quiet in order to encourage the evil spirit to depart from the person's body by:

1. startling the evil spirit with frightening masks, blood-curdling yells and deafening noises.
2. jolting the evil spirit by shaking, biting, pinching, kicking and pummeling the patient.
3. ferreting the evil spirit out with obnoxious odors.
4. driving out the evil spirit by giving the patient vile-tasting concoctions to drink, which included purgatives and emetics.
5. annoying the evil spirit by plunging the patient alternately into hot and cold water baths.
6. enticing the evil spirit to enter an animal (kept at the side of the sick person for that person) or an inanimate object, such as a figurine.
7. pacifying the evil spirit by making sacrifices (usually animal).
8. placating the evil spirit by using amulets.
9. employing objects with magical powers such as *fetishes*, primitive carved figures presumed to carry supernatural power, which were regarded frequently as idols and were deified.
10. encouraging the evil spirit to come out of the body by chanting a rhythmic incantation.

When the evil spirit remained within the person and the symptoms did not subside, the shaman resorted to an operation called *trepanation*.[3] Trepanning consisted of boring a hole into a person's skull with a sharp stone in order to permit the imprisoned devil, demon or evil spirit to escape (Fig. 1–1). This was performed to relieve headaches or to alleviate other conditions, such as epilepsy. The patient did not always survive the treatment.

When a woman in labor was ready to deliver her baby, techniques for scaring the baby from her body were used. Horses galloped toward a woman who had been strapped to a tree, or a fire was placed between her spread legs in the hope of hastening the delivery process.

[3]"Trepanation, the making of an opening in the skull with sharpened flint or shark's tooth, is now considered an obsolescent term; the modern surgeon prefers the term trephining, the cutting out of a cranial disk. The object of trepanation was to give the demon confined within the skull a chance to escape; the object of trephination is to remove intracranial pressure. Since trephining stems directly from trepanning, and the ancient and modern operations are fundamentally identical, medical historians cling to the elder word." Robinson, Victor: "Trepanation after Lister," *Ciba Symposia*, 1:192, 1939.

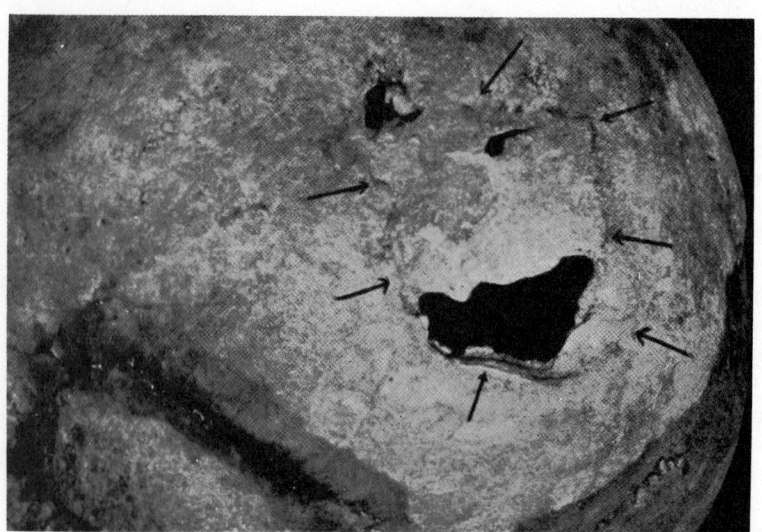

Figure 1–1. A trepanned skull from eastern Arkansas. *Arrows* indicate the original extent of the operation. The healing process can be seen. (Dolan collection.)

PRIMITIVE TREATMENTS

The primitive human cured his minor ailments through empirical techniques. It was believed that affliction of the mind or body should not be separated and that the body (natural spirit) and soul (vital spirit) must remain together for good health to be achieved. When the soul left the body, illness or death could result. Hallucinations, delirium and shock were feared because the primitive human believed that such states occurred when the vital spirit or soul had been stolen and was wandering. Special carved bone charms were used by *soul catchers* to entice the lost soul back into the body.

Sympathetic magic employed medicines that resembled the hoped-for cure for the affliction being treated. For example, the supple bark of the willow tree was used to relieve stiffness in a person suffering from arthritic problems. The medicine was found to be successful, and chemical analysis later found that the bark is an excellent source of salicylate, the main ingredient in aspirin.

SUMMARY

The early functions of the nurse and physician, and the knowledge and practice they involved, were separate and distinct. Nursing originated independently of medicine but provided complementary services for the good of a healthy citizenry.

An essential ingredient in the total health care delivery system over the centuries has been the *faith* of the client in the knowledge and treatment methods of the care givers.

THE HERITAGE OF NURSING

Initial Image of the Nurse Figure

From the inception of the history of the human race, the nurse role has been fulfilled by independent practitioners who:

1. emerged in intuitive response to the desire to keep people healthy, to create a healthful environment and to provide comfort, care and assurance to the sick.
2. were capable, concerned and compassionate persons whose practice encompassed "wellness" in addition to an illness component.
3. used problem-solving skills as well as intuition in assessment of human needs.
4. developed a body of knowledge and utilized intellectual, interpersonal and psychomotor skills in meeting human needs.
5. carried out a sound, practical, essential role that epitomized *caring for, caring with* and *caring about* as well as *curing* a person.
6. shared their knowledge and skills beyond family and neighborhood bounds by teaching individuals, families, communities and their own successors.
7. enjoyed freedom of action to be creative and innovative by discovering new knowledge and enriching the scope of nursing practice.
8. were composites of nurse, nutritionist, dietitian, pharmacist, physical therapist and social welfare worker.
9. possessed a role and function separate and distinct from those of medicine men.
10. worked with the first nurse extenders—the "physician figures"—to achieve the goal of a healthy citizenry.

Thus, the nurturing skills of nurses have been essential to the preservation of life and vital to human welfare from the dawn of civilization.

REFERENCE READINGS

Auel, Jean M.: *The Clan of the Cave Bear*. New York, Bantam Books, Inc., 1980.

Baker, W., and Risse, M.: "Delusions of Witchcraft: A Cross-Cultural Study," *British Journal of Psychiatry, 114*:963–972, 1968.

Baker, W., and Risse, M.: "Clinicopathologic Conference, Case Presentation," *Johns Hopkins Medical Journal, 120*:186–199, 1967.

Bessey, Maurice: *Magic and the Supernatural*. London, Spring Books, 1966.

Douglas, Mary (Ed.): *Witchcraft: Confessions and Accusations*. London, Tavistock Publications, 1970.

Galvin, James, and Ludwig, Arnold: "A Case of Witchcraft," *Journal of Nervous and Mental Disease, 1933*:161–168, 1961.

Gillin, John: "Magical Fright." *Psychiatry, 11*:387–400, 1948.

Gillin, John: "The Making of a Witch Doctor," *Psychiatry, 19*:131–136, 1956.

Haggard, Howard W.: *Devils, Drugs and Doctors*. New York, Harper and Brothers, 1929.

Hill, Douglas: *Magic and Superstition*. London, Hamlyn Publishing Group, 1968.

Lomas, Peter: "Taboo and Illness," *British Journal of Medical Psychology, 42*:33–39, March 1969.

Middleton, John (Ed.): *Magic, Witchcraft and Curing*. New York, The Natural History Press, 1967.

Payne, George H.: *The Child in Human Progress*. New York, G.P. Putnam's Sons, 1916.

Redgrove, Stanley: *Bygone Beliefs*. London, William Rider and Son, Ltd., 1920.

Rosenthal, Ted., et al.: "Social Strata and Perception of Magical and Folk-Medical Child-care Practices," *Journal of Social Psychology, 77*:3–13, 1969.

Simmons, Leo W.: *The Role of the Aged in the Primitive Society*. New Haven, Yale University Press, 1945.

Snell, John: "Hypnosis in the Treatment of 'Hexed' Patient," *American Journal of Psychiatry, 124*:311–316, September 1967.

Health maintenance associated with nurturing skills is represented by this figure of the goddess Selket found in the tomb of Tutankhamen (1334–1325 B.C.). (Dolan collection.)

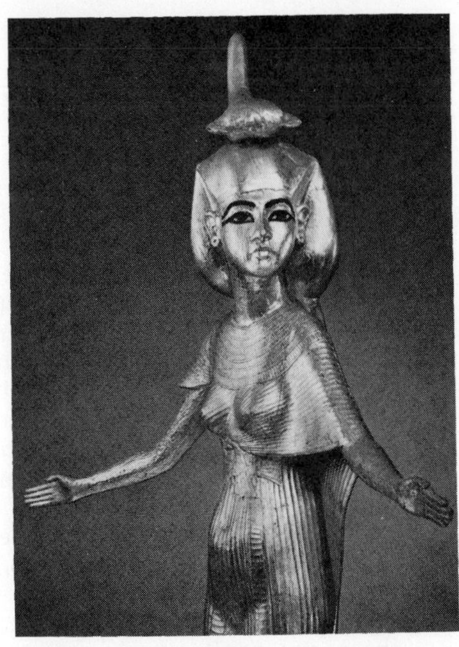

2 Influence of Ancient Cultural Practices on Health Care

PART I

Archeological findings provide information on the early existence of the human and allow for scrutiny of the past. History has been recorded through time in hieroglyphic inscriptions, cuneiform tablets, papyri, books, documents, and figurines, as well as through oral transmission and perpetuation by tradition. Art work has played an important role in the presentation of data. Scenes change because of the differences in social and ethnic styles, but creative thinking is observed and ingenious solutions to crucial problems are evident.

Ethnologists have noted that, with the development of each race and nation, the importance of the healing arts in the lives of people varied greatly from community to community.

Biblical scholars emphasized reverence for the creation of the human and considered him fearfully and wonderfully made. Their teachings have been supported by *paleopathologists,* who have established the antiquity of disease. Skeletal remains indicate infectious and inflammatory processes, and ancient artistic representations portray evidence of disturbances in growth, development and metabolism as well as of the presence of tumors.

As the form of community living changed from tribal groups to empires and, thence, into urban settlements, some cities and nations thrived, while others faded into obscurity. Many of our current problems—overcrowding, slums, high crime rates, gradual inadequacy of water supply, disease outbreaks and economic losses—plagued ancient peoples as well. One wonders how great a role disease, combined with the lack of health teaching and maintenance, played in the disappearance of the ancient civilized groups.

TEMPLES OF HEALING

The theory of *animism* became accepted in many ancient cultures. Strong winds, threatening clouds, violent storms, earthquakes and other sights and sounds in nature were considered visible signs of malevolent gods. Often following such natural displays, disease outbreaks occurred that involved whole communities as well as individuals. Consequently, lack of harmony with nature and natural processes, or *disharmony,* became a theory of disease causation.

As the humans attempted to placate these evil spirits, they came to worship them as gods. They built *temples* to them, hoping to please them so that disease and misfortune would be eradicated. The medicine man became the *priest-physician* who worked in the temple, and medicine began its evolution from witchcraft to craft.

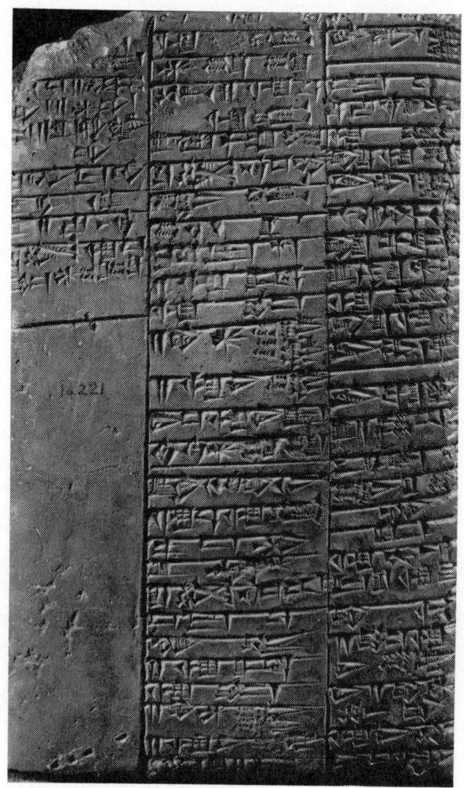

Figure 2–1. The oldest known medical prescriptions written, in cuneiform script on a clay tablet. (Courtesy of the University Museum, Philadelphia.)

ROLE OF THE NURSE

During the time when these ancient cultures flourished, there emerged two types of "nurses." First, there continued to be the well-prepared woman who nursed for hire. She was employed by the wealthy families to provide a high level of health maintenance for a member of the family from birth through life. Her position in the family was recognized as one of authority and importance. Second, and more common, was the nurse whose role regressed from that of the competent and independent nurturer to that of a servant. In the ancient cultures in which a slave economy existed, the nurse assumed a subservient role with the function and image of a slave.

Human lives were not valued by society, and consequently those who cared for them were not respected. In addition to class distinction, sex discrimination was a factor that contributed to the nurse's low status.

The subservient nurse was dependent on the physician, who gave her orders and restricted her sphere of service to the sick. She gave only custodial care, receiving meager rewards and satisfactions for the service. Moreover, because the occupation was often forced upon them, many nurses possessed insufficient preparation and little desire for the role.

THE SUMERIANS

The Sumerians established one of the earliest historic civilizations in the valley of the Euphrates River in present-day Iraq. Their language has been preserved on clay tablets. On a 4000-year-old clay tablet in Sumer, the world's oldest known medical prescriptions were scratched. The ancient physician wrote on both sides of such a tablet with a reed stylus sharpened to a wedge-shaped edge. In 1953 the tablets were translated (Fig. 2–1). Unfortunately, they do not contain the names of the diseases for which the remedies were prescribed.

THE BABYLONIANS

The origins of medical malpractice laws can be traced to the time when Hammurabi, (*ca.* 2000 B.C.) the ruler of Babylonia, produced a medicolegal document, as part of his famous *Code of Law.* To understand this development, one must have knowledge of the societal setting of this great Middle East civilization.

The Babylonian society was quasi-feudal, with the upper stratum made up of wealthy landowners, merchants and priests; the middle class of less wealthy merchants, peasants and artisans; and the lower class of slaves. The religion of the Babylonians revolved around the worship of Bêl, later called Marduk, who was identified with the planet Jupiter. Marduk was described as a cruel god who exacted human blood, frequently children's, in return for his favor. The temple priests were made eunuchs. Handicapped members of society were used as sacrificial victims. The poor were threatened with brutal punishment for the smallest offenses, for example, dismemberment on the altar of Bêl.

Hammurabi's Code of Law was a compilation of the oldest preserved codes of ancient law. It was intended to be humanitarian, and among other things, it tried to restrict the defrauding of the helpless by outlawing unskilled medical practitioners and unnecessary medical procedures and regulating the cost of medical care. For example, the fee schedules for "gentlemen" and "slaves" were presented clearly:

> If a doctor has treated a man for a severe wound with a lancet of bronze and has cured the man, or has opened a tumour with a bronze lancet and has cured the man's eye, he shall receive ten shekels of silver.
>
> If it was a freedman, he shall receive five shekels of silver.
>
> If it was a man's slave, the owner of the slave shall give the doctor two shekels of silver.

The startling aspect of the code was that a governing body replaced the individual as the avenger of injustice and malpractice (Fig. 2–2). The penalties were severe and resulted frequently in cruel physical punishment. Physicians were responsible to the government; in fact, the Code of Hammurabi regulated the physician's conduct:

> If a physician has treated a free-born man for a severe wound with a lancet of bronze and has caused the man to die, or has opened a tumour of the man with a lancet of bronze and has destroyed his eyes, his hands one shall cut off.

The retributive nature of the punishment follows literally the philosophy of "an eye for an eye"; this philosophy was in opposition to Biblical teaching.

The priest-physician occupied a prestigious position, but the surgeon, because he

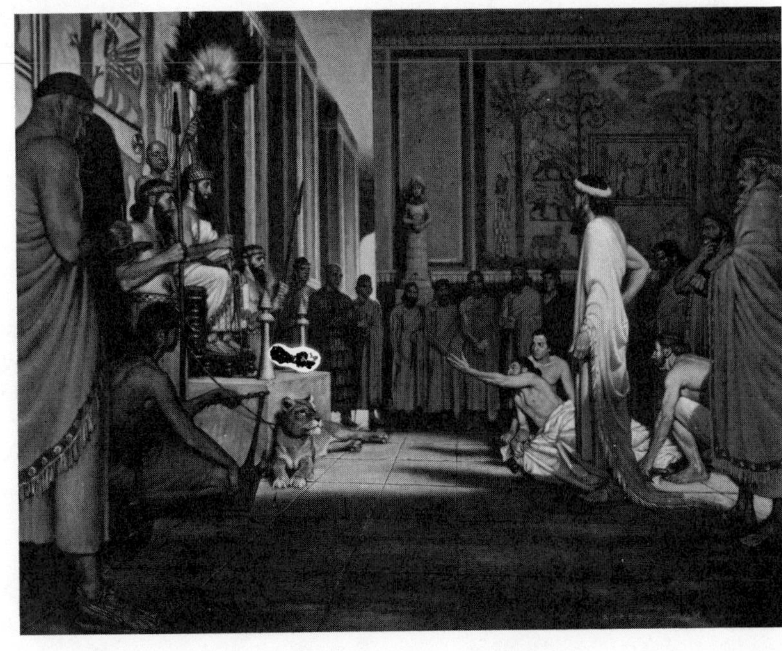

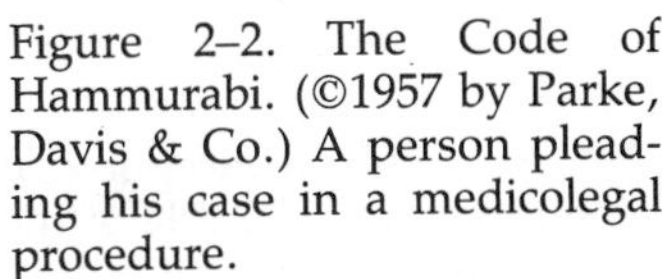

Figure 2–2. The Code of Hammurabi. (©1957 by Parke, Davis & Co.) A person pleading his case in a medicolegal procedure.

worked with his hands, occupied a much lower rank, and it was he who was subject to the malpractice punishments of the code.

Medical treatment in Babylonia was primitive. The notion persisted that illness was caused by sin and by displeasure of the gods; that disease (dis-ease) was inflicted as a punishment for sinning. The sick person was unclean and needed purification, and temples therefore became the centers of medical care. The Babylonians also inaugurated a custom of bringing the sick person out into the busy market place. Here, all who passed inquired about the disease and if a passerby or a relative or friend of the sick person had had similar symptoms, he prescribed a cure. Thus diagnosis and treatment were handled. This practice was probably necessitated by a shortage of physicians.

Principal methods of treatment consisted of ridding the human body of the demons of disease by incantations and by the application of certain herbs. Medicines continued to be vile-tasting concoctions. Many unpalatable ingredients were ingested in the hope of ejecting the evil from the sick person's body. An animal was kept at the patient's side in the hope that the demons would move to its body; then the animal—the "scapegoat"—was sacrificed. It has been mentioned that sacrifices to the gods were frequent and often cruel; human beings were offered on occasion.

Prognosis was determined by the art or practice of divination, carried out by *hepatoscopy*, or the inspection of the liver of sacrificial animals. From hepatoscopy the Babylonians learned the structure of the liver and the gallbladder, and their clay models are excellent anatomical specimens.

In Ezekiel *21*:21, one reads, "For the king of Babylon stood at the parting of the ways, at the head of the two roads to use divination: he made his arrows bright, he consulted with images, he looked into the liver." Why the liver? Because it was believed that the liver was the source of blood and the residence of the soul. By inspecting the liver, the priest-physician could communicate with the mind of God.

In spite of the magico-mystical practices of medicine, the records of obvious *clinical observations*, one of the bases of scientific thought, cannot be ignored. An early Babylonian case study reports:

> The sick one coughs frequently, his sputum is thick and sometimes contains blood, his respirations give a sound like a flute, his skin is cold but his feet are hot, he sweats greatly and his heart muscle is disturbed. When his disease is extremely grave his intestines are frequently opened . . .

In the sickroom scene in Figure 2–3, note the team approach to patient care, with the timeless, independent nurse figure assisting the patient while the physician directs his colleague, the pharmacist, in concocting the medicine. The physician prayed for spiritual intervention. Observe the nurs-

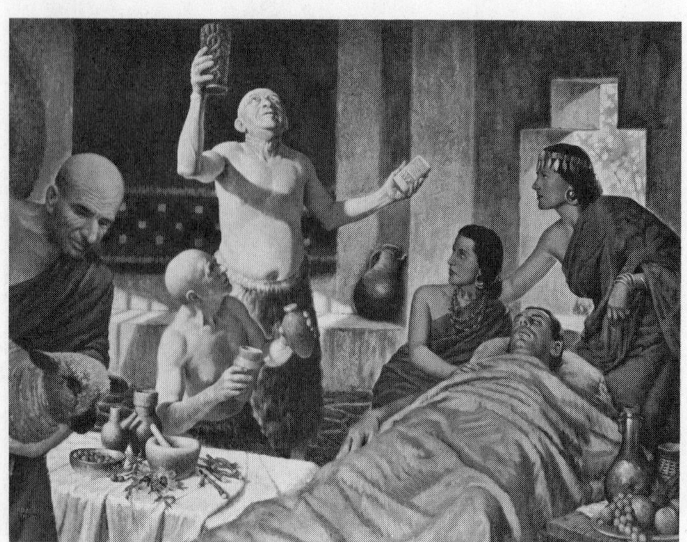

Figure 2–3. An artist's conception of a Babylonian sickroom. The role of the nurse as she assists the patient is portrayed. (©1951 by Parke, Davis & Co.)

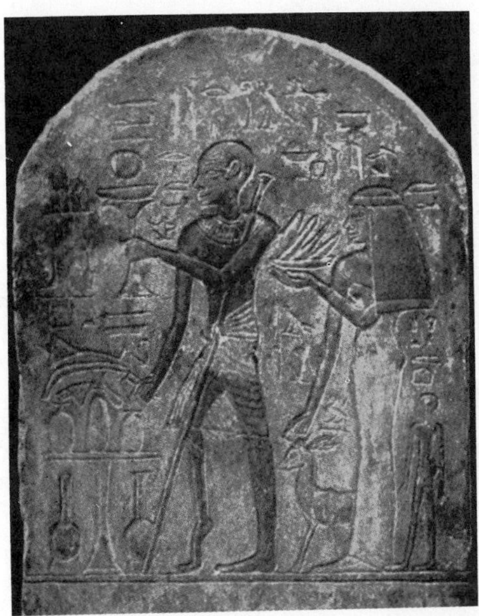

Figure 2–4. Portrayal of a case of poliomyelitis on an Egyptian tombstone. (Dolan collection.)

ing, pharmaceutical, medical and spiritual care of the sick.

THE ANCIENT EGYPTIANS

The Egyptians exhibited careful planning in meeting certain community needs and averting public health problems. Famine and malnutrition have plagued many people throughout history. The Egyptians built irrigation canals and granaries for the proper and provident supply of food.

The pyramids, the best records of ancient Egypt, enable us to understand the burial customs, philosophy and religion. Their representational wall paintings, or murals, provide an unusually clear picture of life in this period and often indicate disease conditions that were prevalent (Fig. 2–4).

Egyptian religious beliefs required that after death the body be prepared carefully and preserved against destruction so that the wandering soul could return to it. Thus the practice of *mummification*, or *embalming*, evolved. The very dry climate of Egypt acted as a natural embalming agent, and many bodies have been found in shallow graves preserved without the benefit of the artificial embalming process. Looking at these bodies and at the carefully preserved bodies in the tombs, we see definite evidences of the diseases of the time.

Bones show signs of malformation and infection. The Egyptians were cognizant of many disease conditions, such as tuberculosis, arteriosclerosis and parasitic infections. Fractured bones were splinted with care.

The position of the physician in ancient Egypt was an interesting one. Like aspirants to other learned professions, he received his preprofessional and professional preparation at the temple of the prevailing deity. The practitioners of the professions were usually members of the lower classes of priesthood; religion and medicine were closely related. Patients came to the temple to intercede with the gods and were treated by the medical practitioners (Fig. 2–5). During the treatment the priest-physician

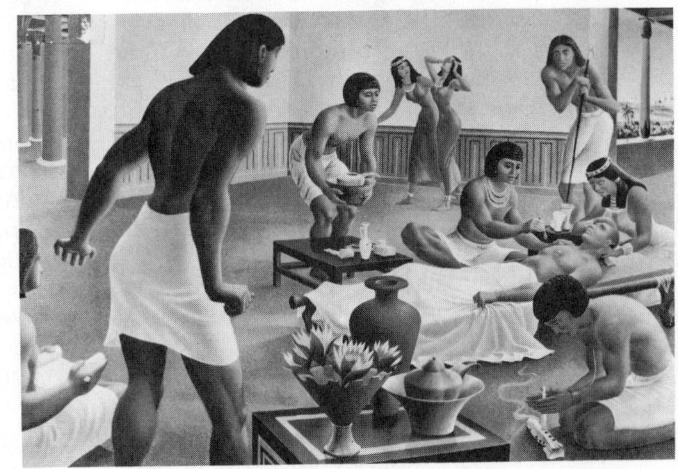

Figure 2–5. An artist's conception of an operation that might have taken place in an Egyptian temple about 2500 B.C. The surgeon is treating an inflamed area with a "fire drill." Note the emotional support and assistance given to the patient by the nurse figure. (Courtesy of *Lederle Bulletin.*)

appealed for assistance from the gods and offered suitable tribute to them.

The *medical area* of the temple is thought to have been somewhat comparable to a large outpatient clinic, with the physicians examining and the medical students observing. There were even medical specialists at this time. Herodotus, the famous Greek historian, writes, "Medicine is practiced among them on a plan of separation; each physician treats a single disorder and no more: thus the country swarms with medical practitioners, some undertaking to cure diseases of the eye, others of the teeth, others of the head, others of the intestines, and some of those which are invisible [internal]." The physician in charge of the intestines gave the enemas and purges. Trepanning operations were performed by the specialist of the head. The physician was also dentist and pharmacist. Because its natural climate and its religious and funerary customs combined to preserve the dead, Egypt has contributed more to our knowledge of the antiquity of disease than any other country up to this time. Data have been gathered by examination, laboratory tests and x-ray of skeletal remains, by scrutiny of artistic endeavors and by analysis of the medical and surgical papyri.

THE ANCIENT PERSIANS

The Persians were a group of Iranian tribes that Cyrus the Great (600?–529 B.C.) welded into a nation. He defeated the Median suzerain Astyages in 550 B.C. and became leader of the Medes and Persians. The conquests of Cyrus were further extended from Egypt to the borders of India under the leadership of Darius the Great (558?–486 B.C.).

The religion of the Persians revolved around the teaching of the prophet Zoroaster. *Zoroastrianism* is still practiced in Iran and in India by the Parsees, who are descendants of the Persians.

The oldest medical records of the Persians are found in the few surviving books of Zoroaster. The Zoroastrian bible, the *Avesta,* contains ceremonial rules relating to the natural laws of birth and death. One of these concerns abortion: To destroy life was to destroy the highest form of creation, and the punishment was the same as that for murder.

Three types of practitioners emerged from the medical centers: those who healed with the knife, those who healed with herbs and those who healed with holy words. The last-named had the most prestige; the surgeons had the least. The Persians, who regarded music as an expression of the good will of Ahura Mazda, the chief Zoroastrian deity, were said to have cured various illnesses by the sound of the lute.

In 330 B.C. Alexander the Great defeated the Achaemenids, demolished the palace of Persepolis and destroyed most of the Zoroastrian literature.

THE ANCIENT HEBREWS

The outstanding contribution of the ancient Hebrews to the cultural heritage of the world was their religion, and the best source of information on their history and culture is the Old Testament of the Bible. This religion of one true God, Yahweh, made them unique among all their contemporaries. His guidance and divine revelation were apparent in the men sent by God to guide His people: "From the time when your fathers left the land of Egypt until this very day I sent you all my servants, the prophets, early and late."[1] The constant, divine guidance kept their religion alive.

Moses was one of the divinely motivated "servants." He was born in Egypt at a time when the presiding Pharaoh was alarmed at the disproportions in population between the Egyptians and slaves (captives from conquests of hundreds of years) on the one hand, and between Egyptians and freemen, such as the Hebrews, on the other. The Pharaoh commanded that the Hebrew birthrate must decrease. The first means tried was to engage the men in a building project at which they were whipped and treated cruelly so that they would become physically exhausted and therefore unable to procreate. When this proved unsuccessful, midwives were ordered to kill all Hebrew male offspring. When the nurse-midwives refused to participate in this genocide, an order was is-

[1]Jeremiah 7:25.

sued to drown all Hebrew male babies in the river.

It was as a result of this order that at birth Moses was placed in the river in a waterproof reed basket, where he was found by the Pharaoh's daughter, who raised him as her son in the best Egyptian tradition of the time.

He received a superior education for his era, and although his learning was obtained in a pagan atmosphere, his natural mother, who had been selected as nursemaid for him, inculcated in him the religious beliefs and traditions of his Hebrew heritage. As a result, years later, Moses responded obediently to God's command to lead his people out of bondage.

God promised the Israelites that if they obeyed His commandments, He would protect them from disease.

> If thou wilt diligently harken to the voice of the Lord, thy God, and wilt do that which is right in His sight, and wilt give ear to His commandments, and keep all His statutes, I will put none of these diseases upon thee, which I have brought upon the Egyptians; for I am the Lord that healeth thee.[2]

On Mount Sinai, God gave to Moses the *Ten Commandments.* The Ten Commandments embody a significant set of rules for ethical human relationships and for mental health. The injunction to "honor thy father and thy mother" has been carried out in the special care provided by families for their elderly. Keeping the Sabbath a day of prayer with freedom from work has remained of vital importance to followers of Judaism. In today's world, work of any kind on the Sabbath is unacceptable to orthodox Jews; thus in hospitals, call-buttons, wheelchairs and elevators will not be used nor will surgical intervention be permitted by Jewish patients unless absolutely necessary. This injunction calls for special consideration on the part of health care deliverers.

The Mosaic Health Code

The ancient Hebrews had a most remarkable history of sound hygienic and sanitary practices. The *Mosaic health code* pertained to every aspect of individual, family and community hygiene and provided a sound basis for "wellness," maintenance of health and prolongation of life.

The code included principles of personal hygiene relating to such things as rest, sleep, hours for work and cleanliness and rules for women concerning menstruation and childbearing. Interest in consumer and environmental protection was evident in the requirements for inspection of food, the detection and reporting of disease, the methods of disposal of excreta, and the disease prevention techniques of isolation, quarantine, fumigation and disinfection after the period of contagion abated. For instance, the Mosaic code directed that when a patient had a communicable disease, such as leprosy, he was to be *isolated* from the community.[3] The rules for prevention of the spread of intestinal diseases (cholera, dysentery and typhoid fever) required that a spade by used to cover excretion after defecation.[4]

The difference between what was clean and what was unclean was delineated very clearly. Moses provided detailed instructions on the correct way to cleanse one's hands: Repeated washings in running water with a time lapse for drying in the sun were recommended.

One of the most remarkably scientific injunctions, in light of current data, pertains to circumcision. The Mosaic code identified the safest time to perform such an *operation,* " . . . and he that is eight days old shall be circumcised."[5]

The Hebrew's knowledge of the importance of animals in the transmission of disease is revealed in the story of the capture of the Ark of the Covenant by the Philistines, who brought it to the temple of their god Dragon.[6] Not only does the story describe the epidemic of bubonic plague, but it also emphasizes the role of rodents as carriers of the disease (Fig. 2–6).

The existence of sanitary legislation has been shown in the accounts of the cases of leprosy in which the afflicted were inspected, isolated and reinspected before being readmitted to the community.

[2]Exodus *15*:26.

[3]Leviticus *13*:46.

[4]Deuteronomy *23*:12–13.

[5]Genesis *17*:12.

[6]Samuel *1*:5–6 (also called I Kings).

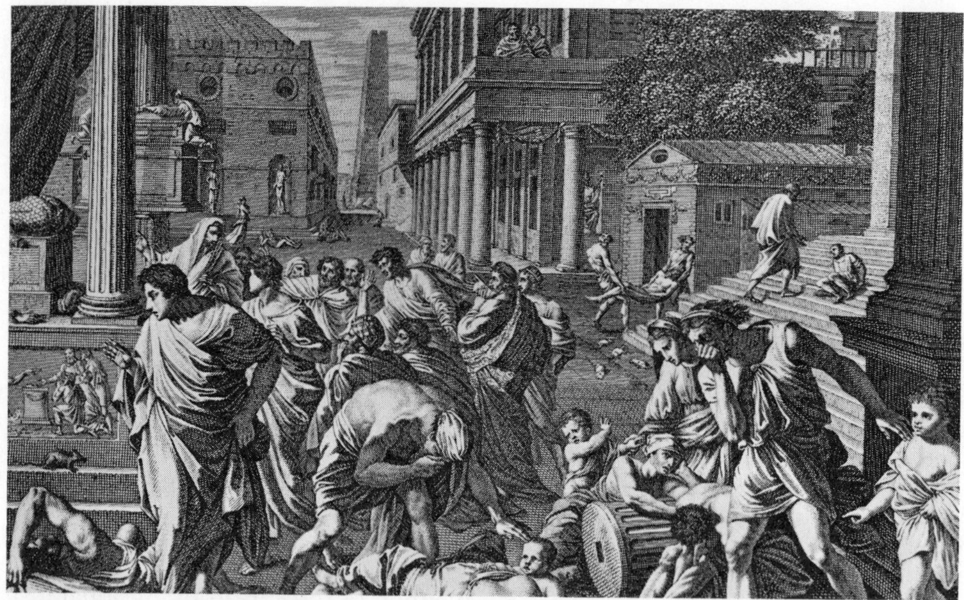

Figure 2–6. The Plague of Ashdod, by Poussin. The picture portrays the sudden onset and fatal nature of bubonic plague. Note the presence of rats. (Dolan collection.)

The high priest was priest-physician and health inspector, and the Hebrew people were admonished to honor him. Persons excluded from the community because of disease were compelled to secure permission from the priest-physician before returning; the cured leper was instructed by these words: "Go and show yourself to the high priest."

Diphtheria was one of the most dreaded diseases, and when it occurred the horn (shofar) was blown to warn the community of this calamity.

Each culture has left some evidence of the diseases with which it was visited, and the Bible furnishes as graphic a picture of the afflictions of this period as do the Egyptian wall paintings and mummies. In

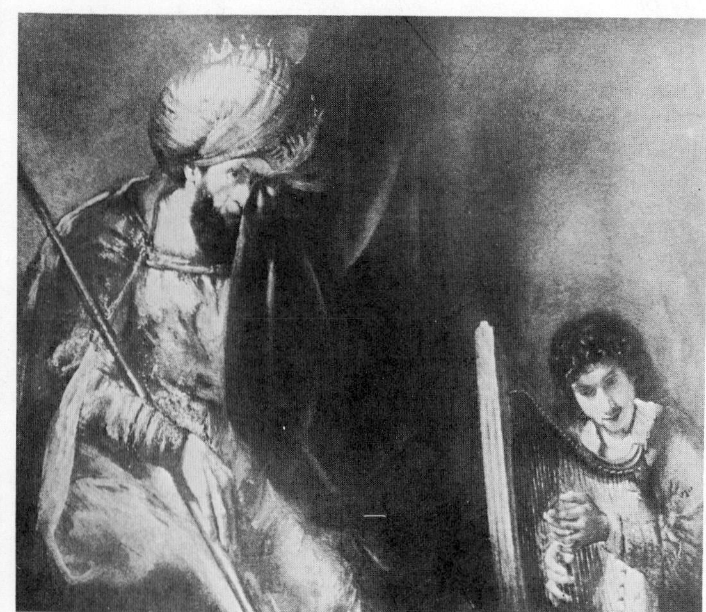

Figure 2–7. Saul and David, by Rembrandt Van Rijn. David playing before Saul to soothe and quiet him. (Dolan collection.)

addition to leprosy and diphtheria, dysentery, dropsy, apoplexy and mental illness are mentioned. Some of the treatments prescribed included fig poultices, artificial respiration and the use of music as therapy for mental illness. David, a gifted harpist, soothed King Saul's melancholy and depression with his relaxing music (Fig. 2–7). In the story of Saul, an abhorrence of euthanasia is evident. When Saul (*ca.* 1013 B.C.) attempted to commit suicide by falling on his sword, the man who answered Saul's call to be put out of his misery was subsequently killed when he reported his murder of Saul to King David.[7]

Houses of hospitality, forerunners of the later inns, hotels and hospitals, were plentiful. The Hebrews were exemplary in the practice of hospitality, and visiting and caring for the sick was a religious duty.

Great respect was accorded the dying and the body of the deceased. Concern and compassion were reflected in the treatment of the sorrowing family. Special persons were assigned to assist the dying and then to care for the body after death. Autopsies were prohibited because they were viewed as a desecration of the dead and because they necessitated postponement of burial.

Dietary laws formed a significant part of the Mosaic Code. Only cloven-hoofed animals that chew their cud and are not scavengers, only birds that are not birds of prey and only fish that have fins and scales were permitted in the diet. Biblical law required that these animals and birds be slaughtered in a precise ritualistic manner utilizing the most humane method. "Kosher" is the term that applies to making things acceptable for human consumption according to Jewish law. To complete the kosher preparation of meat, all blood is removed by salting and soaking.[8]

The Bible presents an interesting description of the foods and the methods of food preparation and preservation used by ancient Hebrews. Grapes and figs were consumed as fresh products, preserved by drying and drunk as juice or as wine after fermentation. Olives were a source of food and olive oil was used as food and medicine. Oil and wine were first-aid remedies. Food restrictions were clearly delineated. The methods of cooking revealed good health principles because they included boiling or roasting.

An early experiment in nutrition was recorded when Daniel requested the steward to feed him and his friends vegetables rather than the rich diet of the king. Daniel and his friends became "better in appearance and fatter in flesh."

The Hebrews appreciated the value of milk, and their description of the promised land was a place "overflowing with milk and honey."

Today, many Jews adhere to the traditional practices laid down so carefully for them in this ancient period. Their fundamental laws of moral and physical conduct are found in the *Torah,* the Hebrew name for the first five books of the Old Testament, which are also called the Pentateuch. The Torah, containing the written law, and the *Talmud,* embodying interpretations of the Bible, are the accepted authority for Orthodox Jews everywhere.

The Ancient Hebrew Nurses

Ancient Hebrew nurses participated in carefully planned programs of visiting the sick in their houses and caring for them. They brought physical and spiritual refreshment for the sick ones and for the family members who were providing care for their ill. The approach to care was family centered.

In response to the Mosaic health code, the ancient Hebrew nurses were active in promoting and maintaining physical, mental and community health, and they continued the nurse's role in health maintenance and health education. The importance and independence of nurses are recorded in the Old Testament story of the nurse-midwives who refused to participate in infanticide.[9]

---

[7]Samuel *1*:5–10.

[8]For a number of years, frozen meals of kosher foods have been available for Jewish patients in hospitals.

[9]Exodus *1*:15–22.

THE HERITAGE OF NURSING

The Image of Nurses in Ancient Cultures: PART I

During the thousands of years when ancient cultures flourished, a positive nurse role in health maintenance and health teaching existed. Nursing continued but role regression occurred, and many nurses were reduced to having only a dependent role in providing health care.

The independent quality of the nurse in this period included:

1. recognition of the importance of health maintenance by certain health-care providers, as in the Egyptian culture.
2. implementation of the Mosaic health code by nurses who promoted physical, mental and community health efforts, thus preserving the positive nurse role in health maintenance and health education while enlarging its scope.
3. continuance of the nurturing skills in the family-centered sphere of practice.
4. the observance of and adherence to a strong code of ethics (e.g., the Ten Commandments) as a motivating guide for practice.
5. documented evidence of the skillful nurse-midwife practitioner who
   a. delivered mothers in the sitting position on obstetrical stools, and
   b. refused to participate in infanticide.

Social forces, fostered class and sex discrimination, forcing "nurses" into a dependent role exemplified by:

1. the nurse's position in a slave economy in which lives were not valued: when her client died, a nurse could be buried alive so she could provide care in the afterlife.
2. nursing as the forced occupation of slaves who possessed neither desire nor preparation for the role.
3. portrayal of the nurse in a subservient role with the image and function of a servant.
4. reliance on the physician for orders and direction.
5. performance of merely custodial care, restricted to sick persons, with meager rewards or satisfactions for the services rendered.

Obviously "caring," the essence of nursing, was minimal for the dependent group, and clients suffered from the lack of personalized health care.

REFERENCE READINGS

Albright, W. F.: *The Archaeology of Palestine*. Baltimore, Penguin Books, 1951.
Breasted, James H.: *The Conquest of Civilization*. New York, Harper & Brothers, 1938.
Elgood, Cyril: *A Medical History of Persia*. London, Cambridge University Press, 1951.
Everyday Life in Bible Times. Washington, D.C., National Geographic Society, 1967.
Grosvenor, Gilbert, et al.: *Everyday Life in Ancient Times*. Washington, D.C., National Geographic Society. (Many excellent illustrations.)
Heaton, E. W.: *Everyday Life in the Old Testament*. New York, Charles Scribners' Sons, 1956.
Leake, C. D.: *The Old Egyptian Medical Papyri*. Lawrence, University of Kansas Press, 1952.
McMillen, S. I.: *None of These Diseases*. Westwood, N.J., Fleming H. Revell Co., 1963.
Moodie, Roy Lee: *Paleopathology, An Introduction to the Study of Ancient Evidence of Disease*. Chicago, University of Illinois, 1923.
Morton, Henry: *Women of the Bible*. New York, Dodd, Mead & Co., 1941.

Oursler, Fulton: *The Greatest Book Ever Written*. New York, Doubleday & Co., 1951.
Renault, Mary: *The Bull from the Sea*. New York, Pantheon Books, 1962.
Renault, Mary: *The King Must Die*. New York, Pantheon Books, 1958.
Smith, C. Raimer: *The Physician Examines the Bible*. New York, Philosophical Library, 1950.
Steuer, R. O., and Saunders, J. B. de C. M.: *Ancient Egyptian and Cnidian Medicine*. Berkeley and Los Angeles, University of California Press, 1959.
Thorwald, Jürgen: *Science and Secrets of Early Medicine*. New York, Harcourt, Brace, and World, Inc., 1963.
Waltari, Mika: *The Egyptian*. New York, G. P. Putnam's Sons, 1949.
Weinreb, Nathaniel: *The Babylonians*. New York, Doubleday & Co., 1953.
Wells, Calvin: *Bones, Bodies, and Disease*. New York, Frederick A. Praeger, 1964.
Woolley, Leonard: *History Unearthed*. London, Ernest Benn Ltd., 1963.

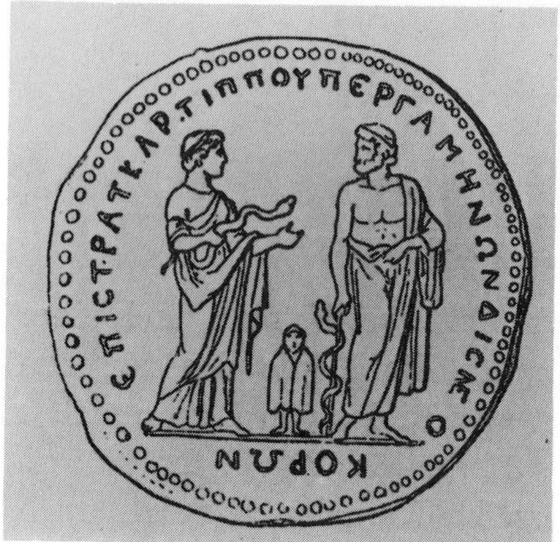

A rare Greek coin presents the close relationship of health maintenance or nursing (Hygeia) to medicine (Aesculapius). (Dolan collection.)

Influence of Ancient Cultural Practices on Health Care 3

PART II

THE ANCIENT AFRICANS

Ancient Africans viewed health as the state that prevailed when the individual was in harmony with himself, with those around him and with nature. Their theories of disease paralleled those ancient theories described in Chapter 1. Illness occurred when there existed a state of disharmony, which could be precipitated by the entrance of bad or evil spirits into the body or by demonic possession. The evil eye influence and the wandering soul (resulting from fright or possession by a restless spirit) were also considered causative factors.

The foundation of the beliefs about health and illness was attuned to the African beliefs about life. Energy was identified as the force that sustains the individual. Healing rites involved a holistic approach to health care and encompassed a unity between physical, mental, emotional and spiritual health. The medicine man not only treated the sick person but encouraged the participation of the family and community. Healing ceremonies were socioreligious in focus and called forth the vital forces of art, singing, dancing and music (Fig. 3–1).

The medicine man endeavored to restore harmony by reestablishing a balance between the forces of good and evil: He attempted to cast out or exorcise the evil spirit, remove the "hex" or the evil eye influence or entice the wandering soul back into the body (Fig. 3–2). The medicine man, the African physician figure, was also known as the shaman, witch doctor, root doctor, obeah man or voodoo doctor.

In addition to understanding the client's needs, the medicine men needed an extensive knowledge of herbs. From earliest times they knew how to inoculate against the dreaded smallpox. Their knowledge and successful technique were utilized by the early colonists in New England during their smallpox epidemics.

Among the means believed to prevent illness was the careful control of one's bodily possessions (such as nail parings, umbilical cord, severed limbs) so that they were inaccessible to another person, who could use them to injure the individual.

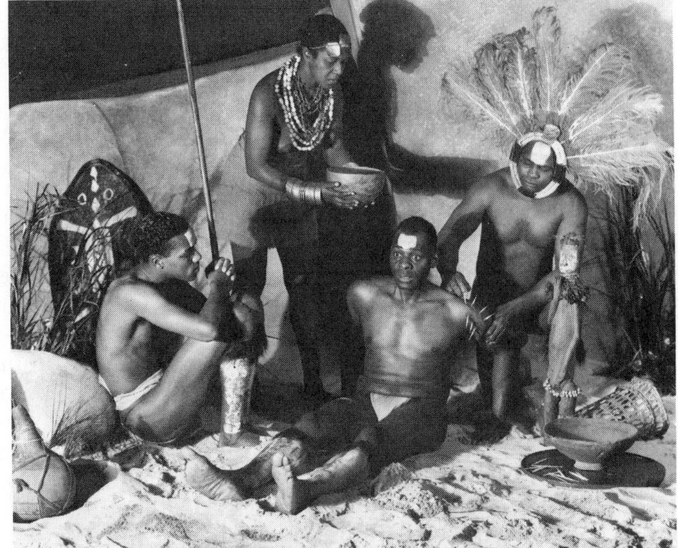

Figure 3–1. The shaman inserts thin, sharply pointed slivers of wood to close a wound. Then leaves are placed over the slivers to serve as bandages. Note the carved wooden figurine at the patient's side. (Courtesy of Davis & Geck Co.)

Deformation of the skull was practiced as well as scarification of the skin in some parts of Africa. (Fig. 3–3).

ROLE OF THE NURSE

The nurturing skills of the African nurses have been recorded. They assumed important roles as nurse-midwives, herbalists and wet nurses in addition to providing child and geriatric care. In the African culture the elderly were treated with great respect.

Modern health care providers can learn from the therapeutic regimen of the shaman. Nowadays we rely on our knowledge of pathophysiology to aid natural repair

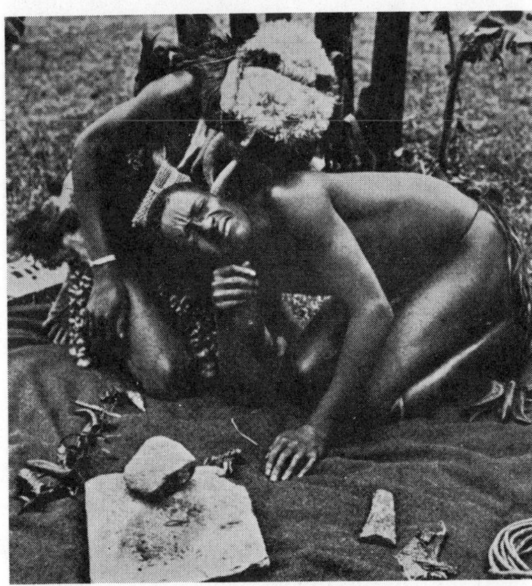

Figure 3–2. A medicine man drawing out the evil influence by means of a sucking tube. (Dolan collection.)

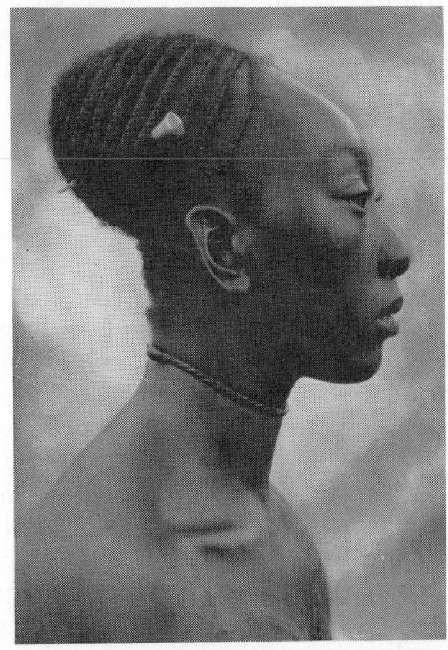

Figure 3–3. The deformation of the head and scarification of the chest of a Mangbetu woman of the Congo. (Courtesy of American Museum of Natural History, New York.)

processes of the body. The shaman, with his attention to psychospiritual aspects, was practicing a type of psychotherapy. A cooperative effort that considers the patient's psychological as well as physical needs might well result in more successful healing.

THE ANCIENT AMERICAN INDIANS

The coming of the Santa Maria, Pinta and Nīna to our shores prompted historians to write books about the "New World," but these books were actually additional chapters in the continuing history of the Americas. We have become aware that highly developed cultures flourished in the Western Hemisphere before the arrival of Columbus, the Spanish conquistadors and the Norsemen. Hermann states that "it may be assumed with some certainty that highly evolved cultures flourished on the soil of the New World from 2000 to 1000 B.C. . . . "[1]

At one time, there were many American Indian nations in North and South America, but the Indian population has since decreased dramatically and tragically. Language and cultural diversity have influenced the traditions of the various surviving tribes. Just as American Indians varied in physical appearance, manner of living and way of life, their systems of healing arts varied from tribe to tribe.

The Mayas

The *Mayan* Indians were supposed to have occupied the Yucatan peninsula from about 2500 B.C. to about 1600 A.D., but the earliest certain date of their occupation is 320 A.D. Mayan cultural artifacts reveal a people who were skilled in astronomy, art and mathematics. They designed a remarkable calendar. Hieroglyphic inscriptions document their achievements, and many of their customs have been perpetuated through oral tradition. Little is known about Mayan health practices, although one custom involved the medicinal use of sweat baths, or temascals.

Mayan religious practices revolved around human sacrifice. One form of sacrifice involved the removal of the hearts of adults, and another involved the sacrifice of children. It has been recorded that in times of community stress, maidens were thrown into the sacred well and youths were put to death on sacrificial blocks. The ceremonies were presided over by either the high priest or members of the priesthood. In addition to this duty, the priests were also soothsayers, medical advisors and herbalists.

The custom of skull deformation was common among the Mayas. Four or five days after birth, a child was placed face downward and one board was tied to the back of the head and one to the forehead. The boards were bound tightly together so that the head was compressed upward. The Mayan stone cutters depict this condition and show the receding forehead that forms a continuous line with the nose. The custom of skull deformation was practiced by many ancient Indian groups (Fig. 3–4).

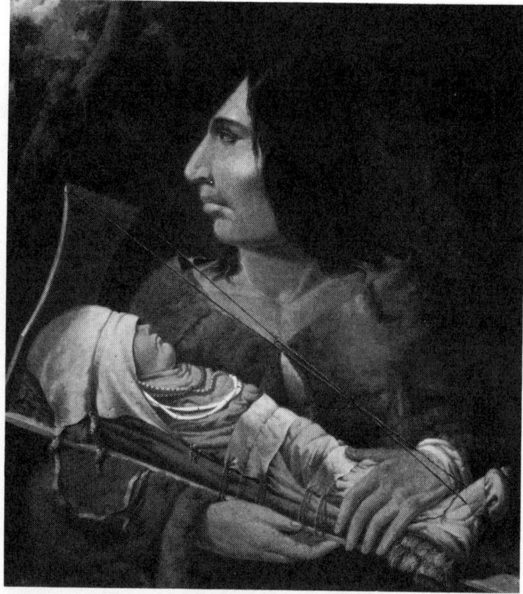

Figure 3–4. Caw-Wacham, by Paul Kane (1810–1872). Note the deformation of the mother's head and the technique employed to reshape the head of the baby. The board used for reshaping is concealed under the chamois that is tied to the frame of the cradleboard. (Courtesy of The Montreal Museum of Fine Arts.)

[1]Hermann, Paul: *Conquest by Man.* New York, Harper & Brothers, 1954, p. 188.

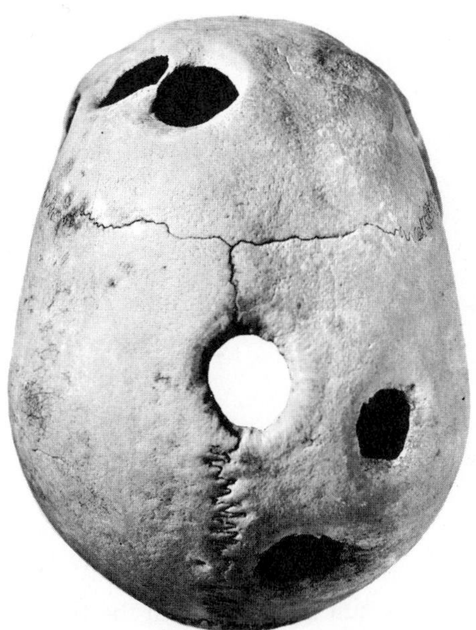

Figure 3–5. A trepanned skull from Peru. (Courtesy of Peabody Museum of Yale University, New Haven.)

The Incas

The *Inca Empire* was located in Peru. The Incas were skilled engineers who constructed a remarkable system of roads and suspension bridges; they also left evidence of medical prowess. They had great skill in the medical technique of trepanation and were noted for their skillful cranial bandaging (Figs. 3–5 and 3–6).

As was common in other ancient cultures, the Incans attributed the many physical afflictions with which man was seized to the displeasure of the gods. Tribute to the gods took the form of a pottery or stone effigy *(huaco)* of the sick person. Many of these effigies have been found, and along with skeletal remains, assist us in understanding the pathological conditions that prevailed in Central and South America.

Remarkably creative case studies have been preserved in these clay figurines, which provide a unique artistic record of patient care. These figurines may well have been used as teaching models to assist persons learning the skills of patient care. They may have been brought to a teaching medical clinic where a diagnosis could be determined (Fig. 3–7). Because of the rugged Peruvian terrain, bringing a patient to a clinic was not feasible, and bringing a figurine was an acceptable solution.

Beds seemed to be individual in design, with canopies for protection from the sun, elevation from the ground and separations in the webbing of the framework to permit the passage of excretions.

The usual posture for delivering babies was a squatting position, which many clay figurines verify.

Diseases were prevalent and treatments abounded. Treatments included bloodletting, cupping or sucking, massage, sweating, splinting, setting of bones, tooth ex-

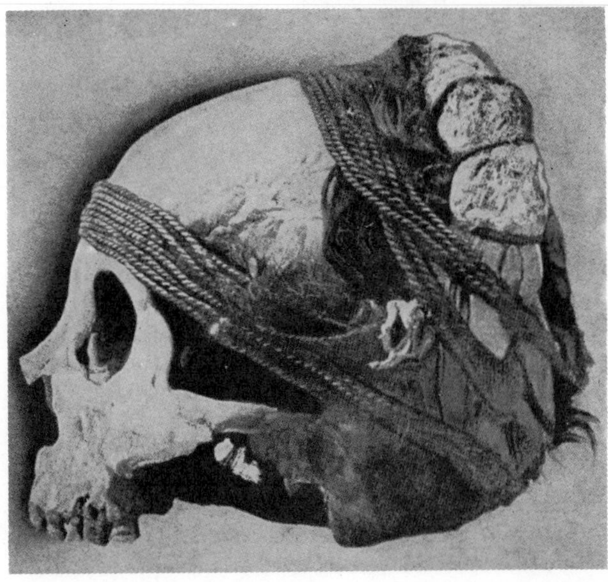

Figure 3–6. An old Peruvian skull showing a trepanation bandage. This specimen is now in the San Diego Museum of Man.

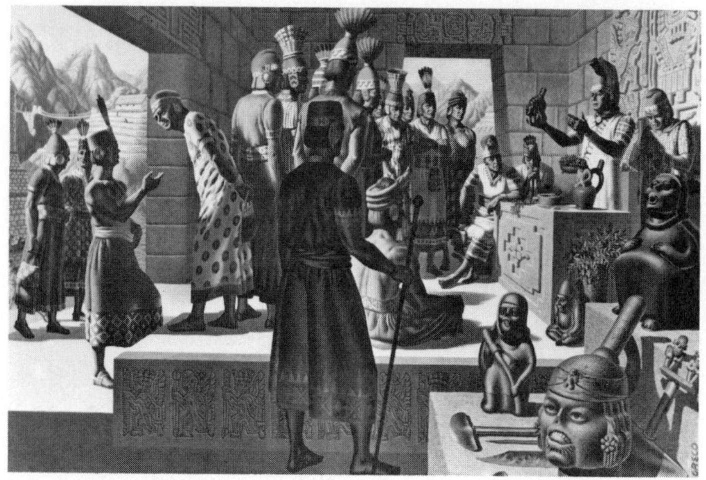

Figure 3–7. An artist's conception of an Inca medical teaching clinic with clay figurines depicting disease conditions. (Courtesy of *Lederle Bulletin.*)

tractions, amputation, suturing, bandaging, poulticing and trepanning.

As mentioned, displeasure of the gods was accepted as the cause of disease. Shamans were active as medicine men. The magic rite of transference of disease to animals was part of the care of the sick.

Herbs were administered as emetics, laxatives, purges, and diuretics and for the relief of respiratory distress. Poisons were known and used. Cobwebs were utilized, very much as they were by the ancient Egyptians, to encourage coagulation of blood in wounds. Cupping was the sucking or drawing out of a foreign object by the use of a hollowed-out horn. Some of these treatments were performed only by the medicine man because they were illness-related.

Heirs of the Ancient Indian Culture

The descendants of the ancient Indians of Latin America—Spanish Americans, Latin Americans and Mexican Americans—inherited the ancient Indian culture while incorporating aspects of the Spanish culture from the fifteenth and sixteenth centuries. These people possessed an extensive knowledge of medicinal plants and herbal therapy using the herbs indigenous to Central and South America as well as those brought to the New World by the Spaniards. Herbs were utilized wisely and efficaciously for centuries. An example is quinine, or "Jesuit Bark," used in the treatment of malaria. This medication was used until World War II, when difficulties in obtaining adequate amounts led to the development of the synthetic medication quinacrine hydrochloride.

The concept of health was one of equilibrium—a proper balance among man, nature and the supernatural. Illness was viewed from a sociocultural as well as a religious perspective. The evil eye influence (mal ojo) and hexing (mal puesto) were considered to cause disease. Children were thought to be particularly susceptible. Thus, folk medicine focused on the whole individual, on the physiological, psychosocial and spiritual aspects in relation to the natural and supernatural environment. The intervention of God was sought to keep one in a state of wellness. Special prayers, blessings, and confession to absolve one's sins provided a catharsis.

Folk healers included a *"wise person"* in each family and others who had folk-healing skills: the *yerbero,* who was a herbalist; the *curandero,* who was skilled in healing; the *sobadore,* who was adept in massage and bone manipulation; the *Spiritualista,* who had spiritualist powers; and the *Brujo,* who controlled malevolent powers. In addition, healing required the use of the healer's own inner energies, which he transferred through the techniques of the laying on of hands and gentle massage. These ritualistic modalities resulted in warmth and tranquility.

Many of these beliefs are still found, in

modified form, among Spanish-speaking peoples in the United States and Latin America.

The use of sweat baths or sweat huts to purify the body and maintain health held a prominent place in the mores of the various groups of American Indians. Methods of achieving the objectives of the bath varied with each group. The most common method consisted of pouring or sprinkling water over very hot stones that were enclosed within an airtight structure or hut. Some groups incorporated the use of aromatic substances in the procedure; others beat their bodies with bunches of twigs to stimulate the circulation of the blood and hasten the sweating process. Many Indians terminated the bath with a quick plunge into cold water or by rolling in the snow.

The sun god was worshiped by ancient American groups, especially the Iroquois, Aztecs and Incas. The therapeutic value of heat as well as light may have been recognized.

Elaborate plans for preventing disease were perpetuated. Protective devices included charms, fetishes, and herbal bags worn around the neck as well as other forms of herbal therapy.

Another therapeutic plan embodied art in the form of *sand painting.* Medicine men were skilled in the creation of these intricate designs, which were made specifically for an individual and a special occasion. They were most useful in the ceremony for healing illness (Fig. 3–8). The medicine man gathered many varieties of colored sand and crushed minerals. He then, by the skillful maneuvering of his thumb and forefinger, permitted a trickle of colored sand to fall on the ground, following the predetermined pattern of the painting. Strange but beautiful pictures developed on the natural-colored sand background. They had great religious significance, and the medicine man endeavored to promote healing through the painting.

In addition to sand painting, a technique of hypnotherapy was integrated into the healing ceremony. The shaman sought to excite the senses: The sand painting appealed to the *sense of sight;* the ritual of the prayerful chant energized the *sense of hearing* (in a manner similar to that of a lullaby); the feathers touched to the patient's body stimulated the *sense of touch;* the sweet-smelling herbs placed in the fire released an incense that was directed to the *sense of smell;* and herbs given to be consumed spurred the *sense of taste.*

During the ceremony the patient was the center of attention: he absorbed this loving interest. Faith on the part of patient, shaman and participating friends was an important ingredient in the ceremony.

The colorful designs of the sand painting were made on the floor of a hogan or a specially built medicine hut. At the end of

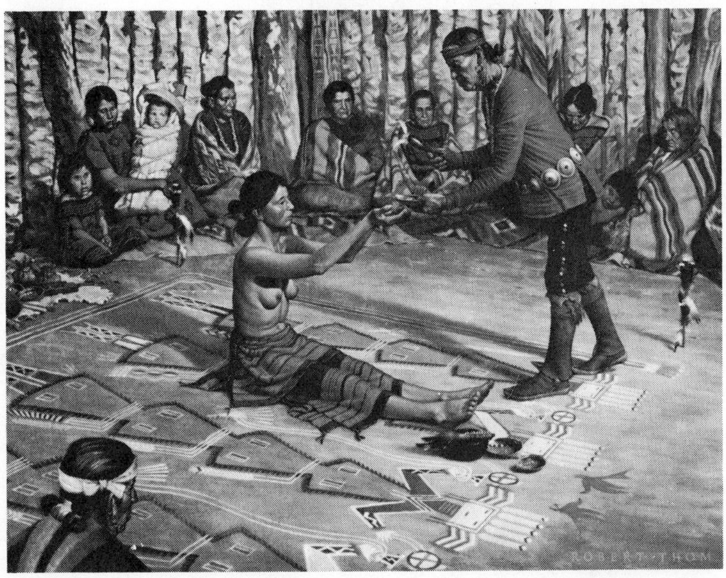

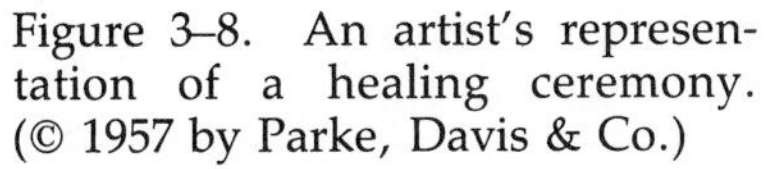
Figure 3–8. An artist's representation of a healing ceremony. (© 1957 by Parke, Davis & Co.)

the elaborate ceremony, the medicine man destroyed the painting, then gathered the sand and scattered it to the four corners of the earth.

Health Care in Modern Indian Cultures

Religion and health care continue to be intertwined. Long years of tradition and trust have produced a remarkable feeling of faith in these cultural health care practices.

The traditional family-centered approach to care includes unified action either through prayer or through chanting and singing by the family or tribal group.

An interesting child care custom is the use of *cradleboards* (Fig. 3–9). Navajo babies have two types of cradles. The first is a canopy cradle, or "face cover," which protects the infant from dust and other disturbing elements. When it appears that the infant will survive, a second and more durable cradleboard is built by the father. Because of Navajo superstitions, it is customary not to make preparations for a new baby until the need is assured.

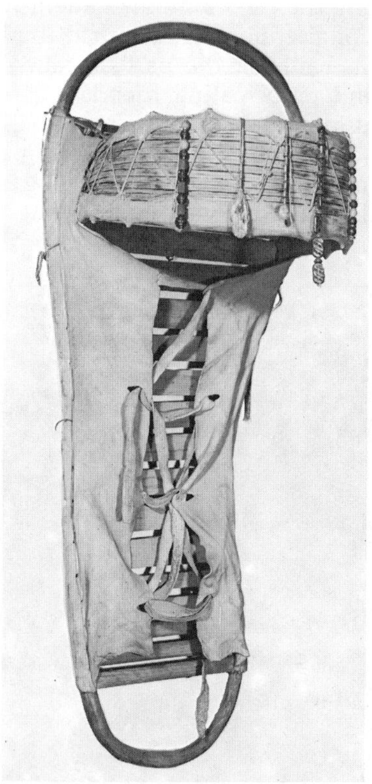

Figure 3–9. An Apache baby carrier or cradleboard. Note the bead and feather charms to ward off evil spirits. (Courtesy of Museum of the American Indian.)

The cradleboard is made to be carried on the mother's back or propped against a sturdy object. This places the baby on eye level with the other members of the family who sit on the floor of the hogan. This establishes his presence as part of the family and increases his feeling of security.

Child care practices encourage independence from early childhood. Discipline does not negate the exercise of judgment and the importance of decision making. This continues throughout one's life and is an important ingredient in the planning for care by health care deliverers.

Great respect is accorded the elderly, and families provide for older members. When death occurs the family receives emotional support and is joined in mourning and grieving by the community.

American Indians were pioneer ecologists. Because of their love and respect for nature and their deep feeling of oneness with it, they lived in harmony with nature.

One of the greatest contributions of the American Indians is their vast knowledge of herbs, some of which have become a significant part of our modern day medicines and medical treatment. The early Indians' willingness to share their knowledge was of vital importance to people who later arrived in North America.

The importance of American Indian health care and therapy continues to the present, and the input of the medicine man should be incorporated as part of the cooperative plan by both nurses and physicians for the delivery of care beneficial to the patient. Respect for the medicine man, whose knowledge and skills are timeless, could be crucial to the welfare of the client and family, could reduce anxieties and could bring about harmonious relationships for all involved in the delivery of care.

In the early nineteenth century, all relations between the North American Indians and the United States government were maintained through the Department of War. It was not until 1849 that the Bureau of Indian Affairs became a part of the Department of the Interior. In July, 1955, the responsibility for Indian health care was transferred from the Bureau of Indian Affairs to the United States Public Health

Service under the Department of Health, Education and Welfare. In January, 1977, Rosemary Wood left her position as executive director of the American Indian Nurses' Association to become the first Indian nurse to serve as chief of the nursing branch of the Indian Health Service.

THE ANCIENT ASIANS

China, the fabled middle kingdom, is one of the oldest and most innovative cultures. Its artistic and technological achievements span a period of several millennia. The exact origin of the Chinese people remains a mystery because of the absence of accurate records predating the Shang dynasty (*ca.* 1776–1122 B.C.).

The three early religions in China had an influence on the development of patient care. *Taoism* and *Confucianism* were indigenous to China; *Buddhism* was imported from India. Underlying these religions was China's *primitive folk religion.*

Taoism, dating from the sixth century B.C., combined magic and mysticism and emphasized the value of charms in combatting the demons of disease. Usually these charms were written on paper, which was then burnt and the ashes were administered in tea, hot water or some medicinal liquid. Then other charms were distributed around the house and carried on the person's body. Later Taoists, searching for the elixir of life and the transmutation of base metals into gold, adopted the study of *alchemy.* Alchemy became the chemistry of the Middle Ages, and from this medieval science, modern chemistry grew.

After Confucius' time (551–479 B.C.), every aspect of Chinese culture and society carried the stamp of his teaching. *Confucianism* stressed family solidarity, respect for elders, village government by elders and veneration of scholars. It encouraged the already existing belief in *ancestor worship,* which prevented the dissection of bodies. It was not until 1913 A.D. that legal permission was granted for the performance of autopsies in China.

Buddhism taught that sin was the cause of disease and was sent by the gods. Thus, one was not encouraged to cure an affliction. In some Oriental countries a devout Buddhist will not eat milk or eggs. The killing of animals or anything with potential for life, such as eggs, is considered sinful. Dogs and monkeys roam the streets and hospital wards unimpeded. Lice are carefully removed from the body but are not killed. Begging is encouraged because it aids a person in working out salvation for a better next life.

These three religions were superimposed on the fundamental Chinese belief in universal animism. Basic to the Chinese healing arts were the practices of sacrificial offerings, frightening evil spirits by beating gongs and shooting off firecrackers and accepting the most bitter medicines offered by the Chinese medicine man.

The female held a traditionally subordinate social position in China, and many female babies were abandoned at birth. A Chinese custom was the practice of foot deformation, done by binding the feet of female babies.

A Chinese woman could not be undressed in the presence of a physician, nor might he examine her. In the homes of the upper classes ivory or alabaster figurines were kept on which the point of discomfort was marked. A marked figurine would be carried to a physician for his diagnosis and recommended treatment (Fig. 3–10). The Chinese physician carried with him a less ornate figurine for patients who did not possess one.

The influence of the *evil eye* on babies

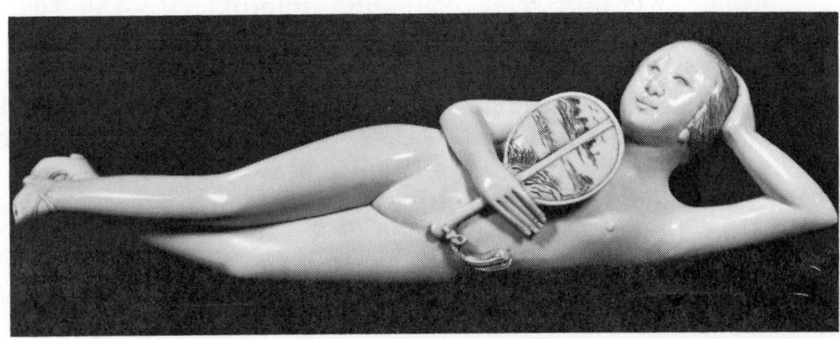

Figure 3–10. A carved ivory figurine, from China, upon which the female patient marked where she had pain. Note the foot deformation. (Dolan Collection.)

was a source of worry for Chinese parents; consequently, male babies were given female names and dressed as girls in the hope that evil spirits would be less interested in them.

Health Versus Illness

In Chinese culture, health has been considered a state of harmony or equilibrium within an individual and in the universe. This state was brought about by a normal flow of energy that was regulated by two opposing forces in nature—the *yang* and *yin*.

The yang and *yin* theory established some scientific basis for disease. The yang was the male principle—positive, desirable, active, fiery and full of life—in contrast to the yin, or female principle, which was negative, cold, weak, dark and lifeless. Life consisted of the interaction of these principles. When they were in equilibrium one was healthy; when there was an improper balance of energy one suffered discomfort and disease.

Health Care

The founder of Chinese medicine is considered to be the legendary emperor *Shen Nung,* said to have been responsible for careful investigation of medicinal herbs. He was supposed to have experimented on himself, thus discovering a large number of drugs, including poisonous ones. The results of his research were allegedly compiled in the *Pen Tsao,* or the Herbal.

Huang-ti, the legendary Yellow Emperor, has been credited with having written *Neiching,* the canon of medicine. According to the Neiching there are four steps in determining a diagnosis: observation, auscultation, interrogation and palpation (look, listen, ask and feel). Palpation referred mainly to examination of the pulse, which was of prime importance. The Chinese were skilled at understanding the pulse's variations in health and disease.

The Pen Tsao and the Neiching were written in lacquer upon strips of bamboo or palm leaves; and both exhibited the ideographic tadpole characters analogous to Egyptian picture writing.

Historians agree that the Chinese were ingenious in developing the field of medical therapeutics. Moxa (see page 271), cupping, cautery, massage and puncture were practiced as far back as the Stone Age. Wong and Wu say that the Neiching stressed that "when the seat of the trouble is in the muscles employ puncture; in the blood vessels, use moxa; in the tendons, apply cautery."[2]

In making punctures, "needles" were used. Needling occupied a rather important position in ancient times, developing into the art of *acupuncture.* Acupuncture originally consisted of inserting needles with a twisting motion an inch or so into designated areas, referred to as meridians, which control the flow of yang and yin (Fig. 3–11). The old method of acupuncture has been refined to a new method of therapeutic acupuncture that consists of hand manipulation of the needles with an up-and-down and concurrent twirling motion between the thumb and index finger (Fig. 3–12). In addition, there has been an increased acceptance of acupuncture as a form of analgesia. Research is being conducted to determine the possible existence of some anatomical structure that would explain the traditional channels, or meridians of energy, that were first described in written and diagrammatic form many centuries ago. Western medicine has been integrated with the traditional arts of acupuncture and herbal therapy in present-day China. What may be the first use of acupuncture for anesthesia in the United States was described, in 1972, in a letter to the editor of the *Journal of the American Medical Association,* reporting on anesthesia for a tonsillectomy.[3]

Massage evolved out of the natural impulse to rub, soothe and stroke an injured or painful spot. The Chinese developed this ability to an extraordinary degree and, using a modern vocational rehabilitation approach, employed blind masseurs (Fig. 3–13). Two modern modalities—*acumassage* and *acupressure*—have been regarded as highly effective. They involve the laying on of hands with a gentle motion over specific energy channels.

---

[2]Wong, K. C., and Wu, Lieu-Teh: *History of Chinese Medicine.* Shanghai, China, National Quarantine Service, 1936, pp. 2–3.

[3]Liu, Wei-Chi: Acupuncture anesthesia: a case report, *J.A.M.A., 221*:87–88, July 3, 1972.

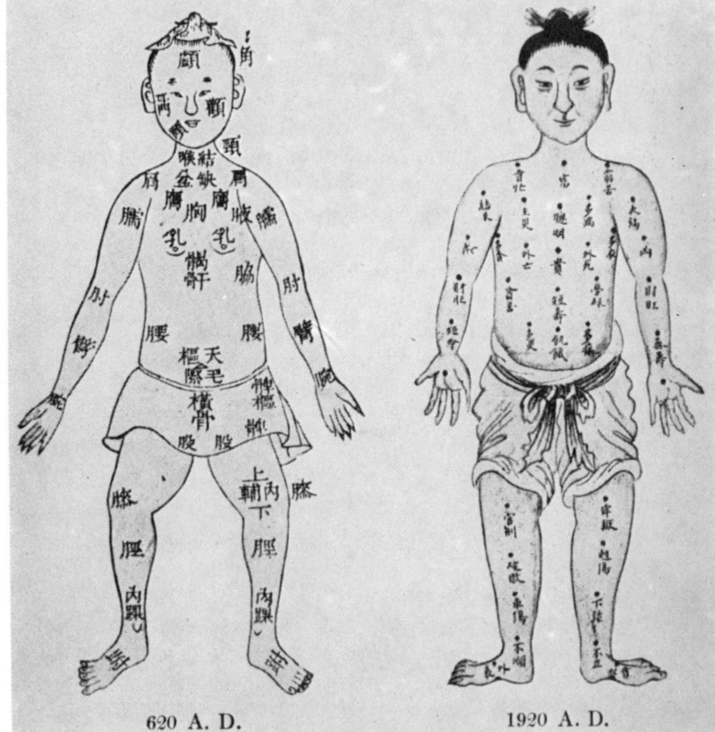

Figure 3–11. Chinese acupuncture diagrams. (Courtesy of Dr. E. V. Cowdry.) (Dolan collection.)

Moxa, a form of counterirritation, involved the application of ignited cones of mugwort to the skin. The smoldering fire burned the skin gradually, causing blisters to form.

Specific medicines and treatments were devised for prevalent diseases. *Smallpox* was described in the third century A.D, and a method of *vaccination* was devised. Smallpox scabs were ground into a powder and blown through bamboo tubes into the nostrils. Frequently the undergarment of a child afflicted with smallpox was worn by a healthy child for two or three days. Concomitant with the scientific advancement of

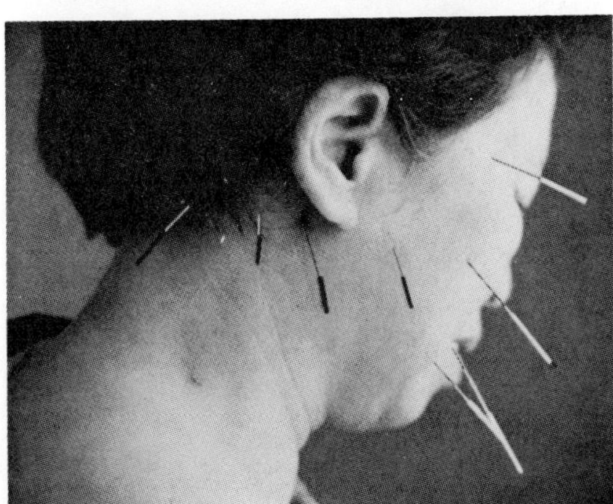

Figure 3–12. Acupuncture being used to relieve facial paralysis, in Japan. (Dolan collection.)

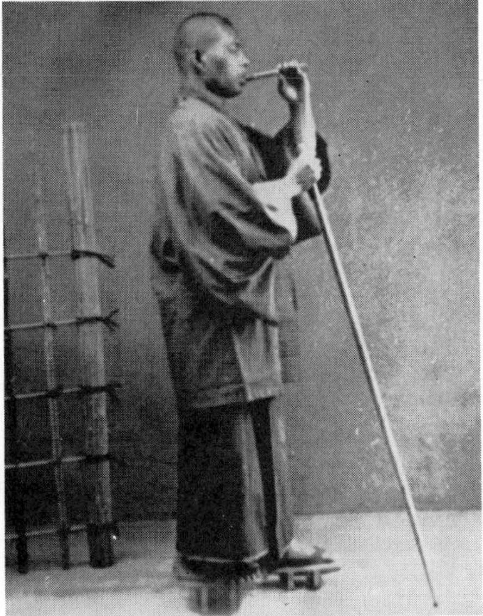

Figure 3–13. A blind man who performs massage blows a whistle as he goes through the street to announce his presence. (Courtesy of Peabody Museum of Salem, Mass.)

smallpox vaccination was the superstitious practice of having a child wear an ugly mask to ward off the deity of smallpox.

Leprosy has been known from earliest times, and chaulmoogra oil was used in its treatment. Medicinal seaweed, rich in iodine, was mixed with bouillon to combat goiter. Animal organs such as liver and thyroid glands were used. The poppy gave up its precious content of opium owing to the careful study by the Chinese. The herb ma huang was found to possess an important alkaloid, ephedrine. An ingenious method of extracting the potent medicinal components of herbs and drugs employed the *Chinese medicine cooker.* The herb or drug was placed in the center section of the cooker, and around it was banked live charcoal; the heat released the beneficial properties.

Opium and its derivatives have long been used to relieve pain. Widespread drug abuse plagued China until well into the twentieth century. In recent years the Chinese Communists have sought, with much success, to eliminate the social use of opium and other narcotics.

"Spirits of hartshorn" (ammonia water) was another contribution of the Chinese. Originally, spirits of ammonia was obtained by the distillation of the horns and hoofs of animals.

The most famous herbal medicine is derived from ginseng, a plant so rare and highly valued that it has been reported as selling for more than $4000 a pound.[4] It can be distinguished from similar vegetation only by its glow in the dark.

A form of divination, to determine the prognosis of a patient's condition, used the *witch ball* (Fig. 3–14). This is an intricately carved ivory Cantonese magic ball that reveals rare beauty and ingenious and skilled craftsmanship. As many as 12 ivory balls fit inside one another, and the stars, constellations and astrological influences are incorporated into their design. By inspecting this work of art, a prognosis was made.

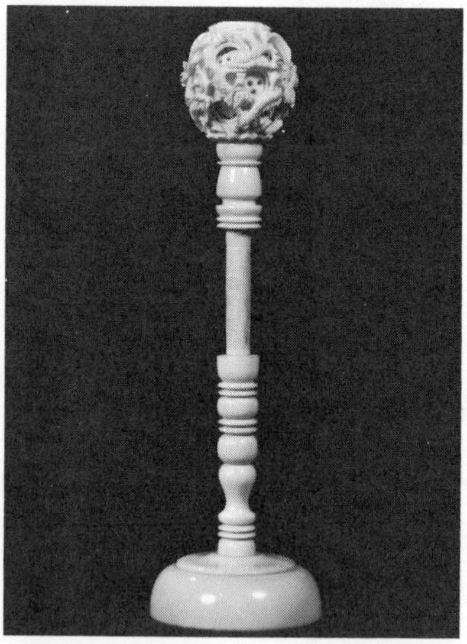

People in the East also recognized the value of moist heat. Hot mineral baths as well as hot sand packs in which patients were buried up to their necks were popular.

Figure 3–14. A carved ivory witch ball used for divination. (Dolan collection.)

Drugs were carried in an *inro,* a box consisting of several compartments or sections, each of which contained vials of medicine (Fig. 3–15). These were fastened to the belts of the medicine men.

Many of these practices were also repre-

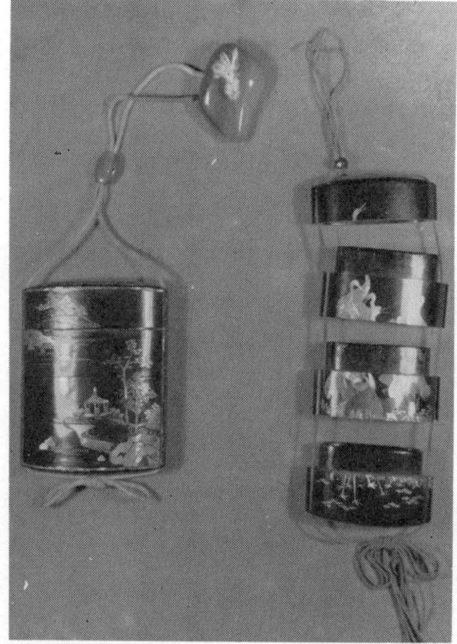

Figure 3–15. Two inros—medicine boxes—one opened to show the drug compartments. (Courtesy of Peabody Museum of Salem, Mass.)

[4]Durdin, Peggy: "Medicine in China: a revealing story," *New York Times Magazine,* p. 76, February 28, 1960.

sentative of the health practices and care of the Japanese, the Koreans and other Orientals. In later years missionaries to the Orient brought back concepts of care as well as knowledge of herbal remedies to Europe.

China's vast body of traditional medical lore is among the most ancient. Today, Chinese doctors have revived an increasing number of ancient health care practices.

Very little mention has been made of the counterpart of the hospital in ancient China. Wong and Wu list the founding of so-called *Halls of Healing* by 651 B.C.; Berdoe[5] explains the absence of such institutions by the fact that the Chinese people would consider themselves remiss in their duty to their family if they did not take care of their relatives at home.

THE ANCIENT HINDUS

The triangular subcontinent of India has been host to civilization for thousands of years. Natural barriers of mountains and seas have isolated India from the rest of the world and encouraged the growth of an indigenous culture. As early as 2000 B.C., tribal Aryans from the Iranian plateau settled on the plains of India and established themselves in the valley of the Ganges.

Between 1000 and 800 B.C. there was a struggle between the ruling class and the priestly caste for supremacy in India. Thence evolved the idea of Brahma, the eternal spirit, and the religion of *Brahmanism* (also called Hinduism) which affirms the doctrine of the transmigration of the living soul—the belief that the body passes into a higher or lower form after physical death according to past conduct. Hinduism has been the most widely accepted of the religions of India. In common practice, worship or devotion is directed to one or more of the deities composing the Trimurti, or divine Triad: Brahma, source and giver of life; Vishnu, the preserver; and Siva, the destroyer.

The territory of the Jumna and Ganges Rivers is sacred to the Hindus, and every 12 years on certain days selected by astrologers, the faithful come to these rivers to bathe and wash away their sins. When a person feels the approach of death, it is his or her greatest desire to go or to be taken to Benares, a city on the Ganges, to participate in this religious bathing. At death, the bodies are placed on funeral pyres in Benares and cremated and the ashes sprinkled on the Ganges.

This religion encourages ancestor worship. Since Hinduism advocates reverence for animals, especially cows and monkeys, it has been a sacrilege to eat products from these animals.

The oldest scriptures of Hinduism are Vedas (*ca.* 1500 B.C.) written in Vedic, the parent language of Sanskrit; these are the historical documents of India and are also of religious significance. The Hindus say that these four books, Rig-Veda, Yajur-Veda, Sama-Veda and Atharva-Veda, were given to Brahma originally. The Rig-Veda (*ca.* 1500 B.C.) contains suggestions for medical treatment by the use of herbs and incantations.

Two of the best-loved Hindu scriptures are the Bhagavad-Gita (Song of God) and the Upanishads, a group of poetic dialogues on metaphysics written after the Vedas and largely as commentaries on them. The Upanishads are meant to impart knowledge of ultimate reality.

Temples are of importance in the life of the people of the East, and they have been masterpieces of artistry. *Contemplation* and *meditation* have occupied much attention, and there have been many followers of the monastic way of life.

Yoga is a method of "yoking" an individual's soul to the Supreme Being. This mystical experience of spiritual detachment from one's surroundings involves certain exercises. Bodily purity, attained by purgation and bathing, is followed by concentration on one subject with the purpose of excluding worldly diversions. The values of certain yoga postures, breathing exercises, breath control and meditation as well as relaxation have been noted by health authorities in recent years.

Siddhartha Gautama (*ca.* 566?–483 B.C.), the son of a northern Indian warrior-king, attained enlightenment (*ca.* 531 B.C.) and as Buddha ("the enlightened") introduced a new religious philosophy which came to be

[5]Berdoe, Edward: *The Origin and Growth of The Healing Art.* London, Swan, Sonnenschein & Co., 1893, p. 130.

known as Buddhism. *King Asoka* of India (269–237 B.C.) became a convert to Buddhism, but he was unsuccessful in fostering its acceptance on a permanent basis. He has been credited with the construction of hospitals, especially for pilgrims.

There were two renowned physicians in ancient India, Charaka and Susruta. Both of these men collected medical information into a compendium, or samhita. *Charaka,* in the second century A.D., presented in a clear, understandable fashion the ethical standards required for those who cared for the sick. Volume I, Section xv of his samhita emphasized that the men who were assistants should be "of good behavior, distinguished for purity, possessed of cleverness and skill, imbued with kindness, skilled in every service a patient may require, competent to cook food, skilled in bathing and washing the patient, rubbing and massaging the limbs, lifting and assisting him to walk about, well skilled in the making and cleansing of beds, readying the patient and skillful in waiting upon one that is ailing and never unwilling to do anything that may be ordered." There was a realization of the need for a skilled person to be at the patient's side.

Susruta, who lived about the fifth century A.D., described diseases, medicinal plants, procedures relating to surgery and some 121 different surgical instruments. Among those mentioned were scalpels, lancets, scissors, saws, needles, forceps, catheters and syringes. Hindu surgeons were familiar with amputation, cauterization (with boiling oil and pressure), delivery by cesarean section, and removal of cataracts and brain tumors (Fig. 3–16). They were especially skilled in such plastic surgery as skin grafting and rhinoplasty (nasal reconstruction). According to Susruta, a surgeon would cut a leaf of a tree to the size of the missing nose, apply this pattern to the cheek and cut a piece of skin of the same size. This tissue was then sewed to the stump of the nose. To facilitate breathing a tube was inserted into each nostril (Fig. 3–17).

Susruta also described the plastic surgery operation for the correction of an ear lobe deformity. Plastic surgery was carried out by specialists who belonged to a caste of potters known as Koomas. They were skilled at reconstruction and used their hands as sculptors and pottery makers did; thus the public associated them with these working groups.

The method of teaching students of surgery is presented most interestingly by Garrison:

> Realizing the importance of rapid, dexterous incision in operations without anesthesia, they had the student begin by practising upon plants. The hollow stalks of water-lilies or the veins of large leaves were punctured and lanced, as well as the blood-vessels of dead animals. Gourds,

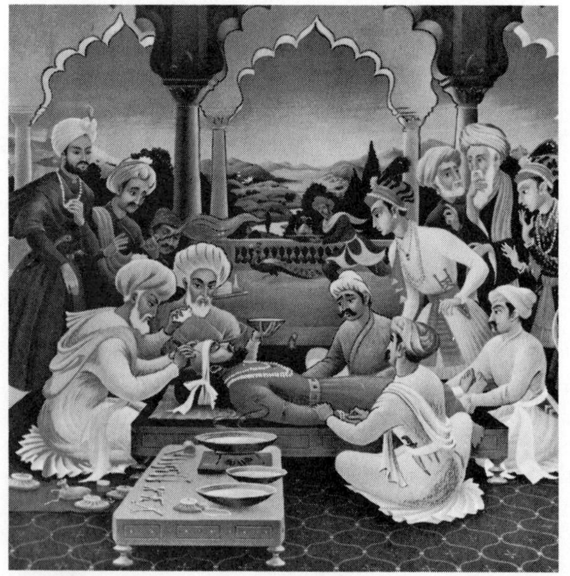

Figure 3–16. Artist's representation of Hindu surgeons performing a trepanation on King Bhoja of Dhar. A brain tumor was removed and the patient survived. The patient was sedated or under the effect of tranquilizers. (Courtesy of *Lederle Bulletin.*)

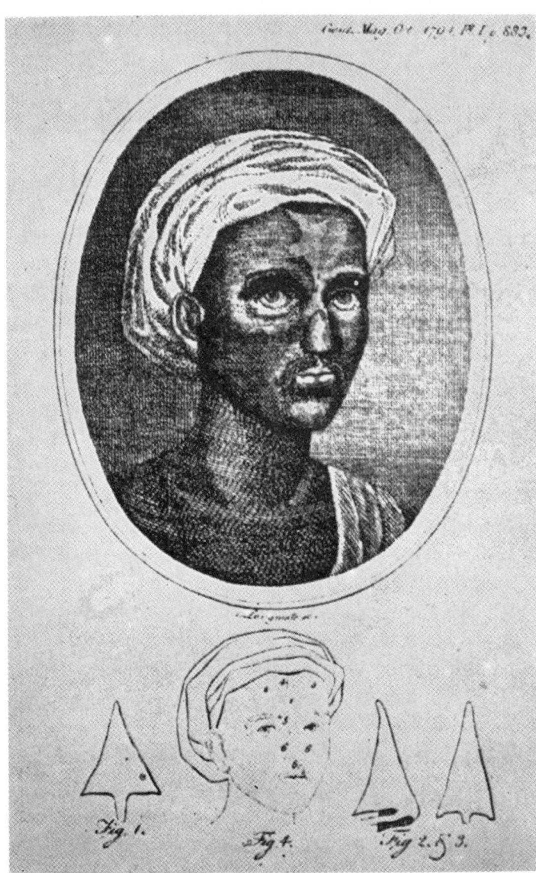

Figure 3–17. Indian rhinoplasty. Details of the technique of nasal reconstruction are shown. (Dolan collection.)

cucumbers and other soft fruits, or leather bags filled with water, were taped or incised in lieu of hydrocele or any other disorder of a hollow cavity. Flexible models were used for bandaging, and amputations and the plastic operations were practised upon dead animals. In so teaching the student to acquire ease and surety in operating by "going through the motions," the Hindus were pioneers of many recent wrinkles on the didactic side of experimental surgery.[6]

Another reason for this careful practice might have been the fine a doctor was compelled to pay if he caused injury to a patient.

Many diseases such as diabetes and tuberculosis were described, as were the transmitters of certain diseases, such as rats in plague and mosquitoes in malaria. Marco Polo described the Hindus' use of mosquito netting to forestall the spread of malaria. Vaccination was employed to prevent smallpox, and the narcotic effects of certain drugs such as hyoscyamus and cannabis indica in surgical anesthesia were noted.

There has been a resurgence of interest in the Ayurvedic (Indian) medicine, and many aspects of this type of medical care have been taught with so-called modern scientific methods. Several herbs that have been mainstays in the medical regimen of the medicine man have become modern discoveries in other parts of the world. One such remedy prescribed by ancient Hindu medicine men for hysteria and nervousness was the plant rauwolfia, from which is extracted the modern drug reserpine, popularly known as a tranquilizer.

By 1774 Great Britain had established colonial preeminence in India, having checked French aspirations to that end during the preceding decades. Many native customs were forbidden by the British and gradually disappeared because of legislation. Several of these customs pertain to women. The Sarda Act, passed by the Indian legislature in 1930, penalized marriages of girls under 14 years of age. *Purdah,* the practice of keeping women in seclusion, which served to retard social, physical and mental development and, *suttee,* or the burning of a widow on her deceased husband's funeral pyre, were forbidden, as was the practice of throwing infants into the Ganges.

It is in the area of teaching methods and surgery that the ancient Hindus made their greatest contribution to medicine. Health care deliverers today are studying and assessing the effects of ancient Hindu meditation and relaxation procedures on the promotion of health. The relation of biofeedback techniques to relief of stress conditions and the influence of these meditative stages and other aspects of yoga on bioenergy are also being examined.

THE ANCIENT GREEKS

Clinging to tradition, many of the ancient empires failed to introduce innovations and improvements of old methods, for instance, of agriculture, into their soci-

[6]Garrison, Fielding: *An Introduction to the History of Medicine.* Philadelphia, W.B. Saunders Co., 1929, p. 72.

eties, and as a result, the societies disintegrated. An infusion of new ideas was needed to release stored energy and channel it into constructive ways of improving the health of society.

The Greeks took the important step forward and provided leadership in many creative areas, including art, philosophy, nursing, medicine and the biological sciences.

The records of ancient Greece are greatly intertwined with such legends as one finds in Homer's *Iliad* and *Odyssey*. A combination of facile pen and vivid imagination was believed responsible for these epic poems until the German archeologist Heinrich Schliemann (*ca.* 1876) excavated the site of ancient Troy and brought a sense of reality to the well-known tales.

The Olympic games furnished a unifying force for the Greek civilization, because producing participants with healthy bodies became the aim of every family in Greece.

The Nurse In Greek Life

Among the glorious elements of the "Golden Age" of Greece was the emphasis Greeks placed on health maintenance. Nurturing for a high quality of life was again identified with nurses who carried out this function.

Probably the most complete picture of the role of the nurse in an ancient culture has been presented in a doctoral dissertation by a Greek scholar, Sister Mary Rosaria.[7] She notes that "the frequent mention of the nurse in connection with the child and the family and the numerous descriptions of her in Greek art have suggested the investigation of Greek classical literature and the inscriptions with the purpose of ascertaining and presenting the position and characteristics of the nurse as a contribution to the private life of the Greeks." Her study included the whole range of Greek literature from Homer (10th Century B.C.) to Plutarch (*ca.* 46–120 A.D.).

The poems of Homer deal with the life of the upper classes of Greek society. The wisest and most capable nurses, who were selected, acquired or captured during conquests, were given positions with wealthy families. Although most of these nurses were slaves, their position appeared to be one of respect and independence. A nurse was engaged to care for a child and then continued to provide health maintenance for that person as an adult. In the *Odyssey*, a nurse, *Eurycleia*, held such a revered position. Not only did she have the general supervision of fifty female slaves, but she assisted the mistress of the household in teaching them, presumably, principles of health education. According to Homer, "she is treated as a member of the family, is the friend and confidante of the mistress who shows her great deference."[8]

In the Homeric *Hymn to Demeter*, the duties of the goddess when she assumes the role of a nurse are identical to those performed by Eurycleia in the *Odyssey*. She is not treated as a slave of the people for whom she works but is promised such compensation for her services as would make her an object of envy to the women of the household.[9] It is assumed that she was exposed to a wealth of learned discussion, which enriched her own background.

Not all nurses were slaves. Certain women offered their services in times of personal financial stress and were hired if found to be skillful. Conversely, there are accounts of nurses who were given their freedom because of the efficient way they executed their duties. Even after emancipation, some remained in the service of their masters and received wages.

Sister Mary Rosaria comments on the respect and gratitude accorded many nurses. A master who cared for his Phrygian nurse during her lifetime set up a monument in her honor when she died so that posterity might see how an elderly nurse received "thanks for her nurture."

The Greek Nurse and Child Care

From a painstaking scrutiny of literature, art and inscriptions, Sister Mary Rosaria not only gleaned the important position

[7]Sister Mary Rosaria, The Nurse in Greek Life," Ph.D. Dissertation, Catholic University of America, 1917.

[8]Homer *Odyssey* 23. 24.

[9]Homer *Hymn to Demeter*. 166 ff.

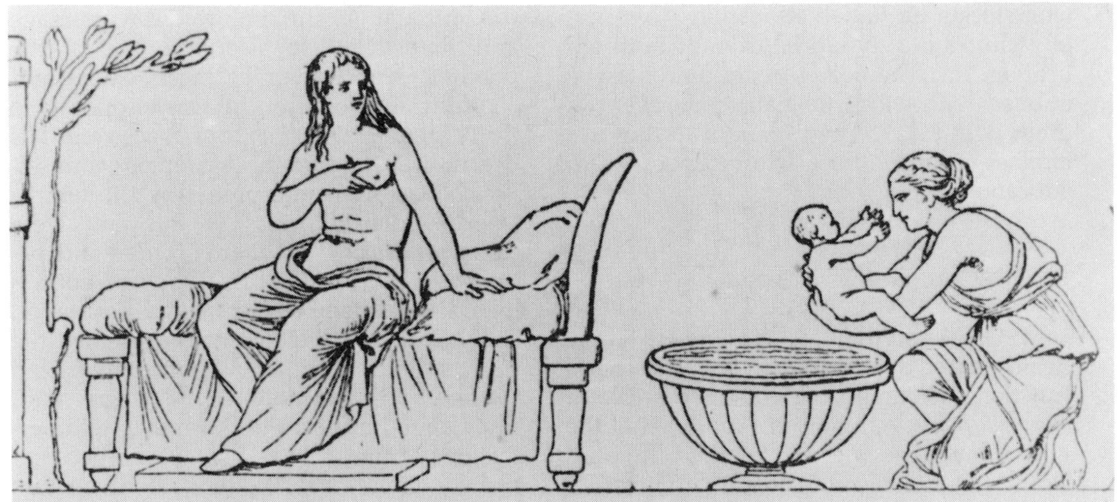

Figure 3–18. A scene on a vase portraying the life of Achilles shows the nurse giving a bath to the infant son of Thetis. (Dolan collection.)

the nurse held in the family, but noted the delineation of the roles she assumed.

Among the principal duties of the nurse in infant care is the giving of the bath. On a vase portraying the life of Achilles one of the scenes shows the nurse giving the infant son of Thetis his first bath (Fig. 3–18).

Children were wrapped in *swaddling clothes,* which are long narrow strips of cloth that were bound like bandages around the child's body, leaving nothing but the child's face uncovered. Homer refers to these bands as white, whereas Pindar mentions purple and saffron. Plantus records that the nurse caring for Hercules reported her inability to swathe him because he was such a large infant. Plato indicates that children were bound in this manner until they reached two years of age.

In *De Liberis Educandis,* Plutarch advises mothers to nurse their own children and describes the advantages. He opines that only if the mother is unable to nurse should a wet nurse be hired. In the same work he inveighs against the practice of entrusting children to any nurse and emphasizes the need for utmost care in the selection of nurses.

Plato refers to definite laws regarding the nurture of children. Aristotle associates infantile maladies with the physical condition of the nurse. He may be referring to Greek nurses' custom of first chewing food before giving it to the child.

The emotional support given by nurses when needed is well documented in classical literature. In the idyllic scene in the *Iliad,* in which Hector bids farewell to Andromache and his little son, it is to the familiar and soothing arms of the nurse that the child turns when frightened by his father's glancing helm.

The nurse's ability to soothe anxious children involved personal skills which included the use of music and motion, as Plato details. Nurses rocked children to sleep while singing lullabies to them. "An external agitation is employed to calm and counteract an internal (stress)." Sr. Rosaria says that "Plato recognized the principle only as it applied to music and to the useful art of nursing." Storytelling played a part in the daily activity of the nurse. This challenged the mind and influenced the spiritual development of the child. After children were lulled to sleep, they were placed in a variety of cradles. An example is the little two-handled basket shaped like a shoe in which the infant Hermes slept.

Nurses amused children with the various kinds of toys in use in antiquity. Sometimes the nurses made toys for children. Amulets and charms were used by nurses to ward off witchcraft and the evil eye.

The Greek Nurse as Educator. It is a tribute to the preparation and ability of the nurse that, together with the mother, she was entrusted with the education of the child. Quintilian quotes the treatise of

Chrysippus on Greek education: "No part of a child's life should be exempt from education. . . . The minds of children may be imbued with excellent instruction even by them [nurses]."[10] The same author advises families to hire nurses who are women of education.

Health Care Deliverers

In Greek mythology there were three health care deliverers whose roles and functions circumscribed distinct areas of service. *Asklepios*[11] (son of Apollo) was the god of medicine who represented the physician figure; *Hygeia* was the goddess of health maintenance, or the embodiment of the nurse; while *Panacea* was described as the goddess of medications, the preparation of which was the purview of the pharmacist. These three figures emphasize the importance that the Greeks placed on nursing, medicine and pharmacy in the health care delivery system.

The Greeks had implicit faith in the gods and before making important decisions consulted them at one of the Oracles. The shrine of Apollo at *Delphi* was one of the most famous Oracles. The gods were supposed to communicate their answers in one of four ways: deliver them orally through priests and priestesses; make them known by signs; present them in the form of dreams; or communicate them directly through spirits.

Asklepios gave his counsel in the form of dreams, which were interpreted by the priests in the temple. One of the chief temples erected in his honor was *Epidaurus,* a famous health center of Greece, which was similar to a very fashionable present-day health resort. The temple was an architectural masterpiece, built on a high hill with a magnificent view. The grounds afforded scenic walks, an outdoor theater, gymnasia and baths of invigorating mineral waters. On arrival, the patient sacrificed an animal to Asklepios, received a purifying bath in the mineral spring followed by massage and then went to sleep on one of the porches, surrounded by sweet odors and soothing music. Then he was supposed to drift into the *incubation* or *temple sleep.* His dream was to contain Asklepios' counsel, which was then interpreted by the temple priests. The followers of this cult were called *Asklepiads.* Pregnant women and patients with incurable diseases were not admitted to the temples for medical assistance.

Greek artists and sculptors presented the human body in action. They emphasized the muscles in motion under the skin. They aimed at perfection, removing imperfections from view; however, the preserved stone slab votive offerings that hung on the temple wall at Epidaurus were exceptions. These replicas of aspects of illnesses indicate cures and were left by grateful patients.

It is paradoxical that in these unscientific surroundings there emerged a distinguished leader who extricated the care of the sick from magic and superstition and inbued it with scientific spirit. This leader, born on the island of Cos in the year 460 B.C., belonged to a renowned Asklepiad family and was referred to by Aristotle as "the great Hippocrates" (Fig 3–19). *Hippocrates* deserves his title of "Father of Medicine." By stressing that there is a *natural cause* for diseases, he liberated the care of the sick from the influences of the mythical deities and magic; by teaching *accurate observation* of the sick and keeping careful records of treatment, he laid a foundation for clinical medicine; by reporting unsuccessful as well as successful methods of treatment, he presented a modern scientific approach; by emphasizing the importance of constant and skilled care at the patient's bedside, he prepared the way for the position of the professional nurse (he dismissed the slave and insisted that his medical students observe and administer bedside care); by instructing at the bedside, he demonstrated the value of clinical instruction by precept and by example; by practicing the high principles embodied in the Hippocratic Oath he laid the cornerstone of an excellent ethical code for medicine.

Hippocrates' care of the sick was *patient-centered,* and he used the scientific method

---

[10]Quintilian *Institutiones Oratoriae* 1. 1, 16.

[11]Asklepios has been portrayed with the staff of a traveler around which a serpent of wisdom is entwined. This has become the symbol of the World Health Organization.

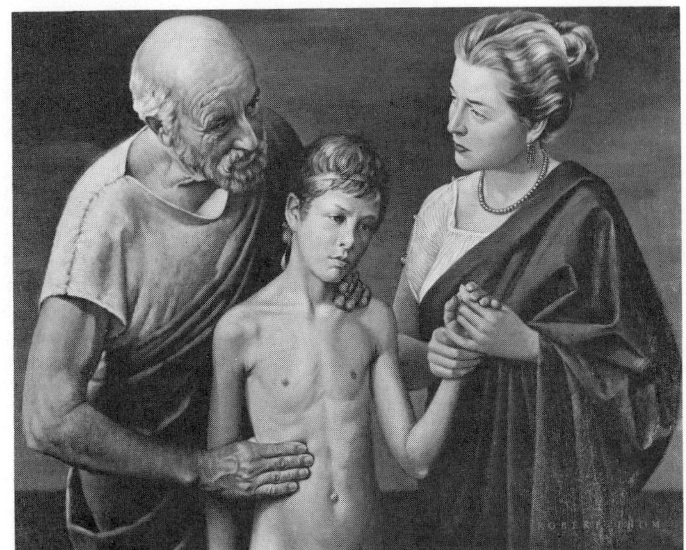

Figure 3–19. Hippocrates: Medicine becomes a science. (© 1958 by Parke, Davis & Co.)

in the solution of the problems of his patients.

He emphasized treating the whole person—the holistic approach. In endeavoring to do this, he indicated that disease was not inflicted by the gods but was a condition related to the laws of nature, and that a physician must understand, in addition to the specific illness, the person who was ill and the surroundings from which he came. Hippocrates stressed "Health depends upon a state of equilibrium among the various internal factors which govern the operations of the body and the mind; this equilibrium in turn is reached only when man lives in harmony with his external environment." A famous quotation of Hippocrates asserts ". . . it is well to tend the sick to make them well, to care for the healthy to keep them well." In describing Hippocrates' regimen for patient care, Plato wrote, "To heal even an eye, one must heal the head, and indeed the whole body."

One of Hippocrates' contributions, the clinical case history, became one of the most important tools of scientific patient care. In his analysis of the needs of the patient, he coupled the information about the person who was ill with details of the patient's environment and the results of the complete examination. The plan for care that Hippocrates outlined was direct and concise.

In a period when intellectual skills took precedence over manual skills, Hippocrates combined the two skills successfully to achieve good patient care.

This great teacher of clinical medicine, using a scientific approach to solve medical problems, reported his lack of success in order to assist others in avoiding similar mistakes: "I have written this down deliberately believing it is invaluable to learn of unsuccessful experiments and to know the causes of their failures."

Thales, who was born about 640 B.C., was the first of the great Greek philosopher-scientists. He stressed that although one must find solutions to problems, one must also discover the principles on which these solutions are based.

Aristotle, another famous natural scientist and an Asklepiad, contributed to the field of medicine. His interests were in the fields of botany, zoology, physiology, embryology and comparative anatomy, and he taught by dissecting animals. He stressed, "Of all the wonders of the universe the greatest is man."

In the *Iliad,* mention is made of the presence of army surgeons on the field of battle. First aid was administered. The art of bandaging was depicted on a famous antique vase that shows Achilles bandaging the wounded arm of Patroklos (Fig. 3–20). Homer may well have been a surgeon with one of the regimental armies. His descrip-

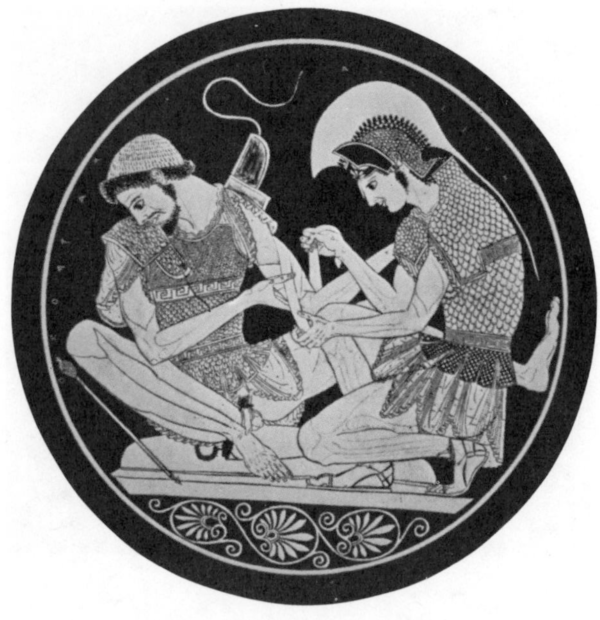

Figure 3–20. Vase painting (*ca.* 520–510 B.C.). Achilles bandaging the arm of his friend Patroklos. The arrow at left may have been removed from wound. (Courtesy of Metropolitan Museum of Art.)

tions reveal an extensive medical orientation if not a skilled practitioner's background.

Description of Disease

Some of the Greek words for symptoms of disease in Hippocrates' day were still in use many centuries later. The word cynanche, in the form kynanche, was used to identify the difficult swallowing and often the suffocation that accompanied diphtheria. Cynanche was recorded as the cause of George Washington's death. It has been reported that the doctors merely looked at George Washington's throat. When Hippocrates inspected a throat, however, he recorded the following observation: "In cases of ulcerated tonsils, the formulation of a membrane like a spider's web is not a good sign." He stated further that "ulcers on the tonsils that spread over the uvula alter the voice of those who recover." Obviously some patients recovered from diphtheria but suffered the accompanying diphtheritic paralysis that resulted in a raspy voice. This is another example of the combination of clinical observation and reason on the part of Hippocrates.

The Role of Environment in the Spread of Disease. Thucydides gives a stirring account of an epidemic in Athens during the Peloponnesian War. The occurrence of epidemics has been well documented. Diphtheria and malaria were two epidemics described. Greek physicians associated the outbreaks of malaria with swamp areas but felt that the fever of malaria was due to the consumption of the swamp waters.

Hippocrates emphasized the role of environment in the spread of disease in his work *Airs, Waters and Places.* Rosen reports that for two thousand years this was the basic epidemiological text.[12] It remained an important document until the late nineteenth century when the sciences of bacteriology and immunology made their appearance. Hippocrates understood the roles of climate, soil, water, mode of life and nutrition as factors of *endemy.* He noted that certain diseases were always present and were therefore *endemic;* diseases that flared up at certain periods and involved large numbers of people were *epidemic.*

Humoral Theory

The theory of the four elements—fire, air, earth and water—was advanced at this time. Bodies were thought to be composed of varying quantities of these four elements; when a state of equilibrium prevailed, health resulted. The four elements

[12]Rosen, George: *A History of Public Health.* New York, M.D. Publications, Inc., 1958, p. 33.

also corresponded to the four necessary qualities of heat and cold, dryness and moisture. This theory became the basis of the *humoral theory,* which governed the thinking of medical leaders for centuries.

Hippocrates stated that *health* depends upon a state of equilibrium existing among internal forces that govern the functioning of body and mind. This equilibrium results when man lives in harmony with his external environment.

THE ALEXANDRIAN EMPIRE

Greece was the intellectual center of the western world and continued to enlighten those people who attempted to enslave her.

The first of these conquerors was Philip II of Macedonia, the father of *Alexander the Great.* At Philip's death in 336 B.C., Alexander started his career of conquest, subduing Thebes (335 B.C.) and thus gaining ascendancy over all of Greece. The period from 336 to 133 B.C. is often referred to as the *Hellenistic Age,* since the conquered lands under Alexander the Great became Greek in culture and language; Greece herself, however, suffered an intellectual decline.

Alexander, who desired to rule the world, conquered Greece, Asia Minor, Egypt and Persia as far east as northern India. *Alexandria,* on the Nile delta in Egypt, became the new capital of his empire and replaced Athens as the center of learning and culture. At Alexandria were located a thriving seaport with docks, lighthouses, rich palaces, a celebrated museum and an outstanding library from which shone a beacon of intellectual light that beckoned scholars from all over the world. In reality the library was a university where the ancient manuscripts were studied and research was carried out in the arts, literature, physics, mathematics, astronomy and medicine. Medicine remained in the hands of the Greeks, and many outstanding leaders from other nations received their education in Greece.

After Alexander's death, one of his generals, Ptolemy, succeeded him as ruler of Egypt, and thus began the Ptolemaic dynasty (323–30 B.C.). The glory of the Alexandrian Empire was short-lived. Octavian's victory over the Egyptian fleet in the battle of Actium in 31 B.C. unified the Roman world and ended Egypt's proud sovereignty.

THE ANCIENT ROMANS

Rome has been a kingdom, a republic, an empire and a city. About 753 B.C. Rome was a small section of land in the center of which was a hill with a few crude shelters. Four hundred and eighty years later it contained all of the peninsula we now call Italy. By the second century A.D. Rome encompassed the territory we now know as England, Spain, France, Switzerland, Austria, Hungary, Italy, Greece, Turkey, Sicily and North Africa as well as other smaller states and islands. At the present time it is the principal city and capital of Italy.

The Romans borrowed much of their culture from Greece and other conquered countries. They worshiped a similar pantheon of gods and goddesses and built temples in their honor. Ancestor worship was practiced, and gradually the Romans inaugurated the custom of worshiping their emperors.

The populace of Rome was divided into two classes, the wealthy and the poor, with the wealthy becoming wealthier and the poor becoming abysmally poorer. A summary of events at this time would include the following: the exorbitant loss of lives through conquests, a decline in morals because of war, the replacement of simple living by luxurious living for the few, the infusion of Greek culture, the introduction of gladiatorial games, the construction of luxurious baths, a decay in political circles, widespread unemployment and extensive slavery.

The ascension of Julius Caesar to undisputed power following the defeat of his archrival Pompey in 48 B.C. marked the greatest single turning point in the affairs of Rome. Following the assassination of Julius Caesar in 44 B.C., his adopted son Octavian gained control of Italy, and in 27 B.C., he was proclaimed Augustus, first emperor of Rome. During his reign peace was restored, industry flourished, roads were constructed and a census of the whole empire was taken.

Emperors good and bad succeeded Octavian. The records reveal a gradual in-

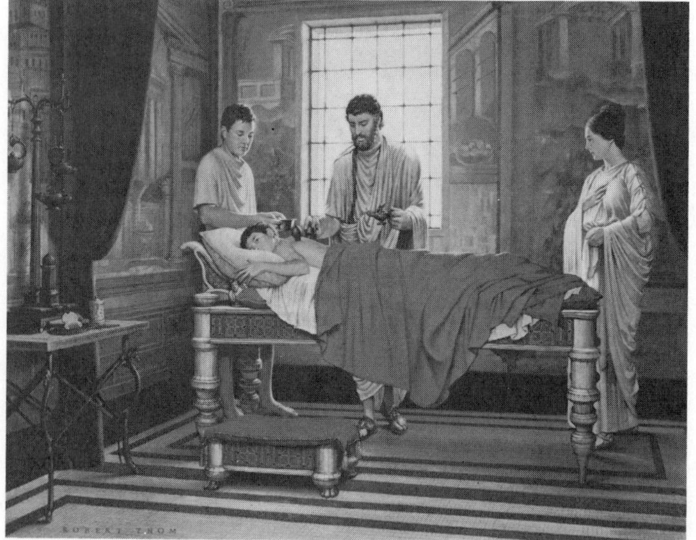

Figure 3–21. Galen: Influence for forty-five generations. (© 1958 by Parke, Davis & Co.) Note that Galen is applying cups, thereby practicing a modality known as "cupping."

crease in deaths by murder, infanticide, burning and being devoured by wild animals, and finally the existence of a dictatorial government that denied the people of Rome liberty.

The Roman family as a unit was not a stable one. Marriages by civil contract were made and dissolved easily, and divorce became a general practice.

The famous Olympic games were replaced as entertainment by the gladiatorial contests.

Nero began persecuting Christians; hundreds of them died in the arenas of Roman amphitheatres.

The value of the individual fell very low, and it is no wonder that the only hospitals of note were built for the military. Nursing homes, *valetudinaria,* were established for sick slaves because they were considered valuable property. Nursing was done by the slaves, and the practice of medicine was under the aegis of captured Greek physicians. The most skillful physicians were granted Roman citizenship.

Galen (Fig. 3–21) was the most renowned of the Greek physicians during this period and for many centuries afterwards. Born about 130 A.D. in the famous city of Pergamum in Asia Minor, which had been colonized by Greek settlers, Galen had an excellent general and medical education for this period. His major contributions included the reintroduction of the famous works of Hippocrates for use in medical thinking and study; the selection, use and compounding of drugs, many of which are referred to as "galenicals"; and the writing of voluminous works used in the teaching of medical science for many centuries after his death in 201 A.D.

Galen also noted that occupation played a role in illness. He reported that certain diseases were due to inhalation and that pallor could be associated with employment in the mines.

It is to *Aulus Cornelius Celsus,* who lived during the reign of Tiberius Caesar (first century A.D.), that we are most indebted for leaving an accurate account of the importance of Greek physicians in Roman medicine. Celsus wrote the first organized medical history, which is considered one of the great Latin classics. He translated works from Greek into Latin and described the four cardinal symptoms of inflammation—*rubor et tumor, cum calore et dolore* (redness and swelling, with heat and pain).

His writings included information on dietetics as well as pharmacy, medicine, surgery and psychiatry. Forms of therapy that he recommended were sea voyages, changes of scene in the form of trips, moderate exercise, exposure to sunlight, massage and warm baths.

Pedanius Dioscorides, a Greek physician of the first century A.D., was a famous leader in the field of pharmacy and author of *De Materia Medica,* which remained for 1500 years the definitive text on botanic medicine. He used his keen powers of observation to broaden the knowledge about plants that were usable for drugs. He accompanied the Roman armies, observing, recording and collecting drugs.

The beneficial contributions of the Romans were in the fields of engineering, public health, sanitation and law. *Aqueducts* were built to supply the city with water from mountain springs many miles away. This water was carried in pipes through tunnels and across lowlands. In addition to the fantastic system of aqueducts, the city plans included the employment of a water commissioner. The first accounts of the duties of an administrative public health official appear in *De Aquis Urbis Romae*.

At the height of the Roman Empire, when the population totalled one million people, about 40 gallons of water per person were used per day. To improve the quality of the water, the Romans encouraged the use of settling basins from which slaves removed the sediment. Reservoirs, properly enclosed and protected, helped maintain a pure water supply.

Marshes were drained, a sewage system was established and plumbing was introduced into the houses. Records show warnings against the use of polluted water. More precise knowledge of pollution in swampy areas has been revealed in a remarkable Roman note of caution that stated that "there are bred certain minute creatures which cannot be seen by the eyes, which float in the air and enter the body through the mouth and nose and there cause serious diseases." Malaria, typhoid fever, dysentery as well as diphtheria and tuberculosis plagued the Romans. A bubonic plague epidemic of historic significance occurred during the reign of Emperior Justinian (483–565 A.D.). The crowded slum areas acted as breeding places for physical and social diseases.

The public baths became quite fashionable. The Baths of Caracalla (186–217 A.D.) in Rome were expansive, palatial and costly. The baths were named for Caracalla, the emperor who was purported to have ordered the mass murder of 20,000 people. Covering acres of land, the baths accommodated thousands of persons in the most grandiose manner. The spacious interior had high arched ceilings and was beautifully ornamented with marble and exquisite inlaid mosaics. There were auditoria, gymnasia, reading rooms, patios with cool fountains, soft music and swimming pools to delight the patrons and provide diversional therapy.

When taking the therapeutic tour of the baths, a person would first undress in the apodyterium and receive a massage; the person would then go to the tepidarium, with its warm refreshing waters; then to the sudadorium, where increasingly warmer water was provided; afterwards he would bathe in the hot waters of the calidarium; the person would complete his tour in the cold waters of the frigidarium.

The heat of the baths was controlled in the basement beneath the floor where open hearth furnaces, manned by slaves, sent the heat through a flue system and pipes to the pools above. The pipes were made of soft flexible lead. This may have caused lead poisoning, which, in turn, may have contributed to the physical decline of the Romans. (Another possible cause of lead poisoning was the process used for preserving and sweetening wine. The wine stood for long periods in lead vats during the so-called sweetening process.) In the frigidarium the clear, cold water came from the aqueduct system.

The sun was so important in the Greek and Roman philosophies of life that Apollo and Helios were revered as sun gods. Heliotherapy (sun bathing) was used in classical times, and Caelius Aurelianus, a Roman physician during the fifth century A.D., advocated its use for the treatment of rickets, bone and joint diseases and skin ailments.

A large swampy section of land was drained by a great arched sewer called the Cloaca Maxima, which emptied into the Tiber River. The land became the basis for the foundation of the famous Roman Forum, the public market place. It was so well constructed that it has withstood the ravages of time and is used today.

THE IRISH CELTS

Ireland was a site of civilized activity as early as 1000 B.C. The story of its beginnings is embellished with interesting legends and sagas. Ireland was called Hibernia by the Romans, Ireland by the Norsemen and Erin by its natives.

The Gaelic-speaking Celts migrated from Europe to Ireland during the middle of the fourth century B.C. It is interesting to note that centuries later, when the Irish discontinued the use of their native language and adopted English, they used the mode of English pronunciation of the Elizabethan and Jacobean period, exemplified in Shakespeare's writings.

It is a matter of record that when the Roman spirit was decaying and the light of civilization was waning, the Irish preserved the spirit and contributed to it, creating literature and poetry, melodious music and gorgeous works of art. The Irish maintained an interest in Latin and Greek and were intrigued by Greek philosophy as well as Greek literature.

In pagan Ireland there were three learned orders: the *druids*, the *brehons* and the *bards*. The druids studied physical and theological science and possessed knowledge of divination and magic. The brehons were lawyers, and the bards were poets who preserved much of the fascinating history and traditions of the country.

Because of the clan system under which they lived, the Irish provided dutifully for the needs of the less fortunate. In 300 B.C. Princess Macha built a hospital in Ireland called *Broin Bearg*, or the House of Sorrow.

The Irish were advanced in medical treatments and in the establishment of laws regulating the practice of medicine. They recognized the benefit of *moist heat* as a clinical treatment. Hot compresses, hot water baths, medicated baths and "sweating houses" are mentioned frequently in records of the time.

The early Irish employed many modern techniques of patient care. For example, they emphasized the importance of peace of mind for the benefit of patients. This was achieved by careful scrutiny of the patient to better understand his needs. Persons and things that were detrimental to the welfare of the patient were excluded from the sick room.

Trepanning operations, as observed in the story of an Irish prince, were performed. Because of a severe blow on the head, the prince had lost his memory, and physicians resorted to a trepanning operation. The prince was said to have lost his "organ of forgetting" as a result of the operation, and his memory was restored.

In a twelfth century Celtic book of *materia medica*, reference is made to mandrake, which was to be used before operations to prevent pain.

The early *obstetrical* practices of the Irish are fascinating. It was an Irish practice to encourage a mother to deliver her baby while in a kneeling position. A feather mattress (burned after delivery to prevent the spread of infection) was rolled up, and the mother knelt on this and leaned against a chair in front of her, helping herself by exercising as she grasped and pushed during the process of labor. The mother's muscles had been kept in good condition by housework and field work. The birth process was not considered a pathological event but rather a normal physiological experience.

A physician was not in attendance during childbirth, but rather there was a "wise woman" or nurse midwife. The Irish mother was out of bed by the third day and back to her chores by the fifth. A hammock arrangement for the baby on the mother's bed permitted her to meet the needs of the newborn. These people practiced an early form of the "rooming-in" method of baby care.

The practice of medicine was regulated by carefully drawn *brehon laws*. One of these laws required that every physician in Ireland keep one door of his house open at all times. The physician's house was to be an open house into which the injured and sick might be brought for treatment.

Every physician was expected to permit four medical students to reside in his home. The physician's duties included teaching these young men by demonstrating the medical care of the patients. It is likely that this prompted doctors to put forth their best efforts as an example to the students. Medical fees were regulated according to the service given to the patient and his ability to pay.

The laws against impostors and people not properly prepared to practice medicine were very strict. The Irish felt that those who were ill could be easily deceived, and anyone who took advantage of this "susceptible" state of mind was punished severely:

> If an unlawful physician treat a joint or sinew without obtaining an indemnity against liability to damages and without a notice to the patient

that he is not a regular physician he is subject to a penalty with compensation to the patient.

Finally, the law of "sick maintenance" required that provision be made for all who needed curative treatment, nourishing food and a place of care. The persons who were responsible for carrying out these needs were clearly and carefully defined by law.

The status of women in Ireland was high. They had legal rights to property, and Irish literature refers to the reverence with which they were treated. One of the outstanding pioneers in the education of women was St. Brigid of Kildare.

CONTRIBUTIONS OF ANCIENT CULTURES TO HEALTH CARE

In pausing to review the achievements and contributions of these ancient cultures, we note that the Sumerians, Babylonians and Egyptians practiced medicine governed by a code imbued with magic principles and did not pursue a scientific quest for the cause of disease; the Hebrews bequeathed a good foundation for hygiene, sanitation and health maintenance; the Chinese laid a firm basis upon which to build the sciences of pharmacology and therapeutics; the Hindus gave inspiring leadership in the field of surgery; and the Greeks were leaders in the theory and practice of clinical medicine and clinical instruction. We notice also, however, that much artistic skill and material wealth accompanied primitive superstition, with its lack of health progress, ruthless brutality and total indifference to the value and equality of the individual.

The Greek spirit of inquiry sparked the use of the scientific approach to problems, the beginning of theoretical science and the health care delivery by nurses. The need for the use of pure reason was extolled. It is evident that the scholarly Greeks respected and appreciated the high quality achievements of nurses.

THE HERITAGE OF NURSING

The Image of Nurses in Ancient Cultures: Part II

Many of the older societies differed in their cultural attitudes toward the sick and toward keeping people healthy, as well as toward the status of women, which influenced the women's role as health care providers. Even amid obstacles to progress, however, the light of nursing still shone.

1. Nursing remained a female societal work assignment.
2. Nursing care was rendered by some women whose status was low in their cultures.
3. In other cultures nurses were competent sustainers of health who practiced their nurturing skills in nurse midwifery, health preservation, herbal therapy, child care and general education.
4. Nurses were healers, using transference of energy through the laying on of hands as well as many folk remedies.
5. Many ancient health care practices have been perpetuated or rediscovered by our contemporary society.
6. Nurses encouraged family participation and emotional support for clients.
7. Nurses cooperated with other health care deliverers in promoting the welfare of their clients.
8. The three health team workers—the nurse, the pharmacist and the physician—were recorded in ancient Greek mythology.
9. Hippocrates pleaded for educated nurses to sustain the lives he

tried so hard to save. (He replaced the "slave nurse" with medical students who lacked the nurses' preparation.)

10. Hippocrates emphasized the need for an ethical base for clinical practice and instruction.

The recognition by Hippocrates, the "Father of Medicine," of the need for an academically prepared, clinically enlightened nurse to "care for, care with, while caring about" the client in order to sustain life was a historic milestone.

REFERENCE READINGS

Adams, Francis: *The Genuine Words of Hippocrates*. Baltimore, Williams & Wilkins Co., 1939.

Branch, Marie Foster, and Paxton, Phyllis Perry: *Providing Safe Nursing Care for Ethnic People of Color*. New York, Appleton-Century-Crofts, 1976.

Buck, Pearl: *The Good Earth*. New York, Pocket Books, 1931.

Bulwer-Lytton, Edward: *The Last Days of Pompeii*. New York, Dodd, Mead & Co., 1834.

Clark, Margaret: *Ethnicity and Health Care*. New York, National League for Nursing, 1976.

Clark, Margaret: *Health in the Mexican-American Culture: A Community Study*. 2nd ed. Berkeley, University of California Press, 1970.

Dechanet, J. M.: *Christian Yoga*. New York, Harper & Brothers, 1960.

Gibbon, Edward: *The Decline and Fall of the Roman Empire*. New York, Viking Press.

Hamilton, Edith: *The Greek Way*. New York, Mentor Books, New American Library of World Literature, 1948.

Hume, E. H.: *The Chinese Way in Medicine*. Baltimore, Johns Hopkins Press, 1940.

Joe, Jennie, Gallerito, Cecelia, and Pino, Josephine: "Cultural Health Traditions: American Indian Perspectives," In *Providing Safe Nursing Care for Ethnic People of Color*. New York, Appleton-Century-Crofts, 1976, pp. 81–98.

Kniep-Hardy, Mary, and Burkhardt, Margaret: "Nursing the Navajo," *American Journal of Nursing, 77*:95–96, 1977.

Lao Tzu: *The Way of Life*. Trans. R. B. Blakney. New York, The New American Library, 1955.

Leininger, Madeleine M.: "Transcultural Nursing: Its Progress and its Future," *Nursing and Health Care,* 2 (7) 365–371, 1981.

Lin Yutang: *Famous Chinese Short Stories*. New York, Pocket Books, 1952.

Lin Yutang: *The Wisdom of China and India*. New York, Random House, 1942.

MacManus, Seymas: *The Story of the Irish Race*. New York, The Devin-Adair Co., 1907.

McKenzie, Joan L., and Chrisman, Noel L.: "Healing Herbs, Gods and Magic," *Nursing Outlook, 25*:326–329, 1977.

Pochin Mould, D. D. C.: *Ireland of the Saints*. London, B. T. Batsford, 1953.

Prabhavananda, S., and Isherwood, C.: *The Song of God: Bhagavad-Gita*. New York, Harper & Brothers, 1954.

Prabhavananda, S., and Manchester, F.: *The Upanishads*. Hollywood, Calif., Vedanta Press, 1948.

Primeaux, Martha: "Caring for the American Indian Patient," *American Journal of Nursing, 77*:91–94, 1977.

Renault, Mary: *The Last of the Wine*. New York, Pantheon Books, 1954.

Rosaria, Sister Mary: *"The Nurse in Greek Life."* Ph.D. Dissertation, Catholic University of America, 1917.

Stirling, Matthew, et al.: *Indians of the Americas*. Washington, National Geographic Society, 1955.

Stobart, John C: *The Glory That Was Greece*. Rev. ed. Boston, Beacon Press, 1934.

"Symposium on Cultural and Biological Diversity and Health Care," *Nursing Clinics of North America,* Philadelphia, W. B. Saunders, *12*:1–84, 1977. (Suggested bibliography on "Cultural Diversities and Transcultural Nursing" by Dr. Madeleine Leininger appears on pp. 85–86.)

Tantaquidgeon, Gladys: *A Study of Delaware Indian Medicine Practice and Folk Beliefs*. Harrisburg, Pennsylvania Historical Commission, 1942.

Von Hagen, Victor W.: *Realm of the Incas*. New York, Mentor Books, New American Library of World Literature, 1957.

Walsh, James J.: *The World's Debt to the Irish*. Boston, The Stratford Co., 1926.

Williams, Joseph J.: *Voodoos and Obeahs—Phases of West Indian Witchcraft*. New York, Dial Press, 1933.

Wong, K. C., and Wu, Lieu-Teh: *History of Chinese Medicine*. Shanghai, National Quarantine Service, 1936.

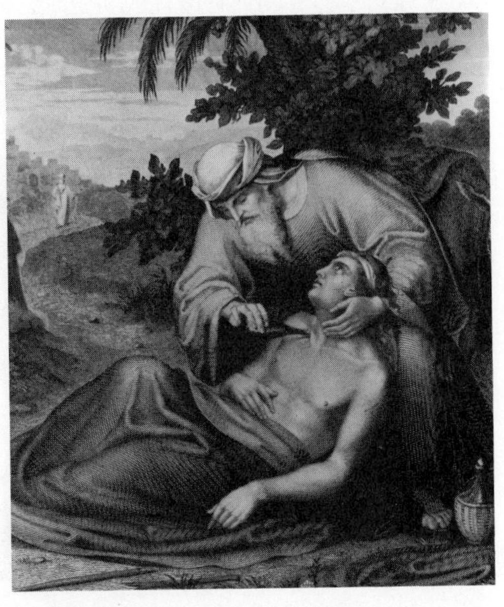

The Good Samaritan. This engraving was ordered by Pastor Fliedner for the Order of Deaconesses of Kaiserswerth in 1854. (Dolan collection.)

4 Effects of Spiritual Leadership on the Enrichment of Nursing

THE INFLUENCE OF CHRISTIANITY

The teachings and example of *Jesus Christ* had a profound influence on the emergence of gifted nurse leadership as well as on the expansion of the role of nurses. Christ stressed the need to love God and one's neighbor. The first organized group of nurses was established as a direct response to His example and challenge.

His philosophy advocated living a life of charity in a world of selfishness and hatred. At the time of His birth much of the world was enslaved, and fear, terror and torture abounded. Poverty, desolation and disease were rampant.

Christ provided the key to His philosophy in His Sermon on the Mount. His way of living reflected His compassion and recognition of human worth. His remarkable deeds evoked a new concept of the innate dignity of each person. His miracles testified to His love, and His attitude toward the sick was a good example in human relations. Instead of "saying the word" and healing the sick, Christ gave individual attention to the needs of all by touching, anointing and taking by the hand (Fig. 4–1).

Christ taught in parables, which was a case method approach. One of these parables describes a man lying by the pool Bethesda who had had an infirmity for 38 years. Because no one would put him into the pool, he could not be cured by Bethesda's healing waters. He continued to have hope for a healing, but time elapsed, and he became a forgotten man. This account epitomizes the hopeless plight of the chronically ill who hope that the humanistic skills of health care deliverers will be used to enable the sick to achieve a richer, fuller life. This is a crucial and continuing problem.

The parable of the Good Samaritan delineated the urgency of Christ's message and example as well as His spiritual reward for caring for anyone in need. "Upon

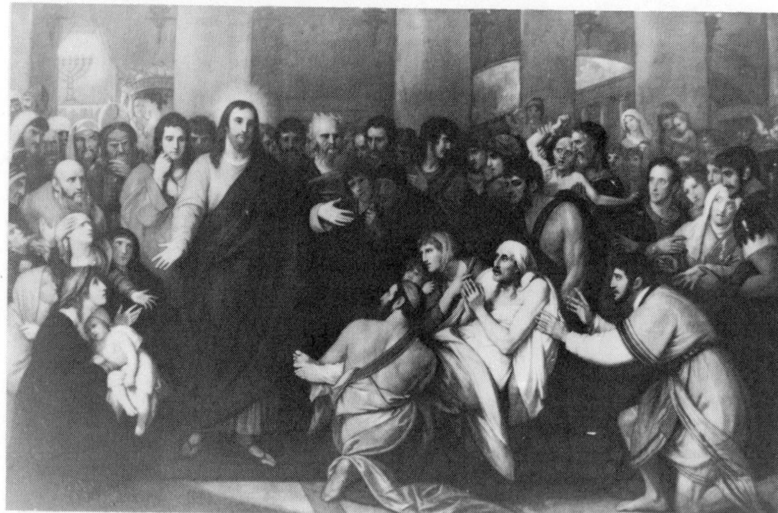

Figure 4–1. Christ healing the Sick in the Temple, by Benjamin West (1845). (Courtesy of Pennsylvania Hospital, Philadelphia.)

my return I will reward you," Christ counseled. "Amen, amen I say to you, as long as you did it to one of these my least brethren, you did it unto me." His followers ministered to those in need and envisioned Christ as the recipient.

At the Last Supper Christ gave to His disciples His final instructions: "A new commandment I give you, that you love one another. That as *I have loved you,* you also love one another." This commandment of love was called *new,* for the world before Christ's coming was a world without love. The object of His coming was that of love, since He explained, "The Son of man came not to be ministered unto, but to minister, and to give His life as a ransom for many"; and before His death He said, "Greater love than this no man hath that he lay down his life for his friends." His command was "Come follow me."

Many historians have recorded stories of the social and spiritual leadership of the Christians as they began to follow in Christ's footsteps. The Carthaginian theologian Tertullian (160?–230? A.D.) wrote:

> It is our care of the helpless, our practice of loving kindness that brands us in the eyes of many of our opponents. "Only look," they say, "how they love one another! Look how they are prepared to die for one another."

Eusebius of Caesarea ("the father of ecclesiastical history," 260?–340? A.D.) described a plague in the time of Maximinus Daza:

> The Christians were the only people who amid such terrible ills, showed their fellow-feeling and humanity by their actions. Day by day some would busy themselves by attending to the dead and burying them; others gathered in one spot all who were afflicted by hunger throughout the whole city and give them bread.

EXPANSION OF NURSING

Charity—love in action—was apparent in the expansive role of nursing, which took root, flourished and expanded in the early Christian period. There were individuals who will be recorded for all time for their example in comforting the afflicted: Solicitously, Veronica wiped the agonized face of Christ, and Mary Magdalene and St. John gave genuine consolation to His Mother.

Not only had Christ's message enhanced the dignity of all persons, but it had two additional significant results: the emancipation of women and the elevation of their status; and the emancipation of men in terms of career choices. Spontaneously, there emerged a freedom for both men and women to engage in humanitarian endeavors. As a result, many men entered the nursing field.

Gifted nurse leadership emerged. Persons who were socially and culturally skilled, intellectually endowed and educationally prepared, including some who were recognized scholars, were recorded as deliverers of nursing care. Well-educated though they were, they recognized the need for educational preparation for nursing in addition to their liberal education base. They were not satisfied with apprenticeship experience or learning by doing at the client's expense. *The nursing care was scholarly.*

DEACONESSES

The earliest "bearers of the lamp" were called visiting nurses. The forerunner of the community health nursing movement of today had its beginning in the first century of the Christian Church. Human suffering had elicited concerned action from individuals down through the years, but the first organized visiting of the sick began with the establishment of the order of *Deaconesses*. They endeavored to practice the *Corporal Works of Mercy*. Note the basic human needs referred to in the Corporal Works of Mercy:

To feed the hungry.
To give water to the thirsty.
To clothe the naked.
To visit the imprisoned.
To shelter the homeless.
To care for the sick.
To bury the dead.

Consider the implications of those works of mercy for the earliest nurses as well as for nurses of today. In addition to the obvious need to provide for those who were underprivileged and culturally deprived, the nurse recognized the needs of those who were malnourished physically, intellectually and spiritually. Besides quenching the thirst for water, they recognized the tremendous thirst for human compassion. They recognized the necessity for clothing a person with the warmth of understanding and love, as well as with garments. They also perceived the importance of visiting the imprisoned in all kinds of institutions, especially those who were confined for long periods, who were neglected or forgotten and who needed to know that people still cared about them.

These nurses incorporated in their care the act of sheltering the homeless, who needed to feel warmth and hospitality in a new or strange environment. Care of the sick merited special attention in the Corporal Works of Mercy.

The importance of giving spiritual meaning to both the care given to patients and the suffering borne by patients was stressed by Christ when He said, "As long as you did it to one of these . . . you did it to me," and "Pick up your cross and follow me." These nurses were following the command of their Master and imitating Him who spent His life ministering to those in need.

There must have been a pattern of organization based on a district plan. The objectives of their service were the provision of care for the sick in their homes as well as the distribution of aid to the needy.

The early Christians sold what they possessed and gave it to the poor. In their thinking charity was synonymous with love. The Church became the central charity organization because there were no other organized charities from which to obtain clothing, food and other necessities. The deaconess, in distributing the food and medicines that she carried in a basket (the visiting nurse's bag of that period), was the forerunner of the social worker and the public health nurse.

The care given by the deaconess probably consisted of bathing patients, especially those who had communicable diseases and were feverish; dressing wounds, including the applications of dressings to burned areas; giving foods and forcing fluids; and bringing physical and spiritual comfort to all patients, especially the dying. There was an overflowing of love, charity and tenderness. Home remedies, using herbs, minerals, diet, bathing and, where possible, fresh air, were relied upon.

The marvels of the structure and beauty of wealthy Rome are well known. It was in the slum sections of the empire, however, that the deaconesses and the Christian Roman matrons carried out their duties. The abysmal poverty of the citizenry has been mentioned, and it was in this setting that Christians labored to bring relief to the suffering and depressed. These patients had few necessities and were crowded into small tenement areas in which little fresh air was available and much sickness, sorrow, want, misery and distress were present.

Phoebe, a friend of St. Paul, was the first deaconess and the first visiting nurse.

From the Bible we learn that she was entrusted with the letters of St. Paul,[1] and he said of her nursing care, "For she also assisted many and myself also." St. Paul referred to nurses as "exemplars of gentleness."

The date of the Epistle to the Romans in which there is reference to Phoebe is about 58 A.D. Note has been made of her education, wealth and important social status and the fact that she had business that necessitated travel to the capital of the Empire.

The writings of St. John Chrysostom (d. 404 A.D.), the Bishop of Constantinople, describe the activities of another deaconess, *St. Olympias*. The daughter of a count of the Roman Empire, Olympias inherited an immense fortune when her parents died during her childhood. She married and held a position of social prestige as the wife of the prefect of Constantinople. Left a childless widow at the age of 18, Olympias erected a convent in which a large number of relatives and friends devoted themselves to works of charity and the

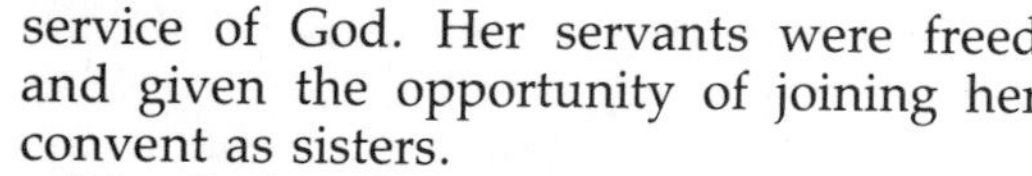

service of God. Her servants were freed and given the opportunity of joining her convent as sisters.

The Order of Deaconesses attained a position of importance for many years, and then gradually died out.

[1]Epistle to the Romans *16*:1–2.

MATRONS

A group of noble *Roman matrons* distinguished themselves in the field of nursing. These were women of wealth, intelligence and social leadership who, having been converted to Christianity, founded hospitals and convents and worked for the good of others.

St. Helena (250–330 A.D.), Flavia Helena, was the daughter of an innkeeper of Drepanum, in Bithynia and the mother of Constantine the Great, the ruler of the Roman Empire (Fig. 4–2). She became the Empress of Rome when she married Constantine Chlorus. She embraced Christianity and dedicated the remainder of her life to the needy. She gave generously to the poor and built shelters and churches for

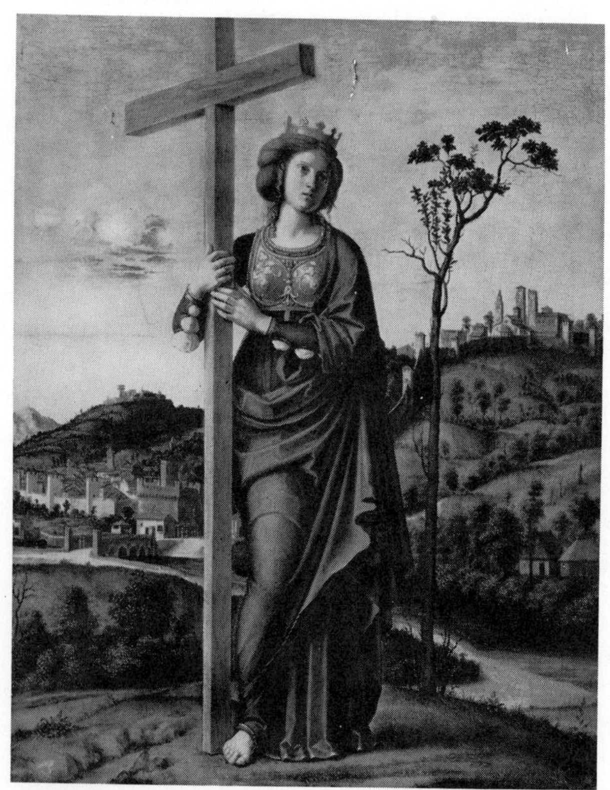

Figure 4–2. St. Helena by Cima Da Conegliano (*ca.* 1459–1517). (Samuel H. Kress Collection. Courtesy of National Gallery of Art, Washington, D.C.)

the pilgrims who were determined to visit the "Holy Places." Her concern and compassion resulted in the construction of hospices, or hostels, called Geroncomion, for the elderly. She encouraged nurses to become specially skilled in what we would now identify as gerontological nursing.

Constantine revered his saintly mother, and her influence over him was quite pronounced. He rebuilt Drepanum and renamed it Helenopolis in her honor; he also bestowed upon her the supreme title of Augusta.

Empress Flacilla, the daughter of Claudius Antonius, the Prefect of Gaul, and the wife of Theodosius the Great (346?–395 A.D.), went to the hospital daily to attend the sick. There she washed and dressed the patients, made their beds, prepared their food and served those who were unable to feed themselves. The Empress was especially interested in assisting physically handicapped persons.

St. Marcella converted her luxurious palace on Aventine Hill into a monastery. A scholar, Marcella encouraged other Roman matrons of intelligence and spiritual depth to join her in studying Latin and Greek literature, Hebrew and the Scriptures. Of her keenness of mind St. Jerome (340?–420 A.D.) wrote: "All that I have learnt with great study and long meditation the blessed Marcella learnt also, but with great facility and without giving up any of her other occupations or neglecting any of her pursuits." Marcella taught the care of the sick to her followers, and her conventual plan encouraged further education for women. Indeed she is considered the *first nurse educator*. Her scholarship and leadership have been recognized by the greatest scholars. Marcella was killed by barbarians during the sack of Rome.

St. Fabiola (Fig. 4–3) was one of the most charming, popular and capable members of Marcella's group. She belonged to the patrician family of Fabian. She had led a very worldly life, but because of the influence of St. Jerome and Marcella, she gave up her earthly pleasures and lavished her immense wealth on the poor and sick. Through her efforts, in 390 A.D. the first general public hospital was built in Rome. St. Jerome describes it as a *nosocomium,* a place only for the sick. Not content with giving her fortune to the needy, Fabiola waited on the patients herself, giving special care to those with repulsive sores. She died in 399 A.D., and the gratitude of her patients and of the people of Rome was manifested at her funeral.

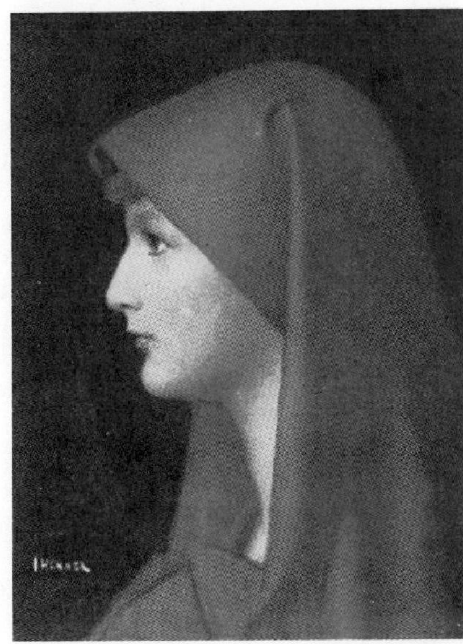

Figure 4–3. Fabiola, by J. J. Henner (1829–1905). (Courtesy of Louvre Museum.)

St. Jerome summed up the contributions of Fabiola in his famous eulogy:

> There she gathered together all the sick from the highways and streets, and herself nursed the unhappy, emaciated victims of hunger and disease. Can I describe here the varied scourges which afflicted human beings?—the mutilated, blinded countenances, the partially destroyed limbs, the livid hands, swollen bodies and wasted extremities? . . . How often have I seen her carrying in her arms those piteous, dirty, and revolting victims of a frightful malady! How often have I seen her wash wounds whose fetid odour prevented every one else from even looking at them! She fed the sick with her own hands, and revived the dying with small and frequent portions of nourishment. I know that many wealthy persons cannot overcome the repugnance caused by such works of charity; . . . I do not judge them . . . but, if I had a hundred tongues and a clarion voice I could not enumerate the number of patients for whom Fabiola provided solace and care. The poor who were well envied those who were sick.[2]

[2]Letter to Oceanus (LXXVII) in *A Select Library of Nicene and Post-Nicene Fathers of the Christian Church.* Second series, Vol. VI, Letters of St. Jerome. New York, Schaff & Wace, 1893.

There have been indications that Fabiola encouraged the construction of a hospice or home for convalescent patients.

St. Paula (347–404 A.D.) was a Roman matron of noble birth, a descendant of the Gracchi and the Scipios, of the line of Agamemnon. A member of a fabulously wealthy family, Paula married at 17 a young man of the illustrious Julian family. She lived in great magnificence on Mount Aventine. She owned the whole city of Necropolis in Italy, built by Augustus. She was one of the richest women of antiquity and belonged to the very highest rank of society in an aristocratic age. She was known for the splendor of her palace and the elegance of her life.

Paula's unusual place in history stems from her friendship with men who were recognized scholars. She enjoyed a definite collegial relationship and was afforded great deference for her "intellectual culture" by these scholars. The historian John Lord, who lived during the Victorian period when women did not enjoy the opportunity of a career choice or of a college education, wrote:

> If to her [Paula] we do not date the first great change in the social relations of man with woman, yet she is the most memorable example that I can find of that exalted sentiment which Christianity called out in the [relationship] of the sexes, and which has done more for the elevation of society than any other sentiment except that of religion itself.[3]

Men and women worked together as equals. They had a spiritual investment, not a vested interest.

Reflecting on the status of women in ancient cultures, Lord wrote:

> The Pagan woman belonged to her husband or her father rather than to herself. She was universally regarded as inferior to man, and made to be his slave. She was miserably educated; she was secluded from intercourse with strangers; she was shut up in her home; she was given in marriage without her consent; she was guarded by female slaves; she was valued chiefly as a domestic servant, or as an animal to prevent the extinction of families; she was seldom honored; she was doomed to household drudgeries as if she were capable of nothing higher; in short, her lot was hard, because it was unequal, humiliating, and sometimes degrading, making her to be either timorous, frivolous, or artful. Her amusements were trivial, her taste vitiated, her education neglected, her rights violated, her aspirations scorned. The poets represented her as capricious, fickle, and false. She rose only to fall; she lived only to die. She was a victim, a toy, or a slave. Bedizened or burdened, she was either an object of degrading admiration or of cold neglect.[4]

Lord opines that the advent of Christianity sparked a new kind of relationship, for "then woman became not merely the gentle nurse . . . but a friend . . . (a colleague)." He states that "the original beatitudes of the Garden of Eden returned, and man awoke from the deep sleep of four thousand years, to discover, with Adam" that woman could be a partner in a real professional sense. This team relationship was apparent in the health care delivery system. These Roman women worked collegially with well-educated men, including physicians, because they were by birth, education and spiritual direction their equals. Lord observes that friendship of this magnitude rarely exists except among equals.

After her husband's death, Paula was attracted to the humanitarian efforts and scholarly program of St. Marcella. Her enjoyment of cultivated society continued, especially her interest in the scholarly discussions of "literary treasures which imperishable art had bequeathed." She spoke Greek fluently. Paula's companions were gifted and learned women closely associated with their mentor Marcella—"a lady who refused the hand of the reigning Consul and yet, in spite of her duties as a leader of Christian benevolence" (and nursing education) was "versed equally in Greek and Hebrew" and was "so learned that she could explain intricate passages of the Scriptures." Paula was one of the most learned women of this period and was a scholar of Hebrew. She assisted St. Jerome (who encouraged each woman to develop her mind through reading and study while increasing her skills in caring for the sick) in his Latin translation of the Scriptures, known as the Vulgate (Fig. 4–4).

---

[3]Lord, John: *Beacon Lights of History*, Vol. V: *Great Women*. New York, Fords, Howard and Hulbert, 1885, p. 63.

[4]*Ibid.*, p. 64.

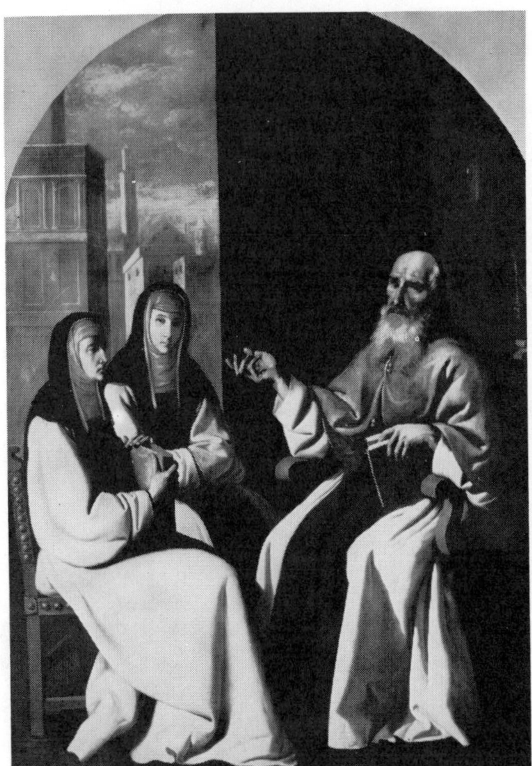

Figure 4–4. St. Jerome with St. Paula and St. Eustochium, by Zurbaran (1598–1664). (Samuel H. Kress Collection. Courtesy of National Gallery of Art, Washington, D.C.)

Accompanied by her daughter, Eustochium, Paula sailed for Palestine about 385 A.D. and settled in Bethlehem. On the road to Bethlehem she built shelters for pilgrims and hospitals for the sick. In the city itself she founded four monasteries and built a hospital in which, it has been said, she and her community of sisters nursed the sick "with untiring zeal." In St. Jerome's story of the life of St. Paula, he said,

> She was marvellous, debonair, and pietous to them that were sick, and comforted them, and served them right humbly; and gave them largely to eat such as they asked; but to herself she was hard in her sickness and scarce. . . . She was often by them that were sick, and she laid the pillows aright and in point; and she rubbed their feet, and boiled water to wash them; and it seemed to her that the less she did to the sick in service, so much the less service did she to God.

St. Jerome provided the inspirational leadership behind the activities and contributions of these Roman matrons. His great spiritual depth was accompanied by a love of learning and an ability to motivate and teach others.

Domenichino is said to have produced a most interesting painting of St. Jerome, in which his soul is leaving his body and he is gazing down upon St. Paula and her daughter as they minister to him. Could this be one of the first examples of a return to life from a "crisis event" that was reported and then recorded artistically? It is of interest in light of recent research and of the fact that St. Paula died 15 years before the actual death of St. Jerome.

In the selfish, indifferent society of Rome the remarkable contrast of these matrons in caring for the sick and less fortunate was strikingly apparent. It was most unusual for women of high social standing to exchange a life of luxury for one of generous service. It is also gratifying to note that high intellectual ability accompanied the practical skill and loving kindness of these women in nursing.

St. Sebastian received the ministrations of these early Christian nurses when sorely in need of compassionate, skilled nursing care. During the reign of Emperor Diocletian (284–305 A.D.), Sebastian became company commander in the Praetorian Guards. In 286 A.D., his religious affiliation with the Christian Church and his public declaration of his faith caused him to be fastened to a stake and shot by arrows. That night *St. Irene,* the widow of his martyred friend St. Castulus, found that Sebastian was still alive, and she and her associates cared for him.

St. Sebastian became one of the most popular subjects in medieval art, and many museums around the world possess an artistic portrayal of him. It is of interest to note that many of these paintings highlight the nursing care given by St. Irene and her associates (Fig. 4–5). They were able to provide both emergency and long-term care as well as assistance and comfort in the dying process. Irene's nurturing skills have been documented and portrayed by many artists.

For many years people prayed to St. Sebastian to prevent or cure pestilential diseases, which they believed were shot into their bodies by invisible arrows.

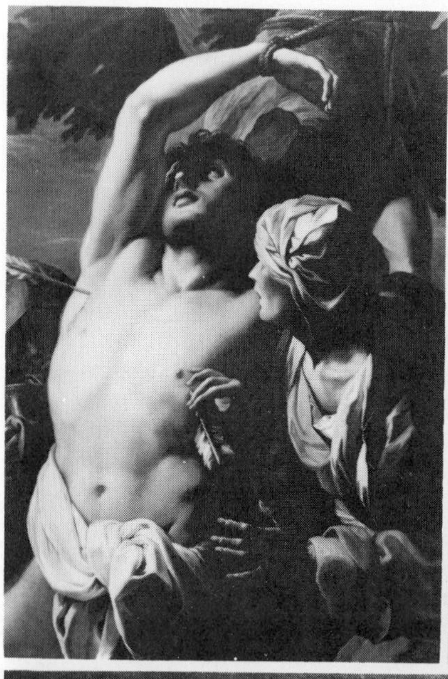
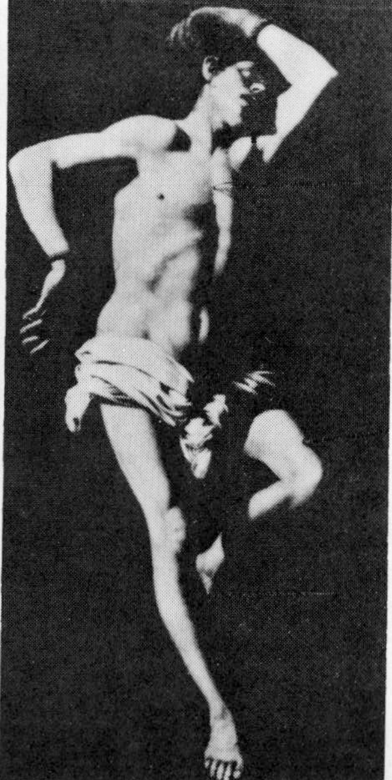

Figure 4–5. Artists' representations of Saint Sebastian receiving care from Saint Irene. *Counterclockwise from top left:* Giovanni Battista Caracciolo, *ca.* 1570–1637; Fogg Art Museum, Harvard. Daniel Seiter, 1640–1705; Mount Holyoke Art Museum. Luca Giordano, 1632–1705; Wadsworth Atheneum, Conn. Georges de La Tour, 1598–1652; Detroit Institute of Art. Jacques Banchard, 1600–1638; Rijksmuseum, Amsterdam. Bernardo Strozzi, 1581–1644; Cleveland Museum of Art.

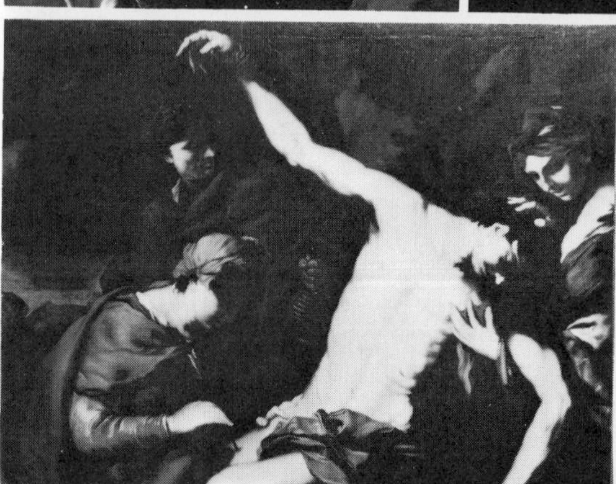
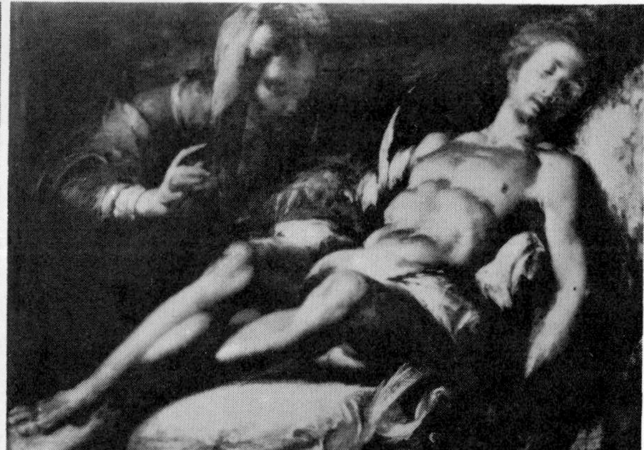
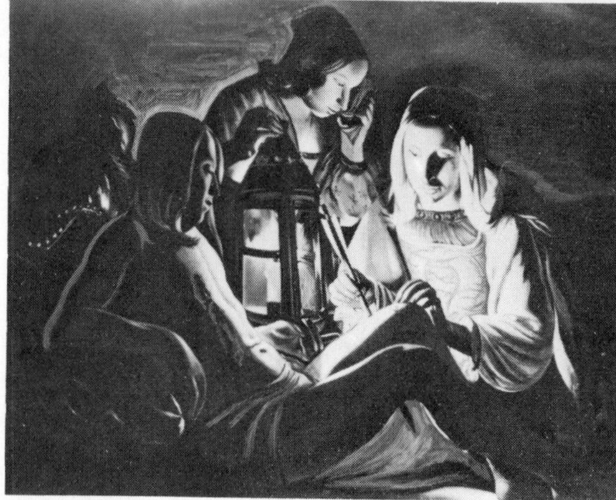
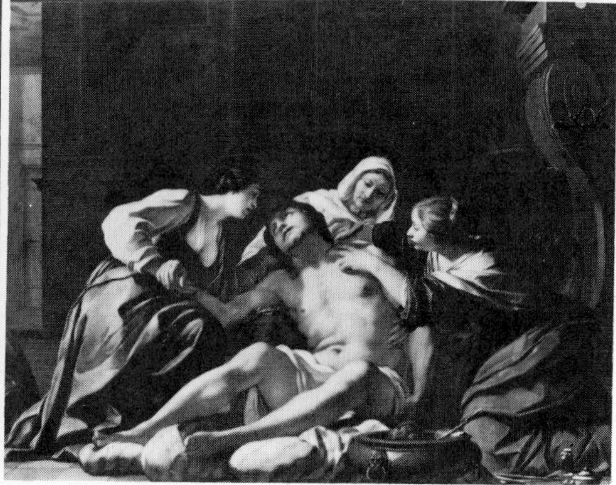

MEN IN NURSING

Members of a brotherhood known as *Parabolani* provided an additional opportunity for male nurses in the early Church period. This brotherhood was organized during a great plague in Alexandria. This group undertook to care for the sick and bury the dead.[5]

ACHIEVEMENTS OF CHRISTIAN NURSES

Christian nurses were not just comforters, they were nurturers—observing, listening, assessing, consoling, teaching, and caring for and about the patient and his family. They provided care for patients' spiritual, mental and physical health. Teaching has been an important duty of Christians since Christ commanded, "Go and teach all nations."

These intellectually and socially skilled leaders of nursing identified the basic ingredients of nursing care through careful assessment of their client's needs. They recognized the dependence of the acutely ill patient on his nurse for maintenance of vital life processes, and they were as scientifically knowledgeable as the time in which they lived permitted.

The nurse role of healer as well as sustainer of health was achieved when possible by cleaning up the filth and squalor and by rectifying human indignities and degradation. Nurses were, in effect, early social reformers. The site of health care delivery was wherever the need existed—in the community, in the hospital, in the patient's home, in the hostel of a pilgrim, in a home for the elderly. The response to human need prompted nurses to care for persons of all ages with all types of illnesses and physical handicaps. The existence of a nurse educator and students of nursing was noted.

Nurses administered the hospitals. When a nursing diagnosis was determined and nursing care indicated, intervention was provided by the nurses. Nurses called upon physicians if medical care was needed and spiritual advisors if spiritual care was warranted. There were strong collegial relationships among the health team members. These early Christian nurses had a high social status, were motivated by a strong spiritual force, were independent practitioners and shared their learning and techniques with interested recruits.

PHYSICIANS

Like nursing, medicine was infused with human warmth and compassion. One of the best known physicians of this period was *St. Luke* the Evangelist, a Greek, of Antioch. He was called the "beloved physician" by St. Paul. Luke's writings indicate an interest in medical subjects and give evidence of medical preparation. Several historians suggest that Luke may have studied at the famous school at Tarsus, the rival of Alexandria and Athens, and that he could have met St. Paul there. As a physician Luke traveled extensively and may have been a physician on board a ship. In addition to his literary ability and medical skill, Luke was a noted artist.

St. Cosmas and *St. Damian* were twin brothers, Arabs by birth and Christians by upbringing, who specialized in the twin professions of medicine and pharmacy. They practiced the art of healing in Asia Minor, attaining an enviable reputation until their careers came to an abrupt end through the persecutions of the Emperor Diocletian. Two other physicians who were martyred during these persecutions were *St. Blaise,* a bishop, and *St. Pantaleon,* the personal physician of Emperor Maximian.

In 312 A.D., during the battle of the Milvian Bridge, Emperor Constantine saw a cross in the sky and the words "In hoc signo vinces." ("In this sign thou shalt conquer".) Winning the battle, Constantine became a Christian, officially recognized the Church and freed it from persecution. Consequently, the Christians no longer had to confine their activities to the catacombs and hospitals; churches and other institutions began to develop.

On the walls in the catacombs muralists painted scenes of significance. One depicts a physician conducting a clinical class for medical students (Fig. 4–6). A student is depicted as he directs a question to the master teacher. The quizzical expression on the faces of the students has been captured by the muralist.

[5]Austin, Anne L.: *History of Nursing Source Book,* New York, G. P. Putnam's Sons, 1957, p. 62.

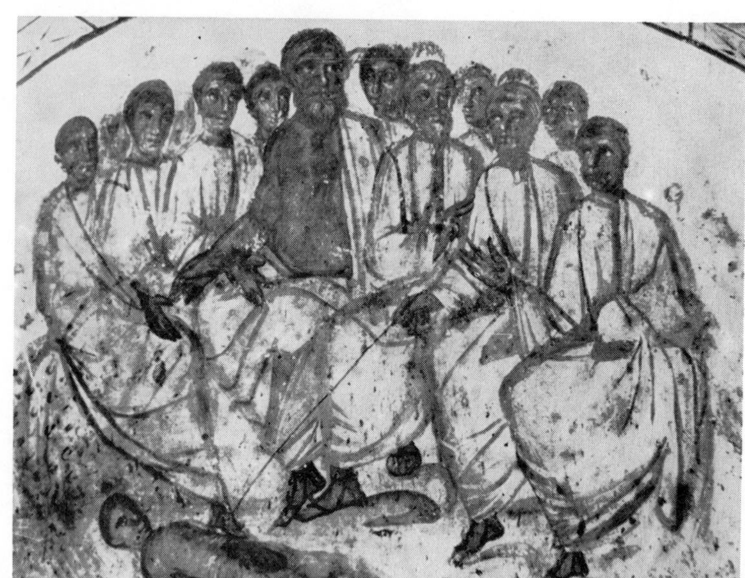

Figure 4–6. Fresco from recently discovered catacombs near the Appian Way. This is a scene of a fourth-century medical class. The instructor and students are listening to one of the students. (Courtesy of Rev. Antonio Ferrua, S. J., Pontifical Commission of Sacred Archeology.)

HOSPITALS

From the moment the significance of Christ's teaching penetrated the thinking of the early Christians, special places were set aside in their homes for hospitality and the actual care of the sick. These were called *Christrooms,* or *diakonia,* reflecting a literal interpretation of the words of Christ: "I was a stranger and you took me in." *Xenodochia* was the name given to shelters built for sick and poor pilgrims, and *nosocomia* the name given to hospitals built by St. Zoticus in Constantinople during the reign of Emperor Constantine.

A hospital planned only for the sick was organized at *Edessa, ca.* 350 A.D., to provide care for the victims of a frightful epidemic. With money presented to him, *St. Ephrem* bought 300 beds and provided care for the critically ill. It is said that he assisted in the care of these sick patients. Later this hospital became the clinical center for a medical school.

One of the most famous hospitals of the period was the *Basilias,* built in Caesarea by *St. Basil* (330?–379? A.D.) and his sister *Macrina,* both of whom are reputed to have studied medicine. The Basilias not only was a hospital for the sick but was also an institution that cared for the crippled and the poor. There was a separate building for children, another for elderly people, a place of hospitality for strangers and a building for the care of patients with leprosy. St. Basil included a special unit where the physically impaired could learn a trade and thus reenter society equipped with the ability to support themselves.

The motive behind the construction of such a hospital is interesting to consider. The plan of religious life was organized on a community basis. One of the first to draw such a group together was St. Basil. When St. Basil gave his monks a scheme for their community life, he established hospitals and schools at the gates of the monasteries. This arrangement was instituted because Basil saw the dangers of the monks' becoming preoccupied with their own salvation and living as hermits concerned solely with themselves in their relation to God; his novel plan provided for both the care of the sick and the practice of the monks' religious duties. In this way he extended the love and service of God to the love and service of one's neighbor. From that time on, nursing, like education, has been part of the religious life and has been one of the principal ways of practicing the worship of God.

SUMMARY

With the coming of Christ and the subsequent advent of Christianity, the value of the individual was emphasized, and the responsibility for recognizing the needs of each individual became apparent. Men and women were inflamed with the fire of Christ's love, and the virtues of sympathy, generosity and service were practiced. The social position of nursing was elevated, and its spiritual foundation was laid during this period.

EARLY MIDDLE AGES

The ancient classical civilization was crumbling rapidly, and an era of restoration and reconstruction was supplanting it. The thousand years that followed the collapse of the Roman Empire, often referred to as the medieval period of history, have been subdivided into the early and later Middle Ages.

The study of the early Middle Ages reveals a deteriorating world. Everything was falling into ruins. Population was decreasing in both numbers and strength. Crime waves terrified the populace. The burden of increasing taxation and the brutality that accompanied the collection of taxes were insufferable; the already hungry and impoverished people were threatened with torture and imprisonment in the hope of extracting concealed possessions. Whenever an increase in taxes was announced, agonized murmurs arose from the people who, in desperation, considered the possibilities of fleeing their country, selling loved ones or even attempting suicide. Many relinquished their freedom and offered their services to a landowner in a bondage relationship. In reality, a great many were becoming slaves.

The once-powerful Roman Empire now faced destruction because of extreme moral decay, increasing sterility among the patrician class, due to lead poisoning from lead drinking vessels, abysmal poverty worsened by high taxation and continuing wars with concomitant indifference to the plight of the victimized peoples. Disorganized and persecuted communities turned to feudalism, monasticism and, in certain regions, to Islam as possible solutions to the chaos they faced.

FEUDALISM

The castle of the feudal lord was a strong stone fortress usually set high in an inaccessible spot. It was enclosed by massive turreted walls and encircled by a moat. The most important fortification of the castle was the keep, which was the innermost tower within strongly constructed concentric walls. The keep was the "civil defense shelter" of the period, because it was the place that offered protection in times of attack.

The noble's wife had charge of the household and attended to the sick and wounded.

The feudal system seemed to encourage the growth of the spirit of *chivalry,* which eventually came to mean the institution of knighthood. Chivalry reflected the spirit of *noblesse oblige,* which required the nobly born to protect and defend the weak.

Although feudalism afforded protection to many, the system had two major disadvantages: a strong central government was not possible, and constant warfare prevented progress.

MONASTICISM

Monasticism offered an opportunity for men and women to live a good Christian life while pursuing an occupational career of their own choosing. The monastic idea is not unique to Christianity; it has been associated with many other religious groups. After the death of Christ, monasteries appeared when small groups banded together in independent units on a conventual plan, such as Marcella had organized.

A well-established form of monasticism, still flourishing today, is the order of Benedictines founded by *St. Benedict (ca.* 480–543 A.D.). Benedict of Nursia was born into a distinguished family. He was sent to Rome for a liberal education and while there was repelled by the moral corruption around him. In disgust he fled to the woods of Subiaco to meditate and pray.

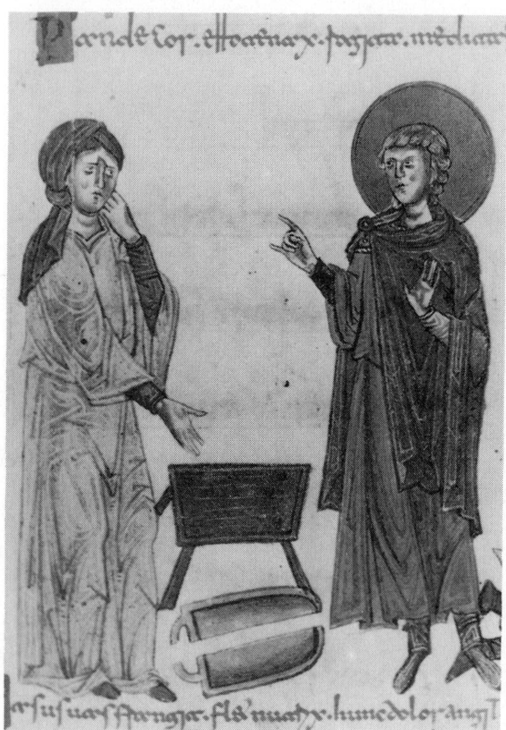

Figure 4–7. St. Benedict with his nurse. (Dolan collection.)

The *Dialogues of St. Gregory the Great* (*ca.* 540 to 604) report that when Benedict left home, he was accompanied by his nurse, according to the custom of the wealthy Greek and Roman families (Fig. 4–7). When Benedict abandoned his studies and went to search for solitude, he and his nurse found shelter at a hospice attached to the Church of St. Peter.

The first miracle attributed to St. Benedict was accomplished to comfort his nurse and is recorded in the *Dialogues of St. Gregory the Great.*[6] The nurse borrowed a tray (a large bowl) for food preparation, leaving it on the edge of a table. The tray slipped off and broke in two. The woman was disconsolate, and when Benedict returned, he felt deep sorrow for the nurse, whose efforts had played a major role in his health maintenance. He took the tray, praying very earnestly. Upon completion of his prayers he noticed that the two pieces were joined together without a mark to show where the break had occurred. Benedict cheerfully reassured his nurse and returned the tray in perfect condition. The news spread, and Benedict received great adulation. Because he preferred prayer to praise, he escaped from his nurse and went into seclusion. Later he complied with the requests of other monks to organize a monastic family. He became their abbas, or father, from which the title abbot is derived.

In pondering the reasons for the emergence of vows of poverty, chastity and obedience, Lord remarks: "It was a protest which perhaps the age demanded. The vow of poverty was a rebuke to that venal and grasping spirit which made riches the end of life; the vow of chastity was the resolution to escape that degrading sensuality which was one of the greatest evils of the times; and the vow of obedience was the recognition of authority amid the disintegration of society."[7]

About the year 528 A.D., Benedict composed his Rule (Fig. 4–8) and undertook the founding of the Monastery of Subiaco in the Sabine Hills near Rome.

His most famous monastery was Monte Cassino (Fig. 4–9), built on a rugged mountain top between Rome and Naples, probably in the year 529 A.D. This monastery, built on the site of one of the temples of Apollo, received great publicity when it became a Nazi stronghold and was bombed by Allied forces during World War II.

Other famous Benedictine monasteries include the one at Fulda in Germany, which became renowned under the direction of Abbot Maurus (776–856 A.D.). This erudite abbot had studied under Alcuin (the teacher of Charlemagne) at the Benedictine Abbey at Tours in France. Abbot Maurus compiled the medical encyclopedia *Physica,* which had a German-Latin glossary of anatomical terms.

The rule of St. Benedict brought a stability and a scheme of organization to an age in which chaos and panic reigned. In this period when men fled to the wilderness in large numbers to practice severe forms of penance, Benedict stressed the need for moderation, fruitful labor and discipline.

[6]Gregory the Great, St.: *Life and Miracles of Saint Benedict, Book Two of the Dialogues.* Trans. Odo J. Zimmerman, O. S. B. and Bernard R. Avery, O. S. B., Bethlehem, Connecticut, Abbey of Regina Laudis, 1981.

[7]Lord, John: *Beacon Lights of History* Vol. V: *Great Women.* New York, Fords, Howard and Hulbert, 1885.

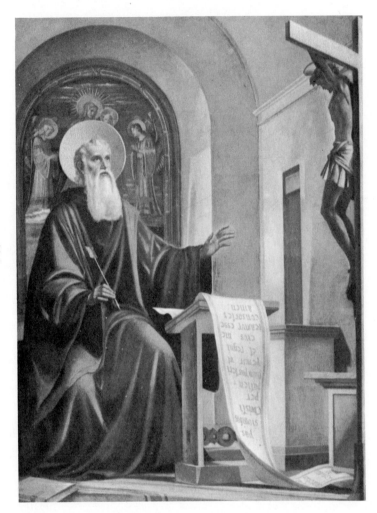

Figure 4–8. St. Benedict composing his Rule. (Dom Agostino Saccomanno, Monte Cassino Abbey.)

His well-known precept, *laborare est orare* (to labor is to pray), has been a guidepost for many Christians through the centuries. He loved the spirit of work, of using hands, head and heart. Peace and charity were so important to the Benedictines that they used *pax* as their watchword. In this atmosphere of peace, love and productive activity, the family spirit was cultivated. The needs of the community were furnished within the monastery walls. Career opportunities were fostered to meet the growing

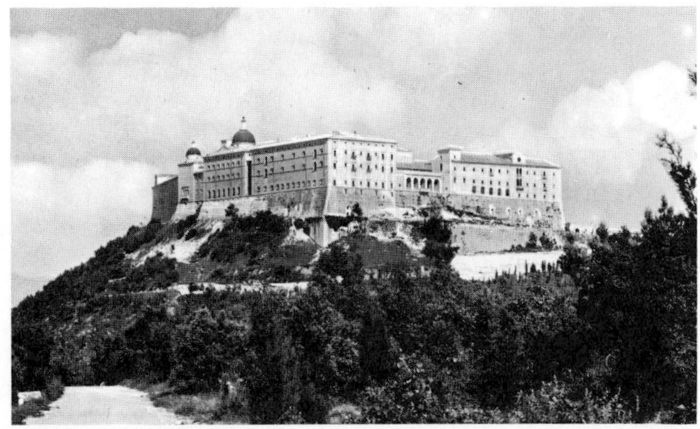

Figure 4–9. Monte Cassino Abbey. (Dom Agostino Saccomanno, Monte Cassino Abbey.)

demands of the community. As workshops of all sorts were erected, the need for teachers became apparent, and the monasteries became centers of learning. Not only did the monks engage in practical skills, but they also cultivated gardens and prepared medicinal drugs, studied music and languages, copied and illuminated precious manuscripts and wrote poetry and drama. The monks were scholars, thinkers, librarians and teachers as well as artisans and farmers. It was the duty of the monk to do for others and share with others. Monasteries offered hospitality and shelter to the homeless, care to the sick and refuge to the persecuted. They were literally survival shelters. In addition, the monasteries equipped each person with the knowledge and skills necessary to provide him with a livelihood. Creative approaches to one's career goals were encouraged.

The *care of the sick* was an important part of the community life, and one of the rules of St. Benedict stressed that the abbot, who was in charge of the monastery, should arrange for an infirmary:

> The care of the sick is to be placed above and before every other duty, as if indeed Christ were being directly served by waiting upon them. It must be the peculiar care of the abbot (or abbess) to see that they suffer from no negligence. The Infirmarian must be thoroughly reliable, known for his piety, diligence and solicitude for his charge.

In *Romeo and Juliet,* the portrayal of Friar Lawrence and his knowledge of medicine was not a figment of Shakespeare's imagination but an accurate portrait of monks at that time. Monastery gardens were the source of plants and minerals used for healing. We are aware that the monks used a combination of mandrake, hyoscyamus, opium and wild lettuce to induce a state of narcosis in which the patient was insensible to pain. Friar Lawrence suggested that Juliet be placed in a state "which shall appear like death."

The monasteries also fostered an opportunity for women to pursue a career in which they could satisfy their intellectual and spiritual aspirations and develop nursing skills. Many of the women who desired conventual life were gifted with qualities of leadership; the abbesses were skilled executives.

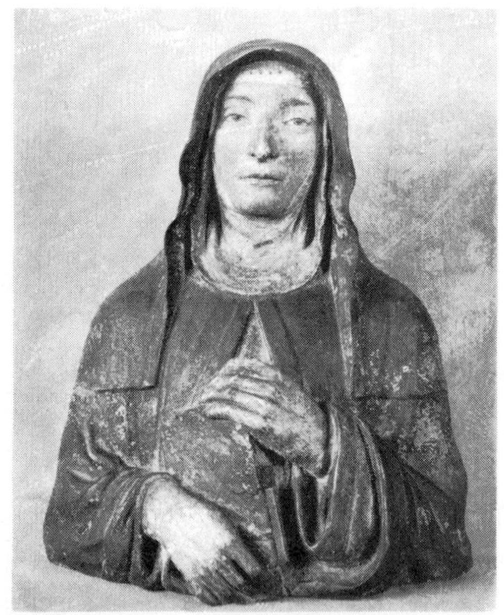

Figure 4–10. St. Brigid. (Courtesy of Isabella Stewart Gardner Museum, Boston.)

Famous Monastic Nurses

St. Brigid (452–523 A.D.), the daughter of a chieftain of Ulster, became a famous abbess in Ireland and a distinguished scholar, counselor, educator and leader in the healing arts (Fig. 4–10). Under her guidance the monastery at Kildare became well known for its culture as well as for its spirituality and was, in fact, an institution of higher learning for women. Brigid founded schools for children and taught in them herself. In fifth century Ireland, when leprosy was an incurable scourge and lepers were free to roam, they came in droves to Kildare to be bathed and treated by Brigid. She tended the sick and gave alms to the poor.

Brigid established within her monastery a school of art in which exquisitely illuminated manuscripts were produced as well as gold and silver work of high artistic quality.

Manuscripts have been preserved, copied and illuminated in these monasteries. One of the best examples of these is the Book of Kells, which can be seen in the library of Trinity College in Dublin.

St. Scholastica (Fig. 4–11), the twin sister of St. Benedict, founded an order for women based on his Rule. This Benedictine community for women was started near Monte Cassino, and Scholastica held

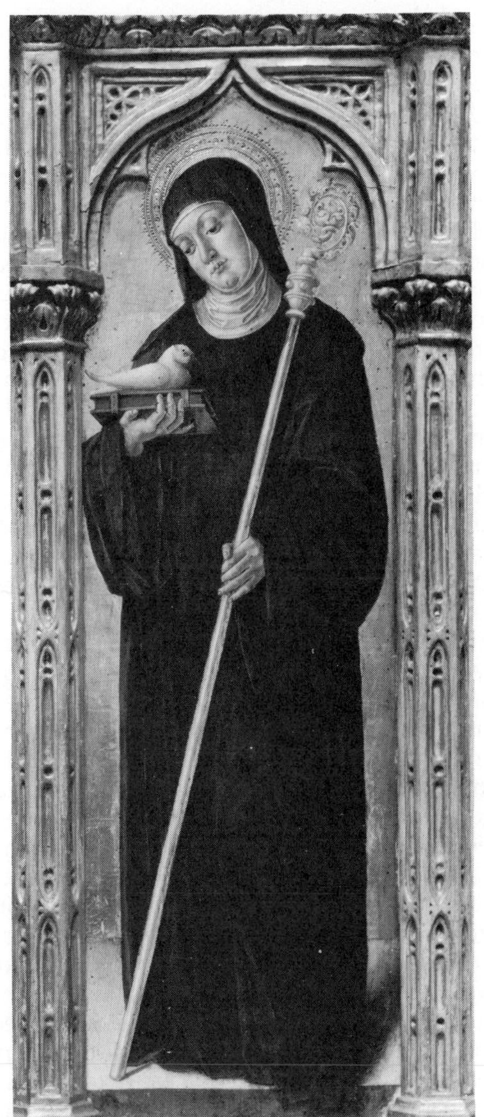

Figure 4–11. St. Scholastica, by Vivarini (1450–1499). (Courtesy of Museum of Fine Arts, Boston.)

the office of abbess. Many other famous women of the Benedictine family have contributed to the field of nursing.

St. Radegonde (ca. 519–587 A.D.), a German princess, the daughter of a Thuringian king and grand-niece of the great Gothic king Theodoric, was a deeply religious, cultured and beautiful girl who had deep sorrow in her life (Fig. 4–12). In her infancy her father was murdered by her uncle; as a young girl she was carried off by Clotaire, the Frankish king of Neustria, when he subjugated her country. She was forced to marry Clotaire and become his queen. She was eventually one of his six wives. The king murdered one of his wives and her son and daughter as well as Radegonde's brother. In revulsion Radegonde fled from him and sought asylum at a monastery.

Radegonde was a scholar and had marked qualities of leadership. After becoming a nun, she founded the Holy Cross Monastery at Poitiers, a religious settlement of 200 nuns. The care of the sick was the chief activity; study ranked next in importance, and two hours every day were devoted to reading literature. The members of her community copied manuscripts and performed dramatic presentations as diversional therapy for the patients. In the hospital she had built, Radegonde bathed the patients herself, giving special care to the lepers. To this group of social outcasts, who were deprived of the necessities of life and of love and affection, Radegonde, a queen and nun, bestowed an embrace of welcome and a "leper's kiss." Queen Radegonde's example encouraged many ladies

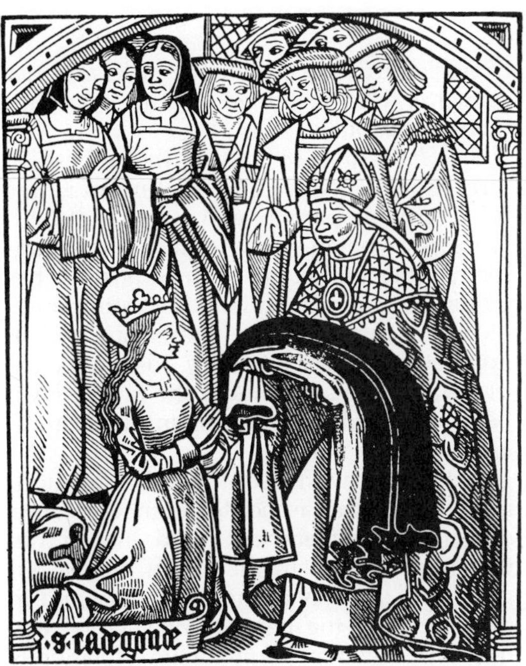

Figure 4–12. St. Radegonde, wife of King Clotaire, receiving religious robes from St. Medard. (From an old woodcut.) (Dolan collection.)

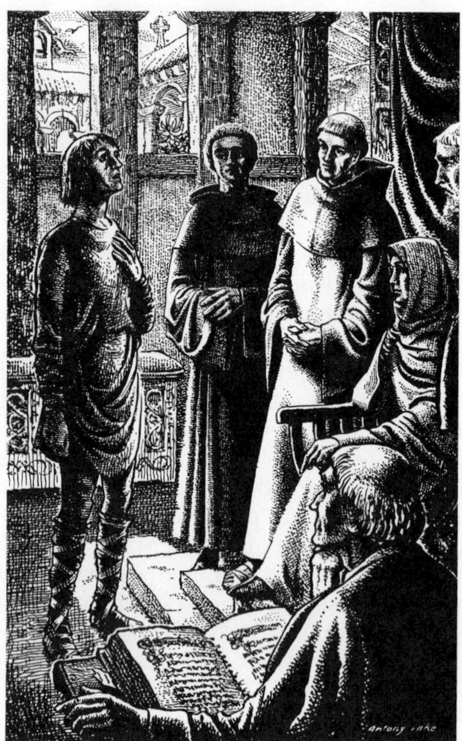

Figure 4–13. Caedmon appearing before Abbess Hilda, who encouraged him to tell his tale in his own words. (From Roche: *Christians Courageous.*)

of noble birth to care for the sick, and her influence also extended to the establishment of hospitals.

St. Hilda (614–680 A.D.), the abbess of Streonshalh (now Whitby) in England, was born of noble parents and was a cultured, scholarly woman and a gifted administrator, teacher and counselor. Because of her guidance and inspiration, her community did more than translate, transcribe and illuminate manuscripts; they fostered creative writing and Caedmon, the first English poet, received encouragement and guidance there (Fig. 4–13).

Associated with each Benedictine monastery were the associate members called *oblates.* These members could live within the monastery or in their own homes but gave their services to the monastery and in turn received the benefits of such a relationship. This type of monastic affiliation is still in existence.

The capable women in the monasteries included not only the abbesses but also the many gifted sisters and oblates who contributed to the monastery in a remarkable way. Such a person was Sister *Hrotswitha* (935–1001 A.D.) of the Benedictine Abbey at Gandersheim. Hrotswitha entered the monastery at the age of 23 and was tutored by the mistress of novices and the abbess. Hrotswitha studied Virgil, Plautus, Horace, Terence and Aristotle. She had great writing ability, and her dramas were given to the literary world through a French translation in 1845. Hrotswitha was one of the great literary personalities of her time.

It is important to realize the part the monasteries played in the preservation of culture and learning. They stood as an oasis in a desert of insecurity, persecution and suffering. These monasteries offered refuge for the persecuted; encouraged manual labor, formerly the duty of slaves; fostered healthy, purposeful lives devoted to personal piety and promotion of human welfare; developed agricultural experimental stations; motivated artists and skilled craftsmen in architecture, music, painting and crafts; provided nurses and physicians to care for the sick; cultivated medicinal gardens; advocated personal and professional growth by studying; preserved manuscripts; and built the foundation for universities by sending copies of manuscripts from monastery to monastery. Lastly, they provided the school teachers of this period. Not only did the monasteries foster new creative expression but they also preserved the ancient cultural treasures. The ancient learning of the classical period would have been lost and forgotten, when the Roman Empire fell, had it not been for the monks of the West.

In the setting of an institution of higher learning, nurses strengthened the scientific, artistic and cultural components of nursing. They were part of a community of scholars.

NURSE LEADERS IN THE COMMUNITY

Nursing attracted many women during the early Middle Ages, and its recruits included several queens. *St. Clothilde (ca.* 474–544 A.D.) was a Burgundian princess who married Clovis I, King of the Franks. Widowed, she spent the rest of her life near the Monastery of St. Martin at Tours where she cared for the sick.

Queen Theodolinde, wife of Agilulf, King of the Lombards, worked conscientiously for the sick among the poor and especially for the lepers. *St. Bathilde (ca.* 634–680 A.D.), wife of Clovis II, King of the Franks, was kidnapped in childhood and became first a slave, then a queen-consort and finally a queen-regent. The founder of the monasteries at Chelles and Corbie, she retired as a widow to her Abbey at Chelles and ministered to the sick poor.

St. Margaret (1045–1093) married King Malcolm[8] of Scotland. Learned, beautiful and deeply religious, she washed the feet of beggars, gave money to the poor, visited hospitals and ministered to the sick. Margaret helped families in distress, especially displaced persons and ransomed captives of every nation, and founded hospitals, churches and monasteries. Her uncle, St. Edward the Confessor, King of England, is believed to have built the Benedictine monastery in London now called Westminster Abbey.

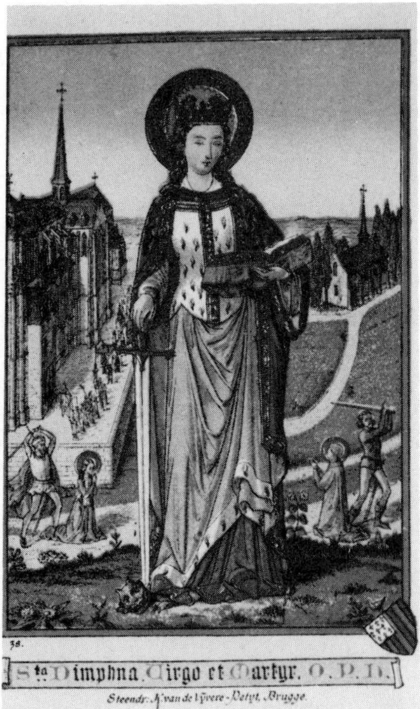

Figure 4–14. St. Dymphna. (Dolan collection.)

SPECIAL CARE OF MENTALLY ILL

The first organized plan for the care of mentally ill and mentally retarded children (other than that employed at St. Basil's in Caesarea) originated at present-day Gheel in Belgium. Tradition says it was begun toward the end of the sixth century by *St. Dymphna* (Fig. 4–14). An Irish princess, she fled the incestuous demands of her demented father, a king of Ireland. He pursued and murdered her in the forests around Gheel.

The fame of the saintly young girl spread as reports were made of miraculous cures, especially of those who were mentally ill and emotionally disturbed, at her tomb. People brought their relatives in the hope of a cure. First, a shrine was built and then a church was constructed and dedicated to St. Dymphna. The alcoves of these edifices could not contain the number of patients who arrived in Gheel on pilgrimages. A building adjoining St. Dymphna's church housed the pilgrims. This structure, called *Sieckenkamer* or *Chambre des malades,* frequently could not accommodate the large number of mentally ill and mentally retarded guests, and the housewives of Gheel accepted these patients as boarders and as foster members of their families. The populace of Gheel developed great skill in caring for these foster members and bestowed love and affection upon them.

Judicious regulations, enacted as early as the fifteenth century by the Municipal Board of Gheel, prevented potential abuses of these people that might have occurred. When France annexed the Belgian provinces, the institution came under local government. In 1852 it was reorganized by the Belgian government and given the title of "Colony."

Today, when a person arrives at Gheel, he is received for observation at the "Infirmary," or central hospital. A plan of care is proposed before he is admitted into the home of a foster family. A home care plan is developed whereby the psychiatrists and psychiatric nurses visit and check out the patients in their new environment at regular intervals.

[8]His father was that "gracious Duncan" whose sad fate has been immortalized by Shakespeare. Macbeth usurped his kingdom.

In spite of their misfortune, the patients entrusted to the Colony of Gheel enjoy all the advantages of freedom and family life, continuous contact with normal persons, voluntary work fitted to their aptitudes and their preferences as well as various forms of entertainment.

In 1957, Gheel had a population of more than 22,000 and contained 5850 families of which approximately 2000 accepted patients. From 1926 to 1950, 8358 patients were admitted to the colony. Of this number 2197, or more than 26 per cent, returned to their families cured or improved.[9]

Gheel is now an institutional town under government control and receives children from all countries. They are put under the care of St. Dymphna and her modern counterparts. Thus, charity in action is carried out by a community of health professionals and kind-hearted people for the benefit of a needy group of individuals, resulting in supervised family care.

Goldin quotes Dr. Harry Shapiro of the American Museum of Natural History, who has made a study of Gheel: "Psychiatrists in this country point out that the treatment is nothing new—but treatment is not the question. What is at issue is the *care* of these people."[10]

The nursing care and supervision has been under the direction of the Soeurs Hospitalières—hospital sisters under the rule of the Augustinian order called Augustinian Sisters. This is the oldest order of nursing sisters in existence.

SCHOOL OF SALERNO

In the transition from monastic to lay medicine the *School of Salerno* played an important part. Although the school's beginnings are not well known, it may have been an outgrowth of the Benedictine Abbey of Monte Cassino; the library of Monte Cassino still contains many valuable medical manuscripts, copies of which may have been sent to the new school. Benedictine monks joined Salerno's faculty, which also consisted of lay men and women. This famous school produced many leaders in the fields of medicine and surgery.

Students were given lectures in the classroom and at the bedside of patients, and discussions were encouraged. Methods of treating the patients included drugs, bloodletting, diet and psychotherapy in the form of soothing words and restful music. It is interesting to realize that the importance of psychotherapy in the process of healing was recognized. *Anthimus,* a physician of Theodoric, wrote a book called *Dietetica* on the importance of nutrition and the selection and preparation of food. In addition to providing an appropriate diet, the book stresses the theory that the food should be attractively served to encourage the patient to eat.

The importance of a good bedside manner was realized, and a physician of Salerno was encouraged to question the messenger who summoned him to the bedside of the patient so that he could consider the patient's condition before seeing him. It is assumed that it was a nurse's assessment that the physician received. A physician was advised to sit and chat pleasantly with the patient so that when he took the pulse it would be a true reading and not elevated owing to excitement or stress.

Because of the influence of the medical leadership at the School of Salerno, medical legislation was enacted. As early as 1140 A.D., a law was passed forbidding anyone to practice medicine without being examined carefully. The essential education required to receive a degree from the School of Salerno and thence to become eligible for the examination for licensure was three years of premedical study in logic, philosophy and literature, five years of study in medicine and surgery, and one year as an assistant to an experienced practitioner.

It is a well-known fact that very early in its history women studied at Salerno. All branches of learning, including medicine, were opened to women, and copies of many medical licenses granted to women can be seen in the Archives of Naples. *Trotula,* a famous woman doctor, is supposed to have written a book on obstetrics and gynecology and to have been head of the department of diseases of women.

---

[9]Gushee, L.: Unpublished translation of brochure obtained by Mrs. Mary Gushee on a visit to Gheel, June 1957.

[10]Goldin, Grace: "A Painting in Gheel," *Journal of the History of Medicine and Allied Sciences,* Volume XXVI (4):400–412, 1971.

MEDIEVAL HOSPITALS

The three famous medieval hospitals built outside monastery walls are extant today.

The *Hôtel Dieu* in Lyons, established in 542 A.D., was organized on the pattern of an almshouse and was under lay management. The nursing was carried out mainly by repentant women, by widows called sisters (though not members of a religious order) and by male nurses called brothers.

The *Hôtel Dieu* in Paris was founded around 650 A.D.; it was also conducted under lay administration and built on the almshouse pattern. The nursing staff was composed of Augustinian Sisters.

The *Santo Spirito Hospital* in Rome was founded by order of the Pope in 717 A.D. and was built primarily to receive the sick. This hospital has inspired the establishment of many others like it.

ISLAM AND ARABIC MEDICINE

A new monotheistic religion called *Islam* arose among the predominantly nomadic peoples of the Arabian peninsula.

Mohammed, the founder of Islam, was born at Mecca in the year 570 A.D. In 610 A.D., he announced that he had been called by Allah to preach a new religion.

Mohammed commenced his work by striving to sway his fellow men from idolatry to the worship of Allah. Gradually his enthusiastic converts extended this invitation by means of the sword. Each convert was called a *Moslem* or "one who submits."

By the time Mohammed died in 632 A.D., Islam had spread with the aid of his military genius, and his followers controlled the territories of Egypt, Palestine, Syria and India. Later, Roman Africa, Spain and even Constantinople were captured. Twenty-one years after the death of Mohammed, the rule of Islam extended over a territory as great as the Roman Empire.

The great contributions of the "Golden Age of Arabic Medicine" were mainly in pharmacology; in the advancement of medical knowledge through diagnosis, description and treatment of disease; in requiring licensure after careful examination of physicians and pharmacists; in providing medical leaders; and in the construction and administration of exceedingly modern hospitals.

Because dissection was forbidden, the Arabs were unable to develop a full understanding of anatomy and physiology. Surgery was frowned upon, cautery being more popular than the knife.

Three famous physicians of this period were Rhazes (860–932 A.D.), Avicenna (980–1037 A.D.) and Maimonides (1135–1204 A.D.).

Rhazes was a Persian scholar and a skilled clinician who added to the medical contributions of Hippocrates and Galen with his medical work *The Compendium.* He described the diseases of smallpox and measles in one of his monographs.

Avicenna, a Persian, was one of the great scholars of the Arabic world. Called the "Prince of Physicians," his writings, especially his *Canon of Medicine,* have been considered some of the most important textbooks in the field of medical education; the *Canon of Medicine* was studied in the medical schools of Europe from the twelfth to the seventeenth centuries.

Moses ben Maimon *(Maimonides),* the third member of the Arabic medical triumvirate, was born in Moslem-controlled Cordova, Spain, of a Jewish family descended from King David. He was an excellent clinician, and his fame spread. He became the court physician to the Sultan Saladin. It has been said that during the Crusades, Richard the Lion-Hearted, learning of Maimonides' great skill, asked him to return to England with him as his personal physician. The greatest rabbinic scholar of his age, Maimonides is remembered for codifying the Talmud and for composing the beautiful prayer that translates:

And now I turn unto my calling;
Oh, stand by me, my God, in this truly
  important task!
Grant me success! For—
Without Thy loving counsel and support
Man can avail but naught.
Inspire me with true love for this my art
And for Thy creatures.
Oh, grant—
That neither greed nor gain, nor thirst for fame,
  nor vain ambition,
May interfere with my activity.
For these, I know, are enemies of Truth and
Love of men,
And might beguile one in profession,
From furthering the welfare of Thy creatures.

Oh, strengthen me!
Grant energy unto both body and the soul,
That I may e'er unhindered ready be
To mitigate the woes,
Sustain and help,
The rich and poor, the good and bad, the
enemy and friend.
Oh, let me e'er behold in the afflicted and the
suffering
Only the human being!

Medical centers at this time were located in Cairo, Alexandria, Damascus and Baghdad. Hospitals were part of these centers and were famous for having beautiful architecture, being well equipped, employing unusual ideas of social service,[11] encouraging study by including lecture rooms and libraries and employing readers and storytellers for the patients.

Alchemy and pharmacology were specialties, and the Arabic scientists, highly skilled in compounding medicines, were interested in finding an "elixir of life." Pharmacists were independent practitioners, and apothecary shops were common in the Moslem countries.

[11]For example, on discharge a patient was given money to permit him to convalesce properly before returning to work.

Moslem women were notably absent in the care of the sick, largely because they were kept in seclusion and shrouded in heavy veils. Polygamy was practiced by Moslem males, and it is said that Islam improved the status of woman only in the sense that it forbade the killing of girl babies, which was permissible in pre-Islamic times.

SUMMARY

Although the early Middle Ages ended amid distress, poverty and political chaos, much progress had been made: Christianity had spread; missionaries brought not only a religious message but civilization as well; benevolent institutions had arisen; and monks and nuns had replaced the deaconesses and matrons in the care of the sick. *Nursing at last had developed roots, purpose, direction and leadership.*

THE HERITAGE OF NURSING

The Impact of Spiritual Leadership on the Image of the Nurse

The first organized groups of nurses were established in direct response to the teaching and example of Christ, which helped to bring about:

1. respect for the dignity of all persons.
2. emancipation of women and elevation of their status.
3. emancipation of men and a new freedom of action for career choices.
4. attraction of socially, politically and intellectually gifted men and women to nursing.
5. a recognition by these well-educated recruits of the necessity for a special education in nursing in addition to their liberal education.
6. the emergence of the role of a nurse educator who was recognized for her scholarship and leadership by the great scholars of that period.
7. the goal of nursing care to meet a person's primary and secondary needs as they were identified in the scientific and humanistic objectives of the Corporal Works of Mercy.
8. a strong teaching program for patients as well as the use of sound rehabilitation techniques and healing therapies such as the transference of energy through the "laying on of hands."
9. an expansion in the role of nursing.
    a. in the *independent* role, nurses:
        (1) founded hostels, hospices and hospitals.

(2) directed these institutions.
(3) assessed the nursing needs of clients.
(4) designed the plan of nursing care.
(5) performed the nursing intervention.
(6) functioned autonomously in all aspects of nursing.
(7) coordinated intradisciplinary nursing team work (freed servants became nurse's aides, hospital housekeepers and home health workers).

b. in the *interdependent* role, nurses:
(1) called upon and consulted with physicians, surgeons, pharmacists and spiritual advisors as colleagues in interdisciplinary team work.
(2) used their nursing diagnoses while physicians added their medical diagnoses using their disease-oriented skills.
(3) were accorded respect and trust, needed for a true collegial team relationship and did not give up their nursing role in order to become physicians' assistants.

c. In the *independent specialist* role, nurses with special interests and skills "cared" for persons with special problems—the elderly, the dying, the mentally ill and mentally retarded and those with communicable diseases.

d. In the *community of scholars* role, nurses in monastic settings strengthened the scientific, artistic and cultural components of nursing.

Ultimately, there emerged gifted nurse leaders, whose names and deeds have been recorded by scholars and portrayed by famous artists.

REFERENCE READINGS

Austin, Anne L.: *History of Nursing Source Book*. New York, G. P. Putnam's Sons, 1957.
Blacam, Hugh de: *The Saints of Ireland–the Life Stories of Saints Brigid and Columcille*. Milwaukee, Bruce Publishing Co., 1942.
Caldwell, Taylor: *Dear and Glorious Physician*. New York, Doubleday & Co., 1959.
Curtayne, Alice: *St. Brigid of Ireland*. New York, Sheed & Ward, 1954.
Eckenstein, Lena: *Women Under Monasticism*. Cambridge, The University Press, 1896.
Gregory the Great, St.: *Life and Miracles of Saint Benedict, Book Two of the Dialogues*. Trans. Odo. J. Zimmerman, O. S. B. and Bernard R. Avery, O. S. B. Bethlehem, Connecticut, Abbey of Regina Laudis, 1981.
Harnack, Adolph: *Luke, the Physician*. New York, G. P. Putnam's Sons, 1909.
Kavanagh, Julia: *Women of Christianity*. New York, D. Appleton Co., 1852.
Kingsley, Charles: *Hypatia*. New York, Lovell, Coryell & Co.
Lord, John: *Beacon Lights of History*, Vol. V, *Great Women*. New York, Fords, Howard and Hulbert, 1885.
Luce, Clare Booth: *Saints for Now*. New York, Sheed & Ward, 1952.
Maynard, Theodore: *St. Benedict and His Monks*. London, Staples Press, 1956.
Merton, Thomas: *The Seven Storey Mountain*. New York, Harcourt, Brace & Co., 1948.
Oursler, Fulton: *The Greatest Story Ever Told*. New York, Doubleday & Co., 1949.
Pond, Marian B.: *Heaven in a Wildflower*. New York, Vantage Press, 1954.
Power, Eileen: *Medieval People*. New York, Barnes & Noble, 1924.
Riesman, David: *The Story of Medicine in the Middle Ages*. New York, Harper & Brothers, 1936.
Roche, Aloysius: *Christians Courageous*. London, Burns & Oates, Ltd.
Sienkiewicz, Henryk: *Quo Vadis?* Boston, Little, Brown & Co., 1896.
Slaughter, Frank G.: *The Road to Bithynia*. New York, Doubleday & Co., 1951.
Smith, C. Raimer: *The Physician Examines the Bible*. New York, Philosophical Library, 1950.
Uhlhorn, Gerhard: *Christian Charity in the Ancient Church*. New York, Charles Scribner, 1883.
Walsh, James J.: *Old Time Makers of Medicine*. New York, Fordham University Press, 1911.
Waugh, Evelyn: *Helena*. Boston, Little, Brown & Co., 1950.
Wheeler, Henry: *Deaconesses, Ancient and Modern*. New York, Hunt & Eaton, 1889.
Wiseman, Cardinal: *Fabiola, or the Church of the Catacombs*. New York, P. J. Kenedy & Sons.

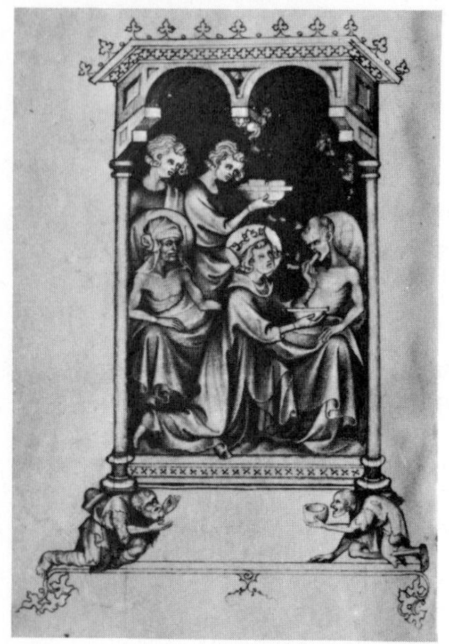

St. Louis administers to the sick in a medieval hospital. This is one of many illustrations depicting scenes from the life of St. Louis that appeared in a small book of prayers belonging to his granddaughter, Jeanne D'Evreux, Queen of France and wife of Charles IV. The illustration by Jean Pucelle (*ca.* 1325). (Courtesy of Metropolitan Museum of Art, The Cloisters Collection, Purchase, 1954.)

5 Social and Spiritual Forces in the Expansion of Nursing (1000–1500)

THE CRUSADES

Toward the close of the eleventh century the Seljuk Turks who had embraced Islam became the most warlike of the Moslems. During their tour of conquest they captured Palestine, among other places, and erected mosques in the Holy City of Jerusalem. Cruel persecutions were meted out to the Christians who had been making pilgrimages there since the death of Christ. The capture of the Holy Places and the harsh treatment of the pilgrims impelled the European Christians to unite to stop the actions of the Turks. Thus were initiated the military expeditions of the religious movement known as the *Crusades,* which lasted for nearly two hundred years (1096–1291).

The Crusades, which served as an avenue of interchange in ideas, customs and disease between the East and West, had both favorable and unfavorable results.

It is difficult for us to envision the ordinary difficulties that beset the Crusaders on their journey. Travel was slow and laborious, adequate and nutritious food was hard to procure and harder to preserve, prevention of disease was impossible and immunity to newly encountered diseases was in most cases low or nonexistent.

Hospitals and shelters had been built for the pilgrims by such persons as St. Helena and St. Paula, but they did not meet the needs of the Crusaders. Fatigue, malnutrition, digestive disturbances from food poisoning, poor sanitary conditions and contact with communicable diseases all contributed to an acute demand for hospitals and providers of health care.

Military Nursing Orders

In response to this demand, *military nursing orders* were formed that drew large numbers of men into the field of nursing. The membership of these orders consisted of knights, monks and serving brothers. Because the recognized accolade of knighthood had to be achieved before membership in one of the military nursing orders was conferred, members of the orders were carefully screened.

The *Knights Hospitallers of St. John* were organized originally to staff one of two hospitals that had been built in Jerusalem by rich merchants of Amalfi in 1050. The hospital for male patients was placed under the protection of St. John (probably St. John the Baptist), and a monk, Peter Gerhard, took charge. The second hospital, for female patients, was dedicated to St. Mary Magdalene and was staffed by nuns under the direction of a capable Roman woman named Agnes. The purpose of these orders was to care for pilgrims who became ill on their journey to the Holy Land. The hospitals extended care to Moslems and Jews as well as Christians. The hospitals in Jerusalem were well equipped. Each patient was provided with a cloak of sheepskin and boots, the forerunners of bathrobe and slippers.

The knights were mainly a nursing order but assumed a military role when it was essential to defend the hospital and its inmates. Their habit, worn over their suit of armor, was a black mantle with a white *Maltese cross* (Fig. 5–1).

Gradually, the knights built additional hospitals, hostels and hospices at strategic points in the mountain passes and at river crossings. When the Knights Hospitallers went to Rhodes, they built extensive fortifications. They set up a health commission that prevented an outbreak of the plague by the strict enforcement of a 40-day isolation period for all those who had come in contact with plague victims.

The order settled on the island of Malta in 1530, and the hospital they constructed there is famous, with many interesting features. As early as 1617, a board was placed at the head of each bed upon which physician's orders were written. The physicians and surgeons were accompanied on their rounds by a secretary who took down the prescriptions as the physicians dictated them. Nurses remained with the patients.

After the knights had settled on the island of Malta, they reestablished the Sisters of the Knights Hospitallers of St. John, who had been forced to flee Jerusalem when that city fell. They had escaped to Europe but came to Malta and remained there after the Knights departed from this area in 1798. This order of sisters, wearing the habit of the Hospitallers, still remains to care for the sick of Malta. It has been said that at first the habit of the order was red with a white Maltese cross, but later the red was changed to black (Fig. 5–2).

The Knights Hospitallers of St. John became known as the Knights of Malta. They have been considered a sovereign power and have had representatives of ambassadorial rank and universally recognized diplomatic sovereignty. Under the Geneva Convention their insignia, the Maltese cross, was awarded the same recognition of immunity by belligerents in war as was the

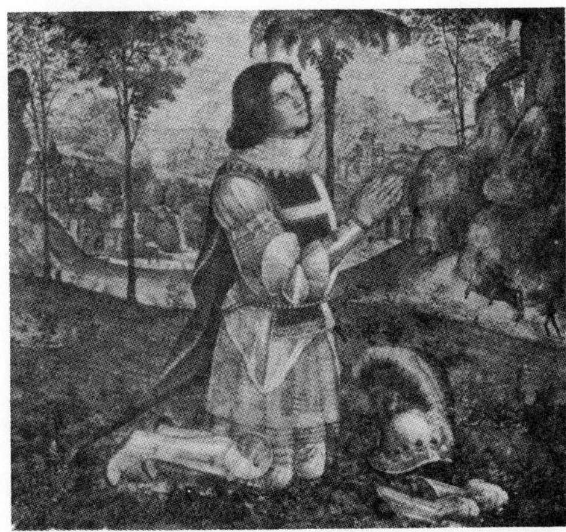

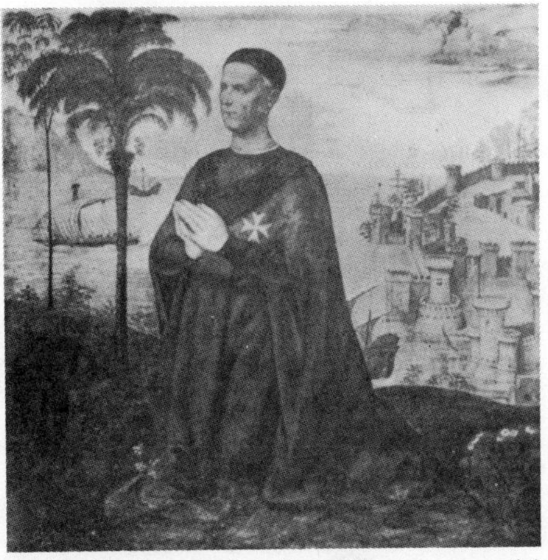

Figure 5–1. A Knight of St. John in armor *(left)* and in the black mantle of a military nurse *(right)*. From frescoes by Pinturicchio in the Cathedral in Siena. (Dolan collection.)

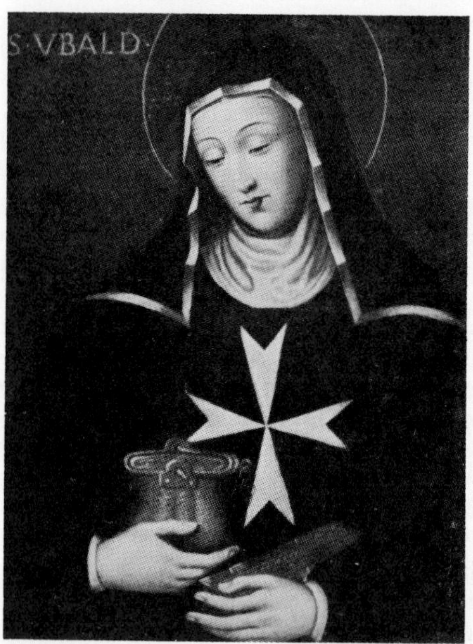

Figure 5–2. Saint Ubaldesca in the military nursing habit of the Hospitallers of St. John. (Dolan collection.)

Red Cross. As Knights Hospitallers of St. John, and later as Knights of Malta, they have given outstanding service in international nursing.

The *Teutonic Knights* came into existence in 1190 during the siege of Acre. This order was composed of German knights, who could be distinguished from the Knights of St. John by the white tunic with a black Maltese cross outlined in gold that each wore over his coat of mail.

The *Knights of St. Lazarus* were devoted especially to the care of lepers; their name was derived from the parable of the leper in the Bible. Many historians think that this is the oldest of all knightly orders. It has been associated with the special hospital for lepers that was part of the Basilias built by St. Basil. Though these knights set a valiant example and gave excellent care, the order ceased to exist by 1830.

The Order of the Most Holy Trinity, more popularly known as the *Order of Trinitarians,* was founded in 1197. Not only did they render first aid on the battlefield and in plague-infested villages, but they also received victims into their monastery hospital. In addition, they ransomed the Christians taken prisoner by the Moslems. This group wore a white habit with a red and blue cross on the breast (Fig. 5–3).

The Crusades afforded a glorious opportunity for cultural interchange and were particularly valuable in broadening the scope of patient care and hospital planning and in developing medical education.

GROWTH OF CITIES

During the late Middle Ages, the feudal system declined in importance, and the groups that had previously lived around

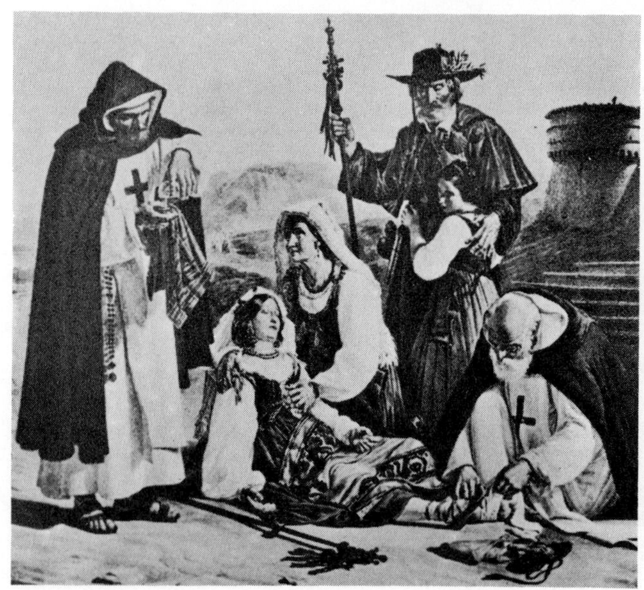

Figure 5–3. Trinitarians giving first aid. (Dolan collection.)

the feudal castles for protection began to build towns and develop a new social structure.

There were disadvantages to this new way of life. Living conditions were overcrowded; houses were ill ventilated and poorly heated; animals shared the family quarters; sewage and garbage were disposed of improperly; and water supply and resources for preservation of food were inadequate. The continuance of these conditions produced serious consequences.

Frequently, when food remaining from the previous day was seasoned highly and served, food poisoning resulted. One historian mentioned a covered casserole that was called "coffin."

Refuse from houses was thrown into the streets. In some cities this refuse was removed every four days, in others every eight days! Where could this garbage and debris be placed? The moat seemed to be a likely place, and so it was used.

This surrounding moat had provided the town with its water, but with its added burden, it was no longer suitable. Fountains and wells became necessities, and communal drinking cups were hung at their sides.

Public bathhouses were constructed, which were used by the sick and healthy alike. It is interesting to note that it was not until the fifteenth century that the sexes were segregated in these baths.

The citizens were concerned about the increase in the disease rate yet were ignorant of the elementary principles of hygiene. They worried about the increase in the numbers of rats and vermin and about inhaling the foul-smelling air. It appears that the problem of air pollution bothered medieval people; a hygienic precept stressed, "The air in which you live must be light, free from poison and should not stink."

LEPROSY

The prevalence of *leprosy*, the fear it engendered and the attempts to isolate it have been documented from earliest times. That lepers have been treated with much cruelty, little understanding and little kindness is also a known fact. Certain persons, however, gave "over and beyond the call of duty" to welcome, befriend and assist these people (Fig. 5–4).

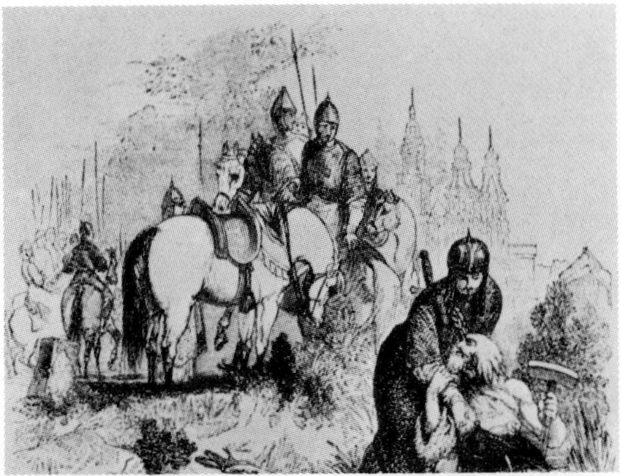

Figure 5–4. The famous Spanish hero El Cid Campeador is remembered for many expressions of concern and compassion. He is here portrayed in the act of saving a poor leper from sinking in a swamp. (Dolan collection.)

In medieval communities it was noted that diseases were increasing, especially leprosy. Because of an inability to diagnose this disease accurately, many diseases of the skin were erroneously considered to be leprosy, and all persons suffering from them were treated in the same way: They were expelled from the community to protect the healthy. Leper houses, lazarettos and finally leprosaria were built to house these patients when they were critically ill. These establishments are reputed to have numbered 19,000 in Europe during the thirteenth century.

Special laws, which demanded that lepers announce their approach by shaking a wooden rattle or blowing a horn, were enacted in the Middle Ages. Lepers were permitted to beg for the necessities of life (Fig. 5–5).

The pathetic plight of the leper has been portrayed in art and literature. It has been emphasized that he was a social outcast. To the rest of the world, the leper was dead. Once he was seen to have the disease, ceremonies for the dead were recited, and he was dispossessed of his fortune, title, money and personal possessions. He was permitted to have only the horn, rattle or bell and his own drinking cup. A white cross was the distinctive mark indicating the dwelling of a leper.

In Norway, churches have doors that were open to permit lepers to observe

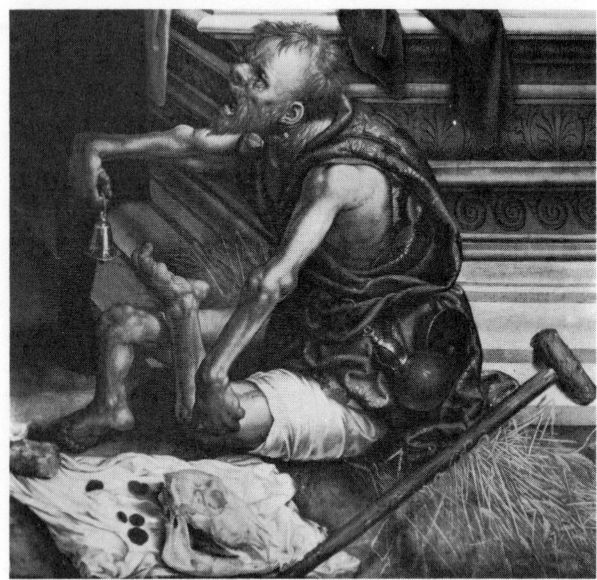

Figure 5–5. A person with advanced lepromatous leprosy. Note the bell and the crutch of the period. From a triptych by Barend Van Orley (*ca.* 1492–1542). (Courtesy of Royal Museum of Fine Arts, Antwerp.)

the service without mingling with the parishioners.

BUBONIC PLAGUE

In the fourteenth century a catastrophic outbreak of the *bubonic plague,* known as the *Black Death,* brought fear and devastation to much of Europe and to the rest of the world. References to this disease appear in the Bible, and mention has been made of the epidemics that occurred in the ancient civilized world. The outbreak of bubonic plague in the fourteenth century was one of the most devastating crises in human history and caused a period of intense psychological trauma.

In 1345, ships returning from a long voyage to China and India reached the ports of the Black Sea and the Mediterranean. The cargo, when landed, included rats from the ships. The stage was set by the unsanitary conditions described previously, and an outbreak of bubonic plague resulted.

A presentation of the clinical picture may help explain this historic tragedy. Plague is an acute infectious disease caused by the bacillus *Yersinia pestis*. Primarily a disease of rodents, particularly rats, the plague is readily transmitted to humans by such parasites as fleas that feed on diseased rodents. The disease can also be transmitted by direct contact with an infected person. There are three different types of plague: the bubonic, the septicemic and the pneumonic. With the bubonic plague, after a brief incubation period of about two days, the following clinical picture is observed: chills, fever (101°-105°F.), severe headache, extreme prostration, vertigo, abscesses called buboes in the lymph glands, and hemorrhage of the superficial blood vessels, which gives the skin a bluish-black color (hence the popular name "Black Death"). Finally death results.

The suddenness of the onset of the disease and the brevity of its duration were responsible for the hysteria and panic that accompanied epidemics.

Medieval people believed that the chief defense against the disease was to flee from the infected persons and from the location of the outbreak. Thus families fled from their loved ones, leaving them to die unattended.

The disease eventually reached pandemic (world-wide) proportions. When the plague ended, India was reputed to have been depopulated; China lost thirteen million persons; Cairo supposedly lost daily from ten to fifteen thousand lives and altogether at least a quarter of the population of the then-known world perished.

THE GREAT POX: SYPHILIS

The other great scourge of the Middle Ages was *syphilis*. Its origin remains a mystery.

Syphilis was known before this time but

under different names. Medieval syphilis was known first as *mal franzoso, morbus gallicus* or *mala napoletana*. After it became epidemic, it was called "the pocks." By the end of the fourteenth century, physicians were already prescribing mercurial ointments, but these were used for many skin afflictions other than syphilis.

On March 25, 1493, the town crier of Paris was directed to order from the city all afflicted with "the greater pox" *(la grosse vérole)* under pain of being thrown into the Seine River.

RISE OF MENDICANT ORDERS—EXPANSION OF NURSING

With the rapid spread of misery and sickness and the fright caused by the plague, religious fervor mounted. A different type of religious ministration was required from that of the period when communities lived around a monastery. The answer to this demand came when St. Francis and St. Dominic each founded three religious orders: the first order was for friars; the second order was for nuns; and the third order was for the laity, men and women who continued to lead secular lives.

St. Francis of Assisi (1182–1226) (Fig. 5–6) is undoubtedly one of the best-loved figures in world history. Francis was a worldly, pleasure-loving youth with extraordinary qualities of leadership. After a serious illness in his early twenties, Francis changed his manner of living, becoming concerned about others and patterning his life after that of his Redeemer.

Disinherited by his merchant father for giving great amounts of alms to the poor, Francis donned a rough brown tunic, bound it around his waist with a heavy white rope and went barefooted around the countryside, ministering to the poor and outcast.

His first real spiritual challenge may have been his encounter with leprosy. St. Francis, who had a marked aversion to leprosy, beheld a leper approaching him and begging for alms. After a brief pause, St. Francis embraced the unfortunate man and gave him what money he had. Becoming the champion of lepers, St. Francis, along with his companions, lived next to the leper hospital and ministered to the pa-

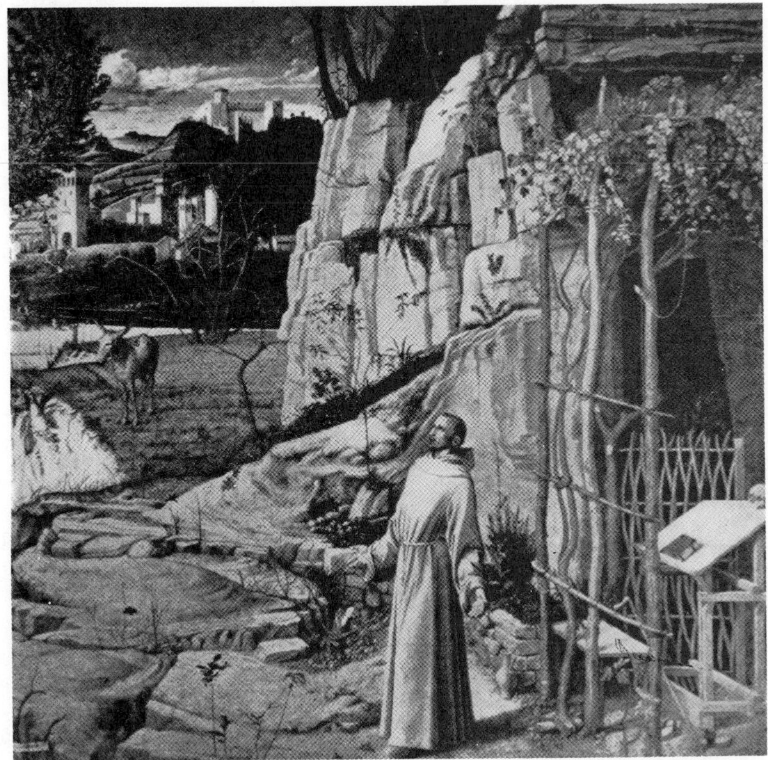

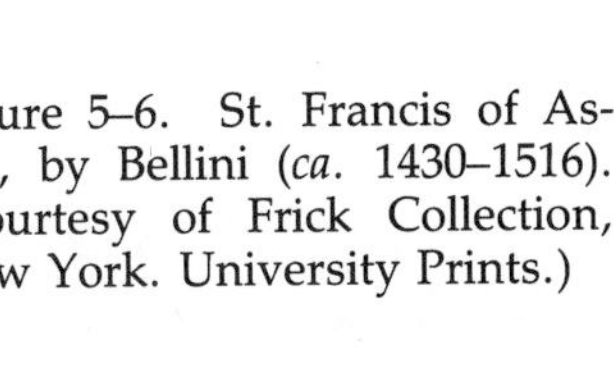

Figure 5–6. St. Francis of Assisi, by Bellini (*ca.* 1430–1516). (Courtesy of Frick Collection, New York. University Prints.)

tients. He made the public acutely aware of the plight of the leper and the problem of leprosy.

Many followers were attracted to this happy, kind and courageous man, and in 1209 the Order of Friars Minor, or "little brothers," was formed. The rule of the Franciscans emphasized poverty and humility; they were mendicants, begging for themselves and for the poor. This obligation of mendicancy forced the friars to receive their daily bread as the fruit of their apostolic labors.

A cruel medical practice of this period was experienced by St. Francis. It became apparent that Francis' vision was failing and that he would soon become blind. The medical treatment selected was to cauterize his eyes with a red-hot iron without even the benefit of a soothing drug.

The spirit that guided St. Francis of Assisi has been summed up in his prayer:

Lord, make me an instrument of your peace.
Where there is hatred, let me sow love.
Where there is injury, pardon.
Where there is doubt, faith.
Where there is despair, hope.
Where there is darkness, light.
Where there is sadness, joy.
O Divine Master, grant that I may not so much seek
To be consoled as to console,
To be understood as to understand,
To be loved as to love,
For it is in giving that we receive,
It is in pardoning that we are pardoned,
It is in dying that we are born to eternal life.

Before his death in 1226, St. Francis' followers numbered in the thousands. One of his well-known followers was the learned *St. Anthony of Padua* (1195–1231), who had been a teacher at the Universities of Paris, Bologna and Padua. Anthony was an eloquent preacher, a benevolent almsgiver and a prison reformer.

St. Clare, the beautiful daughter of a rich and noble family of Assisi, heard St. Francis preach and was motivated to follow his simple life of charity, humility and fervent devotion. Against strong parental opposition, Clare happily exchanged her garb of jewels and finery for a brown sackcloth habit. Then Clare entered a nearby Benedictine abbey; in a short time a special convent was established for her and other young women who wanted to share this life of poverty and simplicity. Her sister Agnes joined the group, and a short time after her father's death, her mother joined them also. This second order of St. Francis became known as the order of *Poor Clares* (Fig. 5–7).

The rule of the Poor Clares was essentially the same as that of the Order of Friars. In times of epidemics, the Poor Clares took care of the sick and opened their convent as a hospital.

St. Clare died in 1253, but her order continues and has been described in *A Right to Be Merry.*[1]

While St. Francis was achieving success

[1]Sister Mary Francis, P. C.: *A Right to Be Merry.* New York, Sheed & Ward, 1956.

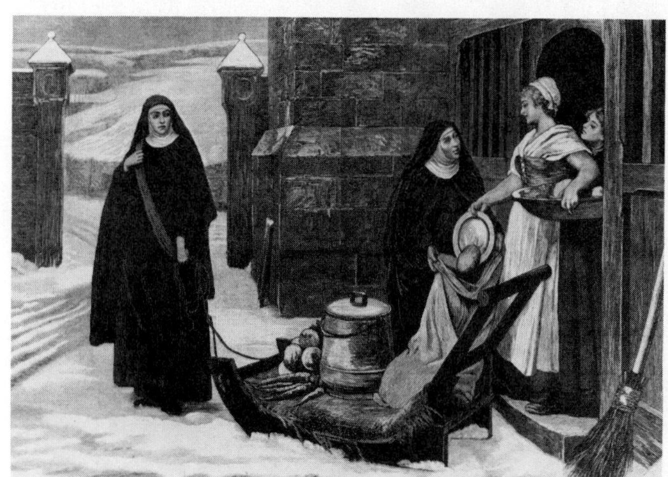

Figure 5–7. For the Poor, a painting by W. F. Yeames (1875). Mendicants begging for food for themselves and for the poor. (Dolan collection.)

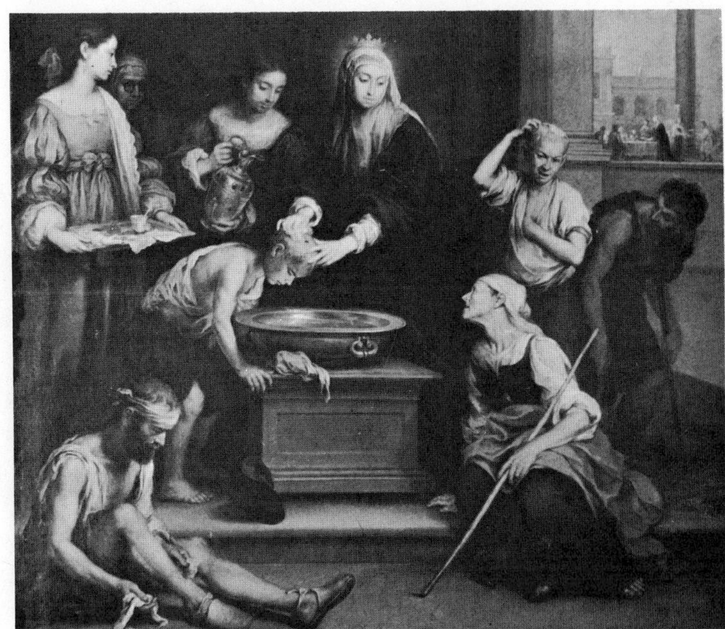

Figure 5–8. St. Elizabeth of Hungary, by Murillo (1618–1682). (Hospital de la Santa Caridad, Seville.) (Dolan collection.)

with his order, *St. Dominic* was establishing an Order of Preachers, more commonly called the Dominicans. Many eminent scholars arose from these two orders at this time: the Dominican Albertus Magnus (1206–1280) and the Franciscan Roger Bacon (1214–1294) contributed to the beginnings of experimental science by emphasizing the value of observation, experimentation and inductive reasoning. Known as the Prince of Scholastics, the Dominican St. Thomas Aquinas (1225?–1274) studied under the Benedictines at Monte Cassino and, sometime after 1265, began his greatest work, *Summa Theologica*.

The *Third Orders* of St. Francis and St. Dominic were established for many distinguished persons whose occupations and obligations could not permit them to live a conventual life but who felt a need for this spiritual bond and wanted an opportunity to share in the accomplishments of the order. Into the Third Order of St. Francis came such well-known persons as St. Elizabeth of the royal house of Hungary; St. Louis IX, the King of France; Dante, the famous poet; and three great scientists in the field of electricity, Volta, Galvani and Ampère.

St. Elizabeth of Hungary (1207–1231) (Fig. 5–8), the daughter of King Andreas II and Queen Gertrude of Hungary, was betrothed at four years of age to Ludwig, son of the Landgrave of Thuringia. They married young (in 1221) and were a devoted couple. Elizabeth was cheerful and fun-loving and exemplary for her goodness, generosity and sympathy. After her marriage, Elizabeth had a turnstile built into one of the castle gates, at which she herself distributed alms daily to the poor and needy. During the famine of 1226, Elizabeth organized a distribution of food, depleting the castle granaries for the purpose. She would take the hour's walk from the castle to the nearby town to visit the sick in their homes, attending the ill and staying with the dying.

Elizabeth joined the Third Order of St. Francis and devoted all her time, strength and energy to the needs of the sick poor. She built hospitals and directed her services especially to the lepers. Prisoners also received her attention, and she bathed the wounds inflicted by their chains.

Before his death during one of the Crusades, Ludwig had cooperated with Elizabeth in her projects, partly in response to having been permitted to witness several instances of her unusual sanctity. After his death, however, Elizabeth was expelled from her husband's castle, the Wartburg, and those to whom she had given so generously refused to assist her. Elizabeth settled at Marburg where she spent the remaining years of her short life (she died in

1231 at the age of 24) nursing the sick in the Marburg hospital that she had founded.

St. Louis IX (1214–1270) was especially interested in the three great needs of humanity—education, justice and charity—and he devoted his life to achieving them for his subjects.

Louis's endeavors in the field of education resulted in the building of the Saint-Chapelle in Paris and the founding of the Sorbonne College of the University of Paris. Louis stressed the need for adequate education for health care deliverers. He himself waited on the sick, bathed them, served them and attended to their needs regardless of their unsightly appearance. Lepers received special care from him. Louis's justice and charity endeared him to his subjects, and when he died on one of the Crusades, he was mourned by Christians and Moslems alike. Under his reign, France enjoyed prosperity, peace and progress.

Members of the Third Order of St. Dominic were known first in Italy by the name Mantellate. These were lay persons who continued to live at home but bound themselves to a more religious life. They wore the Dominican religious habit, which consisted of a white tunic girded by a leather belt, a white veil over the head and a black cloak or mantella.

The first young single girl to join the Mantellate was a blind and deformed girl named *Margaret of Metola* (1287–1320), the daughter of wealthy parents who abandoned her because of her physical afflictions. Margaret spent the majority of her 33 years devoting herself to the needs of others. She visited and nursed the sick and gave special attention to prisoners, who were kept in underground prison cells without sunlight, fresh air, sanitary facilities or heat. These prisoners suffered from lack of food and clothing, from the stench, from "jail fever" and from the wounds inflicted by their chains. Only the few who could afford to bribe their jailors received the bare necessities of life when they were obtainable. Every day, Margaret and her white-robed companions entered the prison armed with bundles of food, clothing, bedding and medicines.

St. Catherine of Siena (1347–1380) (Fig. 5–9) was born Catherine Benincasa, the twenty-fifth child of a well-to-do merchant

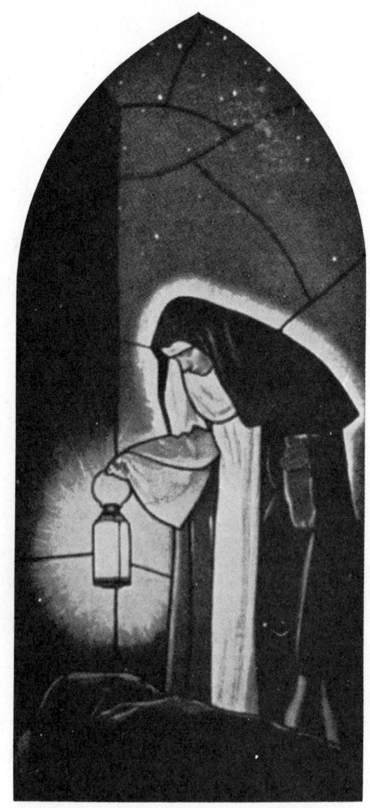

Figure 5–9. St. Catherine of Siena. (Courtesy of Will Ross, Inc.)

and his wife. Catherine became a forceful, gifted, clear-thinking and diplomatic leader and writer. At the age of 18, joining the Mantellate and receiving the habit of the Third Order of St. Dominic, Catherine began her many works of mercy.

St. Catherine has been noted for the kindness and tenderness that she extended to persons with the most loathsome of diseases. When a poor woman with leprosy was refused admission to a hospital, Catherine begged that the woman be admitted, promising to care for her.

During the bubonic plague epidemic, the shadowy figure of Catherine could be seen going around the streets of Siena at night. With a lighted lantern she would look for forsaken victims so that she might comfort them. She ministered to the plague victims who were hospitalized. In her biography of St. Catherine, Curtayne depicts Catherine carrying a bottle of cologne and bringing some refreshment into the stench of the hospital rooms. Catherine rallied her friends, and they, too, "braced themselves to bend close to the livid, swollen faces, choking down the nausea of that pestilential odour."[2] There was very little to be done for the plague victims; to be willing to stay with them and comfort them was a supreme sacrifice.

Catherine of Siena's influence has been great. The nineteenth-century English poet Swinburne praised her accomplishments in his poem "The Laud of St. Catherine":

> Then in her sacred saving hands
> She took the sorrows of the lands,
> With maiden palms she lifted up
> The sick time's blood-imbittered cup,
> And in her virgin garment furled
> The faint limbs of a wounded world,
> Clothed with calm love and clear desire,
> She went forth in her soul's attire,
> A missive fire.[3]

SECULAR NURSING ORDERS

There were other groups of workers who joined together yet were not bound by vows to monastic life. Such groups have been referred to as *secular nursing orders,* and their members visited the sick, took care of foundlings and orphans and brought the sick to hospitals.

The *Order of Antonines,* or Hospital Brothers of St. Anthony, was founded about 1095. This group of laymen specialized in the care of patients suffering from a disease called St. Anthony's fire (ergotism) (Fig. 5–10). Special hospitals were built for the sufferers of this disease, and the Antonines were successful in caring for these tragic victims.

In his book *The Day of St. Anthony's Fire,* which deals with the 1951 outbreak of this affliction that occurred in Pont Saint-Esprit in France, Fuller states:

> In 1089, an observer wrote: "We could see many 'ergotists' in the village, bowels devoured by sacred fire, either dying wretchedly or living with gangrened limbs." When the town of La Motte-au-Bois in the province of Dauphiné, some hundred kilometers from Pont-Saint-Esprit, was stricken by ergotism in the Middle Ages, a nobleman and his son, both afflicted with the disease, called on St. Anthony and were cured by what they thought was the presence of St. Anthony's relics in the town. The relics had been captured by the Saracens in 532 and taken to Constantinople, but they had been brought back to Dauphiné by a conscientious pilgrim. The nobleman and his son then set up a lay society to cure the ill who were smitten by the disease. Even then the disease was nothing new. Ergot in rye had been mentioned in the Bible by the prophet Amos; Pliny had mentioned it in his *Natural History*. It was used in the tenth century in Thuringia for its strange power to hasten childbirth; it is still used under controlled modern medicine for the same thing today. "There is a tingling and burning of the hands and feet," one writer described the symptoms, "and then a frightful heartburn. Fingers and toes are bent nearly doubled and clamped; the mouth is full of foam. Often the tongue is lacerated by the strength of the convulsions. There is a severe secretion of spittle. The sick utter that they are being destroyed by a burning fire. They feel great giddiness, and some of them become blind; the intellectual capacities are polluted, a fog comes over and destroys the mind."

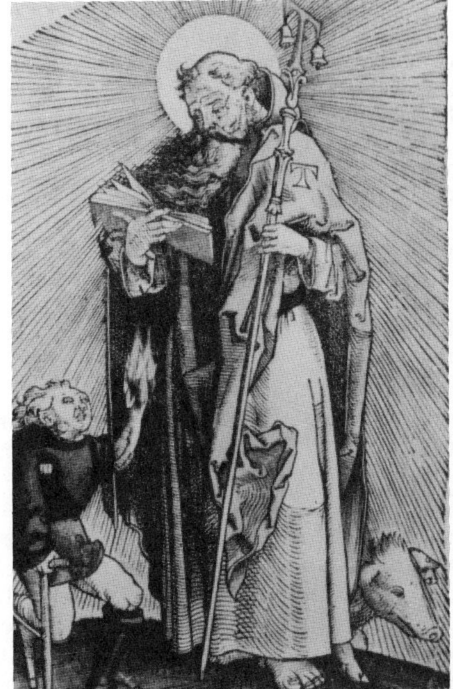

Figure 5–10. The great Egyptian hermit St. Anthony is represented with a victim of St. Anthony's fire, or ergotism. A woodcut by Johannes Wechtlin (*ca.* 1490–1530). (Dolan collection.)

The more sophisticated observations of the nineteenth century recognized that ergot was a

[2] Curtayne, Alice: *St. Catherine of Siena*. New York, The Macmillan Co., 1929, p. 75.

[3] Brown, E. K., ed.: *Victorian Poetry*. New York, Thomas Nelson & Sons, 1942.

parasitic fungus growth on grain, called *Claviceps purpurea*. A dense tissue forms in the ovaries of rye and gradually replaces the entire substance of the grain with a hard, purple, curved body called the sclerotium. This is the commercial source for pharmaceutical ergot, recognized in modern medicine as a very useful but often puzzling drug. It was only in the nineteen-thirties that many of the ergot alkaloids were discovered and defined chemically, but even today many facts are elusive. One thing is certain: All the ergot alkaloids are derivatives of lysergic acid, a chemical that still has much mystery surrounding it.[4]

The hallucinatory manifestations of this disease have been documented in many dramatic references.

The *Beguines* of Flanders, Belgium (1184), was one of the most prominent of the secular nursing orders for women. Lambert le Begue, Bishop of Liège, suggested the founding of this community of women who would live together without taking vows or giving up their property or possessions. They were free to leave the group at any time and to marry.

The Beguines erected communal hermitages known as *Beguinages* on the outskirts of towns. These communities were arranged on a cottage plan, grouped around one large central structure, usually the church. Each cottage accommodated from two to four persons. The Beguinages at Bruges (*ca.* 1184) and at Ghent (*ca.* 1234) are well known (Fig. 5–11).

Each new member received her preparation under a more experienced member on an apprenticeship basis. These women devoted themselves to the needs of widows and orphans of the Crusaders. Because they did not accept payment for services to the sick, they had to pool their resources.

The Beguines devoted themselves to the care of the sick and were praised for their ministrations during war, famine and epidemics. They converted their houses into hospitals and worked as volunteer nurses. They distributed food and clothing during such catastrophic occasions as the Napoleonic Wars and the epidemic that followed, during the cholera epidemics and during the famine and industrial crises of the nineteenth century.

The Beguines built hospitals close to the Beguinages and established an order of sisters called the Sisters of Matilda to staff them. One of the most famous of these hospitals is the Hôtel Dieu at Beaune, which was founded in 1443 (Figs. 5–12 and 5–13). Although the primary work of the sisters was nursing in the hospital, they did give care to the sick in their homes, staying with the dying and consoling the families of the bereaved.

The desire of women to join such a phi-

[4]Fuller, John G.: *The Day of St. Anthony's Fire*. New York, The Macmillan Co., 1968, pp. 117–118.

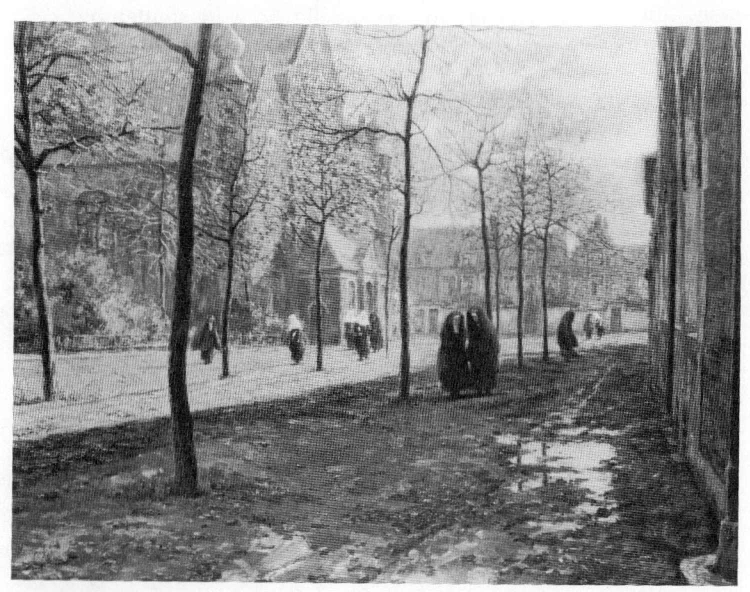

Figure 5–11. Members of the order of the Beguines leaving the Church of St. Elizabeth and heading toward the Beguinage at Ghent in Belgium. A painting by Ferdinand Willaert. (Dolan collection.)

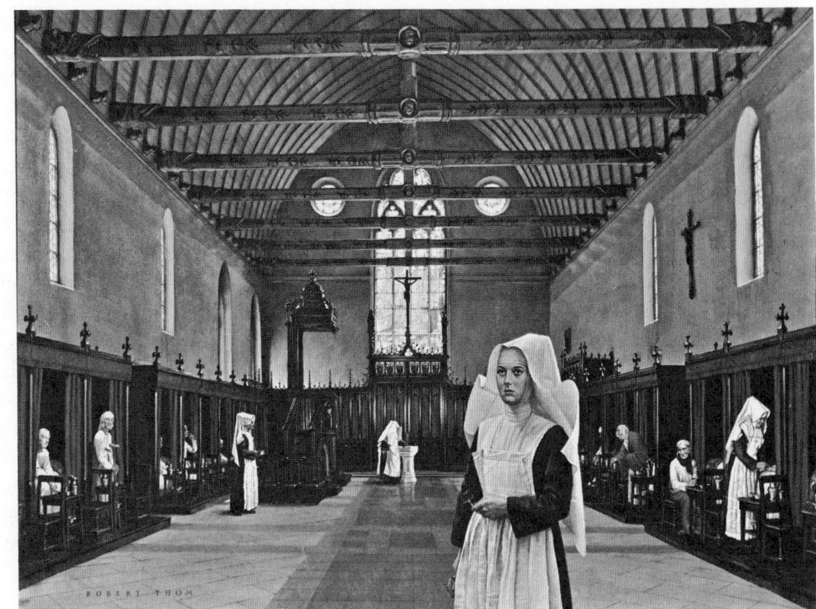

Figure 5–12. Hôtel Dieu, Beaune, France. (© 1958 by Parke, Davis & Co.)

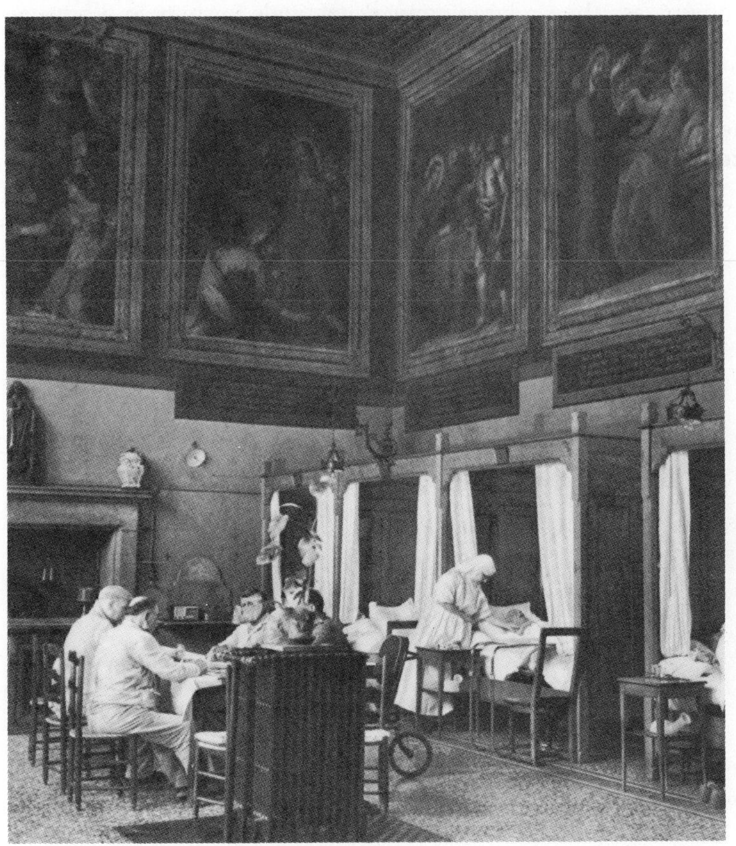

Figure 5–13. A Sister at the Hôtel Dieu in Beaune giving care to a patient in a room compartment. Ambulatory patients enjoy meals at the table in the center. Note the works of art. (Dolan collection.)

lanthropic project is apparent when we realize that by the end of the thirteenth century there was hardly a community that did not have a Beguinage, many of the larger cities having several, and that the Beguines numbered about 200,000.

An order of men, the *Brethren of the Common Life,* was founded at this time by Gerhard Groot. At first, these men devoted themselves to the care of the sick poor and visited them in their homes. They were interested chiefly in teaching children who were bedridden. After a time they became the schoolmasters of the period, and such well-known persons as Erasmus and Thomas à Kempis became members.

The *Sisters of the Common Life* specialized in the care of the sick, of which instruction of sick children was an integral part. These sisters took no vows, lived together in a conventual plan and could leave the group at any time.

The *Misericordia,* founded in 1244, was another group of religious laymen. Their chief contribution to medieval society was the volunteer ambulance work that they carried on in many Italian cities. The Misericordia are sometimes known as the "Masked Brotherhood" (Fig. 5–14). This group seems to have believed that their unique contribution would gain spiritual merit if they prevented themselves (the givers) from being recognized by others. The Italian city of Florence still boasts of the benevolence of the Brothers of Misericordia. In 1961, it was reported that 2500 members devoted at least an hour a week for the charitable purposes of caring for the sick and needy. In their headquarters at the Piazza del Duomo assemble the men of this brotherhood who come from all walks of life: lawyers, students, physicians, civil and public servants. These brothers are prepared to assist the afflicted at any hour, for a carefully planned rotational schedule allows for a staff of twenty men on duty at every hour of the day or night.

The Alexian Brothers, formed during the scourge of the bubonic plague in 1348, was a group of laymen united to care for the plague sufferers. They also undertook the burial of the dead. In 1469 this group was organized under Augustinian rule and took as their patron saint St. Alexius, a fifth-century Roman who nursed the sick in the hospital built by St. Ephrem at Edessa. This order continues to serve the sick. The Alexian Brothers' Hospital School of Nursing in Chicago was at one time the largest all-male nursing school in the United States. The order maintains and staffs several large general hospitals for men and boys as well as a rest home and home for elderly men. Memorial Hospital and Clinic at Boys Town, Nebraska, is also staffed by the Alexian Brothers. Nursing is only one of the many fields in which the brothers serve for the betterment of society.

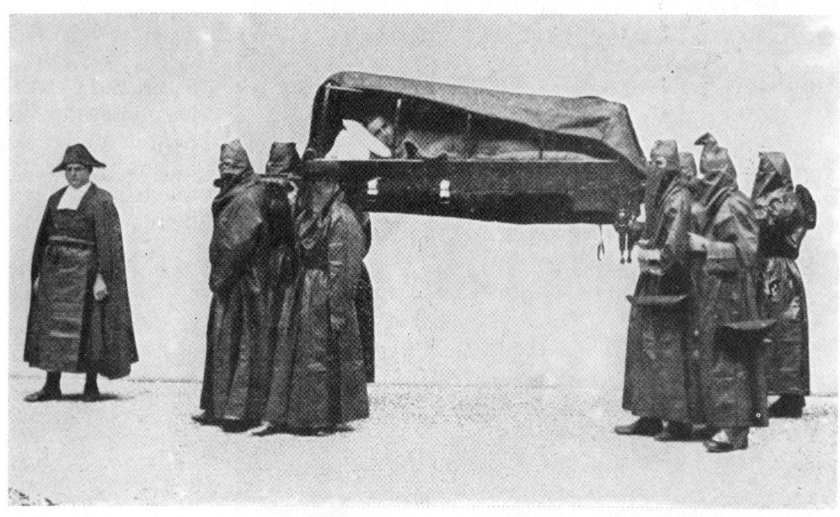

Figure 5–14. The Brothers of the Misericordia taking a patient to the hospital in Florence. (Dolan collection.)

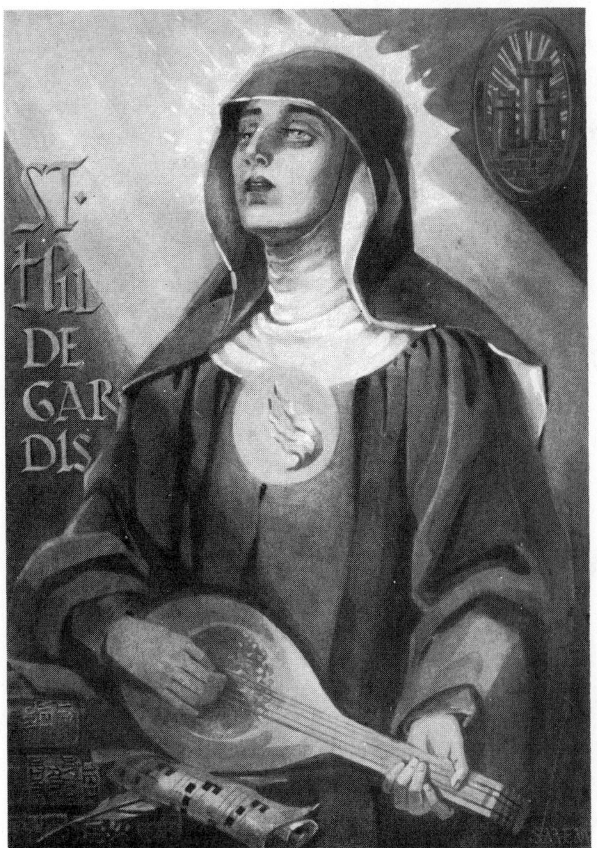

Figure 5–15. St. Hildegarde. (From Bosk, J.: *Patrons of Our Names in Word and Picture*, Neuland Verlag.)

INDIVIDUAL NURSING LEADERS

Besides the part that organized groups played in the nursing achievements of this period, certain individuals were also exemplary in their contributions through research to the field of nursing.

St. Hildegarde (1098?–1179) (Fig. 5–15), one of the most erudite women of the Middle Ages, was born of noble parents and at the age of eight was sent to be educated at the Benedictine cloister at Disibodenberg. After she finished her schooling, Hildegarde entered this monastery and years later became its abbess. She also founded another Benedictine cloister near Bingen on the Rhine.

Hildegarde was a scholar and eagerly absorbed the vast number of scientific writings that had accumulated in the monastery. The fruits of her labors appear in a series of books, some of which are concerned with theological subjects, but at least two of which are related to the field of medicine: *Liber Simplicis Medicinae* and *Liber Compositae Medicinae*. These books are assumed to have been written for the nuns in charge of the infirmaries in the numerous Benedictine monasteries. There was a need for such references, for these infirmarians were responsible for the care not only of the nuns but also of the sick travelers who stayed at the convent guest houses. In the sixteenth century the first of these books was edited under the title *Physica St. Hildegardis*. It contains nine books. The second volume, consisting of five books, presents the general diseases of the human body and their causes, symptoms and treatment. It is a compendium of information based on scientific investigation. Hildegarde discusses the vibration and pulsation of the blood in the veins; the regulation of vital activities by the brain, spinal cord and nerves; and the importance of understanding normal and abnormal psychology.

Her accumulated knowledge encompassed medical science, nursing, music, herb gardening and natural science, as well as a spiritual and religious philosophy of fantastic scope. Her books indicate her constant educational pursuits as well as her original thinking. Her medical works were written between 1151 and 1159, when she was in her fifties.

St. Hildegarde, who knew many things that were unknown to the medical personnel of her day, was both physician and nurse. Her greatest accomplishments, however, were her contributions to the scientific foundation of nursing and medicine. Hildegarde's works prove not only that the monasteries collected and housed intellectual works, but also that their residents were encouraged to peruse these works and to add to the accumulation of knowledge.

Cunegundes, a niece of St. Elizabeth of Hungary, married Boleslaus, the King of Poland. Cunegundes visited the poor and the sick in the hospitals, and she gave special care to lepers. After the death of her husband, Cunegundes entered a monastery of the Poor Clares.

Queen Elizabeth of Portugal (1271–1336) (known also as St. Isabel), a grandniece of Elizabeth of Hungary, devoted her life to charity. She gave food and lodging to the poor, established a house for penitent prostitutes in which they were given special training so that they might reenter society as useful citizens, instituted a hospital for foundlings and nursed the sick in the hospitals. At the death of her husband, Elizabeth joined the Poor Clares and died in the convent at Coimbra, which she had founded.

St. Roch (1295?–1327) was the son of the governor of the city of Montpellier in France. At the death of his parents when he was about eighteen years of age, Roch distributed his large fortune to the poor and set out on a pilgrimage. When he reached Italy, he saw the devastation caused by the bubonic plague and offered his services in nursing the sick. Roch contracted the disease but was miraculously cured, and in the several paintings of him, the "bubo" of the disease can be noted on his leg.

Queen Isabella of Castile married Ferdinand, King of Aragon, in 1469. Isabella has been credited with having introduced the use of tent-type hospitals and ambulances for the injured on the battlefields. She visited and cared for the wounded and showed skill in caring for the sick.

Queen Matilda, affectionately called "Good Queen Maud," was the wife of King Henry I of England and the daughter of King Malcolm III of Scotland and Queen Margaret. In addition to founding hospitals, she gave care to the sick.

MIDWIFERY

Obstetrics and gynecology were practiced by *midwives.* The paintings of this period frequently show the presence of the midwife and the child nurse who cared for the baby. Often the child nurse is shown using either her arm or foot as a thermometer to test the water before bathing the baby. For cases of difficult labor, the midwife asked the advice of the physician, but he did not come to examine the patient or to assume the duties of the midwife. Among primitive peoples, delivery has been carried out in a squatting or sitting position, and in the early days in Europe, the obstetrical chair or V-shaped stool was used (Fig. 5–16). Later, delivery in bed was the accepted method (Fig. 5–17). In the twen-

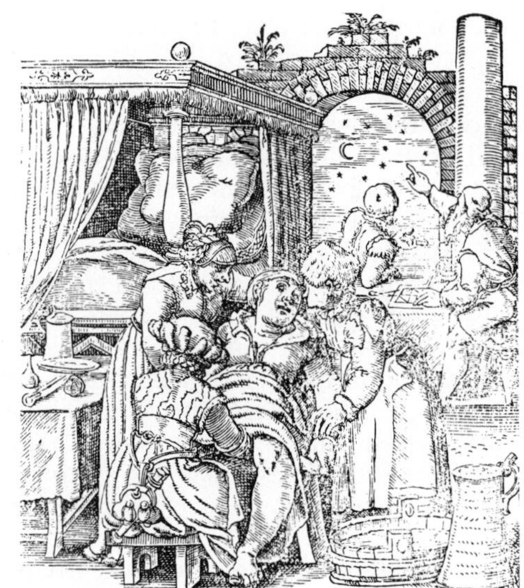

Figure 5–16. A delivery during the Renaissance. Belligerent midwives guard the lying-in chamber against medical interference. The physician-astrologer at the window casts a horoscope of the newborn. An illustration by Jakob Ruff (1500–1558). (Courtesy of National Library of Medicine, Bethesda, Md.)

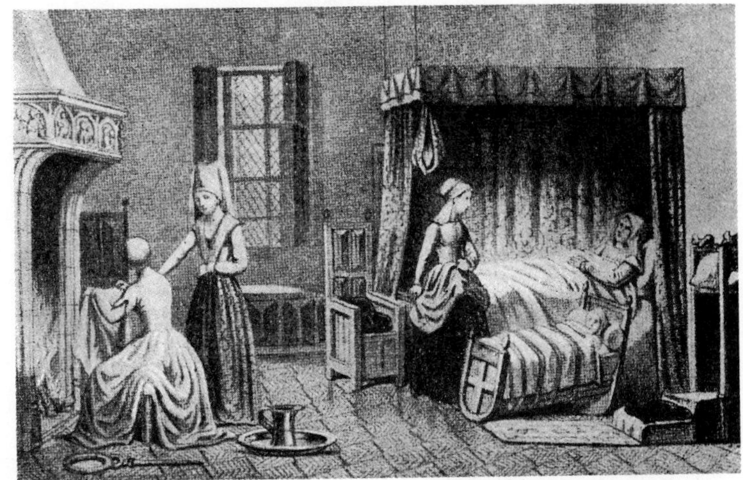

Figure 5–17. Obstetric ward of a Dutch hospital in the fifteenth century. Note rooming-in aspect of child care. (Dolan collection.)

tieth century obstetrical chairs have re-emerged.

ORGANIZATION OF HOSPITALS

It has been mentioned that crowded living conditions and the resulting increase in the spread of disease caused a demand for more hospitals; the existing ones had been organized as almshouses, orphanages and hospices for travelers as well as places to provide accommodations for the sick. *Pope Innocent III* (1116–1216) was a dominant force behind the movement to visit and evaluate existing hospitals and then construct new ones as needed.

The first hospital in England was built at York by Athelstane about 936. This was also a poorhouse and had a ward for lepers. Queen Matilda founded *St. Giles' Hospital* in 1101 to care for forty lepers. For many years this leper hospital was the most important of its kind in the British Isles. She also was the motivating spirit behind the building of the *Hospital of St. Katherine* in London in 1148. The charter of this hospital included the opportunity for nursing the sick poor in their homes. Many centuries later, the Jubilee Institute for District Nursing adopted this charter. Women of noble birth did both the nursing in these hospitals and district work in the homes of the poor.

St. Bartholomew's Hospital in London was built in 1123 with the encouragement of Rahere, formerly the king's jester, who had become an Augustinian monk. *St. Thomas' Hospital*, also in London, was founded by Richard, the prior of Bermondsey, in 1213. This hospital and St. Bartholomew's were the only ones spared during the closing of religious monasteries, convents and hospitals during the Reformation.

The *Hospital of Santa Maria della Scala* in Siena is of special interest because it was here that St. Catherine of Siena gave such valiant care to the plague sufferers. Her major efforts were directed to the patients who were in the attached house for lepers. This hospital's beautiful interior frescoes and artistic paintings continue to attract visitors.

It was the custom of this period to display paintings in the hospitals to provide diversional therapy for patients. This was done at *St. John's Hospital* at Bruges in Belgium, which was founded in 1118 by Augustinian monks and nuns as a hospice for travelers. The older buildings are preserved as a museum. Six masterpieces of the Flemish painter Hans Memling have made this hospital the envy of the world's art galleries. A fascinating account of this hospital and Johannes Beerblock's painting of the great hall has been presented by Goldin.[5]

The Hospital of the Innocents in Florence was built as a foundling asylum for the large number of abandoned children, who either died or became the property of the person who found them (Fig. 5–18). The

[5]Goldin, Grace: "A Walk Through a Ward of the Eighteenth Century," *Journal of the History of Medicine and Allied Sciences*, Vol. XXII, Number 2, 1967.

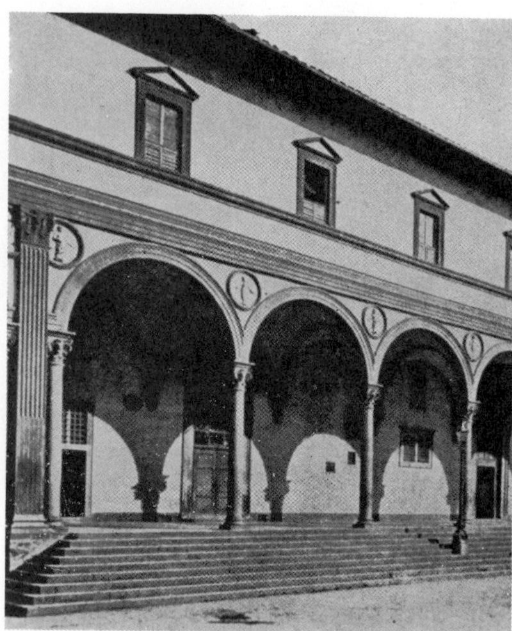

Figure 5–18. Foundlings' Hospital (Innocenti), Florence (*ca.* 1421). (Dolan collection.)

Ospedale Santa Maria degli Innocenti was built in 1451 with the financial assistance of the guild of silk merchants. This hospital exemplifies beautiful architecture and is adorned with the famous medallions of Della Robbia (Fig. 5–19). A type of foster parent plan whereby new parents had to promise to treat orphans as their own children was instituted in the Ospedale Santa Maria. Either the hospital or the new families taught the children trades and provided the girls with dowries. This hospital is administered by the Sisters of Charity of St. Vincent de Paul.

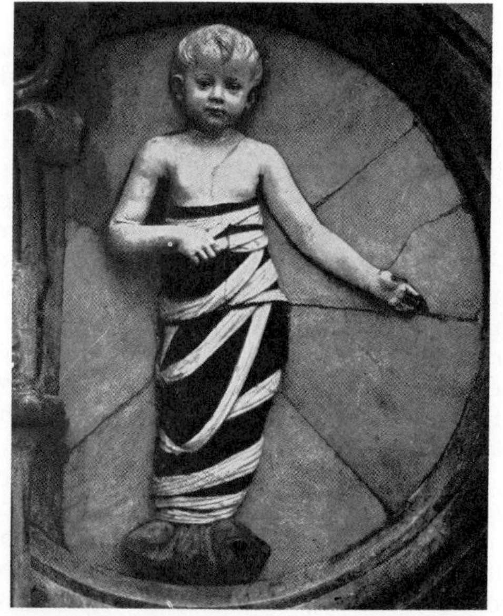

Figure 5–19. Bambino, by Andrea Della Robbia (1435–1525). (Hospital of the Innocents, Florence.) (Dolan collection.)

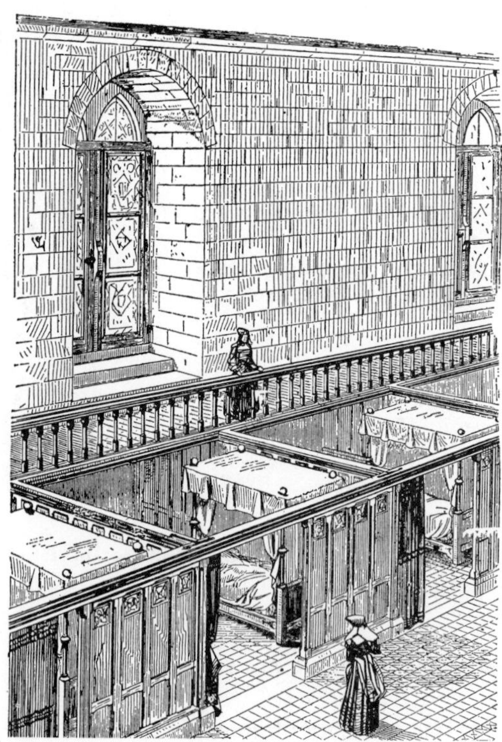

Figure 5–20. A ward in the hospital founded in 1293 at Tounerre in France by Marguerite of Bourgogne, sister of St. Louis IX. It was airy and well ventilated and had richly carved woodwork and beautifully colored stained glass windows. (Dolan collection.)

As Figure 5–20 shows, the interiors of the hospitals in France were light, airy and attractive in appearance.

TREATMENT OF THE MENTALLY ILL

Bethlehem Hospital, commonly known as Bedlam, was originally a hospice of St. Mary of Bethlehem. Later, in addition to providing general care, the hospital made provisions for the care of mentally ill patients. In the fourteenth century, Bethlehem was designed exclusively for the mentally ill, and the *Nursing Mirror* states: "In 1377 it became the first *lunatic asylum* in Britain and the second one in Europe." This article mentions that once patients responded to medical treatment, they were encouraged to go out into the streets and beg for their living. Wearing metal armbands that indicated their mental conditions, these patients were called "Tom o' Bedlams." The article reports that the "violent ones who were interned were kept in chains and cells and treated with considerable inhumanity" because it was believed that they "had neither understanding nor feeling."

Patients who were mentally ill were received into wards for the "insane" in general hospitals or in separate buildings called asylums. The word *asylum* implies security, but these asylums were more for the protection and comfort of the community than for the security of the patients. Centuries ago asylums were in effect prisons; our practice of having a person who is mentally ill committed to a psychiatric hospital by a judge or court is a legacy of these medieval methods. The care of the patient was custodial, and attendants were chosen for their physical strength.

Mentally ill patients were treated as animals, often being half-starved and kept in filthy conditions. For centuries their treatment was based on the idea that they felt neither heat nor cold. People had a fixed idea that the mentally ill were possessed by devils or that they were being punished for their sins. Iron manacles and chains were used for restraint, and there was a time when it was thought that fright and torture were useful in driving out "madness"; this was the "shock therapy" of the period.

In the eighteenth century, Bedlam was one of the tourist attractions of London. Visitors paid admission fees to see the antics of the inmates (Fig. 5–21). These fees were a source of revenue for the hospital.

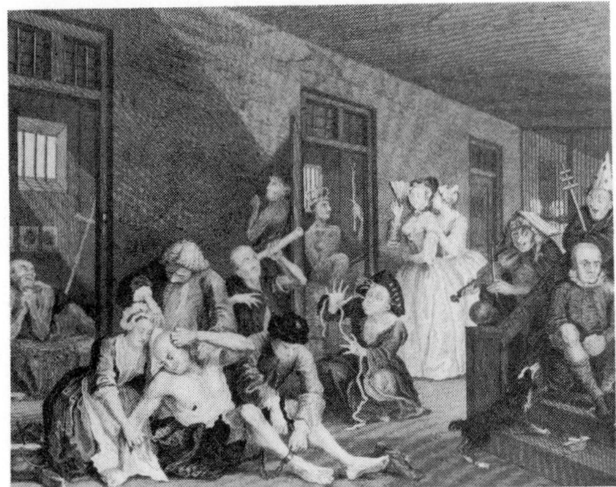

Figure 5–21. Bedlam. An engraving by William Hogarth (1697–1764) from *The Rake's Progress,* London, 1735. (Dolan collection.)

HOSPICES

The hospice movement reemerged and was essential in providing sustenance to the homeless and starving. An example is the *Hospice of St. Cross,* which was built on the ruins of a church that was erected before the Norman Conquest and destroyed by the Danes. A young bishop launched the reconstruction of the edifice between 1133 and 1136 and established the hospice, which is claimed to be Britain's oldest existing charitable institution.

The idea for such an establishment was that of Henry de Blois, grandson of William the Conqueror and brother of King Stephen, who desired to make a home for men too weak and too poor to exist by their own efforts. In addition, the hospice was obliged to provide food for travelers. The "wayfarer's dole" consisted of bread and beer for many years (Fig. 5–22)

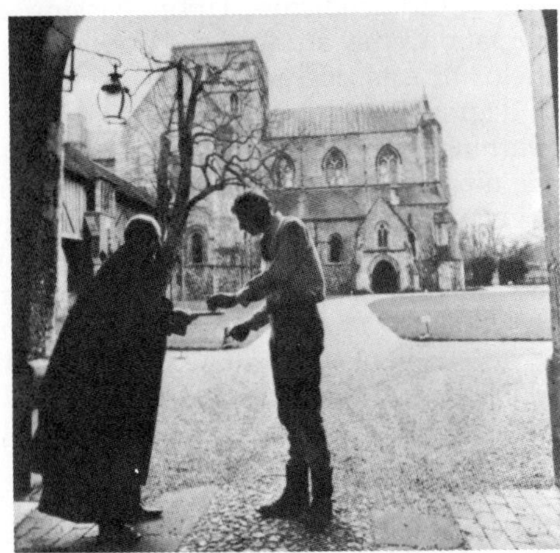

Figure 5–22. A "traveller" receives his dole at the Hospice of St. Cross. (Dolan collection.)

GUILDS

The *guilds,* associations for workmen and tradesmen, were important in the Middle Ages. Each guild divided its workmen into the three categories of apprentice, craftsman and master craftsman and protected the worker, the product and the public.

The apprenticeship method of learning a skill was stressed and expanded. Higher standards of work were encouraged, wages were set, unethical practices were forbidden and certain social insurance was provided for the worker and his family.

UNIVERSITIES AND LEARNING

The founding of universities was a cultural achievement of monumental significance. As there were few institutions of learning, students traveled great distances, first to the schools connected with the monasteries, then to the cathedral schools[6] and finally to the universities.

Latin was the universal language, used for teaching in all schools. Thus, it was easy for teachers to give and students to accept knowledge, regardless of their nationality.

The curriculum in the universities emphasized the seven liberal arts: rhetoric, grammar, logic or dialectics, mathematics (including geometry), astronomy, music and metaphysics. These universities had graduate departments of philosophy, law, theology and medicine. Upon passing an examination, the student was awarded a bachelor of arts degree; master's and doctor's degrees were also conferred.

Learning flourished and an intellectual awakening was occurring. This movement was given added impetus by the invention of movable type by *Johann Gutenberg* in 1438. Previous to this, books were laboriously copied by hand, but with the printing press, books became more readily available.

[6]These schools were attached to the great cathedrals and were started by Charlemagne and his teacher Alcuin. The most famous of the cathedral schools were those of Chartres, Notre Dame, Lyons, Metz, Tours, Rheims and Orleans.

A renaissance occurred in the fields of literature and art. Petrarch, Dante, Boccaccio, Cervantes and Chaucer wrote their literary masterpieces; thousands of singing poets, or troubadours, roamed the countryside; and religious plays based on the life of Christ and on the lives of the saints were performed.[7]

Two visual media used for teaching were beautiful tapestries and magnificent stained glass windows; many were picture chronicles that told a story with liveliness and exquisite color.

MEDIEVAL TREATMENTS

The importance of the four bodily humors in keeping a person healthy remained the prime health concept at this time. To prevent or cure disease it was essential to withdraw the corrupt humors from the body by *purging, bloodletting, leeching* and *cupping.*

A powerful purgative was frequently given followed by the withdrawal of a small amount of blood. This procedure, called bloodletting, was one of the functions of the barber.[8] Leeches were also used for this purpose. These treatments were repeated as frequently as it seemed necessary.

Often, cups were applied to the skin; the cups adhered to the skin by means of suction, the air having been quickly withdrawn from the cup. These applications acted as counterirritants. At the height of ancient Greek and Roman medicine, metal cups were used. The ancient American shamans used sucking tubes made of hollow deer bones for cupping. Glass cups eventually replaced the metal ones.

Many extraordinary medicines came into vogue at this time, such as one called the *horn of the unicorn.* An animal's horn that

[7]The famous Oberammergau Passion Play is supposed to have started when the bubonic plague was carried to that city by a visitor. Untold havoc was caused, and the townsfolk promised to produce the play every ten years if the plague ended. See Crawford, R.: *The Plague and Pestilence in Literature and Art.* London, Oxford University Press, 1914.

[8]The red and white barber poles are symbolic reminders of this early practice.

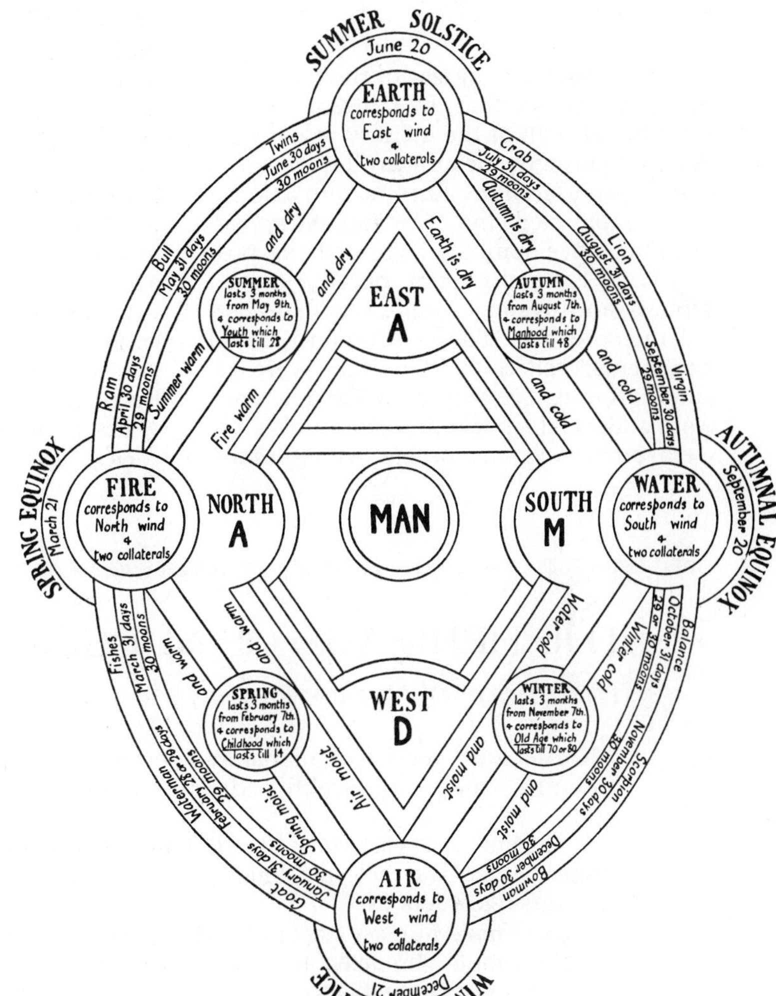

Figure 5–23. A translation of the Macrocosm as conceived in 1011 A.D. by Byrhtferth of Ramsey. (From Grattan and Singer: *Anglo-Saxon Magic and Medicine.*)

was supposed to have the properties of an antidote was hollowed out and used as a cup. The portion of the horn that was removed was powdered and taken as medicine. This was one of the miracle drugs of the Middle Ages and was considered a panacea.

The chief diagnostic aid was *water casting*, or *uroscopy*, which consisted of the examination of urine. Pictures of this technique abound in medical books of this period. Indeed, the urine flask became the symbol of medicine.

MEDICINE

A renaissance did not occur in the field of medicine as it did in literature and art because physicians still had implicit faith in the ancient *humoral theory*.

Many scholars of this period were also firm believers in alchemy and astrology, the latter being based on the belief that the celestial bodies influenced the lives of men. The humors were supposed to be controlled by the planets, and one decided when to take medicine or when to be bled according to the astrological signs (Fig. 5–23).

The guild system penetrated into the field of medicine. Many surgeons had delegated certain aspects of their work to barbers and midwives, a fact officially recognized by King Charles V of France in the fourteenth century when he granted barbers the right to do bleeding and minor surgery.

SUMMARY

In viewing the progress of the later Middle Ages, we see that the Crusades stimulated the growth of the military nursing orders, unwittingly encouraged the spread of disease and brought Europe into contact with Arabic medicine. The sudden spread of urban developments increased the possibility for cultural growth, but also caused sanitary and hygienic conditions that abetted the spread of disease. Certain medical treatments, beliefs and practices were retained from earlier periods while new ones were added. Hospitals of historical interest were built; religious orders were formed and contributed many well-known leaders and groups specializing in the care of the sick. Travel and commerce flourished and acted as cultural media for the development of new tastes and interests. Educational institutions were organized and learning flourished. Although there were great accomplishments in such fields as art, architecture and literature, no striking achievements were noted in medicine.

It has been documented that nurses responded to the needs of society in times of persecution, warfare and pestilential crises. Recruits to nursing continued to be individuals of high intellectual and social backgrounds.

THE HERITAGE OF NURSING

The Image of Nurses During the Late Middle Ages

Nurses with good educational and social backgrounds and strong motivation responded in a health leadership role to social and political crises.

1. In times of warfare, crisis intervention was demonstrated in the response of specially selected knights who formed the first organized military nursing orders of:
    a. male nurses, later joined by female nurses.
    b. men who acted as soldiers or nurses according to necessity.
2. In times of pestilence nurses became extremely adept in caring for persons with communicable diseases such as leprosy and bubonic plague.
3. In times of social distress nurses reflected in their practice:
    a. an understanding of social problems.
    b. an ability to develop ways of alleviating these social problems.
    c. a desire to emulate strong leaders (St. Francis of Assisi) in including promotion of social welfare as an essential ingredient in nursing.
    d. the attraction of nursing for lay people (both men and women) of high educational and social (even royal) backgrounds, who became nurses and provided community health and welfare services.
    e. a continuance of the hospital movement in recognition of the need for emergency relief.

Fortunately, the strengths of the previously identified aspects of nursing continued. Motivation was largely spiritual and humanitarian, and the artistic and humanistic aspects remained strong, and the scientific aspects were as sound as the knowledge of the period permitted.

REFERENCE READINGS

Bedford, W. K. R., and Holbeche, Richard: *The Order of the Hospital of St. John of Jerusalem.* London, F. E. Robinson & Co., 1902.
Bonniwell, William: *Margaret of Metola.* New York, P. J. Kenedy & Sons, 1952.
Chesterton, Gilbert K.: *St. Francis of Assisi.* New York, Doran Co., 1924. (Available as an Image Book, 1957.)
Clay, Rotha Mary: *Medieval Hospitals of England.* London, Methuen & Co., 1909.
Crawford, R.: *The Plague and Pestilence in Literature and Art.* New York, Oxford University Press, 1914.
Curtayne, Alice: *St. Catherine of Siena.* New York, Sheed & Ward, 1935.
Cushing, Richard J.: *St. Catherine of Siena.* Boston, Daughters of St. Paul, 1957.
Fuller, John G.: *The Day of St. Anthony's Fire.* New York, The Macmillan Co., 1968.
Giordani, Igino: *Catherine of Siena.* Milwaukee, Bruce Publishing Co., 1959.
Grattan, J. H. G., and Singer, Charles: *Anglo-Saxon Magic and Medicine.* New York, Oxford University Press, 1952.
Hoff, Hebbel E.: "Nicolaus of Cusa," *Journal of the History of Medicine and Allied Sciences, 19*:101–108, 1964.
Murphy, Dennis G.: *They Did Not Pass By.* London, Catholic Book Club, 1957.
Ogden, Brother Daniel: *Of Valiant Men—A Chronicle of the Congregation of Alexian Brothers.* Wisconsin, The Novitiate Press, 1957.
Robeck, Nesta de: *Saint Elizabeth of Hungary.* Milwaukee, Bruce Publishing Co., 1953.
Schermerhorn, Elizabeth: *On the Trail of the Eight Pointed Cross.* A study of the heritage of the Knights Hospitallers in feudal Europe. New York, G. P. Putnam's Sons, 1940.
Sister Mary Francis, P. C.: *A Right to Be Merry.* New York, Sheed & Ward, 1956.
The Hours of Jeanne D'Evreux, Queen of France. New York, The Cloisters, Metropolitan Museum of Art, 1957.
Thomas Acquinas, St.: *Basic Writings.* New York, Random House.
Walsh, James J.: *The Catholic Church and Healing.* New York, The Macmillan Co., 1927.
Walsh, James J.: *Old Time Makers of Medicine.* New York, Fordham University Press, 1911.
Walsh, James J.: *What Civilization Owes to Italy.* Boston, The Stratford Co., 1923.
Wohl, Louis de: *The Quiet Light.* Philadelphia, J. B. Lippincott Co., 1950.
Wohl, Louis de: *The Last Crusader.* Philadelphia, J. B. Lippincott Co., 1956.
Wohl, Louis de: *The Joyful Beggar.* Philadelphia, J. B. Lippincott Co., 1958.
Wohl, Louis de: *Lay Siege to Heaven.* Philadelphia, J. B. Lippincott Co., 1961.
Ziegler, Phillip: *The Black Death.* New York, John Day Co., 1969.

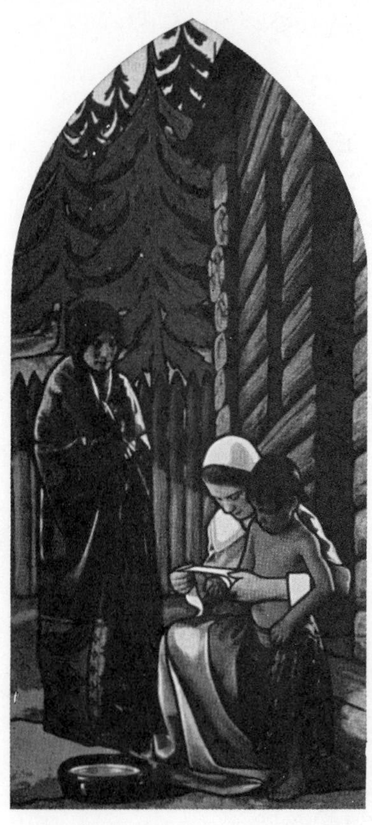

Jeanne Mance ministering to a little Indian girl while the mother watches. (From *They Caught the Torch.* Will Ross, Inc.)

6 Expansion of Nursing Leadership During the Renaissance (1500–1700)

The 200 years between 1500 and 1700 witnessed tremendous economical, political, social and intellectual expansion. The extension of trade encouraged technical innovations involving labor-saving devices, with a concomitant rise in the standard of living. Skilled craftsmen broadened the use of textiles, metal and glass. Improvements in magnification and vision, combined with the spirit of inquiry, led to the construction of microscopes and telescopes. The urge to experiment with these instruments, together with the utilization of mathematical procedures, allowed for the development of a good scientific base for new dimensions in patient care.

Aids for the improvement of vision, in addition to *Gutenberg's* invention of the printing press, opened new avenues of learning. Formerly education was available only to the wealthy. Books had been laboriously handwritten and painstakingly copied; therefore, few had been available. A renaissance occurred in the centers of learning, with an explosion of knowledge and a blossoming of creative thinking within the university setting. Medical education found its way into the university framework. The preparation for nursing was not established under the aegis of an institution of higher learning, but careful selection of candidates and a planned program of nursing education were initiated during this period.

THE NEED FOR IMPROVED HEALTH CARE

The sixteenth century also witnessed another movement—the *Reformation,* which started as a church reform movement and ended as a revolt producing a cleavage in Christianity. As the "reformers" suppressed the Catholic religious orders, hospitals became places of horror, and a period of stagnation ensued. Much has been written about the squalor of the hospitals and the inadequacy of their attendants at this time. During the bubonic plague in London in 1665, the attendants were described as "dirty, ugly, unwholesome hags."

When *Henry VIII* of England closed the monasteries in 1535, it was the aged, the sick, the orphans and the dispossessed who suffered most. The English government wiped out the monastic relief organization without planning for or providing a replacement.

Many died of starvation; the homeless and destitute resorted to begging. A statute against vagrancy was issued by *Edward VI,* who succeeded Henry VIII in 1547. A person discovered begging had the letter B branded on his chest with a red hot iron. If a person reported a vagrant to the authorities, the vagrant became the slave of the informer. The owner was granted the right to beat or chain his slave or force him to labor in whatever manner he desired. Orphaned children could be retained as apprentices by whatever person found them. These children could be chained if the master so desired.

In 1552, a committee was appointed to study the problem of poverty in London. Records reveal that some people were so poor that they ate mice.

In 1557, rules were formulated by which the charitable institutions for the sick poor were to be managed. Under this system, many hospitals became "houses of correction." Any patient able to work was recruited for service, and the work day extended from five o'clock in the morning to eight o'clock in the evening.

Queen Elizabeth I passed the first English Poor Law imposing a compulsory poor tax on every parish. The relief of the poor was no longer an individual problem dependent for solution upon voluntary acts of Christian charity but a national duty exacting a compulsory contribution toward its alleviation.

In 1597, the poor laws were revised because the problem of vagrancy continued. In an attempt to rectify this situation, for a first offense, vagrants were whipped until their bodies were bloody. For a second offense, they were sent to the galleys to be chained in boats as oarsmen. The philosophy of seeing Christ in the least of these brethren had been forgotten. Even the sick poor in hospitals were referred to as objects of charity.

Armed conflict, such as the *Thirty Years' War* (1618–1648), famine and plague still ravaged Europe. Devastating outbreaks of typhus and bubonic plague occurred. As a result of the latter, Germany lost from one-half to three-quarters of her population. It was during this period, in 1665, that the bubonic plague reached England (Figs. 6–1 and 6–2).

When a person contracted the plague, the person's house was boarded up, and the well members of the household were forced to become prisoners with the sick one. Fires were ordered to be kept burning continuously in the streets, one before every sixth house, for three days, to purify the air.

A plague physician wore a long red or black leather gown, leather gauntlets and a mask with glass-covered openings for the eyes and a long beak filled with fumigants and antiseptics, and he carried a pomander container filled with sweet-smelling spices (Fig. 6–3). Many satirical comments and caricatures described the appearance of the physician and the costume he wore to protect himself. Indeed, Hecker commented, "Human science and art appear particularly weak, in great pestilences, because they have to contend with powers of nature, of which they have no knowledge."[1]

Elaborate precautions were taken in the burial of the dead, which was done at night. Dog catchers prowled the streets, killing stray dogs and removing their bodies for burial. Huge mounds of earth were mute testimony to the plight of the English during this scourge. In one of these mounds 50,000 bodies were said to be interred.

The emotional trauma must have been

[1]Hecker, J. F. C.: *The Epidemics of the Middle Ages.* London, 1846, p. 50.

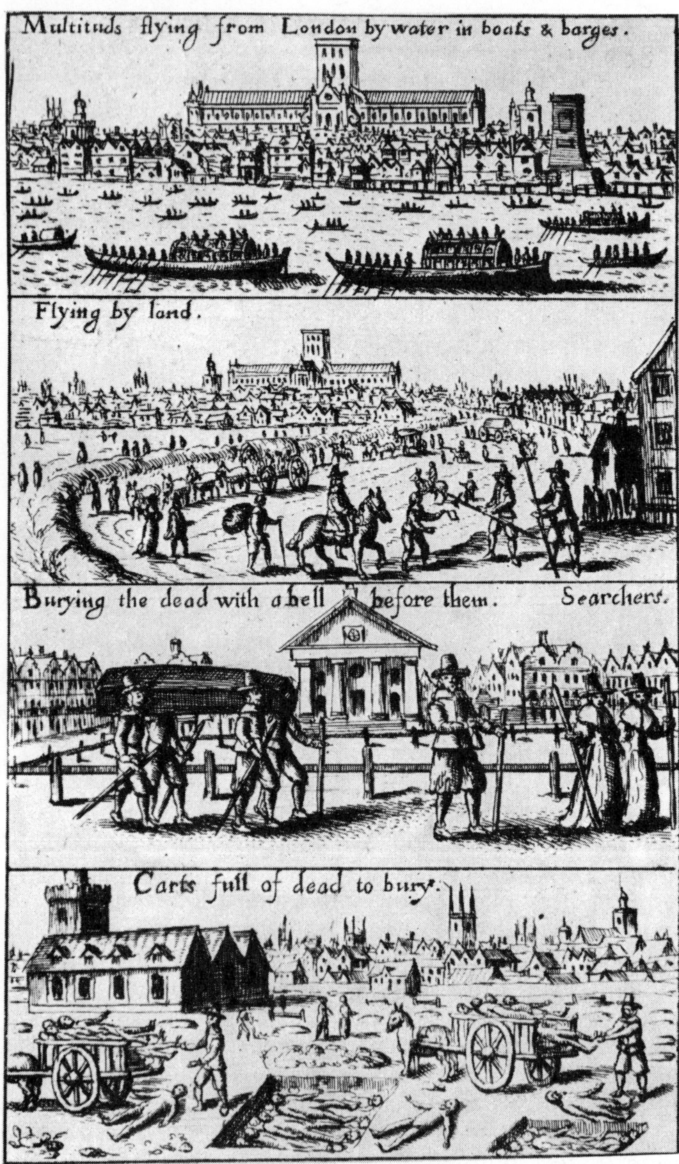

Figure 6–1. Plague scenes in London, 1665. (From Caraman, Philip: *Henry Morse, Priest of the Plague*.)

devastating. Loved ones were abandoned. Hospital service was inadequate; many people died on the street. There was a need for organized charity. The plague subsided in 1666 when a severe fire in London brought destruction to the rats' breeding places.

In France, no longer could workers carry on their trades in their own homes. The artisan now lived on back streets or slept in the attic of his master, often going to bed hungry. His working day was long, sometimes seventeen continuous hours.

In this period of marked intellectual enlightenment and achievement, the knowledge of hygiene was poor. People bathed infrequently, although there were many famous medicinal baths. The value of fresh air was not understood or appreciated; when someone was ill, the doors and windows were closed for fear of colds and draughts. Another unfortunate occurrence was the *window tax*, which was levied in England on all windows above the number eight in houses in towns and cities. This tax fostered the spread of disease because windows in hospitals and homes were blocked up or bricked over to save money. There were those persons, however, whose standard of living was much higher, whose

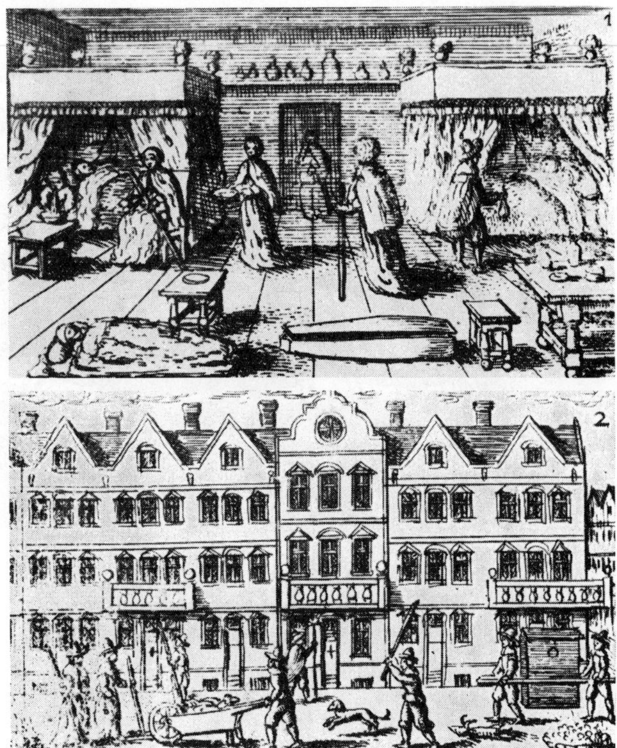

Figure 6–2. Plague scenes. *Top,* a room in a plague-infested house. Several sick patients are in bed, one walks around the room and, in the foreground, a corpse is ready to be placed in the coffin. *Bottom,* a row of London houses boarded up with red crosses on the locked doors. This is an example of enforced quarantine. Two bearers are carrying a sick person to the pest house in a sedan chair. Dog catchers are killing dogs and loading them in wheelbarrows. (From Caraman, Philip: *Henry Morse, Priest of the Plague.*)

homes were comfortable and less unsanitary and whose diet was better balanced.

In the sixteenth century, infants were commonly breast-fed, but wet-nursing was available, and baby farming was a notorious evil. The exceedingly high infant mortality rate was due to very poor public and personal hygiene. Cities had no drainage, filth and infection were rampant and medical knowledge was meager. An example of a medical treatment of this period is shown in Figure 6–4.

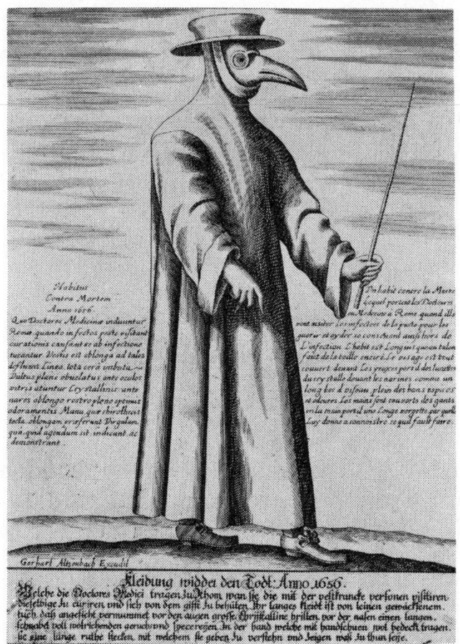

Figure 6–3. The Plague Doctor. A seventeenth-century engraving by Gerhart Altzenback. (Courtesy of Yale Medical Library, Clements C. Fry Collection.)

Of course the people that suffered most during this general misery were the poor, both the peasant in the country and the artisan in the city. There was a need for social reform; a solution was forthcoming that would revolutionize the care of the sick.

COMMUNITY NURSING

St. Francis de Sales (1567–1662) envisioned a group of women forming a voluntary association for friendly visiting of the poor and nursing of the sick. The organization that materialized might be considered one of the early visiting nurse associations. St. Francis de Sales encouraged and motivated influential women to give money and time to an organized service for the sick poor. They were to visit the sick daily, bathe, dress and care for them and take home

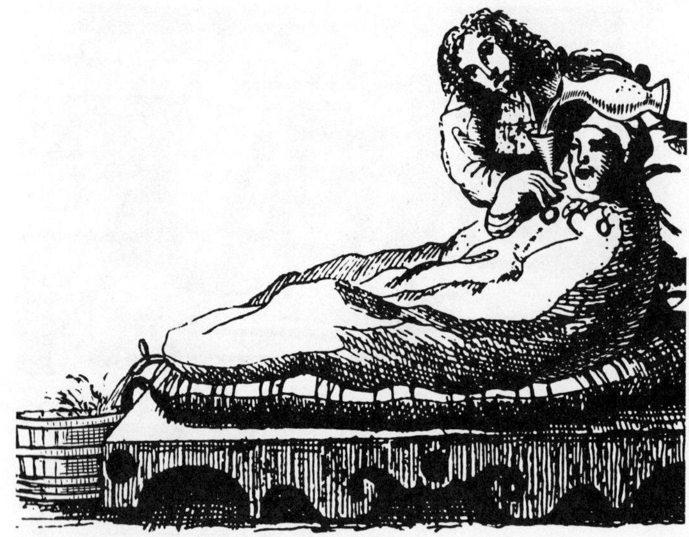

Figure 6–4. A seventeenth-century method of reducing the body temperature of a patient with a fever. The patient is placed in a leather sack and cold water is poured into a funnel. The water runs over the body and is collected in a wooden tub at the foot of the couch. (Dolan collection.)

their linen to be washed (Fig. 6–5). It was his desire that this order of women should be without external vows, so that they would be free to visit the sick in their homes and minister to their needs.

The association was called the *Order of the Visitation of Mary*. The cofounder and director of this order was Madame de Chantal, widow of Baron de Chantal. She was experienced in community nursing.

Madame de Chantal and the members of her group visited the sick in their homes, cleaned and dressed their wounds, made their beds, gave them clothes and took home their linen for boiling to remove impurities and for mending and returned it to the patient. They assisted the dying and washed and prepared the bodies of the dead for burial.

EDUCATION FOR NURSING

It was *St. Vincent de Paul* (1576–1669) who introduced the modern principles of visiting nursing and social service. His concept of charity was a new one for that period: He believed that not only the rich and influential but also the poor and humble could contribute to the relief of the distressed by giving sympathy and personal service. He taught that indiscriminate giving was harmful and that one must investigate the condition of the poor: find out their needs, ascertain the causes of their poverty and, whenever possible, remedy the situation, for example, by finding work for the unemployed. He emphasized the concept of "helping people to help themselves." This was an advanced step and ex-

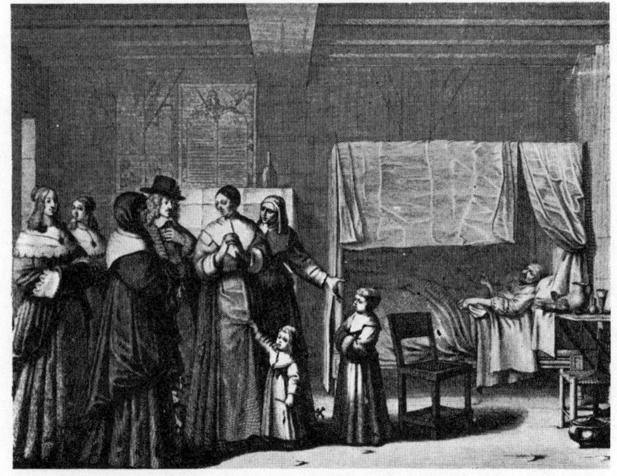

Figure 6–5. Visiting the sick in the seventeenth century (From Brainard, Annie M.: *The Evolution of Public Health Nursing*. W. B. Saunders Co.)

tremely modern thinking. He recognized the right of the poor to their family life, and the benefit to be derived from the recognition of the family unit. He urged that the family be kept together, even if rent had to be paid by an outside group for a time; this, too, was certainly a modern idea.

St. Vincent longed to help and comfort his brothers, but he recognized his ineffectiveness as a single field worker. He believed that, with the participation of others, he could establish an organization that would gain followers and grow until it had members throughout the world.

St. Vincent de Paul founded and directed various charity organizations. He motivated others with his enthusiasm. In 1617, he formed the Society of Missioners, priests trained for special work among the poor; they renewed their vows annually.

It was also in 1617 that he conceived of the idea of the *Dames de Charité.* When he heard of a family's needing assistance, he asked his congregation to supply aid. He got such response that he realized that improperly guided charity could do more harm than good. He suggested to a few women that they form an organization based on the same general plan used by St. Francis de Sales; these women were called Dames de Charité, and their work was mainly community nursing. They went from cottage to cottage visiting patients and making them as comfortable as possible, giving food, preparing medicine and consoling the dying and distressed. This new organization spread throughout France.

St. Vincent felt the need for a person who could teach, direct and coordinate the work of the Dames de Charité. Madame Le Gras became the first supervisor of these community nurses. Louise Le Gras (later known as *St. Louise de Marillac),* a woman of noble birth, was a widow when St. Vincent presented his plan to her, which she accepted.

She would receive directions and counsel from St. Vincent. Then, when she arrived in a village, she would give the Dames de Charité instructions. She accompanied them on their rounds, advising them, assisting them in their duties and making suggestions about other ways of giving care to their patients. The Dames de Charité continued for ten years. Unfortunately, the enthusiasm of these women gradually lessened, for their husbands objected to their absence from home for such lengthy periods.

In 1633, a secular nursing order of superior character was founded. They were called Les Filles de Charité, or the *Sisters of Charity.* Young, single girls who were interested in this program were recruited. They were required to be intelligent, refined young women who were sincerely interested in the sick poor. A systematic educational program, which consisted of gaining experience in the hospital, visiting in the homes and caring for the sick, was established. The program was a combination of social service to the poor and nursing of the sick. The sisters were given a carefully planned program of education before practicing as nurses. Overwork was forbidden by St. Vincent.

St. Louise de Marillac was well-prepared to supervise this program. She had an excellent educational background, which was rare for a woman in this time.

Applications came from great distances, and St. Louise selected her class with care, as noted by the following letter written toward the end of 1639:

> I have no wish to receive any persons except such as are suitable to our life, as regards both health of body and sanity of mind. You know how important this is to a community. I must, therefore, beg you to ascertain whether their desire to come here is prompted by a wish to see Paris, or a desire to make a living for themselves.

Good health, a sound mind, a respectable background and a desire to serve God in the field of teaching, nursing or social service and to labor unceasingly at her own perfection was the only dowry required of a girl who wished to become a Daughter of Charity.[2]

The costume of the Sisters of Charity consisted of the gray-blue gown and apron of rough woolen cloth worn by the French peasant of the period and a stiff white collar and a headdress called a cornette (Fig. 6–6).

Into this dark period of nursing came these young, enthusiastic, well-prepared

[2]*Then—and Now with the Daughters of Charity.* Normandy, Mo., Marillac Seminary, 1946, p. 20.

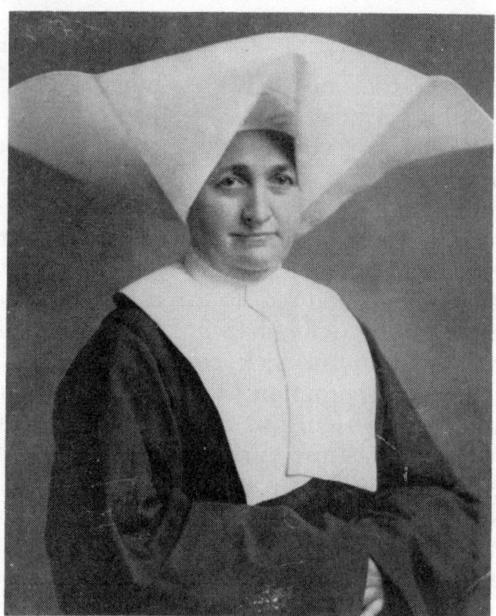

Figure 6–6. Sister Josephine Aloysia Ryan, a Sister of Charity of St. Vincent de Paul. (Dolan collection.)

nurses called Sisters of Charity. Their zeal became infectious, many recruits joined them, and this flourishing order encircled the globe. They have performed every work of charity: nursing in hospitals and homes, teaching in schools, taking charge of orphanages, giving heroic service during such wars as the Napoleonic Wars, the Crimean War and the Civil War in the United States, and since its inception, giving courageous care to the patients in the National Leprosarium in Carville, Louisiana.

St. Vincent de Paul encouraged the Sisters of Charity to expand their role and develop special skills in caring for abandoned children. In 1640 he established the Hospital for Foundlings. He had been dismayed that the so-called receiving institution for abandoned children, La Couche, gave the children to anyone who asked for them. Not infrequently, professional beggars claimed the children and mutilated their bodies in order to arouse pity and collect more money.

Thus arose the second religious order to be founded by St. Vincent de Paul. St. Vincent taught the Sisters of Charity to find the presence of God in the service of the afflicted. The ideas of human brotherhood, of love of one's neighbor and of responsibility for the bodily and material needs of one's fellow creature, originating in Christian love, was being revived.

St. John of God was born in Portugal in 1495. For some reason, he disappeared from his home when he was eight years of age and grew up in Spain, spending the greater part of his first 22 years as a shepherd. The next 18 years were filled with the duties of a soldier, which hardened him in both body and soul. The life of the soldier of this period involved revelry, drunkenness, cruelty to the poor and suffering, looting expeditions and the gathering of booty.

At the age of 40, he left the army and entered the employ of a gentleman farmer who assigned him the task of caring for his horses. The best of care was lavished upon these animals, in sharp contrast to the desperate plight of starving human beings who had to beg for a meager subsistence. Returning to Spain, John again became a shepherd and reflected on the wasted life he had lived. He made a pilgrimage of repentance to Granada.

On the journey to Granada, he encoun-

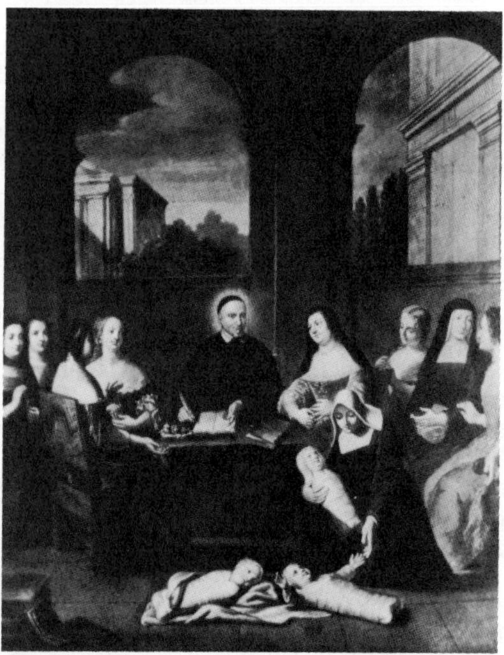

Figure 6–7. St. Vincent de Paul, with St. Louise de Marillac, entreating the Ladies of Charity to continue their efforts on behalf of foundlings. A Sister of Charity is caring for three abandoned infants. Note that the infants are swathed. (Dolan collection.)

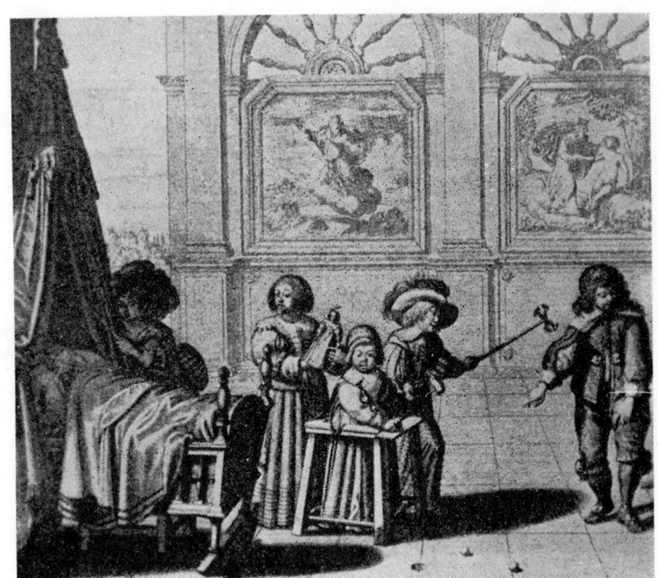

Figure 6–8. Seventeenth-century nursery, from an engraving by A. Bosse (1602–1676). Children learned to walk by means of a walking frame (Dolan collection.)

tered a child weary from walking. St. John carried this little one on his shoulder until the end of the journey. When John placed him on the ground, the child said, "John of God, Granada shall be your cross."

He heard a sermon at Granada that stressed the glory of being made a fool for the sake of Christ. John's most unusual reaction to this sermon resulted in his being hustled off to what was then referred to as a lunatic asylum. The care of the mentally ill of that period was gruesome. The typical treatment was the whip. St. John was stretched out on the floor and was flogged with a double knotted cord, after which he was locked in solitary confinement.

When he was released, St. John returned to Granada, gathered all the homeless vagrants and crippled persons into a house that he rented and gave them special care. It was then the custom to display one's infirmity in order to beg for charity. When he found those who were too deformed to crawl to his abode, he carried them on his back (Fig. 6–9). St. John of God begged for alms in order to feed and purchase medicines for these derelicts. Thus was laid the foundation for the famous *Hospital of St. John of God* at Granada. In this hospital, each patient had a private bed, which was unique in this era when beds contained three or more patients. Patients with contagious diseases were isolated, and an outpatient department was instituted.

St. John had a special interest in abandoned children, admitting them to the hospital until foster or adoptive parents could be found. All patients received superior care, but the ones who were mentally ill were lavished with tender love and understanding. There was an acute need for kinder and more enlightened care of the mentally ill and mentally retarded.

The *Brothers Hospitallers of St. John of God*, the order he founded, grew and thrived and adopted the Rule of St. Augustine. It opened hospitals at Madrid, Cordova, Toledo, Naples and Paris (Figs. 6–10 and 6–11). Less than 50 years after the death of its founder, the order had spread to every Christian kingdom in Europe and other continents. Wherever explorer ships happened to go, the Brothers of St. John of God followed to open hospitals for the natives.

An ambulance unit staffed by the brothers accompanied the forces of King Philip II of Spain and Don Juan in their campaign against the Turks.

In many provinces of the Order of Hospitallers of St. John, the brothers are physicians, surgeons, dentists and pharmacists; however, the greater number are registered nurses. They have been the personal infirmarians to the popes as well as directors of the Vatican Pharmacy. Nursing homes for the aged and for patients with long-term illnesses have been under the

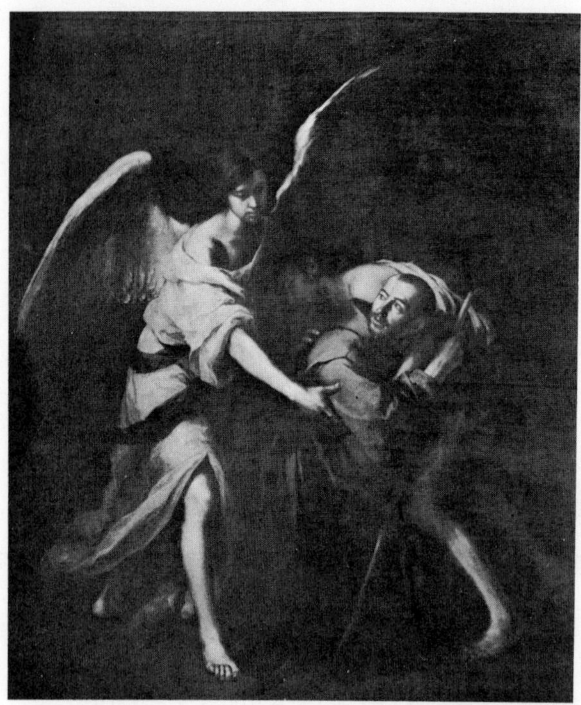

Figure 6–9. St. John of God by Murillo (1618–1682). Hospital de la Santa Caridad, Seville. (Dolan collection.)

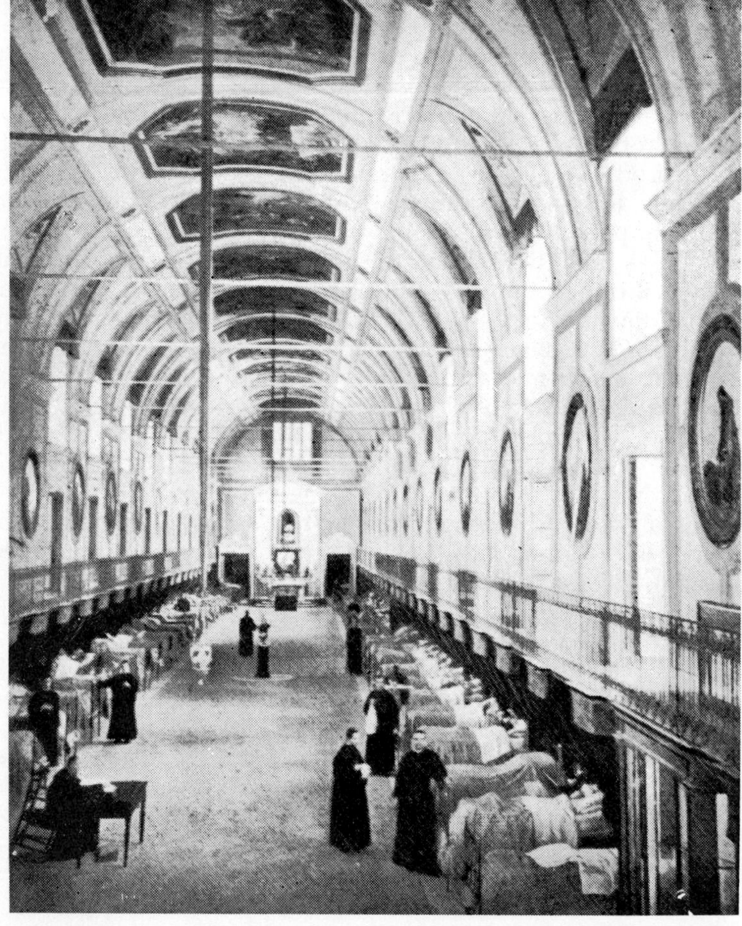

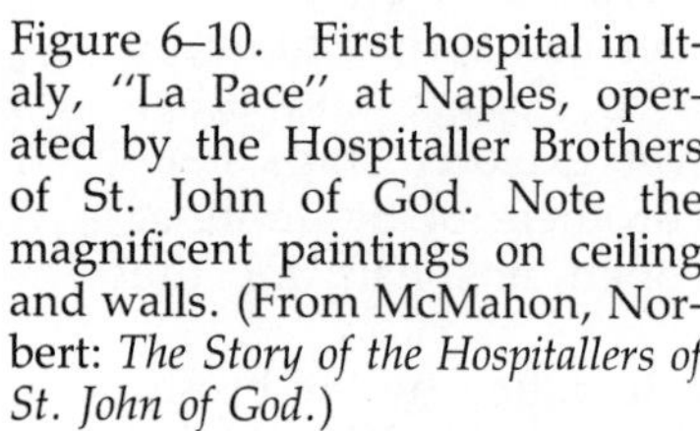

Figure 6–10. First hospital in Italy, "La Pace" at Naples, operated by the Hospitaller Brothers of St. John of God. Note the magnificent paintings on ceiling and walls. (From McMahon, Norbert: *The Story of the Hospitallers of St. John of God.*)

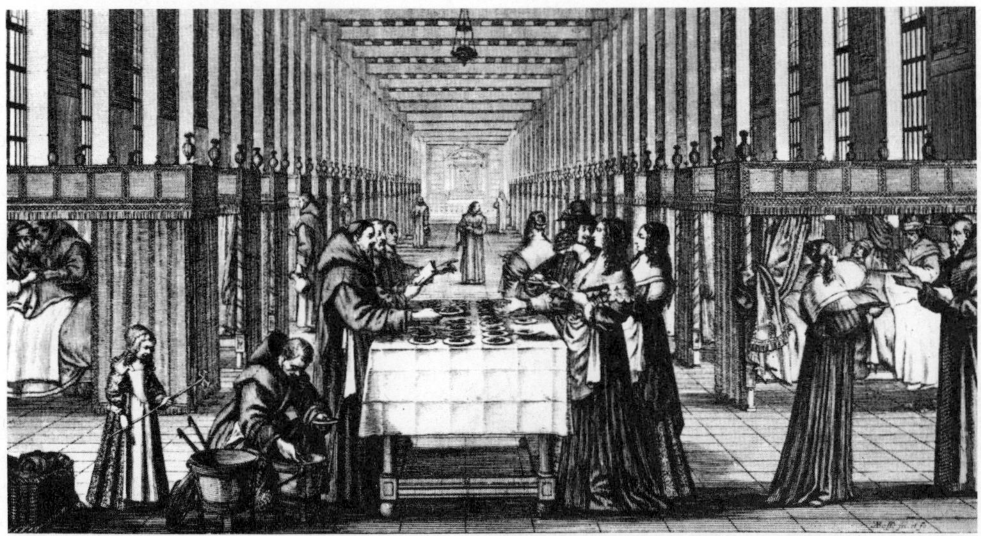

Figure 6–11. The Queen of France and ladies of the court serving the sick at the Brothers' Hospital in Paris. (Courtesy of Metropolitan Museum of Art, Harris Brisbane Dick Fund, 1926.)

aegis of this order. It has maintained residences for homeless men, utilizing opportunities to assist in their rehabilitation and eventual return to society. Even leper colonies were staffed by these brothers. This order of well-educated brothers has a long record of devoted nursing service to the needy.

A most enlightening picture of a hospital and the care of patients in Portuguese Goa (an enclave on the western coast of India) in the seventeenth century is presented in Blunt's portrayal of the translations of the "Viaggi," the travels of Pietro Della Valle.

> Perhaps the most remarkable institution in Goa was the Royal Hospital for men, founded by Albuquerque and subsequently in the charge of the Jesuits, which in many respects seems to have been at least three hundred years ahead of its time. Pyrard, an impartial and accurate observer, spent several weeks as a patient there in 1608. The building, which was surrounded by spacious gardens where convalescents could wander at will, seemed to him more like a palace than a hospital. Everything in the wards was spotlessly clean. The elegant beds were of red lacquer, chequered or gilded, with fine white cotton sheets and silk coverlets that were changed twice a week. Each new patient on his arrival had his head shaved by a barber, and after being thoroughly scrubbed was issued with pajamas, cap and slippers. He was further provided with a fan, a bottle of drinking-water, a little table and a chamber-pot. Lanterns glazed with oyster-shell glowed gently throughout the night. The food was excellent, patients on full diet receiving for supper a whole fowl each, served on a plate of Chinese porcelain, and being encouraged to ask for a second helping. But wine was only allowed when specially prescribed.
>
> The higher officials of the hospital were all Portuguese, the servants native Christians. The doctors, who visited their fifteen hundred patients morning and evening, were accompanied on their rounds by servants bearing baskets of lint and other medicaments or diffusing incense, and by an apothecary and kitchen clerk, notebooks in hand, who jotted down prescriptions and special diet. Male visitors were allowed from 8 to 11 and from 3 to 6 o'clock and might eat with their friends who could apply for extra rations; they were searched at the gate for arms, and to see that they were not bringing unsuitable food or drink to the sick.[3]

St. Camillus De Lellis (1550–1614), born in Naples of a noble family, led a very colorful life. He became, like his father, a soldier adventurer. While he was a soldier, he injured his leg. He went to Rome to the San Giacomo hospital, where he asked for work in return for treatment of his leg. For four years he remained there, finally receiving an appointment as superintendent of the servants, which, in that period, included nurses—all male. He labored tirelessly and began to love those he served.

---

[3]Blunt, Wilfred: *Pietro's Pilgrimage. A Journey to India and Back at the Beginning of the Seventeenth Century.* London, James Barrie, 1953, pp. 255–257.

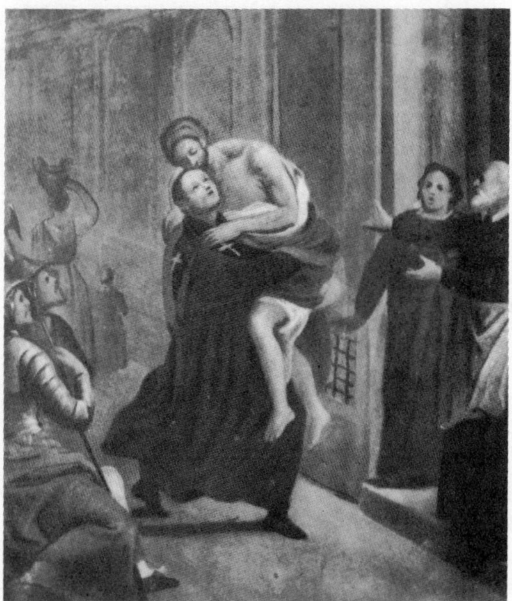

Figure 6–12. In this painting St. Camillus expresses his love and concern for suffering humanity. He carries a beggar into the Hospital of the Holy Ghost and ministers to him. (Dolan collection.)

He realized that good nursing was dependent on love and also that the duties of a priest were carried out best where love was present. He determined to encourage others, both nurses and priests, to join him in this task. In order to prepare himself, St. Camillus studied for the priesthood and was ordained.

He selected a house in the slum area where pestilence was most abundant and gave his service to the sick poor (Fig. 6–12). At first his efforts were directed toward preparing and providing hospital nurses, but he learned that the sick poor outside the hospital and in the slum areas were desperately in need of care. He achieved remarkable success in tending the dying, and from this service, his order, the *Nursing Order of Ministers of the Sick,* evolved. The members of this order wear a red cross on their cassock.

A hospital for alcoholics was opened in Germany by St. Camillus. His love for patients drew him to the prisons, where he gave special care to those condemned to die.

The order, popularly called the Camillian Fathers and Brothers, gave service as army nurses during several wars, including World War I. Some worked in the hospital trains organized by the Knights of Malta.

St. Charles of Borromeo (1538–1584) was a wealthy, well-educated young man who became Archbishop of Milan. When his family died, Charles distributed his wealth to the poor. He spent his free time bringing food and clothing to the poor and visiting the sick. During the plague that devastated Milan in 1575, he nursed the sick and ministered to the dying.

Jeanne Biscot (1601–1664), the daughter of a respected citizen of Arras in northern France, performed outstandingly good nursing work in wars, famines, emergencies and pestilences. In 1640, when her home town was attacked, many sick and wounded needed care. Jeanne set an example, which others followed, of dressing wounds, of feeding and reviving the sick and needy and of assisting the dying. Jeanne and the energetic young women who followed her requested the right to use a building for a hospital and obtained it. They cared for patients as long as care was needed.

Jeanne was talented in detecting and developing the special abilities of her patients. Her hospitals became workshops where community residents of all ages learned to enrich personal skills. She is credited with having initiated a program of occupational therapy.

MEDICAL CARE FOR THE POOR

Medical as well as nursing care was becoming available for the poor. Physicians not only gave their services freely but their lives as well in times of epidemics; they were not equipped to protect themselves and others from infections.

Medical charities were directed by Theophrastus Renardot, who had established an association for this purpose in 1612. By 1640, the king recognized the value of his work and gave him free rein to assist the poor.

Soon, several physicians joined him and set aside two days a week to visit the sick poor and prescribe remedies. Now there were physicians diagnosing cases, nurses giving care and charity associations available to investigate social conditions and give material relief.

LIFE IN THE NEW WORLD

South and Central America

The new routes of trade and travel of the period beckoned the Spanish and Portuguese colonists, who settled in Mexico and Peru. They brought with them many members of religious orders, who were to become the teachers, nurses and physicians in the colonies. The members of these orders taught the Spanish language and the Christian faith to the Aztec and Inca Indians.

European ideas were carried to the New World, and to the Old World came a wealth of information from the Americas. On Columbus' second expedition, Dr. Chanca, the royal physician to King Ferdinand and Queen Isabella, was appointed physician to the 1500 members of the group. He was a well-educated gentleman who had been professor of medicine at the University of Salamanca. During his sojourn in the Americas, he studied the native medicines and was able to introduce remedies, such as balsam of Peru, balsam of Tolu, cascara sagrada and quinine, to Europe.

In 1521, Tenochtitlán, the capital of the Aztec civilization, was conquered by Cortés. By 1524, the Hospital of the Immaculate Conception, the *first hospital* on the American continent, was built in the capital, renamed Mexico City, by Cortés. In 1528, Bishop Zumárraga founded the continent's first library with 200 volumes, and by 1534 the first printing press was built. In 1531, another hospital, the Hospital of Santa Fe (Holy Faith), was built in what is now New Mexico. Mission colleges were founded in 1531 at Queretaro and in 1546 at Zacatecas; in 1536, the College of Santa Cruz was established. The Universities of Mexico and Lima, founded in 1551, possessed departments of theology, scripture, canon law, civil law, arts, rhetoric, grammar and medicine. The *first medical school* on the American continent was established at the *University of Mexico* in 1578; the second medical school was affiliated with the University of Lima, in Peru, before 1600.

North America

From the time Jacques Cartier sailed up the Saint Lawrence River in 1535, tales of the fascination of *New France* lured the adventurous. In 1605, the first settlement, the Habitation, was colonized at Port Royal in Nova Scotia. The famous explorer Samuel de Champlain and the surgeon-apothecary Louis Hebert were two members of this pioneer group. The first nurse in the French colonies was *Marie Hebert Hubou,* widow of Louis Hebert. Marie took care of the sick patients who were recommended to her by Jesuit Fathers.

The reports of life and the need for aid in New France, published in the Jesuit bulletin, prompted religious nursing sisters to answer the call for help. On August 1, 1639, three sisters of the Order of St. Augustine (Augustinian Sisters) arrived in Quebec and staffed the Hôtel Dieu in Quebec, built by the Duchess of Aiguillon, a niece of Cardinal Richelieu (Fig. 6–13). These Augustinian sisters belonged to a cloistered order, and they had been prepared to care for the sick. Their habit consisted of a white woolen dress with a black leather belt and black veil. These sisters gave heroic service during the bleak, cold winters, during the Indian wars and during the epidemics of smallpox and typhus.

Ursuline sisters who were teaching at the mission school were given emergency classes in the care of the sick during the epidemics. Thus instruction in the care of the sick had commenced in the New World.

Jeanne Mance (1606–1673) was born the daughter of well-to-do French parents and was educated at an Ursuline convent. While at the convent school, the stories of heroism from the New World reached France and inspired Jeanne to join the courageous band leaving for the New World when her age permitted. In 1638, during a severe epidemic, an organization of Ladies of Charity (probably those of St. Vincent de Paul) was formed to care for the sick. Jeanne joined the group and in this way received instruction in nursing care.

On May 17, 1641, Jeanne Mance arrived in Montreal, sponsored financially by the wealthy and philanthropic Madame de Bullion, who asked her to erect a hospital. Jeanne Mance cared for the Iroquois Indians as well as the colonists, and the Hôtel Dieu in Montreal, founded in 1644, stands as a testimonial to her.

In 1657, Jeanne Mance returned to France to recruit personnel. The Hospitallers, or

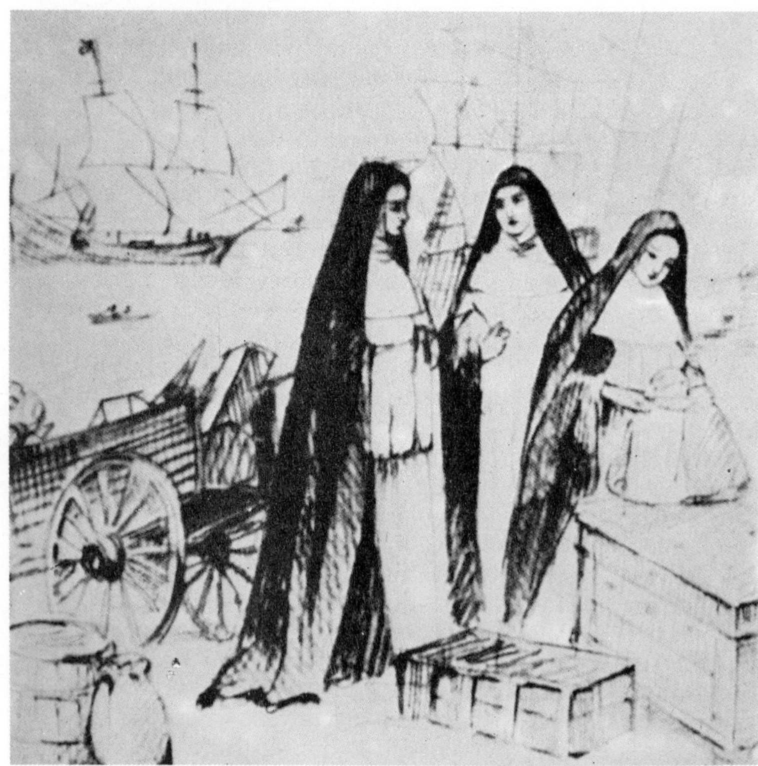

Figure 6–13. Arrival of the first three Augustinian Sisters at Quebec, 1639. (Courtesy of the Hôtel Dieu, Quebec.)

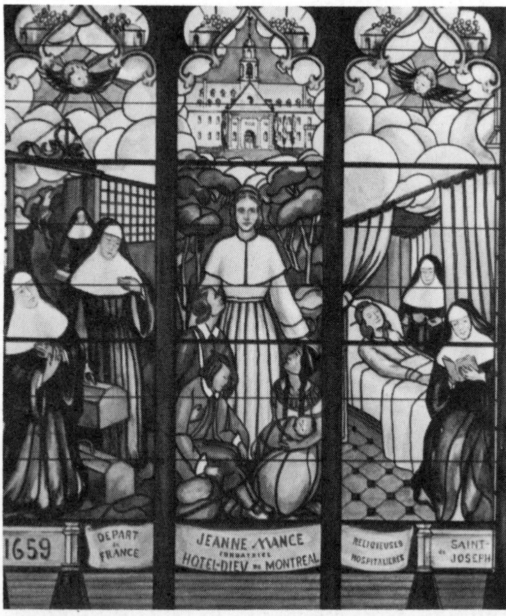

Figure 6–14. In the central panel of a stained glass window in Notre Dame Cathedral in Montreal, Jeanne Mance is surrounded by her patients. On the left the first three sisters, Hospitallers of St. Joseph, are leaving France in 1659; on the right, they are caring for their patients in Montreal. (Dolan collection.)

Nursing Sisters of St. Joseph de La Flèche, came over to staff the Hôtel Dieu in Montreal, with Jeanne Mance as administrator (Fig. 6–14). From France they sailed on the Saint André, a hospital ship that had terminated its role as such without benefit of fumigation or quarantine. An outbreak of sickness spread throughout the ship. Jeanne Mance and three of the sisters were infected with the disease but survived.

Health Problems in the Colonies. The care of the sick in colonial America is a fascinating chapter in the history of the colonists. The settlers were poor, life was difficult in the new land and the lack of medically prepared persons was a serious problem. Outbreaks of smallpox, scurvy and yellow fever killed many of the colonists.

Sir Walter Raleigh sent an expedition to the Roanoke Islands off the coast of North Carolina. The colony obtained no supplies during the period of warfare with the Spanish Armada (1588). In 1591, relief ships were sent out only to find that the settlers had disappeared.

The settlers in the Jamestown colony

faced a rugged existence. During the first three years at Jamestown, all but 60 of the 500 colonists died from malnutrition or from one of the dietary deficiency diseases such as beriberi and scurvy.

In 1620, a type of hospital was constructed that could accommodate 50 persons if at least two patients shared one bed.

The men who practiced medicine in Virginia had great faith in the humoral theory. Medical treatments included withdrawing excessive amounts of humors from the body by using emetics, purges and bloodletting.

Early colonial records speak of certain persons, both men and women, who were chosen on account of their skill and fitness to care for the sick. In the Massachusetts colony at Plymouth, Samuel Fuller, a deacon of the church, acted as physician, using prayer as part of routine treatment. His wife was the first midwife of the colony; Anne Hutchinson and Ann Eliot, wives of prominent men, also practiced midwifery.[4]

In 1630, the Puritans founded the Massachusetts Bay Company. The influence of the Puritan clergymen was great. In the New England settlements, the clergymen were often the physicians. They were called "preacher doctors."

[4]*Male* midwives were fined!

With the absence of medical schools in North America, the clergy had the best educational preparation to practice medicine, although some laymen performed this task without benefit of education or license. The Rhode Island General Assembly is purported to have granted a degree and a license to practice medicine to a Captain John Cranston for his skill and ability in medical care. It seems an unusual procedure to receive a degree from a group of men not associated in any way with an institution of higher learning and to receive a license to practice a professional skill without benefit of an examination.

The first governor of the Massachusetts Bay Colony, *John Winthrop* (1587–1649), and his son, John (1616–1676), who became governor of Connecticut, were enlisted as physicians (Fig. 6–15). They received preparation for this task largely through correspondence with friends in England, and in like manner, they carried on their care of the sick through letters to patients since they could not visit all of them. These men were two of the many who assumed the duties of apothecary and physician. Usually they had a chest of medicines and a guide book of suggested remedies for different ailments (Fig. 6–16).

A minister, Reverend Thomas Thacher, "though no Physitian, yet a well-wisher of the sick," felt compelled to write a leaflet

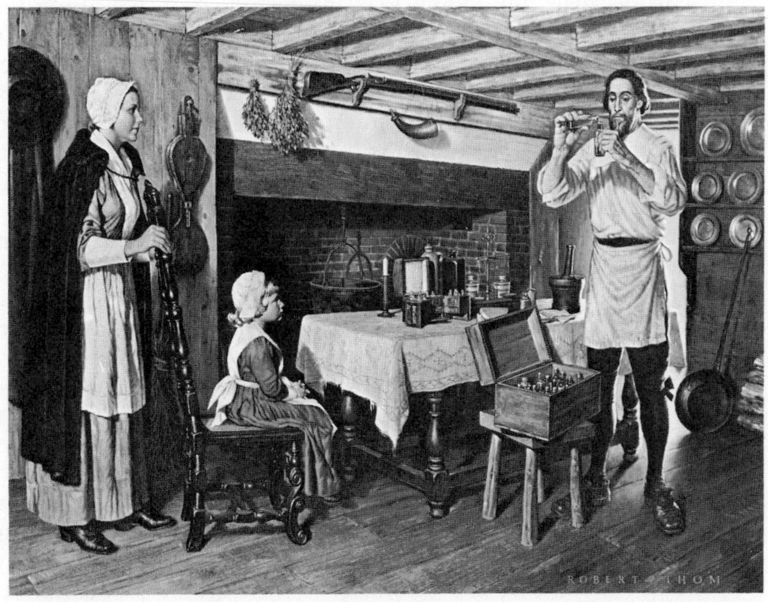

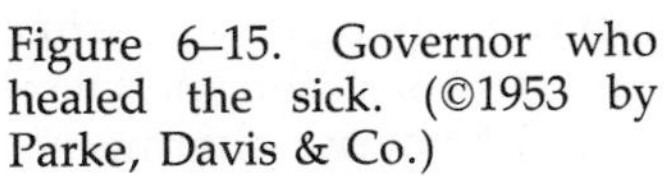
Figure 6–15. Governor who healed the sick. (©1953 by Parke, Davis & Co.)

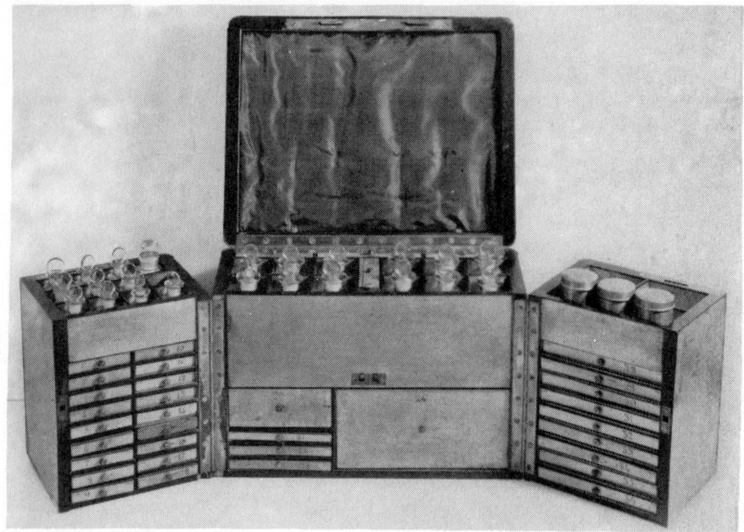

Figure 6–16. A medicine chest of the type used by the colonists and on board ship. Each drawer and section is numbered, and an accompanying leaflet gave directions for a person who was not medically trained as to what to give for each ailment. (Courtesy of Peabody Museum of Salem, Mass.)

for the community to be used during the many troublesome epidemics of smallpox. The title of this discourse, published in Boston in 1677, was: "A Brief Rule to Guide the Common People of New England how to order themselves and theirs in the Small Pocks, or Measles."

Institutions of higher education were needed in the colonies. In 1636, Harvard College was founded, and in 1693, the College of William and Mary in Williamsburg, Virginia, was established. The legislature of the Massachusetts Bay Colony was responsible for the inception of Harvard College because the colony was interested in the promotion of learning and wanted to provide an educated ministry. For the first fifty years the president of the college did all the teaching; students interested in receiving a medical education went to England or France to study.

In 1623, colonists from *Holland* settled in what they called New Netherlands (New York). The *first hospital* in this area was built by the Dutch on Manhattan Island in 1658, with the financial assistance of the West India Company. This was the beginning of New York's Bellevue Hospital, which cared for the sick, the poor and the mentally ill.

Toward the close of the seventeenth century, the *witchcraft* persecutions in Salem, Massachusetts (from January 1692 until May 1693) provided an additional emotional trauma for the colonists. Witchcraft was considered a cause of disease or injury. In the colonies and elsewhere it was believed that sickness was punishment for sin.

DEVELOPMENTS IN BIOLOGICAL SCIENCE AND MEDICINE

A renaissance took place in the field of *pharmacy* in the year 1240, in England, when pharmacy was legally separated from medicine. By 1498 the first official pharmacopoeia was published and became the legal guide for all pharmacists. In 1617, King James I of England granted a charter to the newly formed society of pharmacists known as the "Society of the Art and Mystery of the Apothecaries of the City of London." This extricated pharmacists from the control of the Guild of Grocers; drugs, spices and herbs, used by apothecaries, were brought from many lands and sold by grocers. This association had placed pharmacists under the influence of the merchant group; after 1617, however, pharmacists emerged as a distinct group of craftsmen.

In the field of *general medicine,* two men, Paracelsus and Sydenham, were preeminent. Phillippus Theophrastus Bombastus von Hohenheim, better known as *Paracelsus,* was one of the most unusual men in medical history. He is credited with igniting the fire of new thinking in the field of medicine. A successful alchemist who was well versed in astrology, Paracelsus formulated many unscientific medical theories as well as many that showed marked ability in guessing, intuition or clear reasoning. He opposed the humoral theory of disease, advocated the use in medicines of many chemicals, and overthrew the old medical authorities by publicly burning their books and denouncing their authority.[5] Paracelsus said, "Medicine is not only a science, it is also an art. . . . It deals with the very processes of life which must be understood before they may be guided."

Thomas Sydenham (1624–1689) contributed to the field of general medicine. Sydenham was a true follower of Hippocrates, stressing the need for careful observation of the patient and his symptoms and treating each person's illness on an individual basis. He did not follow the current medical practices completely but used independent thinking. Sydenham advocated fresh air in sickrooms, for windows not only were kept closed at this time but were concealed by heavy draperies; he recommended the simplification of prescriptions (which sometimes filled two and three pages with lists of ingredients) and discarded the useless ones; and he gave a detailed description of prevalent diseases. Sydenham was an eminently able practitioner who used the best of the past in his treatments.

Another area of expansion was in the development of the *fine arts*. Christian idealism motivated the arts of sculpture and stained glass, in addition to music. This was one of the greatest periods in the history of art. It was a productive period in medical art because of the interest of artists in human dissection. A very distinguished group of artists laid this foundation and presented accurate knowledge in the fields of anatomy and physiology. These artists surpassed their predecessors, the classical sculptors, not only by presenting correct external proportions and appearances but also by dissecting bodies to broaden their knowledge. Three of the greatest and most innovative artists of the Renaissance were *Dürer*, *Raphael* and *Michelangelo*.

One of the most versatile figures in this period was the Florentine *Leonardo da Vinci* (1452–1519). Leonardo was also a sculptor, inventor, mathematician, architect and engineer. It is small wonder that Leonardo's keen powers of observation were turned to

[5]Medical science and medical teaching continued at this time to be based on the teachings of Hippocrates, Galen and Avicenna.

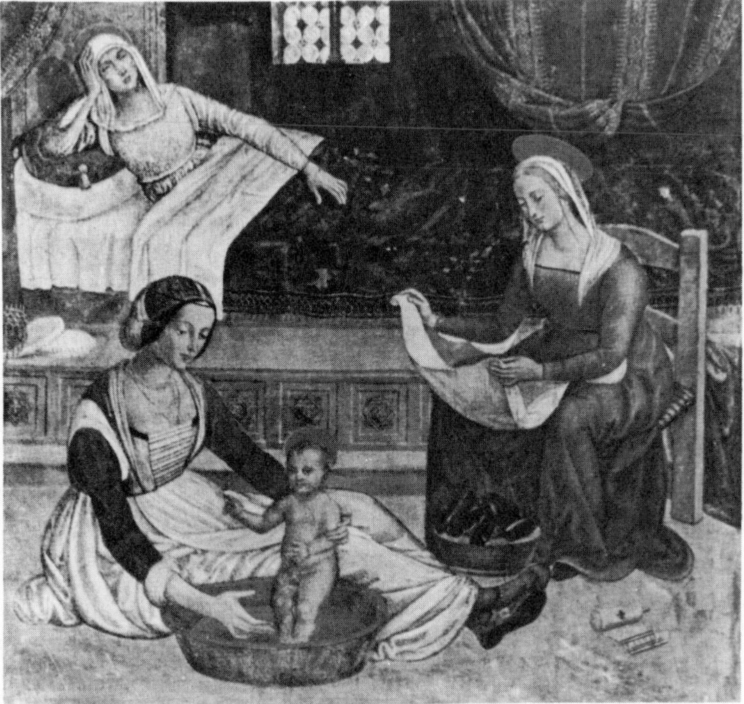

Figure 6–17. The Birth of St. John the Baptist, by Pinturicchio (*ca.* 1454–1513). The continuance of the strong role image of the nurse in health maintenance is portrayed. (Dolan collection.)

the structure and function of the human body. He dissected the body, and the findings that he recorded in his notebooks were masterpieces of accurate observation that expanded the knowledge of the human body in a remarkable fashion. Leonardo's art was natural and lifelike. He not only portrayed man in a realistic fashion, but also revealed the person's reaction of fear, pain and frustration as well as happiness and joy.

Andreas Vesalius (1513–1564), the son of the court apothecary to Emperor Charles V, was born in Brussels. From boyhood, Vesalius was inordinately fond of dissecting, and his first attempts were upon animals. In later life, this interest seemed to increase, and cemeteries and places of execution yielded him the needed bodies. Although the civil courts permitted the bodies of condemned criminals to be taken by artists, it was not so easy for would-be medical scientists to obtain cadavers; therefore, a close association developed between medical men and grave robbers, or "resurrectionists."

The results of Vesalius's painstaking research were presented in *De Humani Corporis Fabrica Libri Septem* in 1543. This book was a masterpiece of care and accuracy and presented in clear readable as well as visual form the representations of the dissected parts of the human body. Vesalius established the position of scientific dissection and corrected previous inaccuracies, especially those of Galen. In his work one notes the confrontation of medieval Galenism with the bases of modern science. A notebook of a student who was present and watched Vesalius's dissections has been discovered and has been an excellent primary source of information.[6]

In the field of *surgery*, the name of *Ambrose Paré* (1510–1590) was a prominent one. Starting his career as a barber's apprentice, Paré became an assistant at the Hôtel Dieu and then a surgeon in the army.

Gunshot wounds were routinely treated with boiling oil at this time. Paré, realizing the injurious effect of this cruel treatment, discontinued its use and searched for a substitute. He invented many new surgical instruments, made amputation less traumatic by reintroducing the use of ligatures to tie off the blood vessels instead of cauterizing them or sealing the vessels with boiling oil, introduced ingenious artificial limbs and belittled the value of powdered mummy and unicorn's horn as medicines. Paré is credited with saying, "I dressed him, God cured him."

The first recorded successful blood transfusion on a human being was performed in June, 1667, by *Jean Baptiste Denis,* physician to Louis XIV, in Paris. The patient was a youth 15 or 16 years old who had some obscure fever. The boy is reported to have made a remarkable recovery following the administration of nine ounces of blood from the carotid artery of a lamb.

The status of barber-surgeons improved in England and France during this time. The climax was reached in 1540 when Henry VIII of England united the Barber Company with the Guild of Surgeons to form the United Barber-Surgeon Company, with Thomas Vicary, the anatomist, as the master. The surgeons, however, were not so fortunate in obtaining status as the pharmacists were in being separated from the Guild of Grocers.

The first *obstetrical forceps* were devised by Peter Chamberlen in 1630 in England. For many years, the Chamberlen family told no one of the forceps' existence, but the secret of their construction was ultimately released and thereby benefited all women who needed them.

William Harvey (1578–1657) was the major contributor to the field of *physiology*. Harvey grew up in Elizabethan England, and in 1628, he announced his discovery of the *circulation of the blood* with the publication of his *Anatomical Disquisition on the Motion of the Heart and Blood of Animals.*

Before Harvey's time, there existed many erroneous notions concerning the blood. His conclusions can be summarized as follows: The blood moves in a continuous onward direction from the right side of the heart, through the purification system in the lungs, to the left side of the heart whence it is pumped in one direction through the arteries of the body and back to the heart through the veins. Harvey did not recognize the interlacing network of

---

[6]Ericksson, Ruben, Ed.: *Baldasor Heseler: Andreas Vesalius' first public anatomy at Bologna: 1540. An Eyewitness' Report.* Uppsala and Stockholm, Lychnos Bibliothek 18, 1959.

capillaries that form the connecting link between the arteries and the veins.

Scientists were describing nature as accurately as possible in the hope that man would adapt himself to it more effectively. Galileo needed instruments to observe natural phenomena; lens grinders devised telescopes. When Sir Isaac Newton described the planets, educated people lost their faith in astrology. Astrology and horoscopes lost their importance in medical care.

The lens grinders also produced *microscopes.* One of the earliest microscopists was Johannes Jansen of Holland, who was reputed to have used one about 1590.

Marcello Malpighi (1628–1694), using the newly discovered microscope, reported his observations of the *capillary circulation* in the lungs and mesentery of the frog. This was the important link needed to understand the circulatory system of the body. Another achievement of Malpighi was his discovery of the *red blood corpuscles* in the blood stream in 1665.

Athanasius Kircher (1602–1680), born in Germany, was educated at Fülda and became a Jesuit priest. His interests were many, as seen in his literary works, over forty in number. His literary works covered a wide range of subjects. One of them described the wonders of nature revealed to him by means of the microscope. He noted the innumerable "worms" in vinegar and milk and the countless "animalcules" in pus and blood that were invisible to the naked eye. Father Kircher was very likely the first scientist to use the microscope in investigating the causes of disease.

Anton van Leeuwenhoek (1632–1723), born in Delft, Holland, is noted for improving the microscope and for identifying certain types of bacteria. Leeuwenhoek did not receive a university education or any preparation in medicine. In his leisure he ground lenses, constructed microscopes, studied the objects of nature and drew diagrams of what he observed; in doing this, Leeuwenhoek established the basis for the development of the field of bacteriology. Although "animalcules" still needed to be identified and classified as bacteria, these "devil spirits" had at last been seen.

Scientists of this era were debating and studying the theory of *spontaneous generation.* An Italian naturalist, *Francesco Redi* (1626–1697), contradicted the idea that living matter such as maggots could spring from nonliving matter. He carried out a controlled experiment by placing meat in jars, some uncovered and others covered with parchment and gauze. In a short time, maggots appeared in the uncovered jars of meat but not in the covered ones. However, Redi's testimony was not accepted by his contemporaries.

SUMMARY

The thread of continuity of leadership in providing nursing care was apparent during the Renaissance. Specially prepared nurses, both women and men, delivered nursing care to people of all ages, in varying degrees of health and illness and in a variety of settings. Nurses expanded their knowledge base while continuing to use intellectual skills and judgment in the execution of the physical as well as the psychosocial aspects of nursing care.

THE HERITAGE OF NURSING

The Image of the Nurse in the Period of the Renaissance

In this period of marked intellectual reawakening, the major step forward in nursing was the recognition of need for sound educational preparation in nursing.

St. Vincent de Paul, the creator of a program for nursing education, was renowned for his scholarship, creative leadership and altruism. The director of the program was chosen because of her educational and social background and nursing and teaching ability.

1. The program was built upon:
   a. a sound philosophy of nursing and education.
   b. stated objectives.
   c. carefully delineated teaching methods.
   d. painstaking selection of a variety of learning experiences to expose students to factors promoting health as well as illness.
2. The students were:
   a. admitted if stated requirements were met (i.e., intelligence, culture)
   b. not permitted to remain if unqualified.
   c. allowed to undertake only a specified amount of study and practical experience.
   d. taught that assessment of needs and intervention should aim toward total care, including social welfare.
   e. encouraged to "care with" and thus "help people to help themselves."

This educational philosophy provided a flexible framework on which to build a well-planned program of nursing education in an autonomous setting. The products of this dynamic education endeavored to recognize the family as the unit of service, encouraged rehabilitation and realized their responsibility to upgrade their knowledge to keep pace with current discoveries.

During the period of discovery and colonization in the New World:

1. settlers found opportunities for cultural interchange, including knowledge of health care, with the ancient Americans.
2. male nurses, members of religious orders from Spain, were the first nurses to arrive.
3. many nurse sisters who were members of religious orders settled in Canada.
4. the lay women of the colonies were again faced with building the practice of nursing as independent practitioners.

REFERENCE READINGS

Bertrande, D. C., Sister: *A Woman Named Louise.* Normandy, Mo., Marillac College Press, 1956.

Caraman, Philip: *Henry Morse—Priest of the Plague.* New York, Farrar, Straus & Cudahy, 1957.

Cather, Willa: *Shadows on the Rock.* New York, Alfred A. Knopf, 1946.

Cooper, P.: *The Bellevue Story.* New York, Thomas Y. Crowell, 1948.

Damel-Rops, Henri: *Monsieur Vincent.* New York, Hawthorn Books, 1961.

Defoe, Daniel: *A Journal of the Plague Year (1721).* New York, Penguin, 1966.

Foran, J. K., and Morrissey, Sister Helen: *Jeanne Mance;* or, *The Angel of the Colony.* Montreal, Sisters of the Hôtel Dieu, 1931.

Gibson, John M., and Mathewson, Mary S.: *Three Centuries of Canadian Nursing.* Toronto, The Macmillan Co., 1947.

Goldin, Grace: "Juan de Dios and the Hospital of Christian Charity," *Journal of the History of Medicine and Allied Sciences, 33*:6–34, 1978.

Heagney, Anne: *God and the General's Daughter.* Milwaukee, Bruce Publishing Co., 1953.

Martindale, Cyril G.: *Life of St. Camillus.* New York, Sheed & Ward, 1946.

McMahon, Norbert: *The Story of the Hospitallers of St. John of God.* Westminster, Md., Newman Press, 1959.

Maynard, Theodore: *Apostle of Charity: The Life of St. Vincent de Paul.* New York, Dial Press, 1939.

Merejkowski, Dmitri: *The Romance of Leonardo da Vinci.* New York, Random House, 1902.

Newcomb, Covelle: *St. John of God*. New York, Dodd, Mead & Co., 1958.
Pachter, Henry: *Paracelsus: Magic into Science*. New York, Collier Books, 1961.
Paget, Stephen: *Ambrose Paré and His Times*. New York, G. P. Putnam's Sons, 1897.
Pepys, Samuel: *Diary (Selections)*. New York, Random House.
Repplier, Agnes: *Mère of the Ursulines*. New York, Doubleday, Doran & Co., 1931.
Shellabarger, Samuel: *Captain from Castile*. Boston, Little, Brown & Co., 1945.
Van Loon, Hendrik W.: *R.V.R.: The Life and Times of Rembrandt*. New York, Liveright Publishing Co., 1931.

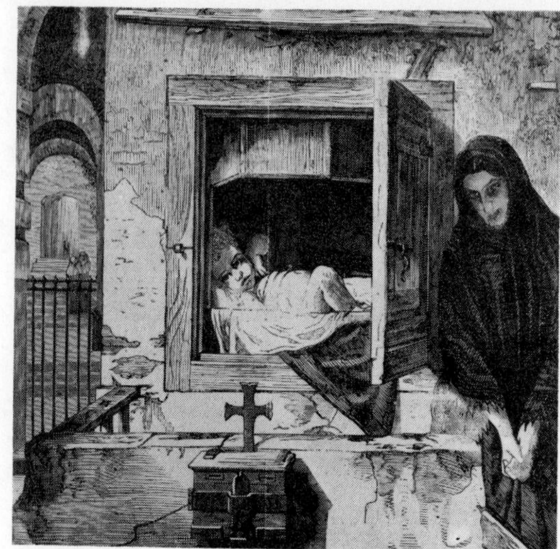

A turnstile of the Foundling Hospital in Florence, Italy, where a mother places her baby. (Dolan collection.)

Nursing and the Pressures of the Eighteenth Century 7

The accomplishments of the eighteenth century must be viewed against a background of outbreaks of political strife. Several of these outbreaks ended in armed intervention and revolution in an endeavor to create more democratic forms of government. Three revolutions, the Enlightenment (a revolution in thought), the American Revolution and the French Revolution, sought to spread a doctrine of independence and to emphasize the rights of man—that all men were born free and equal and were to be entitled to life, liberty and the pursuit of happiness. The thirteen colonies became the United States of America, "a new nation conceived in liberty and dedicated to the proposition that all men are created equal."

There was need for legislation to improve the sanitary and living conditions of the poor. There had been no attempt at preventing disease or at teaching the poor the principles of hygiene and sanitation. Epidemics took a fantastic toll in lives and occasioned severe psychological experiences.

In 1720, when England was threatened with an epidemic of cholera, the government encouraged *Dr. Richard Mead* (1673–1754) to publish a book entitled *A Short Discourse Concerning Pestilential Contagion.* This was an attempt to advise and teach prevention of disease. He stressed that, instead of penalizing infected families,[1] a reward should be given to those persons who discovered and reported a case of infectious disease. He stated further that instead of imprisonment of the family, the sick person should be removed, preferably to a place in the country where care could be provided. Dr. Mead did not believe in fumigation, although he felt the acrid smoke of sulphur effectively penetrated a contaminated area. He advocated that all public gatherings be cancelled.

During the colonial period in America, the means of communication were limited. People traveled by stagecoach, on horseback or on foot. There was no regular stagecoach line between New York and Philadelphia until 1766, at which time the trip took three days. Mail was delivered irregularly.

The colonies in the eighteenth century

[1]The former custom, during the times of the plague, required houses in which infected persons resided to be quarantined with a mark of the sign of the cross on the door and the well persons to be shut up with the sick. The imprisonment lasted at least a month after all trace of the disease had disappeared.

witnessed distressing outbreaks of disease in epidemic proportions. Dr. Caulfield has given a brilliant presentation of one of the catastrophic epidemics that occurred in New England between 1735 and 1740.[2] The epidemic was referred to as "the throat distemper," but was actually three separate epidemics—one of scarlet fever and two of diphtheria. Ultimately, the whole of New England was involved. It was a new disease to that generation, and at one point, nearly one-half of the children died. In the period of five years, five thousand persons died, mostly children and young people.

The best-educated man in any New England town was the minister, and he often assumed the role of physician. Many of the physicians of this period had no medical school training and frequently received their preparation by being apprenticed to men who also had no formal medical education.

Lacking an understanding of bacterial infection, its cause and method of transfer, all these people ignored even the most elementary precautions. Ministers and physicians assisted in spreading disease, carrying infection on their hands and clothes to other patients as well as to their own families. Caulfield states "One of the very noticeable characteristics of the 'throat distemper' epidemic is the frequent occurrence of many deaths in the families of ministers and physicians."[3]

Each family in New England was a self-sustaining unit and had its own supply of milk, water, produce, salted pork and poultry. The occasions when the community grouped together were for church meetings, socials, funerals and protection. Thus, one would expect that the spread of infection would be most unlikely. In the seventeenth century, however, the law decreed that towns with more than fifty families must provide for the education of the children. By 1735, public schools were established throughout New England. The schools were one-room, poorly ventilated buildings, which meant close contact among the children. Another custom contributed to the spread of the infectious disease. When a child died, the neighboring children acted as pallbearers, and in addition to coming in contact with the corpse, which in this period was not embalmed,[4] they associated with the dead child's family.

It was with thanksgiving and deep gratitude that the New England colonists welcomed the end of the "throat distemper" (Fig. 7–1).

In 1755, in New York, the first quarantine law was passed. At Bedloe's Island, vessels were quarantined if persons suspected of having contagious diseases were aboard. Legislation in 1784 enabled the state government to appoint a health officer to the port to enforce quarantine measures. The first New York City death records were filed in the year 1795, and these reported hundreds of deaths due to the yellow fever epidemic. *Dr. Richard Bayley*, a health officer, attributed this epidemic to the filthy conditions of the city and the crowded living conditions of the poor. The following year, in 1796, physicians were compelled to report infectious diseases. Ordinances required the disposal of garbage and refuse.

A new threat evolved with the eruption of wars. The Colonies decided to fight their War of Independence but had no organized army, since the states were not united. Each state had an army that was the spontaneous reaction to patriotism.

During the Battle of Bunker Hill, the need for a medical department for the army was recognized. The Provincial Congress of Massachusetts hired private houses and assembled medical supplies to be used for the sick and wounded, whose needs were great. They lacked shelter, bedding, clothing and adequate food. Infectious diseases were rampant.

[2]Caulfield, Ernest: *"A History of the Terrible Epidemic Vulgarly Called The Throat Distemper, Which Occurred in His Majesty's New England Colonies Between 1735–1740,"* New Haven, Yale Journal of Biology and Medicine, 1939.

[3]*Ibid.*, p. 5.

[4]The body of a person who had died was placed in a coffin, and prior to burial, buckets of ice were placed under and around the coffin to assist in preserving the corpse. As the ice melted, the water was thrown out in the yard and could have been a source of infection. The impossibility of burying a body during the cold New England winter months when the ground was frozen presented a source of contagion as well as psychological trauma. When the receiving vaults were unable to accommodate any more coffins, the coffin had to be kept in the coldest place, usually the barn or attic, until the spring thaws.

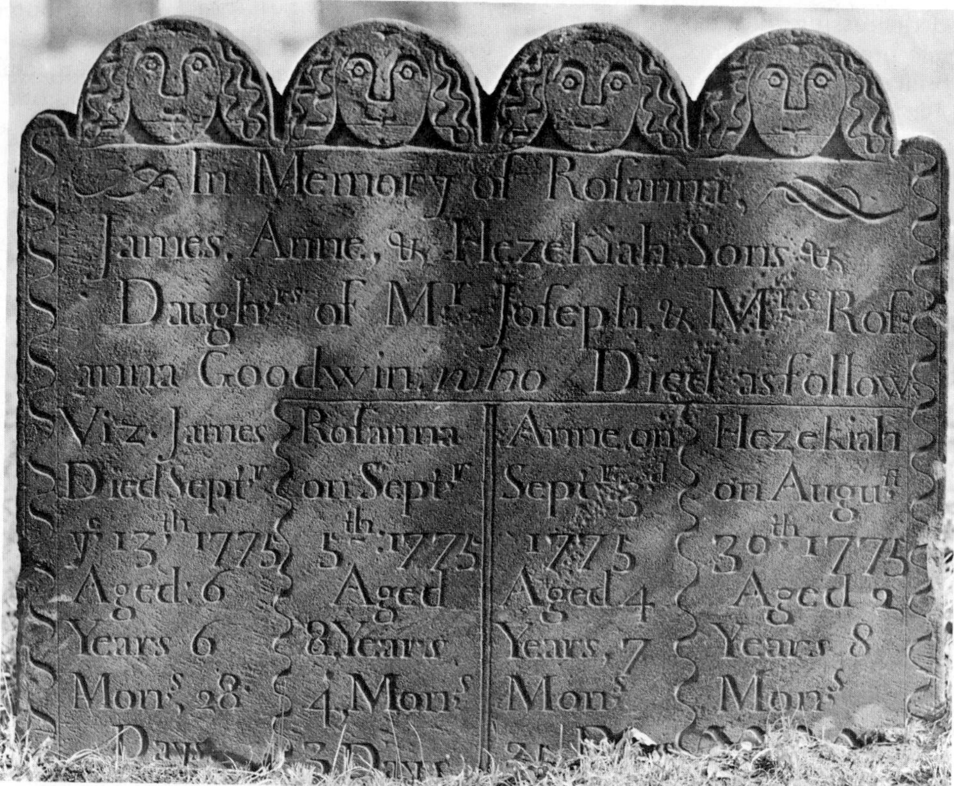
In Memory of Roſanna,
James, Anne, & Hezekiah Sons &
Daughrs of Mr Joſeph & Mrs Roſ-
anna Goodwin, who Died as follows
Viz. James
Died Septr
ye 13th 1775
Aged 6
Years 6
Mons 28
Roſanna
on Septr
5th 1775
Aged
8 Years
4 Mons
Anne on
Septr 3d
1775
Aged 4
Years 7
Mons
Hezekiah
on Augst
30th 1775
Aged 2
Years 8
Mons

Figure 7–1. A tombstone depicting the tragedy that befell a family in Bloomfield, Connecticut, in an epidemic. (Courtesy of Dr. Wendell C. Hall.) (Dolan collection.)

Despite the growing pains of the new country and the trials and tribulations of the older ones in the eighteenth century, contributions were made in the health fields.

PROGRESS IN NURSING

Many social problems as well as physical ills existed at this time. The need for social legislation to relieve afflictions was apparent.

The person who assumed the role of nurse, keeping people healthy as well as caring for them during illness, was the capable woman in the community. Her care was as good and patient-centered as her personal qualities, her inventiveness and her applied knowledge could provide. With science still not established, and in the face of political problems and medical misinformation, she continued her work as an independent practitioner. Her skills at providing care and, in many instances, cure were a tribute to her creativity in planning for the comfort and care of her patients. History was being repeated.

The ideas for many articles that were designed to help a person feel more comfortable and get well may have been suggested by the nurses of this period. The number of examples that remain are indicative of the wide acceptance of the comfort measures that were utilized. The importance of nutrition and of keeping a person warm or cool was also recognized.

Women continued to minister to the needs of families and neighbors. To stay alive in the colonies was a challenge; but the women were courageous and heroic. Without central heating, fireplaces were the source of heat. Beds were cold; therefore, long-handled warming pans, usually constructed of brass, were used as bedwarmers. They were filled with live coals and rubbed over the bottom sheet to heat it. When a person was ill, stone jugs filled with hot water and heated soapstones, the forerunners of hot water bottles and heat-

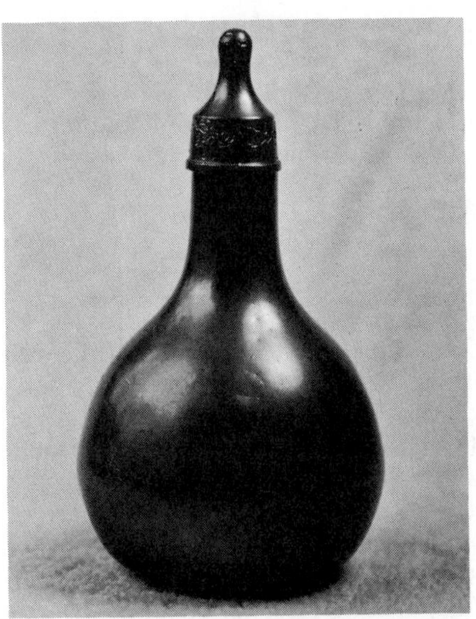

Figure 7–2. Pewter nursing bottle—note the teeth marks. (Courtesy of Miss Kate Hyder.)

ing pads, were utilized. The weight of the soapstones and the stone jugs, however, soon made it apparent that lighter objects were needed. Many uniquely shaped pottery and pewter hot water bottles were designed. The danger of burns, particularly from the pewter ones, does not seem to have been considered.

A mother used a pewter nursing bottle for "dry-nursing." The bottle was heavy. Its top section unscrewed for the milk to be poured into the bottom part. The nipple was part of the pewter top section. The dangers of lead poisoning were not recognized, for children used these nursing bottles for several years and their teething marks are visible on the bottles still in existence. (Fig. 7–2).

The eighteenth-century combination lamps and food warmers were ingenious devices that provided food for the invalid during the long hours of the night (Figs. 7–3 and 7–4). The objective was to keep liquids or nourishing food, principally pap, warm during the night. Pap, a popular substance in the invalid's diet, was made of milk in which oatmeal was cooked and strained. Beaten egg yolks, butter and orange flavor were added. The food was placed in a food pan that fit into a pan of water, much like a double boiler. Beef tea (the extract of the juices in beef made into a broth) was another frequently served dish.

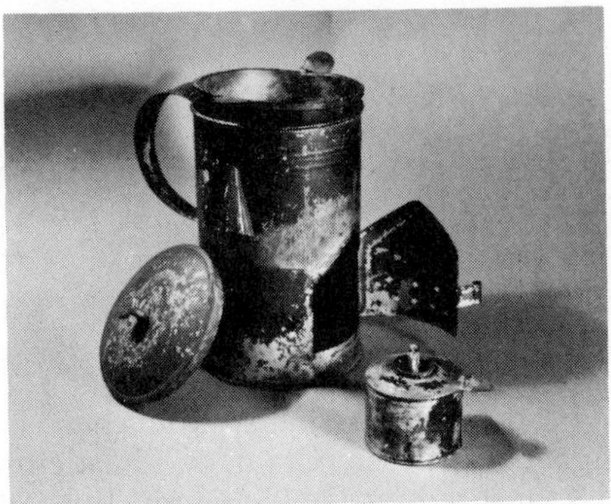

Figure 7–3. Pap warmer. (Photo by DeLores Paul.) (Dolan collection.)

China feeding cups (Fig. 7–5) permitted a patient to serve himself. The sizes of these cups were scaled to meet the personal needs of the patient. Hot water–chambered dishes were designed to keep the food as warm as possible and to serve as trays in which to bring the food.

Invalid chairs were devised during this period. Wheelchairs were called "go-chairs" in the eighteenth century. Gout chairs, rocking chairs and fan chairs were also produced. The fan chair was invented in an attempt to alleviate the sweltering heat

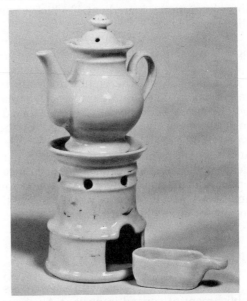

Figure 7–4. A combination night-light and warmer. A wick was floated on whale oil in the small china dish; the ignited wick furnished light and heat to warm the nourishment. (Dolan collection.)

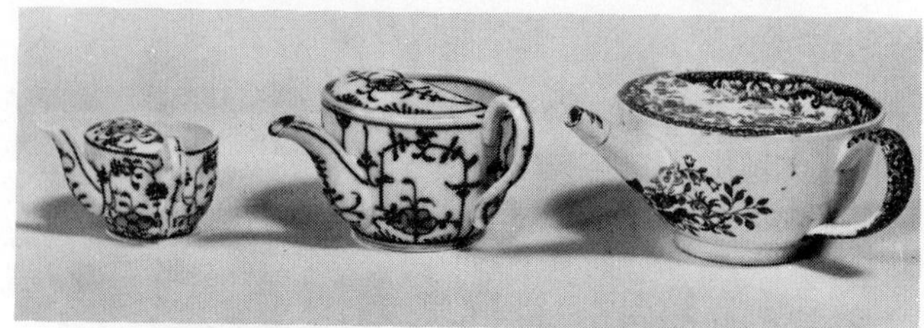

Figure 7–5. Examples of feeding cups. (Dolan collection.)

of Philadelphia summers. The chair was designed by a Mr. Cram of Philadelphia and sponsored by Dr. Benjamin Rush. By stepping on a pedal, the occupant powered the attached fan, which not only cooled the person but also kept flies from annoying him.

Herbs were used extensively as seasoning in food, as air purifiers and as sachets to scent linens and clothes. In addition, nurses concocted many uses for medicinal herbs, which became the basis of medications that are used today. An example is a remedy, found by a nurse in Shropshire, England, that cured dropsy; that herb was foxglove, from which digitalis, a valuable heart medicine, is obtained. *Dr. William Withering* (1741–1799) discovered that this woman was curing patients of dropsy when it was associated with a heart condition. He extracted from her herb mixture the important ingredient, which was digitalis.

Other than the previously mentioned religious nursing groups, there were no specially prepared nurses.

Nutting states: "The eighteenth century saw a deterioration in nursing and hospital organization, and naturally, the surroundings of the sick were also changed for the worse. The large airy halls, the cool springs and fountains, and the sweet green gardens of the mediaeval hospitals of France, Spain and the East now gave place to the small dark wards of the city and state institutions of the eighteenth century."[5]

HOSPITALS

The eighteenth century witnessed the establishment of several important American hospitals.

1731: *Blockley Hospital* (later Philadelphia General Hospital) received the poor, the sick, the insane, prisoners and orphans and was connected with a poorhouse. It was an almshouse and workhouse for the aged and infirm of the city. The care of patients was in the hands of servants, criminals and paupers.

1737: *Charity Hospital* of New Orleans. In 1736, a sailor, *Jean Louis*, died in New Orleans, leaving a sum of money to be used for the founding of a hospital for the care of the sick. His bequest included funds to purchase necessary equipment. The hospital was constructed in 1737 and served both as a hospital and as an asylum for the poor. After several catastrophes, the hospital was rebuilt in 1832; it had high ceilings, spacious wards and verandas, and was put under the aegis of the Sisters of Charity in 1834.

1751: *Pennsylvania Hospital* was founded in Philadelphia through the efforts of Dr. Thomas Bond and Benjamin Franklin, both of whom were Quakers. Its purpose was to admit only those who were acutely ill or had received an injury. Strangers as well as residents of Philadelphia were admitted. It was not an almshouse or a poorhouse, but a hospital in the usual sense of the word. The seal of this institution was that of the Good Samaritan: "Take care of him and I will repay thee."

1770: *Eastern State Hospital*, known as the "Lunatick Hospital," was opened in Williamsburg, Virginia. This was one of the first American state-owned institutions for the mentally ill.

1771: *New York Hospital* came into existence because of the efforts of public-spirited citizens. In 1771, a royal charter was granted by King George III to "the society of the Hospital in the City of New York in America." It was in the New York Hospital that Dr. Valentine Seaman gave the first series of lectures to nurses in the Colonies.

---

[5]Nutting, M. A., and Dock, L.: *A History of Nursing*, Vol. 1, New York, G. P. Putnam's Sons, 1935, p. 251.

1786: *The Philadelphia Dispensary* was established through the influence of the Quakers.

1796: *The Boston Dispensary* was founded by a group of Boston philanthropists. It had the first dental clinic, the first lung clinic, as well as the first evening pay clinic for working people in the nation. Another unusual aspect was that it had the first food clinic in the world.

SOCIAL REFORM

The distressing social conditions existing in the eighteenth century aroused the sympathetic efforts of many persons, including those with political influence. One such person was *John Howard* (1727–1789), who spent years investigating prisons, lazarettos and hospitals in England and on the Continent. In a forceful manner he recorded his observations, much to the consternation of the public. As bad as the prison conditions were, including the horrors of the dungeons, the facilities and care of the mentally ill were worse, and hospitals and nursing conditions were also deplorable. The only praise that he extended was for the work of the Sisters of Charity and the Beguines.

Filth, poor sanitation and an inadequate and unappetizing diet seemed to be universal in these institutions. Windows were not opened for fear of drafts nor were patients bathed for fear of getting them chilled.

One of Howard's recommendations was to keep one ward unoccupied so that patients in a ward could be removed to the vacant one while the one to which they had been assigned was cleaned. This was to be done to each ward in rotation.

Hospital nurses of this period were housekeepers who did the scrubbing and cleaning—when it was done. They were on a low social level, were unable to read or write and were given to drunkenness and, consequently, to drowsiness. These women were more to be pitied than criticized. They had neither desire nor preparation for their job. Fortunately, there were some women serving as nurses who, despite deficient educations, were striving to give devoted service.

Eventually, much progress was noted because of the efforts, courage and endeavors of John Howard.

Conditions in prisons were deplorable.[6] A prison with a pathetic history of torture was Newgate Prison of East Granby, the first prison in colonial Connecticut. Prisoners were not segregated according to sex, type of crime or mental condition; the mentally ill and mentally retarded shared quarters with the most vicious criminals. Screams were heard for quite a distance from the dungeons to which all inmates had to descend every night. Physical, emotional and mental disorders were prevalent, and infectious diseases terminated many lives.

INFANT WELFARE

In the field of infant welfare much needed to be done. St. Vincent de Paul had championed the cause of the abandoned child in the preceding century. The problem had become a more serious one in the eighteenth century. Dr. Caulfield has written of the plight of infants in England during this period and of those who tried to alleviate their sufferings.[7]

On the part of the public, there was an attitude of callousness and indifference in a setting of extensive infanticide. This viewpoint had to be changed before appreciable progress toward reducing infant mortality could be made. Records are replete with evidence of neglect, cruelty and sickness as well as infanticide. The exact statistics are not available, but in the early part of the century, the infant mortality rate for children under five years of age was 50 per cent. In London between 1730 and 1750, 75 per cent of all the babies christened were dead before the age of five. Of 10,272 infants admitted to the Dublin Foundling Hospital during 21 years (1775–1796) only 45 survived, a mortality of 99.6 per cent. Many famous foundling hospitals of the period had similar records. Even Queen Anne, who presumably received

---

[6] *Amelia* (1751), by Henry Fielding, depicts the wickedness of the law courts and the evils of the English prisons of the eighteenth century. It also presents a picture of confinement in debtors' jail.

[7] Caulfield, Ernest: *The Infant Welfare Movement in the Eighteenth Century*. New York, Paul B. Hoeber, 1931.

the best of care, lost 18 children in early infancy.

The greatest cause of death in infancy was neglect. It has been pointed out that the children of the wealthy were neglected because of fashion, whereas those of the poor were abandoned because of poverty. Wealthy women delegated the care of the children to nursemaids. The infant was nursed either by a wet nurse, who could transfer disease to the child, or by "dry nursing," or bottle-feeding, with the possibility of contracting disease from contaminated milk and water. There was a constant supply of wet nurses available because of the deaths of their own babies. It has been stated that "in some cases the infant mortality was the source of the wet-nurse supply; in other cases, the effect." The mortality rate of dry-nursed infants was nearly three times that of breast-fed ones. A common entry into the hospital records was "death from want of breast milk."

In 1761, *Jean-Jacques Rousseau* published his famous book *Emile*. Book I is a popular treatise on pediatrics and deals with the hygiene and nutrition of infancy. The dangers of mercenary wet-nursing and of tightly swaddling infants are emphasized. Rousseau inveighs against women who do not take care of or nurse their own children, much like Plutarch did in his advice to Greek women.

The British painter and engraver *William Hogarth* (1697–1764) used his considerable talent to focus piercing criticism on the social problems of his day. Charles Lamb testified to Hogarth's dramatic gift when he observed that most "pictures are looked at—his prints we read."[8] Hogarth's engravings are picture stories of an intense social ferment and of a world craving the pleasures of life (Fig. 7–6).

[8] "On the genius and character of Hogarth." *Works of Charles Lamb*. Vol. 1, 1818, p. 70.

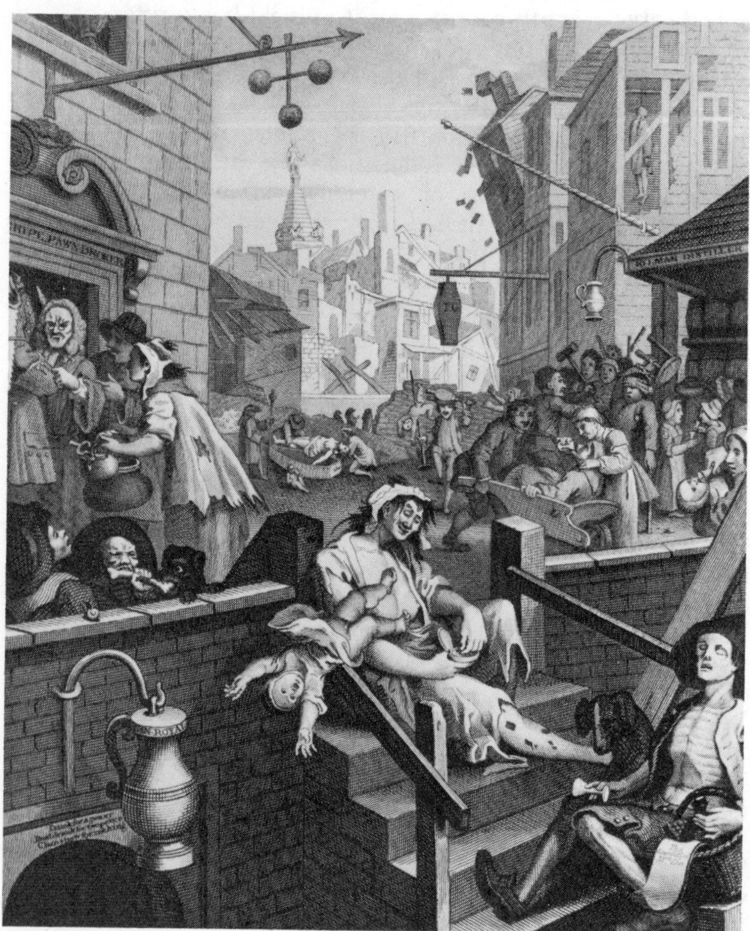

Figure 7–6. Gin Lane. Hogarth's famous picture shows the plight of the child in this period. The frailties of human nature are well displayed in a scene of horrible devastation. (Dolan collection.)

The ARCUTIO.

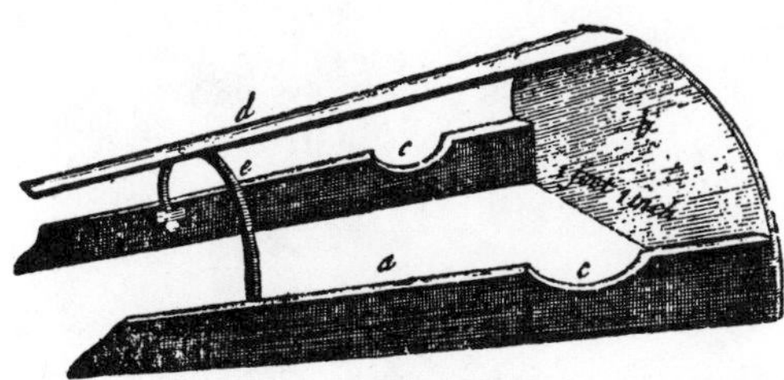

WHEN it is conſidered how many are charged Over-laid in the Bills of Mortality, it is to be wonder'd that the ARCUTIO's, univerſally uſed at *Florence*, are not uſed here in *England*. The Deſign above, is drawn in Perſpective, with the Dimenſions, which are larger than uſual; and is thus deſcribed:

a, *The Place where the Child lies.*
b, *The Head-Board.*
c, *The Hollows for the Nurſe's Breaſts.*
d, *A Bar of Wood to lean on, when ſhe ſuckles the Child.*
e, *A ſmall Iron Arch to ſupport the ſaid Bar*
The Length three Feet, two Inches and a half.

Every Nurſe in *Florence* is obliged to lay the Child in it, under Pain of Excommunication. The ARCUTIO, with the Child in it, may be ſafely laid entirely under the Bed-Cloaths in the Winter, without Danger of ſmothering.

Figure 7–7. An arcutio, used to prevent overlying. (From Caulfield, Ernest: *The Infant Welfare Movement in the Eighteenth Century*.)

"Dropping" of infants was a common occurrence. This meant abandoning the infant on doorsteps of wealthy homes or just leaving them in the street to freeze or starve.[9] Unmarried women occasionally murdered their offspring to earn their livelihoods as wet nurses.

Nurse members of religious orders continued to give nursing care to the well or ill children who were placed in the turnstiles of Foundling Hospitals by mothers who lacked either interest in them or finances to care for them.

Other causes of death as they were reported in this century were *headmouldshot*, or the overriding of the sutures of the cranium, which could cause birth injuries to the meninges that resulted in death; *horseshoehead*, or the separation of the sutures, associated with congenital defects of the cranium; and *overlying*, which was due to the practice of nurses sleeping with infants[10] (Fig. 7–7) as well as to the tightness of the stay (Fig. 7–8). (The stay consisted of

[9]*The History of Tom Jones, A Foundling* (1749), by Henry Fielding, is one of the great realistic novels. The story of Tom Jones begins with Squire Allworthy finding him, an infant, crying in his bed. When the baby was discovered, Allworthy commented, "I suppose she hath only taken this method to provide for her child; and truly I am glad she hath not done worse."

[10]*Pamela* (1740), by Samuel Richardson, describes this practice. It is a domestic novel, and the first modern novel, told in a series of letters. The depiction of scenes common to ordinary life was new to English literature. (Nurses were sometimes paid to overlay babies.)

See also *The History of the Adventures of Joseph Andrews and His Friend Mr. Abraham Adams* (1742), by Henry Fielding, a satire on Richardson's *Pamela*.

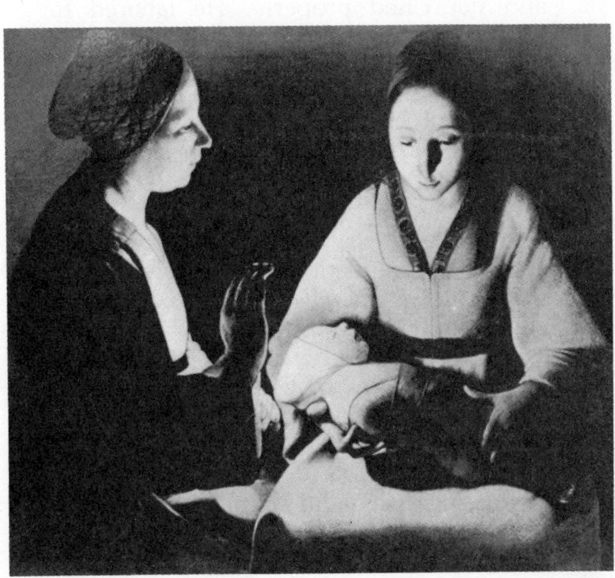

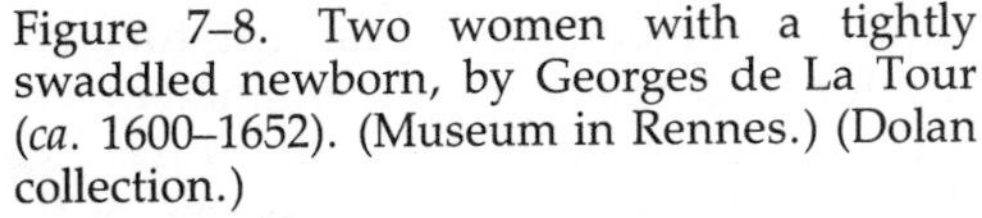

Figure 7–8. Two women with a tightly swaddled newborn, by Georges de La Tour (*ca.* 1600–1652). (Museum in Rennes.) (Dolan collection.)

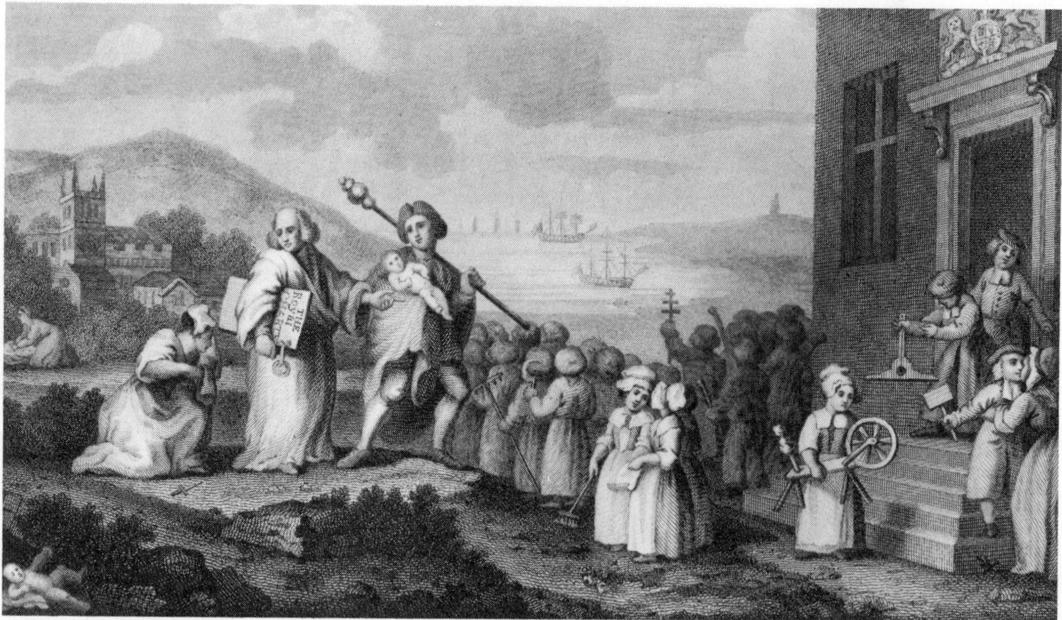

Figure 7–9. The Foundlings, by William Hogarth, was painted to celebrate the establishment of the Foundling Hospital in England in 1739. The Hospital provided an asylum and an industrial training center for youth in a wholesome environment for growth. (Dolan collection.)

the strings attached to a cap, which were tied tightly under the baby's chin; this cap was worn day and night to prevent chilling.)

There were some efforts to alleviate this high mortality rate of children. *Thomas Coram* (1668–1751) of England was instrumental in bringing poor families to settle in America in Oglethorpe's Colony in Georgia. His plan involved erecting huts in which deserted infants were to be cared for and nourished properly. He labored for seventeen years on this project, exhausting his funds, and then appealed to influential ladies for assistance. Thus, in 1738, the Hospital for Foundlings in London came into being (Fig. 7–9). So many children were brought to this institution that admission was by lot. The Foundling Hospital sent printed instructions to all foster mothers on the treatment of minor illnesses.

William Cadogan (1711–1797), who graduated from Oxford on June 20, 1755 with the Master of Arts degree and on June 27, 1755 with the degrees of Bachelor of Medicine and Doctor of Medicine, wrote "An Essay upon Nursing and Management of Children." In this essay he advocated loose clothing and frequent change of clothing at a time when the body and limbs of a baby were cramped in flannels, swaths and wrappers. (Wrapping babies in swaddling clothes had been a custom for ages.) Dr. Cadogan also stressed the value of daily baths during an era when it was thought that washing even a baby's head meant subjecting the baby to a cold.

Jonas Hanway (1712–1786), a philanthropist, was appointed one of the governors of the Foundling Hospital, and he studied its problems. He became interested in parish workhouses, which were outgrowths of the English poor laws. The parish workhouse movement, beginning about 1723, was an effort to provide quarters for the poor who were unable to support themselves and their infants. The populace was astonished at the descriptions by Hanway of the conditions that existed. He was successful in persuading Parliament to enact laws for the relief of the infants of the poor.

George Armstrong (?–1781) was one of the first English pediatricians. He possessed unusual powers of observation and was an ardent advocate of infant welfare. He was the prime leader behind the dispensary movement. On April 24, 1769, he opened the Dispensary for the Infant Poor. Armstrong recorded his rich experiences at the dispensary in *An Account of the Diseases Most Incident to Children,* which was published in 1771, revised in 1777 and revised again in 1783. His diagnostic ability was evident in this early pediatric textbook, in which he wrote about what he saw. Dr. Armstrong was one of the first to realize that many mothers wanted to nurse their infants but were unable to do so. Dry nursing was recommended. He also suggested that rubbing a baby gently was a soothing remedy.

Infanticide continued to be a public problem into the nineteenth century.

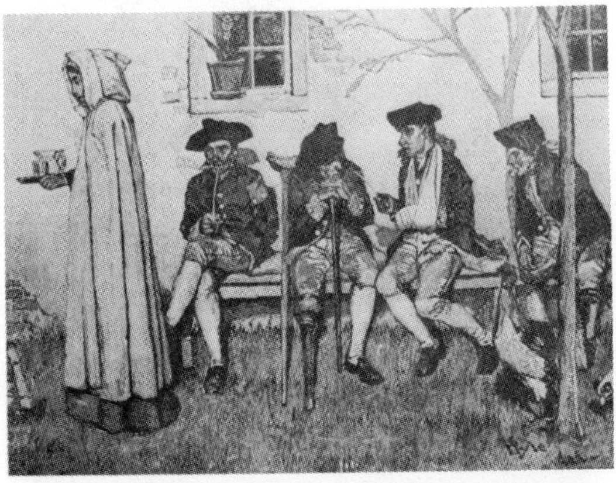

Figure 7–10. A monastic sister at the Ephrata Cloister in Pennsylvania attending the wounded soldiers after the battle at Brandywine. (Dolan collection.)

NURSING IN THE REVOLUTIONARY WAR

One writer says, "At the start of the *Revolutionary War* the tale of the medical department was a sorry one. There was practically no organization nor discipline. Surgical instruments were few. Drugs were few and bad; opium and quinine were scarce and ether was then unknown. Educated nurses did not exist. Blundering assistants called 'mates' were the only help the surgeons had." There were only five hospitals in New England, two in New York and two in Philadelphia. In New England, after the battle of Bunker Hill, several private houses in Cambridge were made into a hospital with Dr. John Warren in charge. The nurses were mostly men with no training in nursing. "Improvised hospitals at strategic points were often only halls, churches or hastily constructed sheds. Sometimes an inn was available. Means of transportation were primitive, and long journeys from the battle front left the wounded in grave condition. . . . Despite the exertions of Dr. Benjamin Rush, one of the most distinguished physicians in the Colonies, hospitals were frightfully overcrowded and unsanitary beyond modern conception. Fever and epidemics ran almost unhindered."

In 1777, General Washington ordered that women be engaged to nurse the soldiers; though many were employed, they apparently cooked and served meals but did little nursing. Some women followed their husbands into war and took care of them if they were wounded or ill.

At Valley Forge, in the winter of 1777, small log huts were used as hospitals. Each contained two double and four single bunks made of logs, a table and a fireplace. The operating room was located in a stone schoolhouse, built by William Penn's daughter Lucy.

A religious sect in Pennsylvania, the German Seventh-Day Baptists, formed a monastic community called the Ephrata Cloister. The habit of the Capuchins or White Friars was adopted by the new monastic community. The brothers wore a long white gown and cowl. The sisters' costume was the same, with the addition of a belt with an embroidered rose pattern on it.

After the bloody battle at Brandywine, during the American Revolution, some 500 wounded soldiers were brought to the cloister to be nursed by the sisters (Fig. 7–10). The buildings that served as a hospital had to be burned following their occupation to stop the spread of typhus fever. A monument in the monastic cemetery marks the graves of the many soldiers who were buried there.

HOSPITAL SHIP

Nurses had served aboard hospital ships for centuries. An eighteenth-century hospital ship in the Mediterranean in 1705 carried five nurses and three laundresses. The duty of these naval nurses was specifically to care for the sick. The work of cleaning and washing was performed by the laundresses, and cooks prepared the food.

An interesting assignment for these women nurses was to participate in an early research project.[11] In a pamphlet entitled "An Account of the Experiment made at the desire of the Lords Commissioners of the Admiralty, on board the *Union* Hospital Ship to determine the effect of the Nitrous Acid in destroying Contagion, and the safety with which it may be employed . . . ," Dr. James Carmichael Smyth described the experiment.

The HMS *Union* served many British naval ships by receiving the sick from them. When a Russian fleet became burdened with typhus fever, which caused a very heavy death rate, as many of the Russian sailors as could be accommodated were brought on board the *Union*. They were cared for by the nursing staff consisting of a matron and at least fifteen nurses.

The relationship of lice to typhus fever, frequently called "jail distemper," was unknown. Dr. Smyth, the ship's doctor, and the nurses carried out a regimen that stressed cleanliness, thorough bathing, the disinfection of clothes and bedding and the shaving of heads and beards. The patients were placed in newly washed bedding. Their sheepskin tunics, with the hair turned inward, were regarded as sources of infection and were removed in order to carry out the "antiseptic" (this word was used frequently) plan of care. Fresh air and the use of a disinfectant referred to as "antiseptic gas," derived from heating crude niter (potassium nitrate) with carbon, which gave off oxides of nitrogen, killed the lice. Another interesting arrangement on the HMS *Union* was the placement of the sanitary facilities so that they projected from the side of the ship instead of being inside it.

Dr. Smyth valued good nursing and opposed such treatments as bleeding and harsh drug therapy.

There were also male nurses assigned to military ships, and they wore a special garb. They are familiar from some of the many pictures of Nelson's death at the Battle of Trafalgar in 1815.

[11]Singer, Charles: "An Eighteenth Century Naval Ship to Accommodate Women Nurses," *Medical History*. Vol. IV, Number 4, pp. 283–287, October 1960.

NURSING IN THE FRENCH COLONIES DURING THE EIGHTEENTH CENTURY

The most traumatic year in the history of the Hôtel Dieu of Quebec was 1703. In that year, a severe epidemic of smallpox occurred in Quebec and eventually in the whole of New France. More than 2000 deaths occurred in Quebec. In 1710, a yellow fever epidemic wrought havoc. *The Sisters of the Hôtel Dieu* labored tirelessly during both epidemics. Several of the sisters died at their heroic task of caring for the afflicted.

A ship docking in the harbor in 1740 brought 241 plague-stricken patients to the Hôtel Dieu. There was a remarkably low death rate, which indicates that skilled nursing care had been given to these patients.

In 1755, another catastrophe confronted the sisters when the Hôtel Dieu was razed by fire. The Bishop of Quebec offered his home and volunteered to be the first orderly.

Two years later the sisters resumed their care of the sick in the newly rebuilt hospital. In 1759 they had a new challenge. The Augustinian Sisters of the Hôtel Dieu were ordered to go to the General Hospital that was outside of the city to nurse soldiers who were fighting in the French and Indian War. The wounded from the battles of the Plains of Abraham and Sainte-Foye were nursed devotedly by the Augustinian and the Ursuline Sisters. When Quebec fell to the British, the majority of the sisters returned to their hospital. They received kind treatment from the new regime.

A description of the two hospitals in Quebec as well as the type of women who joined the nursing orders was written in 1769 by Francis Brooke in *The History of Emily Montague*.[12]

> The Hotel Dieu is very pleasantly situated with a view of the two rivers and the entrance of the port; the house is cheerful, airy and agreeable; the habit of the nuns extremely becoming, a circumstance a handsome woman ought by no means to overlook; 'tis white with

[12]Gibbon, John M., and Mathewson, Mary S.: *Three Centuries of Canadian Nursing*, Toronto, The Macmillan Co., 1947, p. 53.

a black gauze veil . . . the nuns of this house are sprightly and have a look of health.

The General Hospital, situated about a mile out of town, is on the borders of the river St. Charles. The order and habit are the same with the Hotel Dieu, except that to the habit is added the cross, generally worn in Europe by canonesses only; a distinction procured for them by their founder St. Vallier, the second bishop of Quebec. The house is, without, a very noble building; and neatness, elegance and propriety reign within. The nuns, who are all of the noblesse, are many of them handsome, and all genteel, lively and well bred; they have an air of the world, their conversation is easy, spirited and polite.

The nursing sisterhoods in Canada came from France to Montreal and Quebec City in the seventeenth century. By the eighteenth century, the members of the orders were Canadians.

The *St. Joseph Hospitallers of the Hôtel Dieu of Montreal* had a rigorous time during the greater part of their first hundred years there. They were beset by problems: lack of money, supplies not arriving from France, fire destroying the hospital, temporarily having to use a portion of a home for the aged, living through the perilous days of the "cold war" while the Indians armed with tomahawks were preparing to attack the English, struggling to care for an extra 500 patients during a smallpox epidemic, and coping with a malignant fever epidemic brought by one of the king's ships.

In 1738, *Madame d'Youville*, a widow of means who had been responsible for many philanthropic endeavors, organized a group of women with similar interests. These women became the Soeurs Grises, or *Grey Nuns*. Their order was similar to the Order of Visitation founded by St. Francis de Sales. The Grey Nuns differed from the two other nursing order of sisters in that this new order was not cloistered and included in its program the visitation of the sick in their homes, which was community nursing *(visites à domicile)*. The community of the Soeurs Grises, under the title of Sisters of Charity of the General Hospital of Montreal, received from Louis XV a charter to operate their hospital. They wore a gray habit with a silver crucifix on the breast (Fig. 7–11).

When English prisoners who had been sick or wounded were convalescing, Mother d'Youville put them to work at their trades and, in this way, utilized the modern concept of rehabilitation. She sheltered the prisoners from the Indians in the chapel.

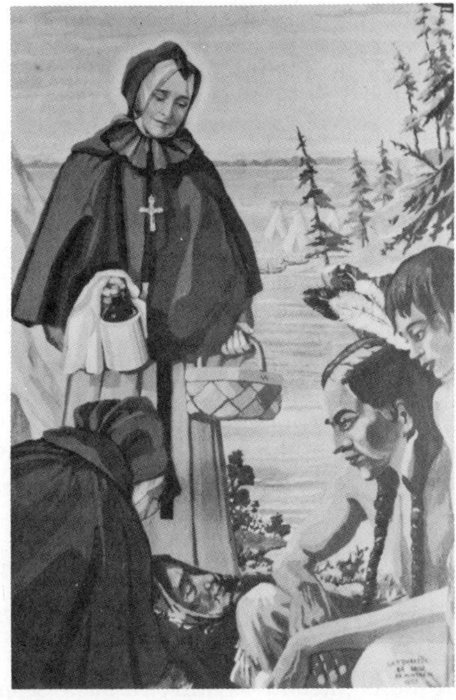

Figure 7–11. In 1755 a smallpox epidemic erupted in Montreal and in the surrounding villages. The Grey Nuns nursed the afflicted Indians in their communities. (Dolan collection.)

When the English captured New France, the various orders of sisters received protection, were not disturbed or prevented from continuing their work and were praised for the care they gave to all soldiers.

In Canada, a home for abandoned children was established and given the name *La Crèche d'Youville*. It was and still is used as a center for the placement of abandoned children with foster parents.

In Acadia (Nova Scotia) between 1629 and 1630, a tiny settlement prospered amid trials and tribulations and came to be known as Port Royal. From its beginnings, it had a type of infirmary for the sick under the supervision of the *Brothers Hospitallers of St. John of God*. Gradually, this infirmary developed into a hospital.

Another hospital was constructed at Louisbourg in Cape Breton. Five members of the Brothers Hospitallers of St. John of God were sent to staff this institution; two male nurses, two surgeons, and an apothecary were also assigned.

The British colonized Nova Scotia, and a hospital was constructed for the citizens at Halifax. The matron of the hospital, Sarah Dunlop, was reported to have worked without pay. This hospital became an almshouse for the poor in 1766.

The English had hospital ships that were described as being utilized when General Howe was moving his army, including sick and convalescing soldiers.

The accomplishments of nursing in eighteenth-century Canada were remarkable. Men and women of nobility who gave superior care in the face of insurmountable odds were recruited.

DEVELOPMENTS IN BIOLOGICAL AND PHYSICAL SCIENCES AND MEDICINE

In the eighteenth century, a basic scientific foundation for the eventual blossoming of the allied health professions was continuing to be laid.

Daniel Fahrenheit (1686–1736) was born in Danzig and later became a maker of glassware in Amsterdam. He was interested in the measurement of temperatures, and his skill in blowing glass led him to produce thermometers of extraordinary reliability. He made his first thermometer in 1714. Fahrenheit used alcohol at first and then changed to mercury. Fahrenheit developed the following temperature scale:

fever heat	112°
human heat	96°
summer heat	76°
temperate	51°
water freezes	32°

Herman Boerhaave (1668–1738), a Dutch physician, was the first to use the mercury thermometer devised by Fahrenheit. It was ten inches in length, required fifteen minutes or more to register and had to be held in place against the person's body. As soon as the thermometer was removed from the body, the mercury fell to room temperature; therefore, it was essential to determine the temperature while the thermometer was in place against the body. Dr. Boerhaave was a clinician who taught his students at the bedside as he made his clinical rounds.

Giovanni Battista Morgagni (1682–1771) was responsible for presenting to the medical world the idea that diseases originate in localized areas of the body, such as in organs or tissues, rather than as a result of an imbalance of humors. In 1761, he published a book entitled *On the Seats and Causes of Disease,* which presented in logical sequence the historical background of each disease, the symptoms, the treatment prescribed and, finally, the pathological findings obtained through autopsies. The data indicate a remarkable amount of knowledge of the previously published literature on the subject.

James Lind (1716–1794) discovered the solution to the problem of scurvy, one of the earliest known nutritional deficiencies, which had bedeviled soldiers and sailors from the days of the Crusades. The disease was known to the ancient cultures but did not become a major catastrophe until long journeys were undertaken and sailors depended on rations that had to be stored for many months. Scurvy took a greater toll in lives than all naval warfare. Many other people developed scurvy when their diets were deficient in fresh fruits and vegetables.

In 1747, Lind carried out an experiment with twelve men who had succumbed to scurvy. The most startling response was noted in the men to whom he gave citrus fruits—oranges and lemons (Fig. 7–12). The results of his careful observations, deliberations and experimentation were reported in his works, *An Essay on the Most Effectual Means of Preserving the Health of Seamen in the Royal Navy,* in 1757, and *An Essay on Diseases Incidental to Europeans in Hot Climates,* in 1768. These writings embodied his suggestions for the care of the patient with scurvy, for the upgrading of the hygiene and sanitary environment of sailors and for better comprehension of tropical diseases.

In addition to the inclusion of citrus fruits in the diet to prevent as well as cure scurvy, his recommendations included baths and issuance of clean clothing for sailors to curtail the spread of typhus, increase morale and aid in recruitment; an organized program of physical exercise to keep the sailors in good condition; a method of distilling salt water to obtain fresh water; a

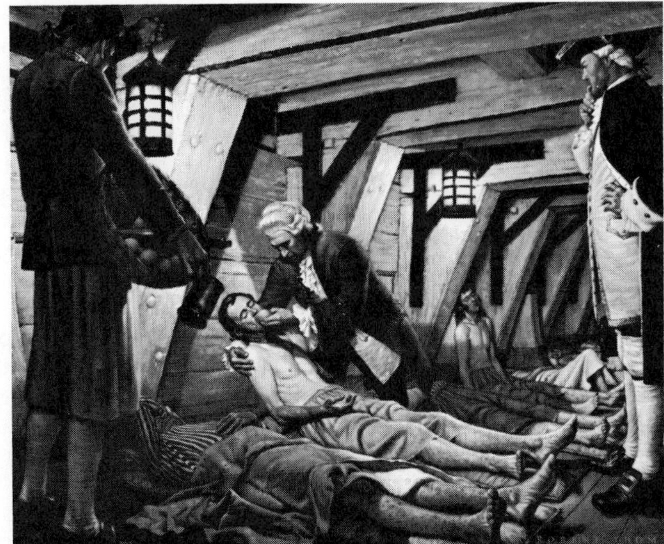

Figure 7–12. An artist's conception of James Lind engaged in his experimental study of sailors with scurvy. (© 1959, by Parke, Davis & Co.)

plan for physical examinations with proper notations on physical record sheets; the use of cinchona bark to prevent malaria; and the inadvisability of going on shore leave in the tropics where malaria was prevalent.

Lind did not live to see his suggestions adopted, but his pioneering efforts in the prevention of disease and in the experimental method of gathering data have been rewarded. Members of the British navy—often referred to as "limeys"—were probably the first group to receive vitamin therapy.

Leopold Auenbrugger (1722–1809), an Austrian physician, became acutely interested in the processes of diseases, especially those of the chest. He noticed that when the chest of a healthy person was tapped lightly it sounded like a muffled drum but that in a sick person, the sounds varied, especially if the person had an infectious involvement of the chest. In 1761, he published a small brochure entitled *On Percussion of the Chest*.

From time immemorial, *smallpox* had been one of the major scourges of society. The method of treatment used by the ancient Chinese has been discussed, as has Rhazes' work describing the disease. *Lady Mary Wortley Montagu* (1689–1762), the wife of the British Ambassador to Turkey, was responsible for introducing to Europe the practice of "engrafting" to prevent smallpox. She described the Turkish method as follows: An old woman would scratch the venom of smallpox into a child's skin. About a week later, the child would suffer a higher temperature accompanied by a pustular rash that left scars or pock marks.

After six condemned prisoners of Newgate Prison volunteered for experiments and won their freedom by being inoculated successfully, King George I permitted his two granddaughters to be inoculated. Thereafter, this preventive treatment was warmly received in Britain.

This method was of dubious value because of the dangers of its spreading smallpox and of keeping the disease condition ever present. The prevalence of this disease was shown by the availability of smallpox scabs with which to inoculate. Parents felt the necessity of exposing youngsters because there was a feeling that contracting the disease was inevitable; thus, to acquire the disease and have it over with was more important than to prevent it.

In 1721, after the infected crew of a vessel from the West Indies landed in the New England colonies, half the population of Boston developed smallpox and about one-fourth of these patients died. This was Boston's sixth smallpox epidemic in a century. *Cotton Mather* (1663–1728) observed that many Africans were not afflicted by the outbreaks of smallpox. By questioning these men, he learned of the knowledge, method and skill of Africans in the practice of inoculation. Subsequently, in 1721, he

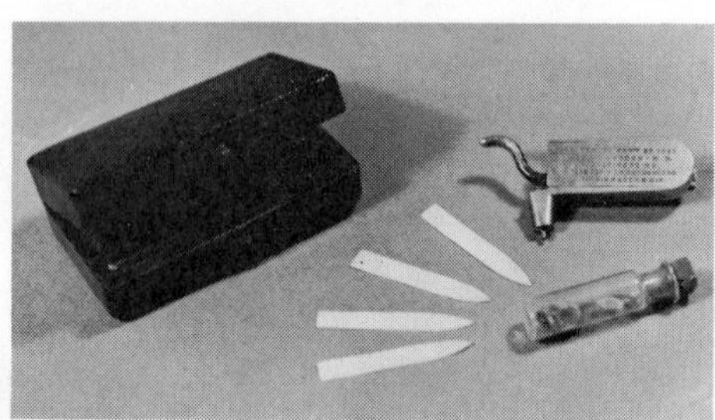

Figure 7–13. A container of necessary ingredients for smallpox inoculation: a bottle of dried smallpox scabs, a metal scarifier to produce the pinprick incisions and the probe-like instruments to introduce the scabs into the superficial pinprick area. (From Mayo Clinic Collection. Photo by DeLores Paul.) (Dolan collection.)

wrote an "Address to the Physicians of Boston" beseeching them to try inoculation.

There were several types of variolation, or inoculation, such as an arm-to-arm inoculation, in which the matter from smallpox pustules was rubbed onto the arm of a healthy person in the hope of conferring immunity. There was always the chance of contracting the disease itself. Another method consisted of making minute incisions into which some of the variolus pus was introduced on cotton (Fig. 7–13); still another method was to dip a thread into the pus and strap it to the arm. Gradually, the methods became more complicated until all were replaced by the vaccination described by Jenner in 1798.

Edward Jenner (1749–1823) started his medical career as a student at St. George's Hospital in London and was apprenticed to and studied under John Hunter, living in his home for two years. Hunter's advice to Jenner to be willing to experiment probably motivated the project for which he received international recognition.

Having noted the similarity between cowpox and smallpox, and the immunity to smallpox among milk maids, Jenner hoped to establish immunity to the more serious disease by inoculation with the less threatening one. In 1796, when cowpox appeared on a farm, Jenner obtained some of the pus from a sore on the hand of one of the dairy maids (Fig. 7–14). He introduced this matter (cowpox virus) by superficial pinprick incisions into the arm of a healthy eight-year-old boy named James Phipps. The vaccinated spot developed a small pustular sore, followed by a scab and a scar. The vaccination proved to be successful when six weeks later Jenner tried to inoculate the boy with smallpox virus. The inoculation failed to take, indicating James's immunity to smallpox. Jenner reported his results in 1798 in a booklet entitled *An Inquiry into the Causes and Effects of the Variolae Vaccinae*. An important milestone had been reached because someone had been willing and scientifically prepared to experiment with this method of inoculation to prevent an infectious disease.

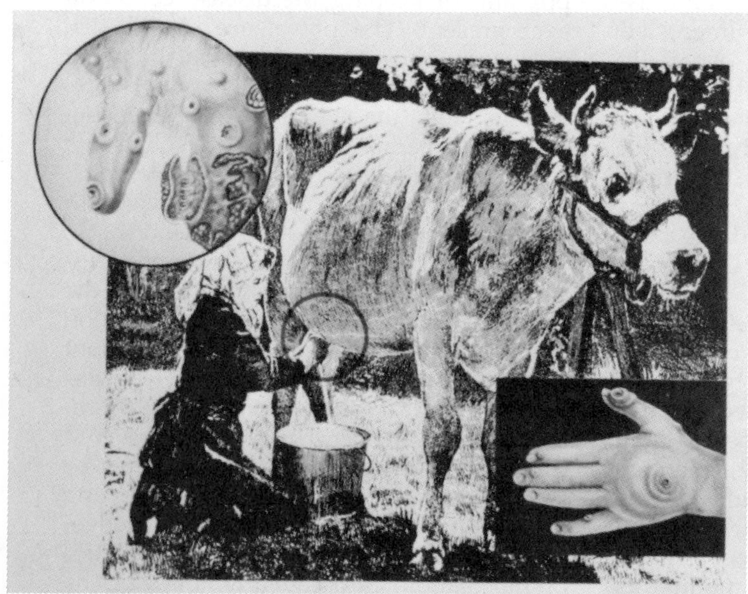

Figure 7–14. Milkmaids contracted cowpox on their hands during the milking process and became immune to smallpox. (Dolan collection.)

In contrast with the scientific foothold that medical theorists were striving to attain, there were many therapeutic fads, and of course, medical practitioners resorted to the time-honored practices of purging, cupping, bleeding and leeching.

Psychiatry

Benjamin Rush (1745–1813) was born in Philadelphia of Quaker parents. At the age of 15 in 1760, he received an A.B. degree from the College of New Jersey (now Princeton). The course consisted primarily of Latin, Greek and mathematics; at that time no science was offered. Medicine appealed to him, and he became apprenticed to a Dr. Redman on the staff of the Pennsylvania Hospital for five and a half years. It is interesting to note that Dr. Redman encouraged Benjamin Rush to keep an educational diary called a "commonplace book" into which he inscribed valuable information about patient care.

Rush went to the University of Edinburgh, from which he obtained an M.D. in 1768. He became professor of chemistry at the College of Philadelphia, then a professor of medicine when the college merged with the University of Pennsylvania.

Politics absorbed some of his time and energies, and he was appointed surgeon-general of the army. In 1777, he wrote a directive *To the Officers of the Army of the United States: Directions for Preserving the Health of Soldiers*. Rush was one of four physicians to sign the Declaration of Independence. In 1783, he joined the staff of the Pennsylvania Hospital, and while there he introduced clinical instruction.

Among the patients assigned to him were twenty-four "lunatics." These patients were given no medical treatment and were subjected to discomforts and dampness. Benjamin Rush protested against this improper treatment until the legislature appropriated $15,000 for the construction of a ward for the mentally ill. At a time when bathtubs were considered a luxury, his request that patients receive hot and cold baths was granted. He called attention to the need for diversional therapy for psychiatric patients; for suitable companions to listen sympathetically to patients; for a plan for recreation and amusement; for personnel to direct these activities; and, lastly, for separation of the mentally ill from those who were convalescing. His requests were eventually granted. In addition to his modern, progressive thinking, however, he also resorted to bloodletting, violent purging and the use of a special type of chair called a "tranquilizer" (Fig. 7–15). In 1812, Rush wrote an outstanding monograph on insanity, *Medical Inquiries and Observations upon the Diseases of the Mind*. His treatments were palliative, but the cause of mental illness remained unsolved.

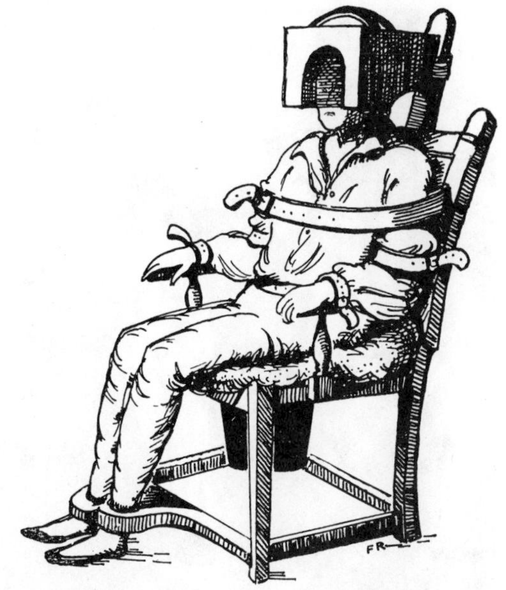

Figure 7–15. Dr. Rush's tranquilizer chair. (Courtesy of Pennsylvania Hospital. In *Some Account of the Pennsylvania Hospital from 1751 to 1938*.)

In 1786, Rush founded the Philadelphia Dispensary, the first in this country.

Philippe Pinel (1745–1826) was born in a small village in central France. During the days of the French Revolution, the citizenry cried for liberty, equality and fraternity. Yet these conditions were absent in the treatment of the mentally ill. Pinel, a timid man, of slight, slender build, demanded justice for these patients.

In 1793, a council of three men was responsible for the administration of the Hospital of Paris. Recognizing the worth and ability of Pinel, this council sent for him and informed him that he was the one man in France capable of bringing order

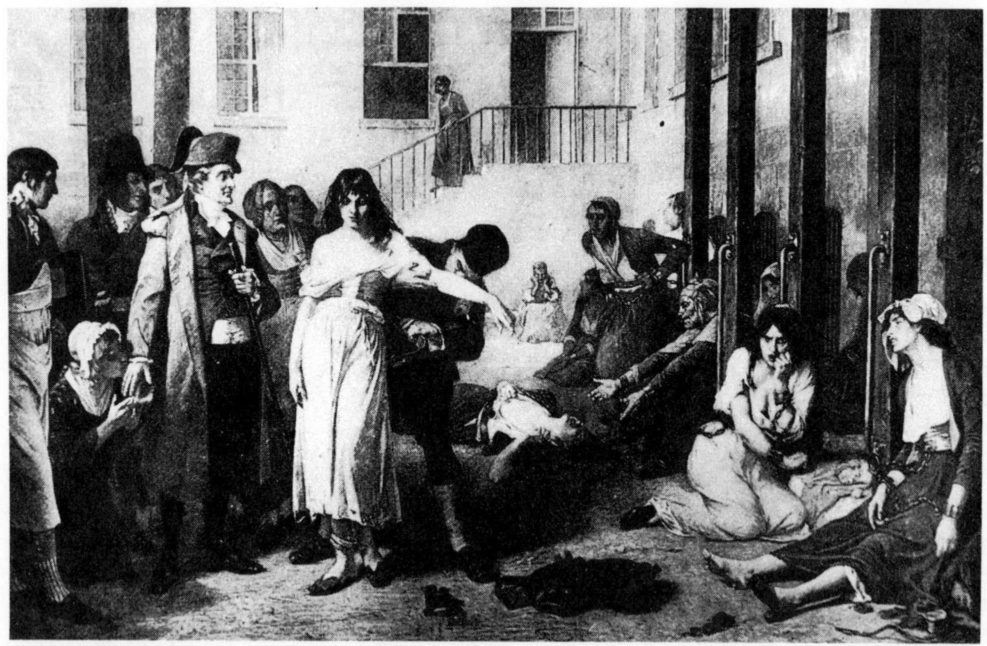

Figure 7–16. The mentally ill at the Salpêtrière are liberated from their chains by Philippe Pinel in 1795. (Dolan collection.)

out of the chaos that reigned in the insane asylums. The patients who were mentally ill were chained to walls, posts or beds. Violence was the only treatment they received. For a fee, curiosity seekers could obtain amusement by watching these sufferers. After assuming his new position, Pinel obtained permission from the proper authorities to remove the chains from these patients (Fig. 7–16).

Pinel advocated separating the patients who were agitated from those who were calm. To Pinel goes credit for systematizing mental diseases according to symptomatology. This gentle man taught compassionate treatment of the mentally ill by his own example.

EDUCATION OF HEALTH TEAM MEMBERS

The field of *pharmacy* continued to benefit mankind. The Marshall Apothecary was established in Philadelphia in 1729 by *Christopher Marshall* (1709–1797), an immigrant from Dublin. His apothecary was the first practical or proprietary school for the training of pharmacists, from which sprang America's first college of pharmacy, Philadelphia College of Pharmacy. His son Charles Marshall became its first president in 1821. In 1804, Christopher's granddaughter Elizabeth assumed the role of *America's first woman pharmacist*.

The education of the members of the health team in this period was sketchy. Apothecaries received little formal educational preparation but had an apprenticeship and much practical training and experience. Many laymen functioned as physicians without having earned the degree of doctor of medicine. The M.D. degree was only of relative significance and required various types of preparation, including a certain period of apprenticeship with an apothecary or a surgeon, a semester or two of university classes, and a course of study at a dissecting or anatomical school or a hospital. Any combination of these preparations sufficed and the gentleman then applied for and received an M.D. degree. There was no medical school in the English colonies until 1765, and it was very costly to go to Europe for medical preparation.

In North America, the pioneer in medical education was *John Morgan* (1735–1789).

Morgan spent several years abroad where he worked with William and John Hunter, studied with Morgagni and enrolled as a student in Edinburgh University, from which he graduated in 1763 with the degree of M.D. He returned to Philadelphia to establish a medical school comparable to those in Europe. It was his firm conviction that a medical school should not be a private venture or proprietary school but rather an integral part of a college or university. He emphasized the need for good premedical preparation, including Latin, a modern language, mathematics and natural sciences. His opinions were presented in *A Discourse upon the Institution of Medical Schools in America,* which logically summarized the needs for housing the school for the profession in an institution of higher learning and for the proper study of sciences, starting with the anatomical structure of the body, in order to understand health and illness and as a *sine qua non* for surgeons. Materia medica, botany, and chemistry were essential to an understanding of diet and medicines and their properties, including the fact that new substances form from the changes resulting within the body.

It was Dr. Morgan's belief that every practicing physician should have a comparable background of planned instruction; this was impossible with the apprenticeship system. He advocated planned clinical lectures to be given in the clinical setting of the Pennsylvania Hospital. A suggestion that his adversaries rebelled against was that pharmacy be separated from medicine and surgery. The practice of combining them had arisen in the Colonies out of necessity. In Europe pharmacy and medicine were separate entities. Morgan stressed that prescriptions should be filled by a competent apothecary.

The College of Philadelphia (later the University of Pennsylvania) opened in 1765, and Dr. Morgan became the first professor of Medicine in the Colonies. Although political strife and warfare disrupted some of the school's plans and activities, the cornerstone had been laid for medical education in North America.

An educational struggle was brewing between those who learned by training and experience and those who were well grounded in the theory of scientific investigation. King[13] presents a letter, written by Oliver Goldsmith in 1759, comparing preparation received in Edinburgh (old type) to that received in Oxford (new type).

The plight of the medical student of the eighteenth century has been well publicized. The diary of a medical student of this century provides an invaluable description of patient care and medical education at this time.[14] A medical student was indentured to a practitioner, and in return for food, lodging and learning, he helped as a servant, performing many nonmedical functions. His opportunity for education depended not only on his resourcefulness, but also on the practitioner's capability and ability to provide a proper milieu for inquiry and research. Frequently the student had to join the groups of grave robbers in order to provide anatomists with cadavers for dissection and instruction. The engraving shown in Figure 7–17, published in 1773, depicts a watchman at the left of the picture holding a resurrectionist who, in turn, is pointing an accusing finger at an anatomist. The wicker hamper contains a recently exhumed corpse.

Medical equipment was costly and scarce (Fig. 7–18). The physician brought his medicines in the medical chest that he carried with him; he also provided the enema equipment for the "clyster" that he administered. A wooden box contained the pewter clyster, which had a nozzle attached to the pewter tubing. The fluid ingredients were poured into the opening beside the plunger; the patient was seated on the nozzle, and when the plunger was released, the fluid was injected with tremendous force (Fig. 7–19).

Another custom of this period was that of the itinerant oculist, who traveled throughout the colonies with boxes of glasses to be tried on and selected for assistance in reading.

The sickroom scene of a famous patient is worthy of consideration at this point. In December of 1799, George Washington developed a cold accompanied by a severe

[13]King, Lester S.: *The Medical World of the Eighteenth Century.* Chicago, University of Chicago Press, 1958, pp. 28–29.

[14]Knyveton, John: *The Diary of a Surgeon in the Year 1751–1752.* Ed. by Ernest Gray. New York, D. Appleton-Century Co., Inc., 1937.

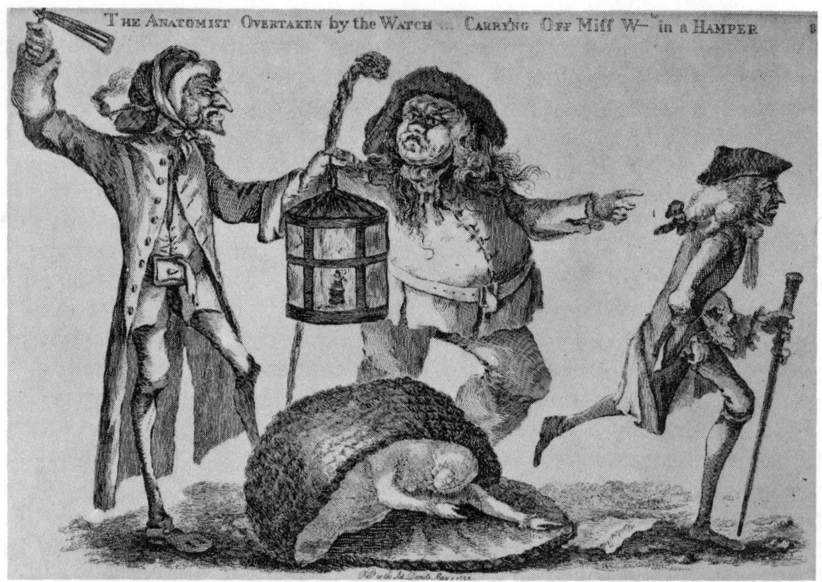

Figure 7–17. "The anatomist overtaken by the watch in carrying off Miss W—in a hamper." Engraving by William Austin (1721–1820). (Courtesy of Yale Medical Library, Clements C. Fry Collection.)

sore throat. Soon he had great difficulty breathing and swallowing. The remedies that were prescribed consisted of giving him mixtures of molasses, vinegar and butter to drink; bleeding, done by the overseer of the farm at least three times, which removed almost two quarts of blood; rubbing a menthol-type preparation on his throat and then wrapping a piece of flannel saturated with this preparation around his neck; applying a poultice of Spanish flies (made from dried and powdered beetles) to his throat; setting up a vinegar and hot water steam inhalation; and giving calomel as a laxative together with tartar as an emetic. Consultants were summoned and a diagnosis was made by observing the external symptoms. The throat was not inspected, nor the chest listened to. The first diagnosis was quinsy, which was the name given to the condition of tonsillar abscess. The final diagnosis was "cynanche trachealis." It is now believed that diphtheria was the disease, but the bacterial infection coupled with the medical care that he received was the cause of death.

One of the physicians called in for consultation wanted to do a tracheotomy to assist him in breathing and also argued against bleeding because he felt this weak-

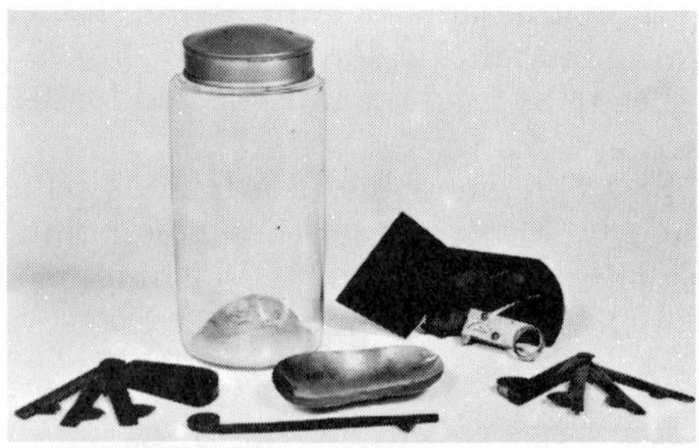

Figure 7–18. Eighteenth-century medical equipment—blown glass leech bottle, small leech basin, scarifier and three sets of bleeding knives, the center one being hand-forged. (Dolan collection.)

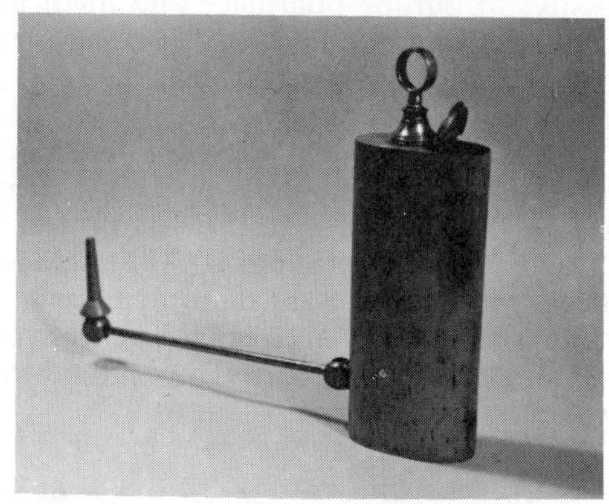

Figure 7–19. A pewter clyster. (From Mayo Clinic Collection. Photo by DeLores Paul.)

ened the patient. Skilled nursing care is not mentioned, because there were no nurses present.

Nurses needed a scholarly leader to advocate proper academic preparation for entry into practice.

SUMMARY

The eighteenth century witnessed struggles to achieve independence on the part of many peoples, to conquer pestilential contagion, to end the marked loss of lives and to improve the standard of living, while laboring under inadequate means of transportation and communication. Achievements were notable in conquering certain diseases, devising diagnostic equipment, developing the beginnings of humane treatment of the mentally ill and expanding the bases of the sciences of chemistry and physics.

The areas needing strengthening were social legislation for public and industrial health, improvement in medical care and in the newly formed United States, the recruitment of persons with leadership qualities for nursing and the provision of educational preparation for them.

THE HERITAGE OF NURSING

The Image of the Nurse in the Eighteenth Century

In this period of constant fear for survival, the role of the nurse was as strong as it had been from the beginnings of time. The image of the nurse as given in Chapter 1 is appropriate to this chapter as well. In addition, warfare and social change called for a nursing response to:

1. the mass devastation of diseases by
   a. devising preventive as well as curative measures.
   b. discovering new treatment methods following nursing assessments.
   c. developing skill in providing care to families during bereavement.
   d. offering nursing skills in a home environment to prevent use of the "pest houses."
2. the plight of the child by
   a. attaining special skills in child health nursing.
   b. aiding the establishment of protective agencies for children to prevent child abuse and infanticide.

Gradually, in response to the crises arising from revolutions and epidemics, male and female nurses assumed essential roles in preventive and curative aspects of nursing. During this period the need for programs to educate nurses for nursing practice was recognized. Leaders in nursing needed to join those in medicine in requiring practitioners to have a sound academic base, provided in a university, prior to entering practice.

REFERENCE READINGS

Andry, Nicholas: *Orthopaedia*. (Facsimile Reproduction of the First Edition in English, London, 1743) Philadelphia, J. B. Lippincott Co., 1961.

Austin, Robert B.: *Early American Medical Imprints 1668–1820*. Washington, D.C., U.S. Department of Health, Education and Welfare, 1961.

Bartlett, Josiah, M.D.: *A Dissertation on the Progress of Medical Science in the Commonwealth of Massachusetts*. Boston, 1810.

Bayley, Richard: *An Account of the Epidemic Fever which prevailed in the City of New York, during part of the Summer and Fall of 1795*. New York, T. and J. Swords, Printers to the Faculty of Physic of Columbia College, 1796.

Caulfield, Ernest: *The Infant Welfare Movement in the Eighteenth Century*. New York, Paul B. Hoeber, 1931.

Caulfield, Ernest: "Some Common Diseases of Colonial Children," *Transactions of the Colonial Society of Massachusetts,* pp. 4–65, April 1942.

Caulfield, Ernest: "The Throat Distemper of 1735–1740," *Yale Journal of Biology and Medicine, 11*:219–272, 277–335, 1939.

Dexter, Elizabeth Anthony: *Career Women of America, 1776–1840*. Francestown, N.H., Marshall Jones Co., 1950.

Dickens, Charles: *A Tale of Two Cities* (1859). New York, E. P. Dutton & Co.

Drinker, C.K.: *Not So Long Ago: A Chronicle of Medicine and Doctors in Colonial Philadelphia*. New York, Oxford University Press, 1937.

Edmunds, Walter: *Drums Along the Mohawk*. Boston, Little, Brown & Co., 1936.

Fielding, Henry: *The History of Tom Jones, a Foundling* (1749). New York, Random House.

Franklin, Benjamin: *Autobiography* (1790). New York, Oxford University Press.

Halsband, Robert: *The Life of Lady Mary Wortley Montagu*. New York, Oxford University Press, 1957.

King, Lester S.: *The Medical World of the Eighteenth Century*. Chicago, University of Chicago Press, 1958.

Kobler, John: *The Reluctant Surgeon: A Biography of John Hunter*. New York, Doubleday & Co., 1960.

Neilson, W., and Neilson, F.: *Verdict for the Doctor—The Case of Benjamin Rush*. New York, Hasting House, 1958.

Packard, Francis R.: *Some Account of the Pennsylvania Hospital*. Philadelphia, The Pennsylvania Hospital, 1938.

Paine, Thomas: *The Rights of Man* (1791). New York, Random House.

Paine, Thomas: *Common Sense* (1776). New York, Random House.

Roddis, Louis H.: *James Lind, Founder of Nautical Medicine*. London, Heinemann, 1951.

Rush, Benjamin: *The Autobiography of Benjamin Rush*. His "Travels Through Life" Together with his "Commonplace Book" for 1789–1813. Ed. by George W. Corner, Princeton, N.J., Princeton University Press, 1948.

Van Doren, Carl: *Benjamin Franklin's Autobiographical Writings*. New York, Viking Press, 1945.

Wardrop, James: *On Bloodletting*. London, J. B. Bailliere, 1835.

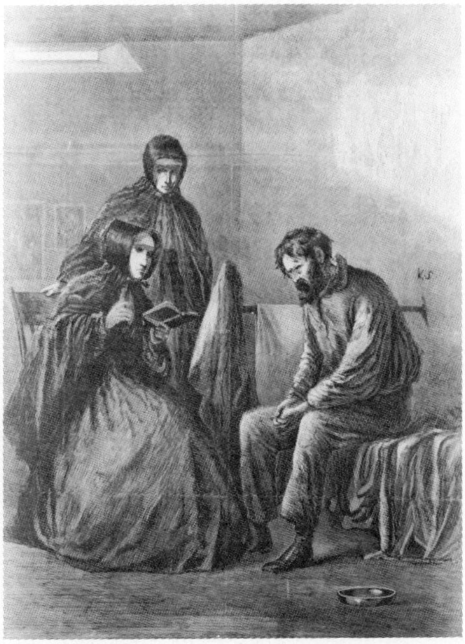

Sisters of Mercy visiting, consoling, and praying with a condemned man in the "Tombs," a famous prison in New York City. (Dolan collection.)

8 Response of Nursing to Health Problems of the Early Nineteenth Century

A survey of the nineteenth century reveals political, geographical, economic, medical and social expansion in a century of inventions, discoveries and creativity in every area of human endeavor. There were revolts, wars and emotional conflicts. In the United States, it was inevitable that the presence of slavery on democratic soil would bring into question the basic beliefs and principles woven into the fabric of the Constitution.

SOCIAL FORCES

There was upheaval in the agricultural and industrial areas because of the application of scientific knowledge to the techniques of production. Power-driven machinery replaced handcraft and human hands; it created mass production, but it also created new problems. The *Industrial Revolution* brought about poverty, overcrowding, disease and many other social problems.

Under the domestic system of manufacture, a man's work was done at home in a healthy country setting, with the assistance of his family. This work might have included carding, spinning, weaving, dyeing and many other skills. The craftsman owned his own tools, purchased whatever raw materials he needed and was in essence a small businessman.

The next step in the evolution of industrial production in England, and gradually elsewhere, was the development of a system of home industry. Under this system, a businessman with capital outlay would purchase large quantities of raw materials at lower prices. Skilled workers at home produced the finished product for the businessman, who had two concerns: purchasing raw materials and selling the manufac-

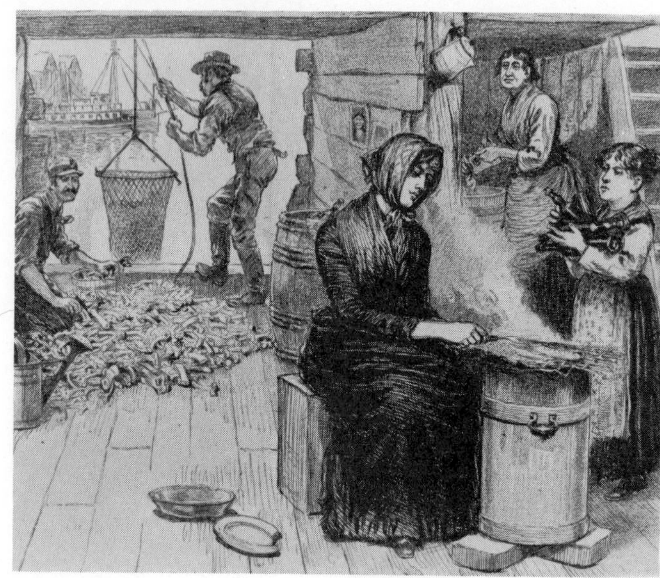

Figure 8–1. Women and children working under extremely unfavorable conditions. (Courtesy of New York Academy of Medicine and New York City Department of Health.)

tured product. The manufacturer was the man who worked in his home, his entire family contributing to his product or service.

In England, toward the end of the eighteenth century, a series of inventions revolutionized production; machinery replaced handcraft and the factory replaced the home as the work center. The manufacturer became a hired hand; his product was skilled labor. He was now dependent for lodging, whereas he once had his own cottage, usually in a rural setting. Factories were noisy and dirty, and the workers had to live close to their work, huddled together in poor, sunless homes. Although ultimately the inventions improved society, initially they caused a change for the worse in living conditions and brought about unemployment, which resulted in poverty, that social disease that is the parent of physical disease.

In England, the whole household worked, for low salaries (Fig. 8–1). Orphans were apprenticed to overseers of factories, and were treated cruelly, as were the "brick-yard children of England" (Figs. 8–2 and

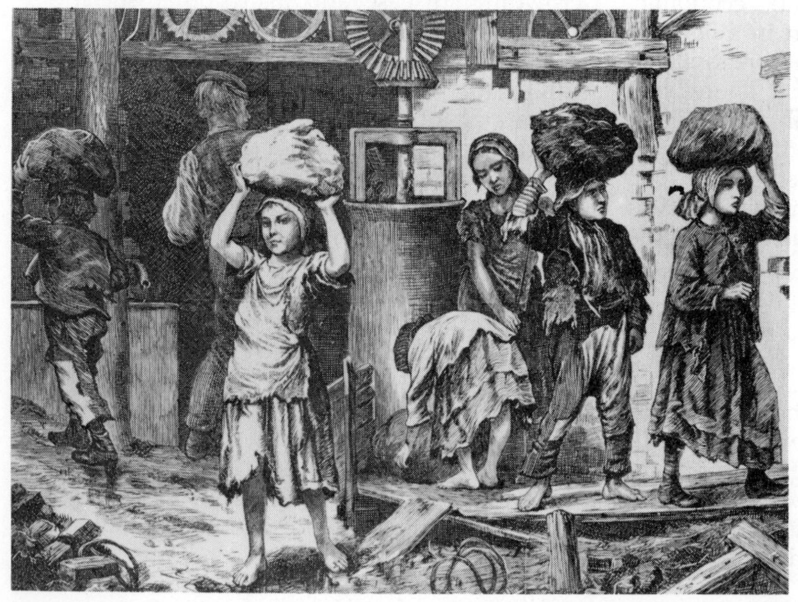

Figure 8–2. The highly publicized "brick-yard children" of England. The moral problems were publicized by the Children's Employment Commission in 1871. (Dolan collection.)

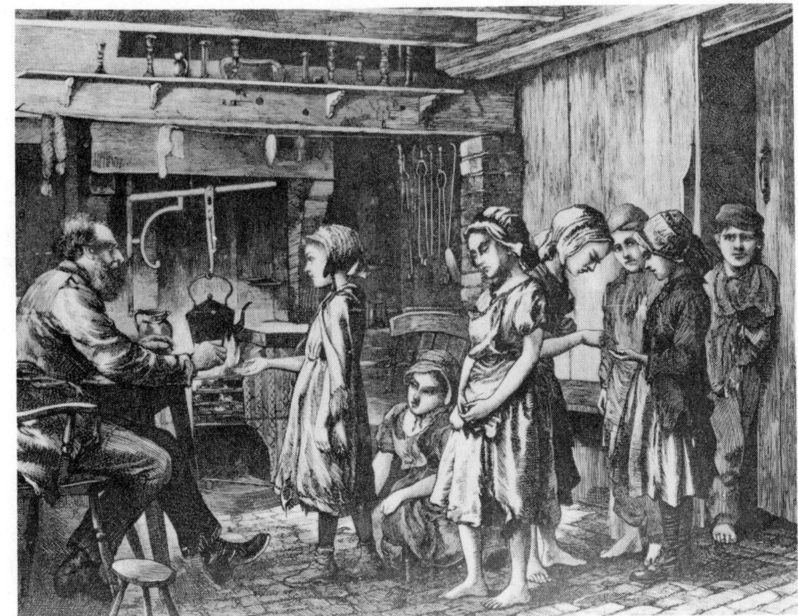

Figure 8–3. The English brick-yard children being paid in an inn where they were forced by their elders to buy beer. (Dolan collection.)

8–3). For wages, they were given poor food and were lodged in an attic or cellar. The same beds were used by two sets of children, one during the day and one at night. The working day was long, 15 to 16 hours even for children of five. The indignation that arose against these atrocities to children was expressed by Elizabeth Barrett Browning (1806–1861) in the poem "The Cry of the Children" (1843):

Alas, alas, the children! They are seeking
  Death in life, as best to have.
They are binding up their hearts away from breaking,
  With a cerement from the grave.
Go out, children, from the mine and from the city;
  Sing out, children, as the little thrushes do;
Pluck your handfuls of the meadow-cowslips pretty;
  Laugh aloud, to feel your fingers let them through.
But they answer, "Are your cowslips of the meadows
  Like our weeds anear the mine?
Leave us quiet in the dark of the coal-shadows,
  From your pleasures fair and fine.

"For oh!" say the children, "we are weary,
  And we cannot run or leap:
If we cared for any meadows, it were merely
  To drop down in them, and sleep.
Our knees tremble sorely in the stooping;
  We fall upon our faces, trying to go;
And, underneath our heavy eyelids drooping,
  The reddest flower would look as pale as snow;
For all day we drag our burden tiring.
  Through the coal-dark, underground;
Or all day we drive the wheels of iron
  In the factories, round and round."

Within the factories, there was little ventilation and no sunlight; these conditions, in addition to poor housing, constituted a serious health hazard, and many infectious diseases took a heavy toll in lives. Trouble was brewing, and riots broke out; unions began to be organized.

Philanthropists toiled to achieve the passage of laws to protect the workers and alleviate their unhealthy situation. In England, in 1819, an act was passed that required that no child under three years of age be employed, that 12 hours a day at work be the maximum for those under 16 years of age, that time for meals be allowed and that walls and ceilings be white-washed at least twice a year. The law was not enforced.

This act was followed in 1833 by the adoption by Parliament of a bill prohibiting night labor by those under 18 years of age and demanding that children from nine to 13 not work more than 48 hours a week, that those from 13 to 18 not work more than 68 hours a week and that children under nine not be employed. The conscience of the public was awakened at last. By

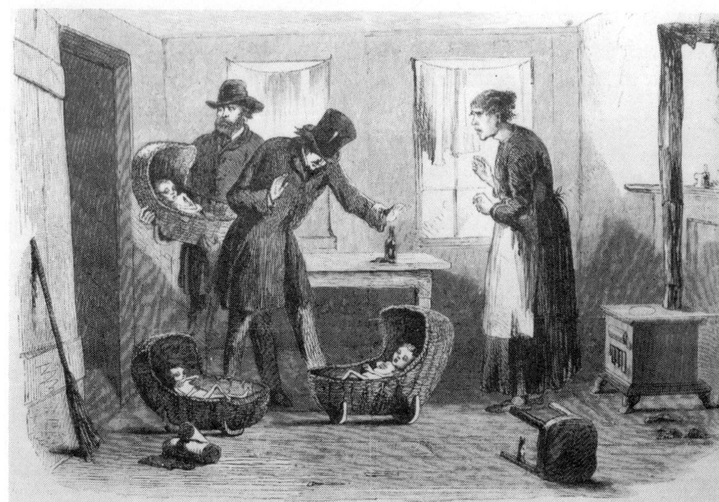

Figure 8–4. Mrs. Carlock and the emaciated and abused infants. (Dolan collection.)

1847, a ten-hour workday became a reality for women and young persons, while men continued to work for 12 or more hours a day.

Other evils, including bad housing, poor sanitation and lack of formal education, were noted. Women and children worked in mines as well as in factories.

Plight of the Child

In addition to the children who were orphaned and left homeless because of epidemics, *foundlings* were being abandoned in many countries, necessitating the construction of institutions to care for them. Public attitudes toward the homeless children were reflected in the names of institutions, such as "Home of the Friendless" and "Home for Little Wanderers."

The plight of children and the shocking treatment they received were highlighted in the infamous Carlock case in New York City (Fig. 8–4). A man who suspected his servant of theft obtained a warrant and went with a warrant officer to search the premises where the servant lived. They found an elderly woman housing three starving almshouse children. The evils of the almshouse system were exposed, including the health and social problems as-

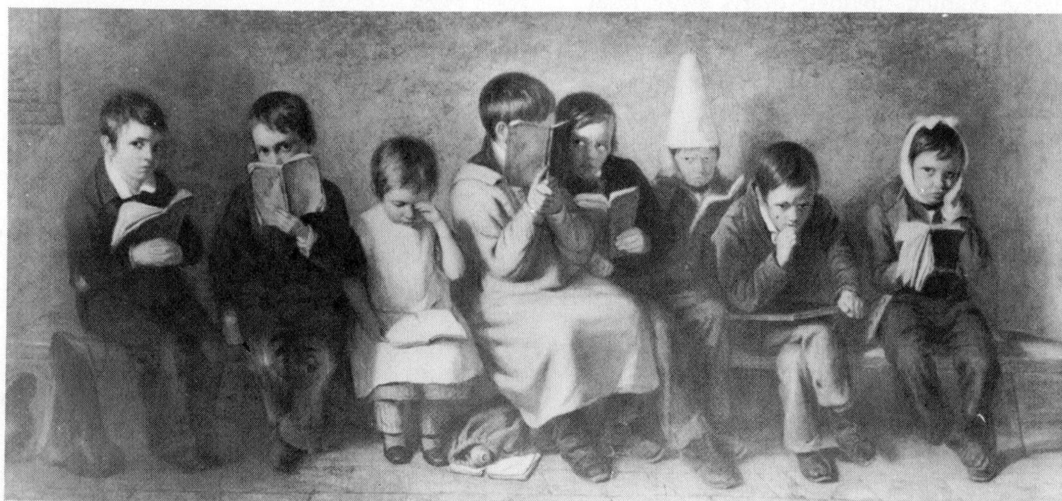

Figure 8–5. "The One-Room School." This setting could have a physically as well as psychologically unhealthy character. Note the presence of a communicable disease (child with mumps at right). (Dolan collection.)

sociated with wet-nursing, the apprenticeship system with its cruel indenture techniques and the high mortality rate of children.

Even when children were raised in their homes, the crowded condition of the one-room school encouraged the spread of disease and high mortality rates (Fig. 8–5).

DISEASE EPIDEMICS

Disease spread in awesome waves through working-class districts. *Cholera* was the devastating epidemic of the nineteenth century, with major outbreaks in 1832, 1849 and 1866 (Fig. 8–6).

Cholera had existed for centuries in India, and the earliest records indicate that Hindus worshipped the goddess of cholera, hoping to placate her so that they would be spared the evils of this dread disease. Other than in India, there was no extensive spread of cholera until the nineteenth century, when records indicate pandemic outbreaks. The disease was associated with abnormal climatic conditions, such as unusual flooding due to heavy rainfall, which were followed by famine and disease.

In England, it appears that the many reports of diseased cattle can be associated with Asiatic cholera. The cattle were slaughtered, and because of lack of public health laws, poor people purchased the diseased meat. Unfortunately, no one knew the real cause of this outbreak of disease. The filth of cities and the overcrowding of the population, together with the impure water supplies, the inadequate sewage disposal and the unhygienic living conditions, contributed to the outbreaks of cholera. It was because of the disastrous effects of cholera, however, that the local boards of health came into being in England, as well as in the United States.

In England, the board of health demanded that quarantine regulations be carried out. A special sign, placed on the front of a house, indicated that it was the dwelling of a person with the disease. Houses had to be "purified" by special methods after the death or recovery of a person suffering from cholera.

Fires were lighted in the streets and tar was burned. Clothes were washed in the river, which helped spread the disease to others, although this fact was not known.

Families deprived of income by the epidemic received food tickets. Soup kitchens were also set up, and records reveal the

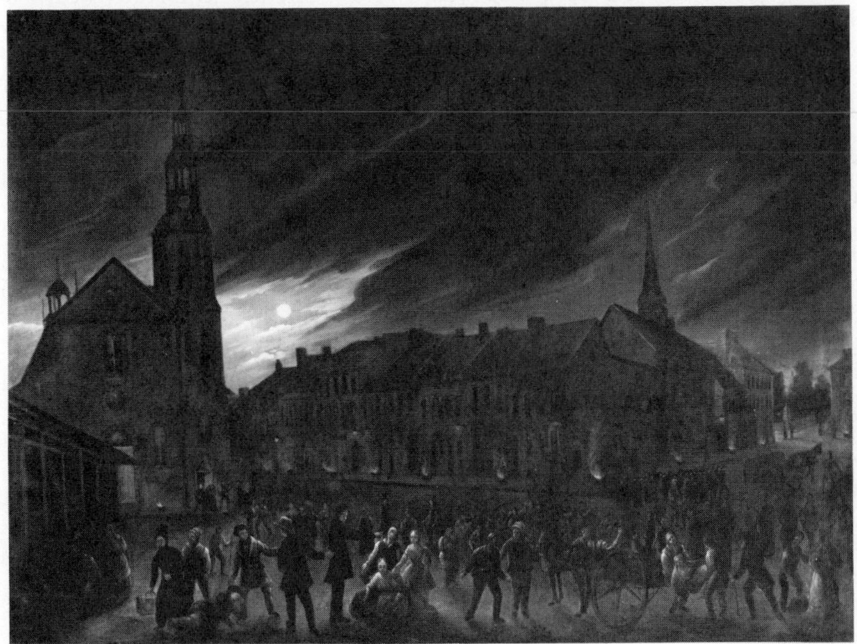

Figure 8–6. Cholera Plague in Quebec, by Joseph Legare (1795–1855). (Courtesy of the National Gallery of Canada, Ottawa.)

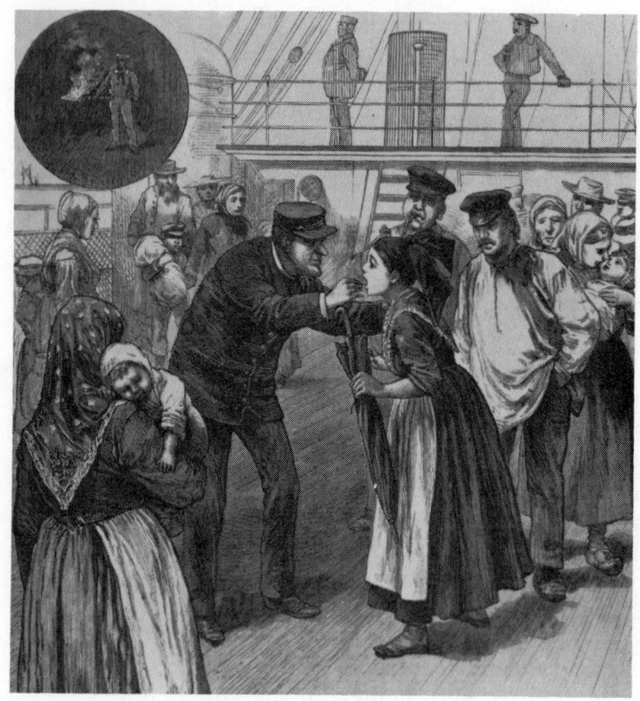

Figure 8–7. An attempt to inspect and quarantine at the immigration ports those who might have a contagious disease. (Courtesy of New York Academy of Medicine and New York City Department of Health.)

kindness and understanding shown by the poor to one another.

The disease was devastating. The best description of it appears on a monolith inscribed during the days of Alexander the Great: "The lips blue, the face haggard, the eyes hollow, the stomach sunk in, the limbs contracted and crumpled as if by fire. . . ."

At the time of the first cholera outbreak in the United States in 1832, it was considered to be the plight of the sinful. The disease seemed to be attracted to large cities, to be allied to poverty and slum dwelling and to be associated with the large numbers of immigrants. The disease spread across the country with the adventuresome forty-niners.

In 1866, when the Metropolitan Board of Health of the City of New York was instituted, clergy, physicians and municipal workers recognized that cholera outbreaks were preventable (Fig. 8–7). Rosenberg's book *The Cholera Years*[1] gives a dramatic and factual account of the panic and terror this disease caused in the United States and points to the continuing need for public health workers, including well-prepared community nursing workers.

Reading about the lack of understanding of the disease and the panic that ensued emphasizes that there was a need for a new science—the study of the life processes.

There was a growing awareness that health was the responsibility of the public and that the state had a definite duty to protect the public by wise legislation.

LIVING CONDITIONS

Providing an adequate or well-balanced diet was difficult. *Francois Appert*'s work on canning helped to add variety to the diet because more foods could be preserved.[2] Appert believed that applying heat to food sealed in an airtight container prevented it from spoiling. He was aware of the necessity of obtaining a proper seal. In America in 1819, the first canning establishment using Appert's technique was set up in Boston. Outbreaks of disease due to food spoilage occurred occasionally.

[1]Rosenberg, Charles: *The Cholera Years*. Chicago, The University of Chicago Press, 1962.

[2]Appert, F.: *Art of Preserving All Kinds of Animal and Vegetable Substances*. London, Black, Perry & Kingsbury, 1811.

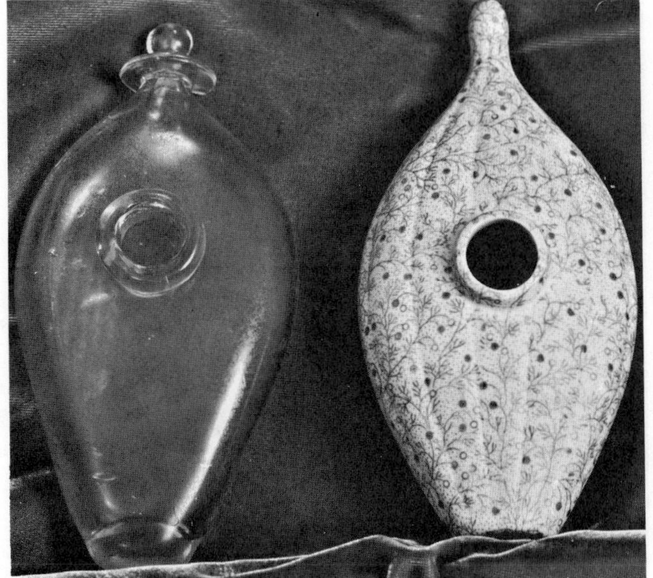

Figure 8–8. Nursing bottles used during the late eighteenth and early nineteenth centuries. One is of blown glass with a glass nipple; the other is of porcelain that probably matched the family's china. (Dolan collection.)

In 1853, Gail Borden perfected the process for manufacturing condensed milk, which was immediately used in feeding babies and was responsible for saving many of their lives.

The steam pressure autoclave was utilized beginning in 1874, and the new science of bacteriology was applied to the food preservation industry. Refrigerators were unheard of, but ice chests or iceboxes were in vogue. Large chunks of ice were placed in these boxes, but the ice melted, and consequently, food spoiled. Frequently, ice was obtained from a contaminated water supply and acted as an avenue of disease transmission (Fig. 8–9).

Proud mothers brought newborn babies to the local grocery shop to be weighed on the same scales that were used for weighing meat and produce thus increasing the risk of contamination (Fig. 8–10).

Keeping a sickroom warm and free from smoke from wood-burning stoves or fireplaces was a difficult problem. Furnaces in which coal rather than wood was the fuel became available around 1850.

The *sanitary conditions* needed scrutiny. Outdoor toilet facilities (privies) were com-

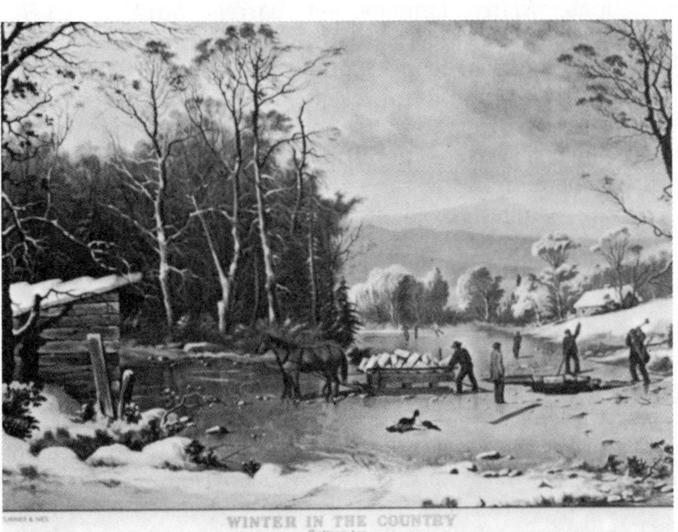

Figure 8–9. A Currier and Ives print of ice cutting from a pond in which the water could have been contaminated. (Dolan collection.)

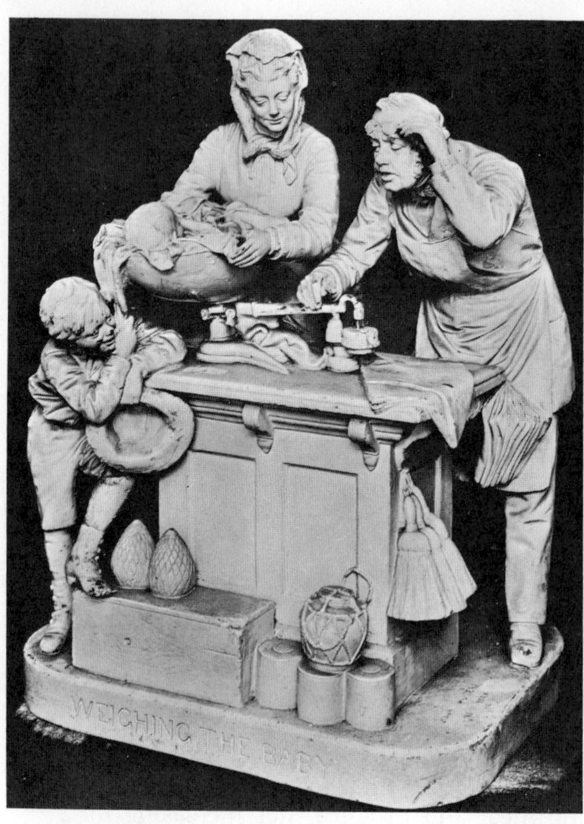

Figure 8–10. Weighing the Baby. A statuette by John Rogers (1877). (Dolan collection.)

monly used. Gradually, these were replaced by indoor flush toilets by those people who could afford this improvement. Indoor plumbing was slow in reentering the historical picture. Water was brought into homes through a water system composed chiefly of hollowed-out wooden logs. Eventually, cast iron pipes replaced the logs. Many families set barrels out in the yard to catch rain water. They realized the value of conservation of natural resources. In outlying areas, wells provided the water for the household. All water supplies served as potential sources for the transmission of infection. The quality of the water needed improving because pollutants came in contact with the water supply and thereby caused contamination.

The removal of sewage was another serious problem. Community water supplies to assist in the removal and disposal of sewage were slow to evolve. This problem was partially solved by draining this water through a system of sewerage pipes. In 1829, a slow sand filtration system to remove impurities from the water was constructed in London. In time, other filtration systems appeared.

Epidemics of cholera, yellow fever, smallpox, diphtheria, scarlet fever, dysentery, typhus and typhoid were devastating to the people of the nineteenth century. Contaminated water played a role in the transmission of disease, as did food, utensils and persons who were disease carriers.

An early public health reformer was *Lemuel Shattuck* (1793–1859), a former teacher who was engaged in the book-selling business. In 1842, he was instrumental in achieving the passage of a law in Massachusetts that resulted in statewide registration of vital statistics. In 1845, he compiled and published a *Census of Boston* that encouraged and stimulated accurate reporting of statistics in the United States. Shattuck's census presented the shocking facts of a high mortality rate, including an unbelievably high infant and maternal mortality rate. His crowning achievement came in 1850 when the results of his efforts were published by the Massachusetts Sanitary Commission. The Shattuck Report, one of the first public health documents in the United States, was a milestone in the evolution of the field of public health. Shattuck recommended the establishment of state and local health departments or boards of health and emphasized the need for sanitary surveys.

PROGRESS IN NURSING

With the dawn of the nineteenth century, the actual care of the sick again became the responsibility of the "wise women" of the community. Tender, loving care was given to friends as well as family. Every bride purchased or received a cookbook that, in addition to rules and recipes to develop culinary skills, always had a section on first aid and the care of the sick. When one became ill, there were instructions such as the following:

> For a sudden attack of Quinsy or Croup, or a cold that is tight on the lungs, bathe the neck with bear's grease and pour it down the throat. Goose grease or any kind of oily grease is as good as bear's grease. Onions stewed in molasses are loosening. Put draughts of wilted horseradish leaves on the feet. A drop or two of skunk's oil or hen's oil on a lump of sugar will loosen up a cold.[3]

This seems to be a period when lubrication of the "bronchial tubes" and the entire respiratory tract was advocated. The major care of the sick was given at home with home remedies; for example, the heart of a baked onion placed in the ear was used to withdraw the "trouble" from the afflicted middle ear. If these remedies were unsuccessful, the local physician was called. Many herb medicines made at home were basic preparations, and treatments such as poultices similar to the one previously mentioned, which was composed of "onions stewed in molasses," were resorted to frequently. Mustard footbaths seemed to be considered good for everything.

The medicines that were not concocted at home were procurable from the patent medicine man as he traveled from town to town, or obtainable as proprietary preparations in the apothecary shops. Burdick's Blood Bitters, Ayer's Cherry Pectoral and Lydia Pinkham's Vegetable Compound were popular examples of patent medicines. Traveling patent medicine peddlers sold such things as Snake Oil and Kickapoo Extract to gullible buyers, then promptly left town.

Most families kept sick members at home. The well-known picture, "The Doctor," presents a sickroom vigil with the members of the family waiting for the crisis to be reached and passed (Fig. 8–11). Pneumonia was one of the most-feared diseases.

The care given to patients in their homes was very different from that given in hospitals. Only the very poor or homeless went to hospitals. Because hospital conditions were deplorable, respectable people believed it a disgrace to send their relatives there.

The most expert person at healing in the family cared for the sick. Neighbors volunteered for "night watching," and although they were unskilled, they ensured that medicines were given and new symptoms were reported. In the early nineteenth century, there were few physicians; therefore, nurses prescribed for those in need.

There were a good many "monthly" (obstetric) nurses in those days whose duties involved midwifery.

HOSPITALS

Hospitals were unattractive in structural design and psychological atmosphere. Pest houses were part of the hospital complex. Most hospitals were crowded and were filled with the critically ill and dying. Having adequate beds and pillows was the exception rather than the rule.

In 1736, *Bellevue Hospital* in New York City had only a small ward for the sick. It was situated where New York's city hall now stands. For some time it was used only as a "pest house."

In 1811, the city purchased a tract of land, named Belle View, on which the cornerstone for the hospital was laid in 1811. The hospital was opened for occupancy in 1816. By a ruling of the Common Council in 1825 the name Bellevue Hospital was adopted. The original plan provided for cells for unruly patients and prisoners, apartments for maternity patients and sixty rooms, forty-one of which were set aside for paupers. Women inmates of the almshouse did the cooking, laundry and gave what nursing care was available. In 1837, an investigation was made that found con-

[3]*The Documtur Housewife—The Fruit of Experience freshly gathered from Elderly Lips, and preserved in print. A Guide to Domestic Cookery as it is practiced in the Connecticut Valley.* 1805, pp. 1–3.

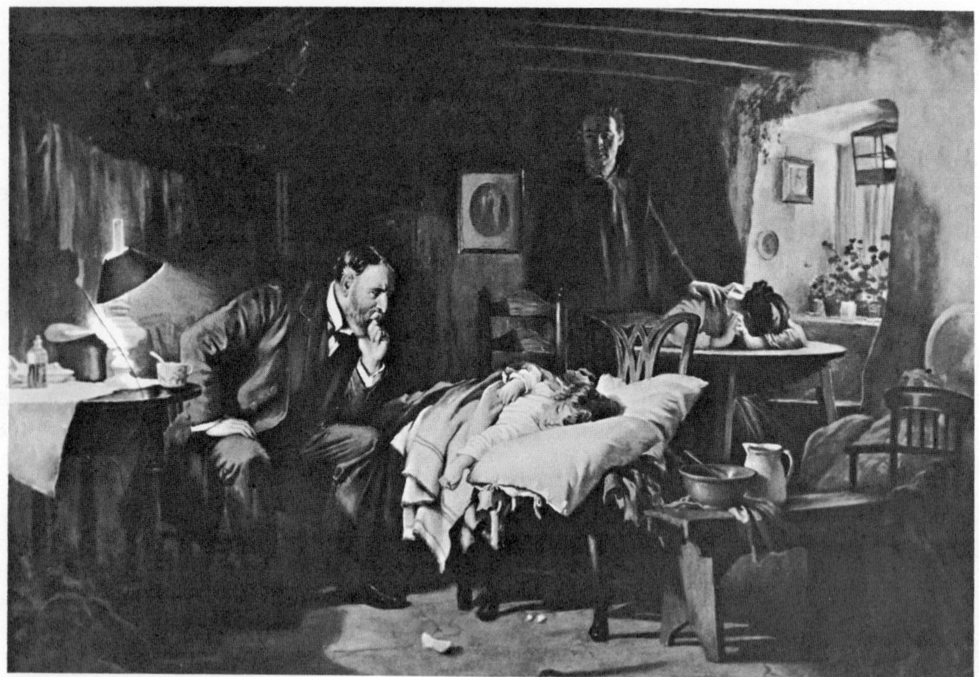

Figure 8–11. The Doctor. (Dolan collection.)

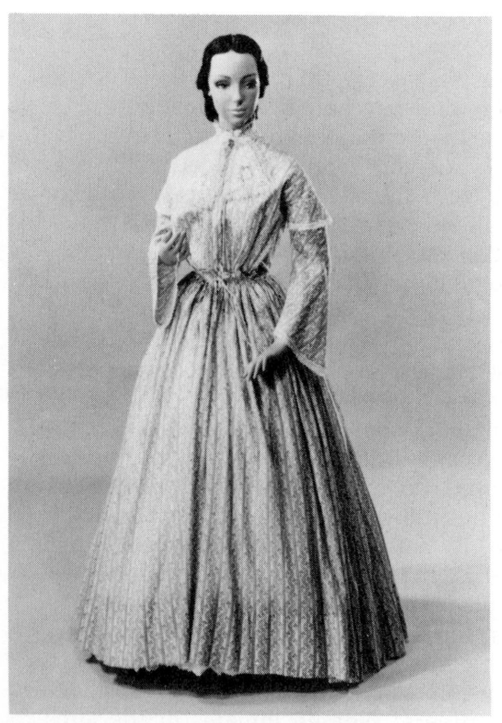

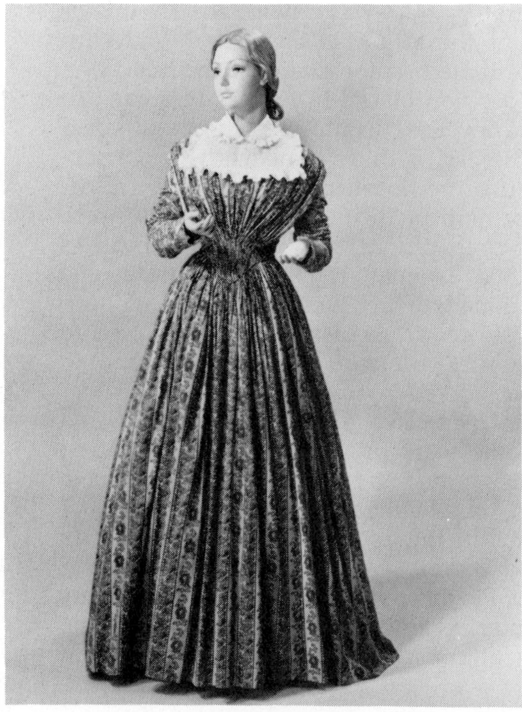

Figure 8–12. Early American (ca. 1840) "maternity dress" *(left)* and "nursing dress" *(right)*. The latter has concealed darts fashioned with hooks and eyes to facilitate nursing. (Courtesy of Wadsworth Atheneum.)

ditions at Bellevue to be unspeakable, and the pest house, prison, and later the psychiatric wards were removed to Blackwell's Island. The poorhouse continued under the same roof with the hospital until 1848. No better attention was given the sick; the dirt and neglect were shocking and the death rate was 25 per cent. Upon the creation of a medical board in 1847, matters improved slightly, but treatment of the sick remained most deplorable.

Blockley Hospital of Philadelphia was also a combination poorhouse, insane asylum and hospital. (During the Revolution the inmates were freed by the British troops.) All the work in the place, including the nursing, was supposed to be done by the inmates. An investigation in 1793 brought to light shocking conditions but did not result in any improvements. In 1832, the problem was reviewed again, and Bishop Kendrick of Emmitsburg was persuaded to send a group of Sisters of Charity to undertake the task of reform. Their work so effectually transformed the hospital that they were asked to remain, but the bishop was not of like mind. After they left, conditions again grew unsatisfactory and remained so until *Alice Fisher*, a Nightingale nurse, arrived in 1884.

Hospital patients were penniless folk, usually homeless and friendless. In most of the city hospitals the nursing was done by inmates usually over 50 years old, many being 70 and 80. Physicians sent elderly people to serve as nurses in the wards, because they could get better food there.

There was practically no night nursing, except for the "night watchers" provided for women in childbirth and the dying.

An article in *Harper's Weekly* in 1859 presents an interesting picture of the *New Orleans Charity Hospital*. Admissions that year were 11,337; 2290 died. During the yellow fever epidemic of the preceding year, 2727 patients were admitted with this disease, and 1382 died. A miasmometer was used for detection of organic impurities.

Dr. James J. Walsh, in *The History of Nursing*, writes:

> Hospitals were as a rule in a disgraceful state of degradation. They were dirty and ill ventilated, they reeked with infection, so that patients who came in suffering from one disease, or from a wound, caught another disease or some virulent infection. The death rate was fearfully high, sometimes actually more than 50 per cent. In the days before Lister, hospital surgery was extremely discouraging. The only nurses that could be obtained for hospitals were women who did the menial work besides caring for the patients.[4]

Prejudice against hospitals arose here, as in Europe, because of the neglect and ill treatment of patients and because the death rate from infections was high. A writer as late as 1877, in speaking of maternity hospitals, remarked, "Experience has taught us that any kind of a home is a safer place for a woman to be delivered in than any hospital; but there are cases with no homes who must be provided for." The change in the attitude of the public toward hospitals indicates how radical has been the change in hospital conditions.

NURSING LEADERSHIP

Religious Nursing Orders

Almost the only good hospital nursing was done by religious orders. "The beautiful order enforced by their gentle discipline, their self-denial, patience, skill and tact, were the effect of Christian charity on the sympathetic hearts of intelligent women."[5] Their gentle manner, dignity and poise were models for all nurses.

At the request of Archbishop Du Bourg of the Order of St. Sulpice, the first American religious order in the United States was founded by Mother Elizabeth Seton in 1809.

Elizabeth Ann Bayley Seton (1774–1821) (Fig. 8–13), who in 1976 became the first American-born person to be canonized, was born in New York at a momentous time in history. Her father, Dr. Richard Bayley, was one of the leading physicians of his day and was the first professor of anatomy at King's College, now Columbia University. He was also the health officer of the Port of New York, was responsible for the development of the quarantine laws of the State of New York and was given authority to administer them. Elizabeth, a beautiful and popular young lady, married

[4]Walsh, James J: *The History of Nursing*.

[5]Wise, T. W.: *Review of the History of Medicine*.

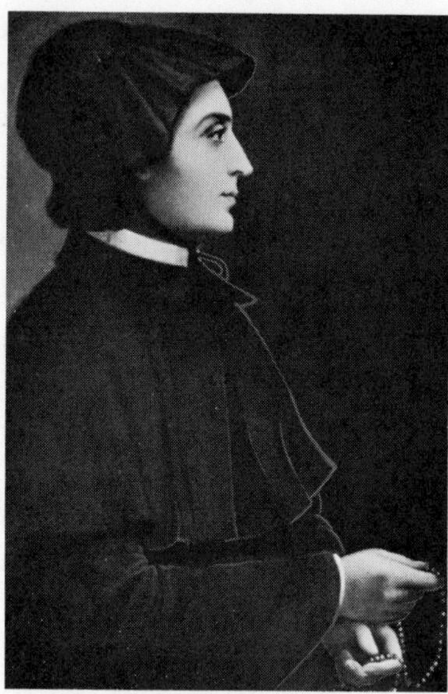

Figure 8–13. Saint Elizabeth Ann Bayley Seton. (Courtesy of St. Joseph's College, Emmitsburg, Md.)

William Seton, a banker, in 1794. The marriage was a most happy one.

Elizabeth Seton demonstrated an interest in helping people in times of need. In 1797, she and other society matrons formed the Widow's Society in New York. This organization, which was dedicated to public charity, was the Protestant equivalent of St. Vincent de Paul's Ladies of Charity. These women raised money for poor widows and visited them in their homes to nurse and comfort them.

The Setons traveled to Italy, leaving New York when an epidemic of yellow fever was raging. On arrival in Italy, all passengers were quarantined in a grim and loathsome lazaretto, or pest house. Mr. Seton, already in a weakened condition, succumbed to a fatal infection. When Mrs. Seton returned to America, she had to face financial ruin and its tragedies. Meanwhile she had joined the Catholic Church.

An interest in teaching prompted her to open a school for girls in Baltimore, which marked the beginning of the parochial school system of education in the United States. A choice spot of land at Emmitsburg was selected for the school. Immediately, applications were received from young women who wished to join her and become sisters in this new teaching order.

In 1809, Mother Elizabeth Seton, with her newly formed religious family attired in a habit that resembled Mrs. Seton's own widow's dress, arrived in Emmitsburg. This group was interested in affiliating with the community of the Sisters of Charity founded by St. Vincent de Paul. Requests from Mother Seton's sisters for nuns to come from Paris to America to explain the Rule of St. Vincent and help them to become established properly was denied by Napoleon. The rule had to be adapted to the needs of the American group.

The Sisters of Charity at Emmitsburg in 1809 was divided into seven different branches. Leadership opportunities were provided in nursing education, delivery of nursing service and parochial education.

In 1850, the sisters at Emmitsburg officially united with the world-wide community of Sisters of Charity of St. Vincent de Paul, at which time the habit of blue with the large linen headdress or "cornette" was adopted. The Sisters of Charity of New York, referred to as the Black Cap Sisters of Charity, wore the headdress and habit originally worn by the founding group. The Sisters of Charity of Greensburg, Pennsylvania, although a separate entity, also chose a black cap and habit. The Sisters of Charity of New Jersey, Halifax, and Cincinnati substituted a veil for the cap but wore the original dress or habit worn before the affiliation with the Paris Sisters of Charity of St. Vincent de Paul.

In 1812, the Sisters of Charity of Nazareth, Kentucky, was founded by *Mother Catherine Spalding*. The sisters incorporated the care of the sick in their homes into their daily work. They went on horseback to the homes of their patients. This order included teachers and nurses.

In 1823, the Baltimore Infirmary, later the University of Maryland Hospital, was established by six professors as a private proprietary school in a clinical setting. There were four wards and two resident students. These medical resident students were required to pay $300 a year, in advance, for board, room and laundry. The visits of the medical and surgical staff men were paid for every day at noon by the institution. Only patients who were acutely ill were admitted, and they were required to pay a fee of $3.00 a week, which included room, meals and care. This hospital did not furnish any material assistance to the visiting doctors or professors. They had to use their own medicines, bandages, instruments and even their own leeches.

Soon after they opened the Baltimore Infirmary, these six professors sent a request to Emmitsburg for Sisters of Charity to staff the hospital. Their request was granted. The sisters had charge of hospital housekeeping and the kitchen and laundry, supervised the wards and administered simple care and medications. Treatments were carried out by the house doctor or resident—this was a learning experience for him.

In 1829, *the Sisters of Our Lady of Mercy,* of Charleston, South Carolina, undertook an unusual assignment—staffing the Hospital of the Society of Working Men. The Brotherhood of Saint Marino, an association of mechanics and laborers, was the motivating force behind the inception of this hospital and assumed its financial support. The society evolved because of the need for a place to house and take care of homeless men.

Demands for nursing care by the various religious orders became very great. Epidemics, though an added burden, were handled with courage and skill, and visiting nurses served an important function. The Sisters of Mercy offered their services to the board of health during outbreaks of cholera and yellow fever. When epidemics subsided, many children were left orphaned, and institutions were needed to care for them. St Vincent's Infirmary in Louisville, Kentucky, was opened mainly to house the orphans left after a cholera epidemic.

Another charitable endeavor was the establishment of homes for unwed mothers (Fig. 8–14).

Sisters staffed psychiatric hospitals, such as the state-sponsored Maryland Hospital in Baltimore, which was under the supervision of the Sisters of Charity until 1840. Then, the Sisters opened a private institution for psychiatric patients that was later called the Mt. Hope Retreat.

Many religious orders contributed their efforts to alleviate the sickness and tribulations of this period. Their efforts are evidenced in the many hospitals constructed and serviced by them.

Sister Mary Aikenhead, who was trained in England, founded the *Irish Sisters of Charity* about 1815. They did social work among the poor and public health and hospital nursing during epidemics of plague, cholera and typhus. At Cork in 1831, during a cholera epidemic, the people were afraid to enter hospitals until they learned that the Sisters of Charity were working there.

Mother Aikenhead wished for a sister's hospital in Dublin and sent three nuns to be trained at the Hôpital de la Pitié in Paris. They remained there a year. Upon their return, a hospital of twelve beds was established, which grew rapidly into an excellent institution. They organized other hospitals and an asylum for the blind. In 1857, they went to Australia and continued their work.

During the early nineteenth century, a gentle but dynamic leader founded a religious community whose contributions to

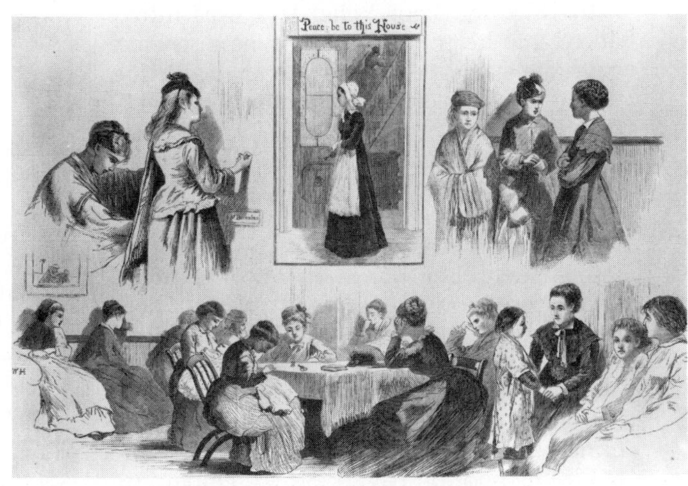

Figure 8–14. Scenes at a home for unwed mothers as depicted by Winslow Homer. (Dolan collection.)

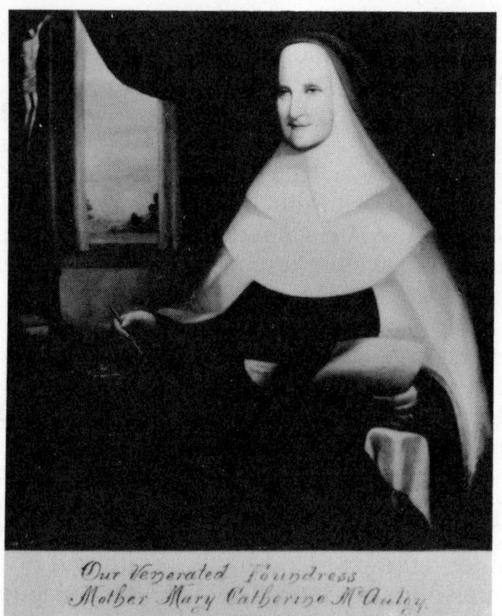

Figure 8–15. Mother Mary Catherine McAuley. (Dolan collection.)

nursing has been of historical significance. *Mary Catherine McAuley* (1781–1841) (Fig. 8–15), foundress of the Congregation of Our Lady of Mercy, was born during a critical political and social crisis in Ireland's history. The Anglo-Irish tensions were being severely felt in every area of life. The political edicts had reduced the majority of the Irish to paupers and had encouraged begging. Manufacture dwindled; hundreds were thrown out of work, food was difficult to afford and personal savings were usurped to pay for the expenses of England's foreign wars. The animosity of the English towards the Irish was obvious.

In 1838, the Poor Relief Law was introduced into Ireland. This unfortunate scheme gave alms but no employment and introduced the despised "workhouse system" that was in force in England. This system compelled the impoverished to live in a workhouse—even those who needed but temporary assistance, all who lived in the workhouse became permanent paupers. Immediately their homes were confiscated, their possessions were seized or sold, their families were separated and their freedom was lost. Both Protestants and Catholics objected to this form of relief.

Conditions were desperate when Catherine McAuley opened a house for the relief of the poor on Baggot Street, Dublin, in 1827. She was uniquely qualified to understand and mitigate the woes of the poor. Catherine became an impoverished orphan at the age of eleven, an heiress at sixteen and then the legal ward of wealthy non-Catholic relatives. In response to her own experiences, she shared her intellectual gifts, her unbounded compassion and her material assets with the less fortunate.

It was Mother McAuley's great desire to provide an organization to visit the sick, instruct youth and protect poor girls of good character. From her plans emerged the order of *Sisters of Mercy* in 1831, which ministered to the poor, the sick and the ignorant. Catherine McAuley was seen in the slums of Dublin providing temporal and spiritual sustenance.

During a severe outbreak of Asiatic cholera in 1832, the Sisters of Mercy were recognized for their excellent nursing care. Their number increased as did the quality of their efforts during the tragedy of the *Great Famine.*

Mother McAuley's order spread to many countries including England, with the foundation of an order at Bermondsey in the year 1839. The Sisters of Mercy have served as nurses in hospitals, homes and prisons and as educators at all academic levels; they have provided superb nursing care in the Crimean War, the Spanish American War, World Wars I and II and the Vietnam War.

Many of the first hospitals in American cities were named Mercy Hospitals and were under the aegis of the Sisters of Mercy. The Sisters of Mercy have been applauded for visiting prisoners in their cells, as Harper's Weekly, in 1868, notes, "they never argue, discuss or theorise about religion, but help the convicts in the only practical, useful and efficient ways. . . . They furnish money to needy relatives and to the men themselves when they come out of prison. They never inquire into a man's crimes; all they ask is to be told of his troubles and worries and to be allowed to do what they can to relieve them."[6]

Many Roman Catholic nursing orders sent members to America for missionary work. Nuns came from Ireland, France, Germany, Italy, Spain and Portugal.

The *Sisters of St. Joseph,* the *Sisters of*

[6]Walsh, James J.: *Those Splendid Sisters.* New York, Sears, 1927, p. 137.

Charity of Nazareth and the *Ursuline* nuns had many houses and hospitals. The *Sisters of St. Mary,* who worked in St. Louis in the 1880s, were called the "smallpox sisters" because of their work with this dreaded disease.

At the time of the Civil War, the larger and better hospitals were those staffed by Roman Catholic nuns. The *Alexian Brothers* were involved in hospital work by 1870.

A social reformer of note was *Mrs. Elizabeth Gurney Fry* (1780–1845), whose work in prison reform has been recognized throughout the world. Elizabeth Gurney was a deeply religious Quaker who married Joseph Fry and settled in London. As an active member of the Society of Friends, she decided to seek admittance to *Newgate Prison* to attempt to reform the criminals; this was an early rehabilitation project.

In 1813, she visited Newgate and was horror stricken at the conditions and the treatment of the poor prisoners incarcerated there (Fig. 8–16). The prison was cold, dark, damp and poorly ventilated. The prisoners were meagerly fed, not properly clothed and not segregated. Thieves, murderers, sex offenders, the mentally ill and the mentally retarded—all were housed together. Many children were inmates of this institution.

Mrs. Fry asked to talk to the women prisoners. Armed men were offered to protect her from this snarling mob. She refused their protection, and her quiet manner, somber dress and genuine interest in them calmed the unruly group. Later, she brought food and clothing and soap and towels for the children as well as the adults; she commenced a program of instruction for the children that was later attended by the women; she provided the women with sewing materials so that they might earn a livelihood when released. She inspired some of her friends to come and read to them as they worked.

Elizabeth Fry was an eloquent and forceful speaker, and after visiting prisons in the British Isles and in Europe, she endeavored to share her findings with the public. She made them aware of the need for reform in nursing and in hospitals as well as in prisons.

Mrs. Fry was an example of human kind-

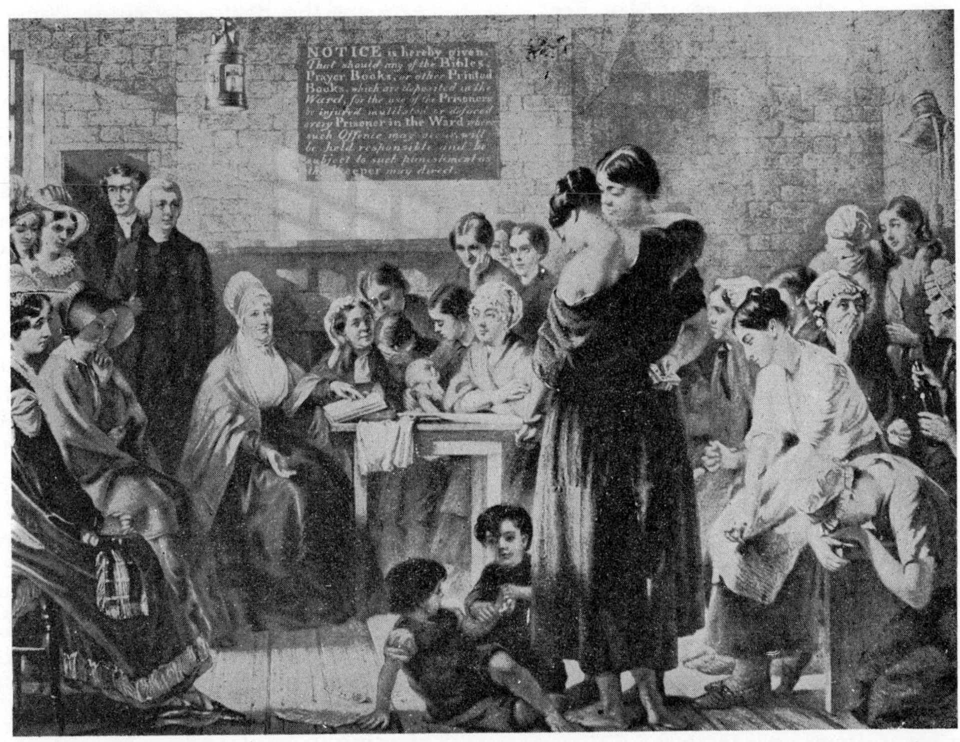
NOTICE is hereby given.
That should any of the Bibles,
Prayer Books, or other Printed
Books, which are deposited in the
Ward, for the use of the Prisoners
every Prisoner in the Ward
such Offence may
be held responsible and be
subject to such punishment as
may direct.

Figure 8–16. Elizabeth Fry reading to the prisoners at Newgate Prison, 1823. (From Whitney: *Elizabeth Fry, Quaker Heroine*. Boston, Little, Brown & Co., 1937.)

ness to people who had received relatively little of it from life. She urged careful trials for offenders, planted the idea for reform schools, stressed the need for psychiatric patients to be separated from criminals and insisted that criminal offenders needed moral assistance in hospitals rather than punishment in jails.

In England in 1840, the group of ardent helpers who assisted her so capably in her crusade were organized and called the *Society of Protestant Sisters of Charity*. Their primary objective was to supply nurses for the sick of all classes in their homes. This group was motivated by deep religious convictions but was secular in organization. They became the *Institution of Nursing Sisters*.

The work of Mrs. Fry had a profound influence on many people, including a young Lutheran minister, *Theodor Fliedner* (1800–1864) (Fig. 8–17). He was appointed pastor of a church in Kaiserswerth, Germany, in 1822. Shortly after his arrival, the main industry of this little community failed, and the people had financial difficulties. Pastor Fliedner set out on a tour to raise funds and returned with money and ideas for a program of social work prompted by the efforts and achievements of Mrs. Fry.

Pastor Fliedner married Frederika Münster

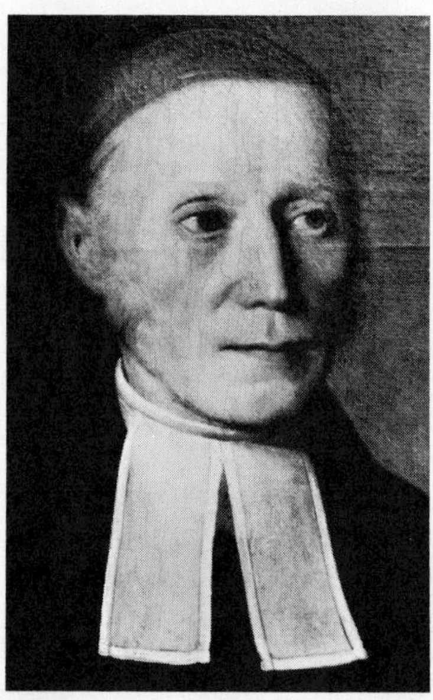

Figure 8–17. Pastor Theodor Fliedner. (Courtesy of Kaiserswerth Institute. Copyright by Hans Lachmann.)

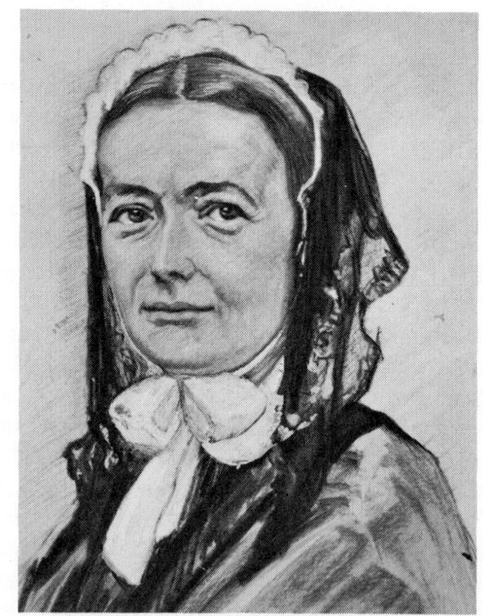

Figure 8–18. Frederika Münster Fliedner. (Courtesy of Kaiserswerth Institute.)

(Fig. 8–18) in 1828, and they raised a family of ten children. Inspired by her husband, Frederika Fliedner organized a Woman's Society for visiting and nursing the sick poor in their homes, but it was inadequate to meet the heavy demand. Women prisoners and children released from jails needed schools and hospitals as well as nursing care. The Fliedners opened their home in 1833 to these released prisoners.

Recognition of the need for the services of women in the Protestant church sparked the restoration of the ancient order of Deaconesses. Pastor Fliedner and his wife became the crusading spirits of this movement and, in 1836, founded the *Kaiserswerth Institute for the Training of Deaconesses*.

They purchased the largest, finest house available in Kaiserswerth, and by the end of the first year, seven hard-working young women were in training. Pastor Fliedner, like St. Vincent de Paul, wanted youthful, enthusiastic girls of refinement with healthy bodies, good moral standards and character, who were twenty-five years of age or over and were desirous of caring for the sick. The daughter of a physician, *Gertrude Reichard*, was the first to become a deaconess. Each woman was consecrated for her work by the laying on of hands and a blessing.

The Fliedners were well qualified to di-

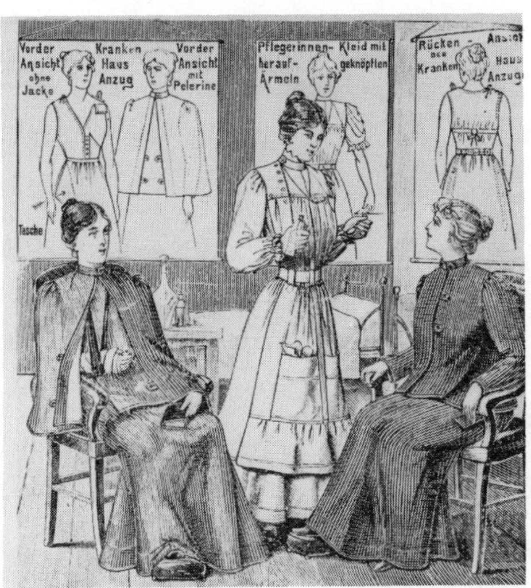

Figure 8–19. The teaching function of the nurse was emphasized by the deaconesses. Clothing was designed to fit the needs of the patients. (Dolan collection.)

rect the educational endeavors of this order. They organized training centers for the teachers of nursery schools (called infant schools), elementary schools, vocational schools and high schools. They opened an orphanage and kindergarten, which provided learning experience for the student teachers. In addition, they directed the school for nurses and the hospital, which also served as a training and practice center for the students.

The dress of the deaconess was a plain blue cotton gown with a white apron, a large turned-down collar and a white muslin cap with a frill around the face that tied beneath the chin with a large white bow. Outdoors they wore long black cloaks and black bonnets over their caps. (Fig. 8–19)

The initial course of instruction consisted of housework, bookkeeping, letter writing and oral reading. The student made a choice between becoming a teacher or a nurse. In addition to her hospital experience, the student was given instruction in visiting nursing in the village under Mrs. Fliedner's supervision. Frederika Fliedner very forcefully assisted her nurses in establishing independence with regard to physicians, the clergy and the hospital governing bodies and authorities.

According to the original plan, these deaconesses took no vows but made a simple promise "to work for Christ"; they received no salary and were taken care of for life. This is the so-called *motherhouse system*, which, like the monastic system, provides its members with a permanent home so that when deaconesses are sent out to private duty, to other hospitals, to do visiting nursing or to distant mission fields, they are always under the protection of their home organization. Their work is chiefly among the poor. Deaconesses may work in almshouses, direct orphanages, teach children, work among prisoners or unfortunate women or do private nursing. They have helped in many epidemics and in many wars.

Early schools for nurses utilized much from the deaconess organizations and borrowed many organizational ideas from Mrs. Fliedner, such as preliminary grouping (long called "probation"), the physician's certificate of health, usually a clergymen's certificate, money allowances, regular classes and lectures, a special etiquette and having a woman superintendent in full charge. They did not admit "lady probationers," as did the English hospitals, but insisted that all nurses be on the same social level. They required that nurses sent out to private duty be treated as members of the family, not as servants, and they saw to it that nurses were allowed proper time for rest.

After Frederika Fliedner died in 1842, Pastor Fliedner married *Caroline Bertheau*, who continued this very worthy project. It soon seemed essential to give brief instruction in the care of the sick to the women of the community. This endeavor had two objectives: helping the women of the community to do a better job of caring for their families and providing a reservoir of lay nurse helpers.

Kaiserswerth remained the motherhouse for many deaconess institutes throughout the world, and the graduates of the deaconess program went to all areas bringing an atmosphere of peace and love to the sick and needy (Figs. 8–20 and 8–21).

Communities and physicians were becoming aware of the value of better-prepared religious as well as lay women in caring for the sick. In 1841, a physician asked for a nurse to work in his dispensary; her work was to be preventive in character. She was to instruct mothers in the care of the sick in homes, to ask if all

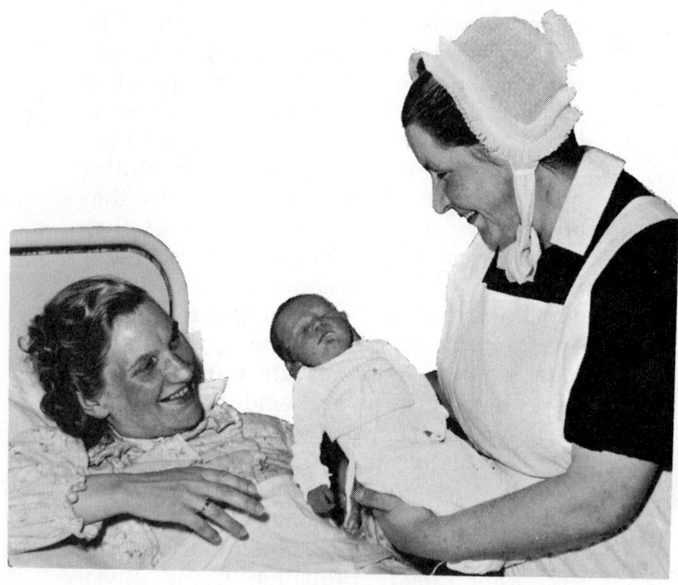

Figure 8–20. A deaconess rejoicing with a mother. (Courtesy of Kaiserswerth Institute.)

members of the family had been vaccinated, to report illnesses and to teach ways of cooking inexpensive foods.

Pastor Fliedner's influence extended to America when in 1849, with four deaconesses, he arrived in Pittsburgh. They were to assume responsibility for the *Pittsburgh Infirmary* (now *Passavant Hospital*). This was the first Protestant church hospital in the United States. *William Passavant,* a clergyman, requested the assistance of Pastor Fliedner in getting permission for the deaconesses to come to this country. Their intent, to establish a motherhouse to educate sisters for this country, became a reality in 1850. The first American deaconess was *Louisa Marthens,* who was consecrated on May 28, 1850.

Jacobs[7] has indicated that Pastor Passavant's plan was too progressive for his parish to undertake; therefore, it was never an extensive project. The quality of the work of the deaconesses, however, was evident in their efficient nursing care of the sick during cholera epidemics and the Civil War. They were able to establish other institutions.

Amalie Sieveking of Hamburg, Germany, whose humane concerns were reflected in many nursing projects, did volunteer nursing during an epidemic of cholera. She and the society she formed, the *Friends of the Poor,* were instrumental in assisting in the development of Kaiserswerth.

Sister Elizabeth Fedde was the first nurse to practice among the Norwegian sick poor of the United States. She came from Norway and was a trained nurse as well as a trained pharmacist. She established the Norwegian Lutheran Deaconess Home and

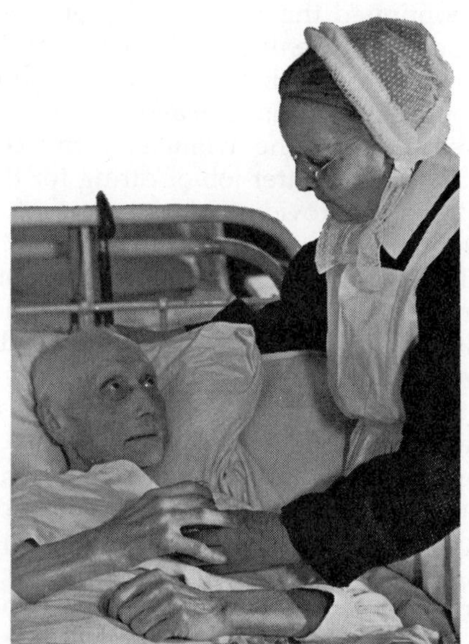

Figure 8–21. A deaconess empathizing with her patient. (Courtesy of Kaiserswerth Institute.)

[7]Jacobs, H. E.: *A History of the Evangelical Lutheran Church in America.* The American Church History Series, Vol. IV, New York, The Christian Literature Co., 1893, p. 387.

Hospital in Brooklyn, as well as the Lutheran Deaconess Home and Hospital in Minneapolis, and she was active in caring for the sick in their homes.

The first nursing order that was established by the *Anglican Catholic Church* was the *Sisters of St. John's House* in England. They were founded in 1848 to give nursing care to the sick in hospitals and in homes. Preparation for this work was given at King's College Hospital.

The *Episcopal Church* in the United States established a group of sisters in the Diocese of Maryland. These deaconesses cared for the sick in a house called St. Andrew's Infirmary.

The *Sisters of the Holy Communion,* founded in 1845, carried out both hospital and home nursing in addition to doing parish work and teaching parish school. *St. Luke's Hospital* in New York City was constructed because of the vision, inspiration and direction of its founder, first pastor and superintendent, *Dr. William Augustus Muhlenberg* (1796–1877). It opened as the Infirmary of the Church of the Holy Communion in 1854 and then became St. Luke's Hospital in 1858. The Sisterhood of the Holy Communion, under the leadership of *Sister Anne Ayres,* accepted the responsibility of providing nursing service at St. Luke's from its inception until 1888.

The architecture of St. Luke's Hospital was most interesting. It was built around the Church of the Holy Communion. "The patients lived in the House of the Lord. St. Luke's, as a church, has the chapel for its nave and the wards for its transept."[8] The prayerful atmosphere, with its soothing organ music pervading the confines of the wards, coupled with the service of the sisters seems to have been of great value in the healing process.

Dr. Muhlenberg emphasized that the patients were guests of the church and stressed the concept that the Christian family should entertain their guests, all of whom were sick. He recommended that the nurses should have "a cheerful spirit, skillful devotion and appreciative interest in the patient individually."[9] The motto of St. Luke's appears on the pin of the School of Nursing: *Corpus sanare, animam salvare*—to heal the body and to save the soul. Religious fervor accompanied scientific progress.

Several anecdotes give a picture of the times. Dr. Muhlenberg taught the nurses that they were to pour the patient's medication and bring it to the patient when it was due rather than follow the then currently accepted method, which was to require the patient to be responsible for taking his own medicine. Muhlenberg believed that this would eliminate many problems:

> Patients cannot be trusted with their own medicine. They cannot be made to understand the fallacy of the argument, that if a teaspoonful of anything will cure a man slowly, the whole bottle will do it immediately. It is not an unheard of thing for an elegantly disguised and flavored medicine to be rubbed on an injured limb, and for the cooling lotion, ordered at the same time, to be faithfully taken in teaspoonful doses after meals. To avoid such gross mistakes as these, it is customary in hospitals for the nurse to administer the medicines according to distinctly marked directions on the bottle. This works well, and mistakes are rare. But to have the medicine given by one who is herself responsible for its proper administration and preparation, who is required by the rules of the Sisterhood to understand its nature, the ordinary dose, and its expected effect, and who is honest and faithful enough to report immediately any mistake which may occur shuts up many sources of error and danger.[10]

Another interesting notation concerned the value of diet in the plan for care of the patient. He stated, "Every physician knows that the only hope for a man in the third week of typhoid lies in the amount of nourishment he can be induced to take. In private practice, he administers food and stimulant with his own hand."[11] Muhlenberg proceeded to discuss the impossibility of the physician's assuming this duty in a hospital and inveighed against any but the best-prepared and most capable of nurses accepting this responsibility.

In the nineteenth and early twentieth centuries it was well-known that only good nursing care brought a patient through a serious case of pneumonia, typhoid fever or other serious afflictions.

---

[8]*History and Alumnae Roster of the St. Luke's Hospital Training School for Nurses.* New York, St. Lukes Hospital, 1938, p. 18.

[9]*Ibid,* p. 20.

[10]*History of the St. Luke's Hospital Training School for Nurses.* New York, 1938, p. 23.

[11]*Ibid,* p. 24.

In 1863, the Sisterhood of the Holy Communion reorganized: some of the sisters remained in the original order; others formed the Sisters of St. Mary; and another segment established the Sisters of St. Luke and St. John.

The *Sisters of St. Mary* engaged in a special field of nursing that needed skilled attention—venereal disease control. They managed a home for delinquent girls and women and built and staffed St. Mary's Free Hospital for children in New York City.

In 1855, another very important Anglican order, *St. Margaret's Sisterhood,* was founded. The Sisters of St. Margaret were invited to come to the United States, and in 1871 they arrived from England. They participated in the nursing service administration of the Children's Hospital in Boston. This community of sisters remained in charge of the hospital for 45 years. Their greatest contribution was effected at this hospital, but they opened and maintained several others through the years.

St. John's Sisterhood and the *Sisterhood of All Saints,* both Protestant orders, worked in Baltimore. It was from the latter that Sister Helen, the first superintendent of nurses at Bellevue, came.

Deaconesses were also found in the *Methodist Church,* and nursing profited by their efforts. Many of the deaconesses' hospitals were maintained under the supervision of these deaconesses.

Still another group of deaconesses was organized by the *Mennonite Church.*

Lay Nursing Leaders

A compassionate young woman, *Annie M. Andrews* (Fig. 8–22), left her home in Syracuse, New York, to assist the victims of yellow fever and their families in Norfolk, Virginia. She worked tirelessly to keep patients alive or to comfort and console them and assist them toward a peaceful death. Her skill and valor were documented.[12]

The Howard Association of Norfolk, grateful for the eminent services of Miss Andrews as well as the noble example she set, presented her with the gold medal usually awarded only to physicians. The *Howard Association* was formed in 1856 to protect those who were sick and suffering because of man's inhumanity to man.

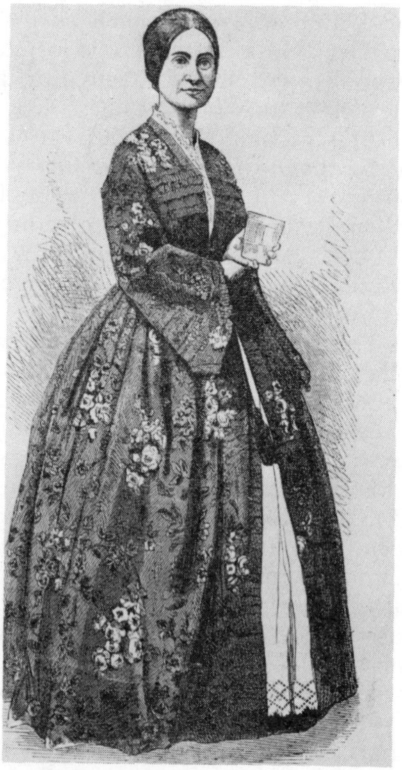

Figure 8–22. Annie M. Andrews, a recognized nurse heroine of the yellow fever epidemic in Norfolk in 1855. (Dolan collection.)

[12]*Harper's Weekly,* 1:353–354, June 6, 1937.

PROGRESS IN PSYCHIATRIC CARE

In the nineteenth century, mental illness was generally thought to be incurable. Few persons realized that mentally ill patients needed humane treatment; the law classed them next to criminals. Until 1820, the mentally ill were exhibited for a fee for the diversion of the public. Iron manacles were used in asylums until 1886. The *McLean Asylum* of Massachusetts, established in 1817, was the first institution of the sort to treat its patients kindly. The *Friends' Asylum* at Philadelphia, of the same period, was one of the few hospitals that appreciated the patient's needs.

In the United States, the pioneer crusader for reform in the treatment of the mentally ill was *Dorothea Lynde Dix* (1802–1887). Her first contact with the mentally ill came in 1841 when a theological student who had been given a class assignment to teach Sunday school at the jail in East Cambridge, Massachusetts, asked if she, a retired school teacher, would be willing to assume his assigned task. She was shocked by the conditions in which the prisoners lived. Many of the prisoners were mentally ill, and the treatment they received ranged from indifference through negligence to brutality. The assumption seemed to be that they were incapable of sensation; therefore no heat was provided for these tragic prisoners. Because of her persistence, logic and forcefulness in the court of East Cambridge, heat was provided in jail. This was the first milestone.

After surveying the needs of the mentally ill in Massachusetts, gathering data, securing the support of influential citizens, presenting the facts and then obtaining the results she desired, she moved on to the state of Rhode Island. Her phenomenal success continued as she gained the financial backing of a wealthy gentleman, Cyrus Butler, who provided for the establishment of *Butler Hospital*, an outstanding psychiatric institution.

The success of Dorothea Dix was due to her painstaking cataloging of the repulsive facts about the treatment of the mentally ill, and her presentation of them to honest, forthright citizens. Such was her presentation of a patient in Rhode Island who had been literally entombed in a six by eight foot stone cell into which no sun, heat or companion could enter. Frost and ice coated the walls of the cell, the bed and the patient. The realization of the existence of this incredible cruelty won support for the patients for whom she fought so desperately. She had found patients "confined in cages, closets, cellars, stalls, pens, chained, naked, beaten with rods and lashed into obedience." Through her efforts, the first state psychiatric hospital was constructed in Trenton, New Jersey; Canada and Scotland as well as the United States elevated their standards of care for the mentally ill. Her fiery crusade continued until, at the time of her death, more than thirty psychiatric hospitals had been established in the United States and other countries.

In the December 2, 1865 issue of *Harper's Weekly*, an article entitled "Dancing by Lunatics" described a dance at the Lunatic Asylum on Blackwell's Island, New York, at which the patients were the dancers (Fig. 8–23). The change in attitude toward the mentally ill at that time was reflected in the editorial: "Occasions of this sort no doubt tend in a great degree to relieve the sluggish melancholy which too close confinement or too monotonous surroundings are apt to produce in our institutions for insane people. It is often the case that isolation renders incurable diseases of the

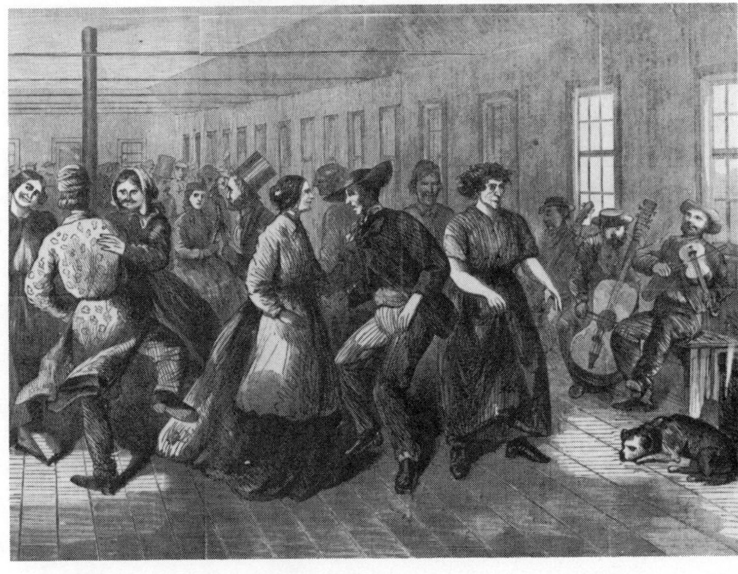

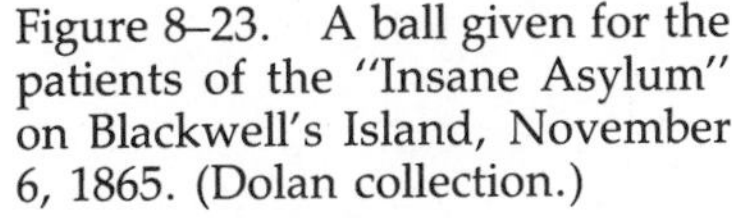

Figure 8–23. A ball given for the patients of the "Insane Asylum" on Blackwell's Island, November 6, 1865. (Dolan collection.)

mind which a more considerate treatment might ameliorate, or perhaps entirely relieve."[13]

SOCIAL REFORMERS

Samuel Gridley Howe (1801–1876), the well-known social reformer and abolitionist, made a major contribution to health care in the course of his work with the blind. Through his efforts, the New England Asylum for the Blind, later called *Perkins Institute,* was chartered in 1829 and was opened in 1832. He directed this famous school for forty-four years. Two famous pupils were Laura Bridgman, who was deaf as well as blind, and Anne Sullivan Macy, who tutored Helen Keller. The education of individuals with the special problems of blindness and deafness was now a reality. Dr. Howe was an ardent supporter of Dorothea Dix in her efforts on behalf of the mentally ill. His wife, *Julia Ward Howe,* joined him in his opposition of slavery.

Louis Braille (1809–1852), another pioneer in the crusade for assistance for the blind, had become blind himself at the age of three as a result of an accident. He was admitted to a school for the blind in Paris when he was ten years of age and later became a teacher there. In order to make the learning situation for his students better, he improved the system of writing with dots that Charles Barbier had devised. The *Braille system of communication,* using this raised-dot method, has been utilized by the blind for printing, writing and making musical notation. Louis Braille developed skill in playing the organ, and he became an organist in a church in Paris.

The facile pen and boundless imagination of *Charles Dickens* (1812–1870) were forceful weapons for social reform in the nineteenth century (Fig. 8–24). He had the rare ability to portray in a startlingly revealing way the social evils of his day, to break the literary barrier by depicting characters from the stratum of society that most needed assistance and to provide detailed and accurate descriptions of many diseases. This was an unusual combination of faculties.

Disease was a constant and often catastrophic problem. It was strikingly in evidence because of the lack of institutions to

[13] *Harper's Weekly,* 9:765, December 2, 1865.

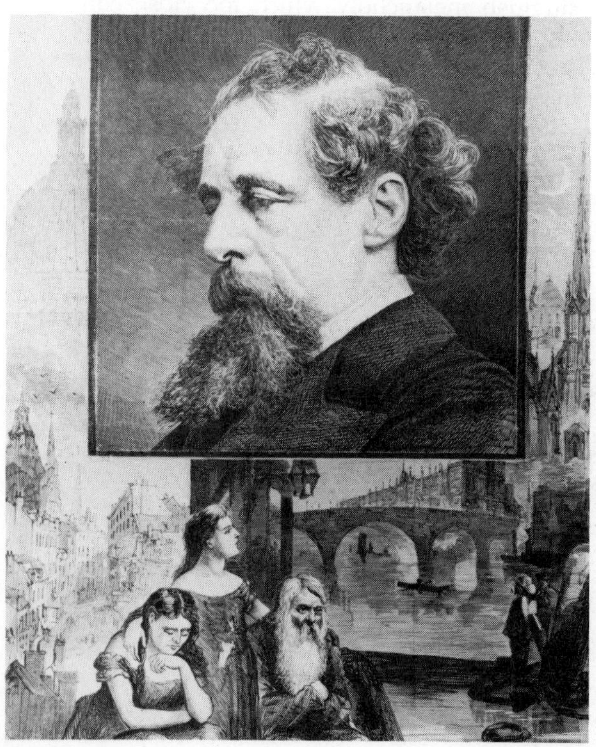

Figure 8–24. Charles Dickens, a catalyst for social reform, which had an effect on nursing. (Dolan collection.)

house people with specific conditions. Dickens' powers of social and medical observation were most acute and rivaled those of the most gifted medical clinicians of the period. Brain[14] describes, in an interesting way, the medical observations and recordings of Dickens.

Dickens waged a powerful crusade to make citizens aware of the need for social change. He portrayed the plight of the orphan and the need for more stringent child-labor laws; he exposed the unfair court trials, with imprisonment for minor offenses and unjust lengths of imprisonment, with members of the family incarcerated with parents, *Little Dorrit* (1857); he wrote of the birth of children in prisons and of their lives there, of life in workhouses, of the evils of the apprenticeship system, *Oliver Twist* (1838), of poor preparation of teachers and educators, of the cruel treatment of the mentally retarded, *Nicholas Nickleby* (1839), of the brainwashing of victims in prison, *A Tale of Two Cities* (1859), of the unscrupulous tactics of lawyers, of the inadequate preparation of doctors, of grave-robbing to sell cadavers to medical students and of the ghastly level to which "nursing" had sunk.

[14]Brain, Russell: *Some Reflections on Genius*. Philadelphia, J. B. Lippincott Co., 1960, pp. 123–136.

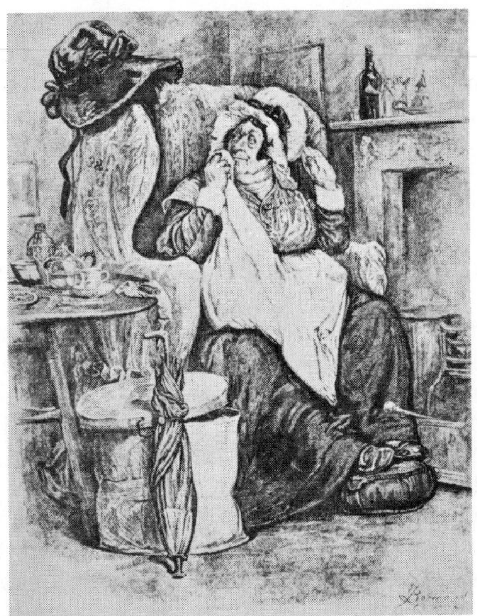

Figure 8–25. Sairey Gamp. (From Dickens' *Martin Chuzzlewit*.) (Dolan collection.)

Dickens' *Martin Chuzzlewit* (1844) focused attention on the "nursing care" given by pardoned criminals, women who were too old for harlotry and women of low moral standards, who lacked interest in or love for their fellow human. His immortal portrait of *Sairey Gamp* (Fig. 8–25) reflects the nature of these unfeeling, unsympathetic, alcohol-imbibing characters who contributed to the sufferings of mankind.

DEVELOPMENTS IN BIOLOGICAL AND PHYSICAL SCIENCES AND MEDICINE

Physiology

It is to *René T. H. Laënnec* (1781–1826) that we owe the contribution of the *stethoscope*.

Tuberculosis, also called the White Plague, was an ever-present affliction in the nineteenth century, and its incidence was very high. It has been stated that one-third of all the patients in Paris hospitals had tuberculosis. The disease seemed to consume a person and, in fact, was called "consumption."

In treating patients with this condition, Laënnec had resorted to palpation and percussion but was dissatisfied with these ineffectual methods of listening to chest and heart sounds. It was the custom in this period for the physician to place his ear over the patient's chest in order to hear these sounds. Many physicians were reluctant to use this method because of the patient's uncleanliness, coughing or obesity (which muffled the sounds).

In 1816, while walking near the Louvre, he observed children on one end of some wooden beams tapping out messages to children who were listening intently at the other end. Immediately, Laënnec had an inspiration; he returned to the hospital, rolled some paper into a tube, placed one end over the chest of an obese patient and rested his ear against the other end. He heard heart sounds more clearly than ever before.

This chest examiner he called a stethoscope. At first, it consisted of the rolled paper tied with string; then he devised a cylinder made of light wood—about twelve inches long—that could unscrew into two parts. (It was Dr. Cammann of New York who developed the binaural stethoscope.)

Laënnec believed that tuberculosis was contagious, that it was curable, and that the disease might be quiescent without manifest symptoms and then later blossom into an actute phase. Laënnec believed strongly that scrofula, called "King's Evil," was tuberculosis of the lymph nodes of the neck. This form of the disease, as well as several other varieties, occurred before pasteurization of milk was introduced.

The cause and cure of this disease still needed to be discovered, but Laënnec contributed to the advancement of medicine and thereby benefited society with his stethoscope.

William Beaumont (1785–1853) was the son of a prosperous farmer in Lebanon, Connecticut. He enlisted in the United States Army as a surgeon's mate and later was assigned to a lonely outpost on Mackinac Island. Here Beaumont met the man who was to become his physiological laboratory. Alexis St. Martin was a young trapper who had been wounded accidentally in the abdomen by a gunshot blast. This injury left an opening through which Dr. Beaumont could study the reactions of the stomach to various types of foods, liquids and emotions. The wound never healed.

In his study of this most unusual affliction, Army Surgeon Beaumont shed much light on one of nature's most baffling mysteries, the process of digestion. In 1833, he wrote *Experiments and Observations on the Gastric Juice and the Physiology of Digestion.*

Claude Bernard (1813–1878) is said to be responsible for introducing the use of the scientific method into the field of medicine. It is recorded that before Bernard, medicine was purely empirical. His skill in the use of the experimental method of scientific investigation led to an expansion of the knowledge of body organs.

The fruits of his labors included studies of digestion, with a concentration on the breakdown of sugar in the body as well as the part played by pancreatic juice; the explanation of the role of glycogen in the liver; the demonstration of the vasomotor mechanism in governing bodily activities, with the conclusion that irritation of the vagus nerve could cause an increase in sugar production, resulting in sugar excreted in the urine (glycosuria); the discovery, through studies of carbon monoxide poisoning and experimentation, that carbon monoxide could displace oxygen in the red blood cells; and the proof, through experimentation, that curare destroyed the contact between nerves and muscles. He found that muscles reacted to artificial stimuli and proved that disease could be produced artificially by biochemical experiments.

Bernard's efforts were published in 1865 in his classic work, *An Introduction to the Study of Experimental Medicine.* His labors enriched the fields of physiology and physiological chemistry.

In 1865, an Augustinian monk, *Abbot Gregor Johann Mendel,* of Brunn, Moravia, announced the results of his research in a publication that went unnoticed for almost half a century. *Mendel's law* of dominant and recessive characteristics has applications in biology, eugenics and in the understanding of heredity, including the hereditary aspects of some diseases.

Hermann von Helmholtz (1821–1894), utilizing his background in physics and mathematics, made practical applications in the field of health, especially in physical optics and acoustics. Among his achievements were the invention of the *ophthalmoscope* and the *ophthalmometer* and an understanding of the transmission of sound through the middle ear to the brain, which he described. He presented a delineation of the law of conservation of energy as well as fundamental principles relating to the overall field of dynamics, including hydrodynamics, thermodynamics and electrodynamics.

Anesthesia

Pain has been one of the greatest ordeals of humanity. There have been many attempts to find soporific potions to deaden pain. Early groups resorted to the use of wine, opium, mandrake and many other substances, which were more merciful than the cruel methods of either rendering the patient unconscious or restraining the patient by force. The world desired something to dull the senses and permit the blissful state of unconsciousness so desperately needed by patients. Relief came with the discovery of *anesthesia,* one of America's greatest gifts to the world.

During the 1840s, the famous circus owner P. T. Barnum sent traveling bands of entertainers around the country to give the "ether frolics." In 1842, young medical friends of Crawford W. Long, a physician from Georgia, inhaled ether for a bit of fun and amusement. Also joining as a participant in this "ether frolic," Long realized that ether gave a person more than a feeling of euphoria, that it created a loss of sensation that might be tried for surgical and obstetrical purposes. This he did successfully, but did not report his results until 1849.

In 1766, Joseph Priestley isolated nitrous oxide. A Hartford, Connecticut, dentist, *Horace Wells* (1815–1848), successfully administered nitrous oxide before extracting teeth. He had witnessed a public demonstration of "laughing gas"; the demonstration was attended largely by young men in the field of medicine as a form of amusement. Dr. Wells obtained permission to give a clinical demonstration before a class at Harvard Medical School. Unfortunately, the patient was not anesthetized completely and screamed during the operation. The medical students jeered and shouted humbug; the demonstration was considered totally unsuccessful, and Wells was humiliated.

A dentist in Massachusetts, *William T. G. Morton* (1819–1868), was present at the unfortunate demonstration of his friend, Dr. Wells, and felt that some substance other than nitrous oxide was needed that would be more reliable. Sulfuric ether had been known and used. In 1846, after experimenting with ether upon himself, Dr. Morton administered ether to a patient of the famous surgeon John Collins Warren, professor of anatomy and surgery at Harvard Medical School and chief of surgical service at Massachusetts General Hospital. When the patient became unconscious, Dr. Warren, turning to the surgical staff, said, "Gentlemen, this is no humbug." It was administered in the operating room amphitheater, later called the Ether Dome, of the Massachusetts General Hospital (Fig. 8–26). The patient was placed in the operating chair, which was upholstered in

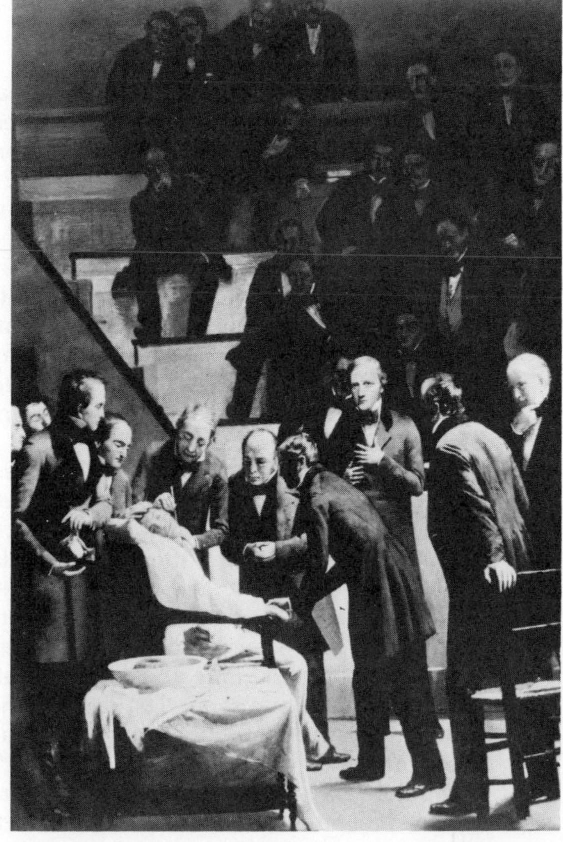

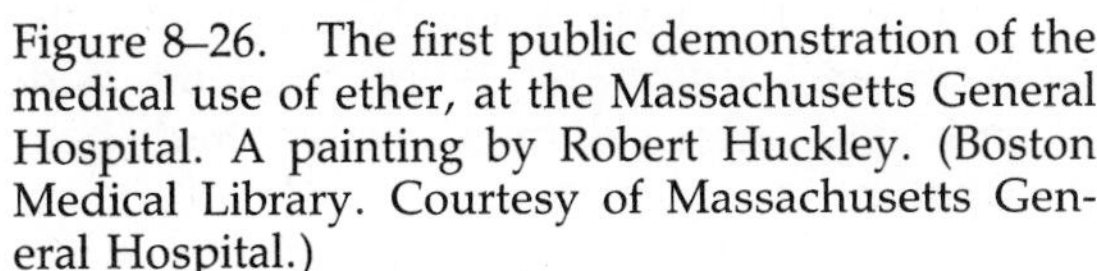

Figure 8–26. The first public demonstration of the medical use of ether, at the Massachusetts General Hospital. A painting by Robert Huckley. (Boston Medical Library. Courtesy of Massachusetts General Hospital.)

red plush with an adjustable back. This operating chair is still in the famous Ether Dome of "M.G.H."

Surgical operations could now be performed that would have been impossible without anesthesia. The terms anesthesia, anesthetic and anesthetist are supposed to have been proposed by Oliver Wendell Holmes.

Obstetrics and Gynecology

The world owes a tremendous debt of gratitude to *Ignaz Semmelweis* (1818–1865), a brilliant Hungarian physician, who was an independent thinker, an earnest and careful investigator and an ardent reformer interested in improving medical practice and thereby saving lives. He earned degrees of doctor of medicine, master of midwifery and doctor of surgery.

Upon receiving an appointment as assistant director of the Obstetric Clinic at the Lying-in Hospital in Vienna, he discovered and was appalled by the high maternal mortality rate due to *puerperal sepsis*, or *childbed fever*. People dreaded going to hospitals at this time because the chances of survival were poor.

He began to use his powers of observation and to analyze patient care. He noted a marked difference in the maternal mortality rate between two of the clinics. In the one in which the midwives practiced, the incidence of childbed fever as well as the mortality rate was decidedly lower than in the clinic in which the medical students practiced. The transfer of infection, Semmelweis determined, was due to the filthy habits of medical students, who dissected bodies on the autopsy table and then went directly to deliver a baby or to examine a prenatal or postpartum patient. He confronted medical students with his observations and indicted them for transferring infection by not washing their hands. He was derided by his colleagues. Nevertheless, he demanded that medical students wash their hands with soap and water, and then chlorinated lime and finally scrub their hands with fine sand. The drop in the death rate of maternity patients was astounding.

Semmelweis also suspected that doctors carried infections from one patient to another. Thus, it was essential to wash hands after treating every patient. In 1861, he published an account of his valuable research efforts in *The Cause, Concept, and Prophylaxis of Childbed Fever*. His theory was revolutionary and was not accepted by his contemporaries. Their treatment of him and his work was responsible for his eventual mental illness. He died in 1865 of a wound infection that caused blood poisoning, a condition he had fought to eliminate.

Another leader in the fight to eliminate childbed fever was *Oliver Wendell Holmes* (1809–1894). After graduation from Harvard in 1829, Holmes abandoned the study of law for that of medicine. In 1842, he wrote an essay on homeopathy that was a forceful exposition of the fallacies of that form of healing. In 1843, he composed a brilliant essay, *The Contagiousness of Puerperal Fever*, which is a medical classic. It was published five years before the work of Semmelweis appeared. His views were bitterly attacked by his medical colleagues, but, like Semmelweis', his opinions and theoretical concepts were correct. In 1855, he republished this paper, adding an introduction criticizing the unjust remarks. Many years later he wrote a letter to a friend with this comment: "I do know that others had cried out with all their might against the terrible evil before I did, and I give them full credit for it. But, I think I shrieked my warning louder and longer than any of them and I am pleased to remember that I took my ground on the existing evidence before the little army of microbes was marched up to support my position."

As may be noted, Pasteur's work (1879) showing the connection between streptococci and puerperal fever received wide publicity after Holmes' letter had been written.

MEDICAL EDUCATION

In early nineteenth-century New England medical practice, more than half of the practicing doctors were not graduates of a medical school. Students learned the practice of medicine by observing, reading and practicing, either in their preceptors' offices or on home visits. There were no formal medical schools in New England until 1782, and as late as 1840 probably no more than one-third of the physicians in practice had graduated from medical schools. The preceptor-apprentice system of medical education was firmly entrenched; it was common practice for a young man to have spent as many as 144 weeks, or almost three years, as an assistant to the preceptor-doctor. This vested interest group, preceptor-doctors, became a powerful force for prevention of progress in medical education and medical care. The medical apprentice helped with farm and home chores and, in addition, paid a tuition averaging $100.

There were no uniform laws in New England governing medical qualifications, practice and licensure. Many physicians expressed the need for a liberal arts foundation, for anatomical dissecting materials, for clinical facilities in which to practice and for a greatly upgraded plan for medical education.

SUMMARY

In this period, reflected against a background of social distress, and a myriad of health problems, the need for well-prepared nurse practitioners for every age group, in a variety of settings, was evident. The contributions of many religious orders as well as of strong individual leaders helped fill this need.

THE HERITAGE OF NURSING

The Image of the Nurse in the Early Nineteenth Century

The backbreaking efforts to build the United States, the plight of poor families, the long work days for many, including women and children, plus the prevalence of disease brought into focus:

1. the urgent need for community health nurses.
2. the crucial demand for well-suited and properly prepared nurses to staff the hospitals that were being established.
3. the demand to end the appalling practice of permitting alleged criminals either to go to jail or to work in hospitals as "nurses" to care for the ill.
4. the critical requirement of an educational program for preparation for nursing.
5. the necessity of sound social and health legislation.

Outstanding contributions to nursing were made by the many religious nursing orders of various Christian denominations. Their image was one of:

1. "caring," resulting from their spiritual calling, or "vocation," and "dedication" to spiritual goals.
2. poverty, chastity and obedience, in accordance with religious vows.

Members of public and certain vested interest groups have over the years tended to undervalue the superb contributions of these religious orders and their special qualities when criticizing all nurses:

1. for their supposed lack of "dedication" when they requested adequate economic security and personal and professional freedom of action.
2. for being unwilling to adhere to rigid discipline and to unquestioningly accept any and all orders.

The plight of the receiver of nursing care and the horrifying image of the "nurse" was communicated by Charles Dickens:

1. in the cruel and abusive treatment of patients by Sairey Gamp.
2. in his warning to nurses and the public of the dangers inherent in permitting poorly motivated and inadequately prepared attendants to assume responsible roles in giving nursing care to patients.

Nurses owe much to the religious orders that perpetuated an important role for the nurse at this crucial period in history. Their heroic contribution and response to the needs of the poor were of great significance in reestablishing a firm base for the emergence of modern nursing. They became members of religious orders in the interests of spiritual rewards and humanitarian service rather than for monetary gain.

REFERENCE READINGS

Armstrong, George: *The Summer of Pestilence—A History of Yellow Fever.* Philadelphia, J. B. Lippincott & Co., 1856.

Bailly de Barberey, Helene: *Elizabeth Seton.* Trans. from sixth French ed. by J. B. Code. New York, The Macmillan Co., 1927.

Bolster, Sister M. Angela: *Catherine McAuley.* Wexford, John English and Co., 1978.

Dickens, Charles: *Martin Chuzzlewit.* Boston, Estes & Lauriat, 1896.

Eaton, Evelyn, and Moore, Edward R.: *Heart in Pilgrimage.* New York, Doubleday & Co., 1948.

Marshall, Helen E.: *Dorothea Dix, Forgotten Samaritan.* Chapel Hill, University of North Carolina Press, 1937.

Packard, Francis R.: *Some Accounts of the Pennsylvania Hospital from 1751 to 1938.* Philadelphia, Engle Press, 1938.

Robinson, Victor: *Victory over Pain.* New York, Henry Schuman, 1946.

Rosenberg, Charles: *The Cholera Years.* Chicago, The University of Chicago Press, 1962.

Slaughter, Frank G.: *Immortal Magyar.* New York, Henry Schuman, 1950.

Thompson, Morton: *The Cry and the Covenant.* New York, Doubleday & Co., 1954.

Thorwald, Jurgen: *The Century of a Surgeon.* New York, Pantheon Books, 1956.

Tilton, Eleanor: *Amiable Autocrat: A Biography of Dr. Oliver Wendell Holmes.* New York, Henry Schuman, 1947.

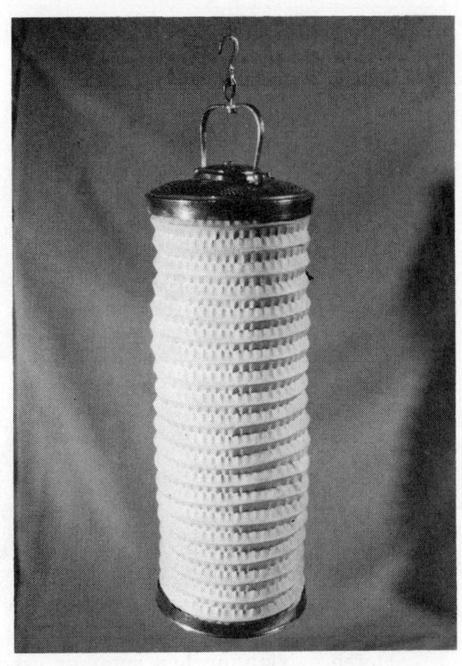

A lamp of the type carried by Florence Nightingale in the Crimean War. The outer case, which acted as a wind shield, collapsed into the brass top and bottom, which held a removable candleholder and a candle. (Photo by DeLores Paul.) (Dolan collection.)

9 The Leadership of Florence Nightingale

The social reformers of the early nineteenth century had focused attention on the plight of the poor and on the need for reform of prisons, hospitals and nursing. Leadership in social welfare and nursing was needed. One person who responded to this exigency was *Florence Nightingale*. Her story is proof of a woman's ability to make important contributions in a male-dominated cultural setting. She demonstrated by precept and example the powers of a woman leader.

Florence Nightingale's parents, Mr. and Mrs. William Shore Nightingale of Lea Hurst, Derbyshire, and Embley Park, Hampshire, were traveling in Italy when Florence was born, on May 12, 1820. They named her for the city of her birth (Fig. 9–1). Her youthful surroundings included many places on the continent as well as nineteenth-century English manors, with their warmth and gaiety (Fig. 9–2). In a period when many young women were subjected to the constricting influences of Victorian society, Miss Nightingale had her father's guidance and under his direction

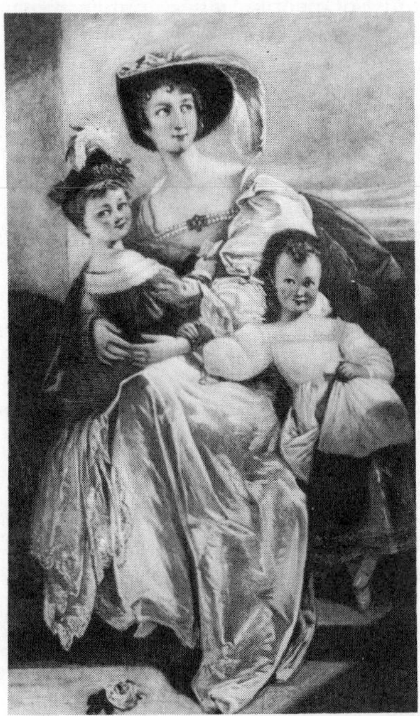

Figure 9–1. Mrs. William Shore Nightingale and her daughters Parthenope and Florence. (Dolan collection.)

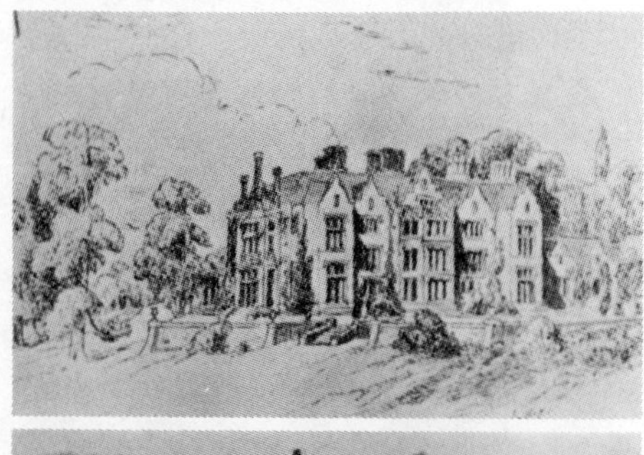

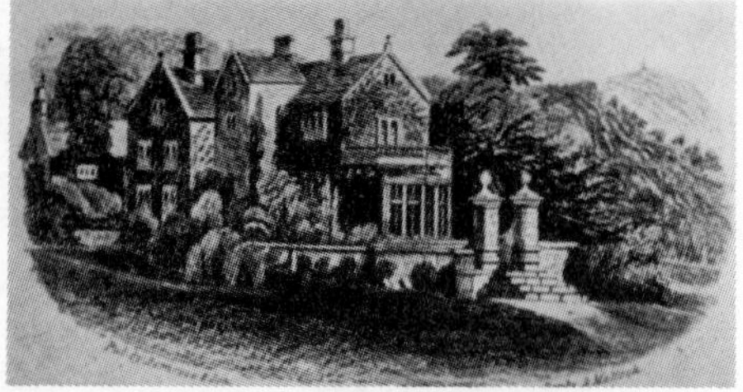

Figure 9–2. *Top,* Embley Park in Hampshire, Florence Nightingale's summer estate, from a sketch by her sister Parthenope. *Bottom,* Lea Hurst, the winter home of Miss Nightingale in Derbyshire, near Mattock. (Dolan collection.)

gained a liberal education, not only by instruction in Latin, mathematics, philosophy, religion and modern languages but also, as one who knew her recounts,

> by the surroundings of life itself—by travel and the study of people, cities, public movements and institutions, and, . . . by intellectual and cultured companionship under the home roof. Those who can remember still look back on the peculiar charm of the family life at Embley and at Lea Hurst; on Embley summer mornings filled with what Walter Scott somewhere calls 'matutinal inspiration'; when the talk over the breakfast-table was so vivid with interests and sympathies that sometimes, before the meal was over, the very bookshelves would be called into requisition to provide statistics and quotations . . . and Blueboks would find their way among the silver and china on the breakfast-table and huge tomes of reference be heaped on the carpet at Mr. Nightingale's feet.[1]

Florence's sister, Parthenope, who later became Lady Verney of Claydon, presents charming descriptions of one of the Nightingales' memorable visits to Paris in 1839–1840, where in the mansion of Mrs. Clarke, the mother of Madame Mohl, the Nightingale family met the best political, literary and scientific society of that period. It is hardly surprising that Florence Nightingale evolved into an attractive, charming, brilliant, cultured, dynamic, gifted and forceful leader whose thoughts and desires were channeled into action (Fig. 9–3). Her intelligence and education were recognized by many of the scholars of the last century. She had the assurance and courage to challenge contemporary political leaders and to seek their advice on a collegial basis.

A meeting between Florence Nightingale and a gentleman from the United States had a profound influence on her decision to pursue the life of a nurse. In 1844, Dr. Samuel Gridley Howe and his wife, Julia Ward Howe, were visiting the Nightingale family at their summer estate at Embley in Hampshire. Florence, at the age of 24, was undergoing a particularly frustrating time in her life: She wanted to be useful to humanity instead of being waited on. She turned to Dr. Howe for counsel:

> Dr. Howe, you have had much experience in the world of philanthropy; you are a medical man and a gentleman; now may I ask you to tell me upon your word, whether it would be anything unsuitable or unbecoming to a young English woman, if she should devote herself to

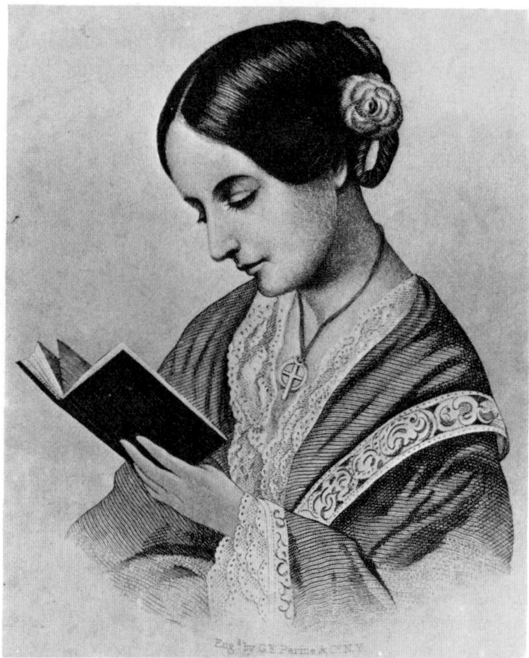

Figure 9–3. Florence Nightingale. (Dolan collection.)

[1]"Florence Nightingale—By One Who Knew Her," *The Nursing Mirror and Midwives' Journal,* August 20, 1910, pp. 311–312.

work of charity in hospitals and elsewhere as the Catholic Sisters do?

My dear Miss Florence, Dr. Howe replied, it would be unusual, and in England whatever is unusual is apt to be thought unsuitable; but I say to you, go forward, if you have a vocation for that way of life; act up to your aspiration, and you will find that there is never anything unbecoming or unladylike in doing your duty for the good of others. Choose your path, go on with it, wherever it may lead you, and God be with you! [2]

This auspicious conversation has been described by Mrs. Howe in her *Reminiscences* and by the Howes' daughter, Laura E. Howe Richards, in two of her books. This discussion seemed to have had a catalytic effect on the inner desires of Florence Nightingale and to have prompted the action she later took.

In 1860, Florence Nightingale stressed that "women should not be excluded by law or usage from the liberty of trying any mode of existence open to men, at their own risk in case of failure." Miss Nightingale emphasized the obligations of women to improve society. Although an advocate of the "rights of women," she criticized women who entered the field of medicine and adapted themselves to the male medical model rather than using their unique qualities to bring about improvement in medical care. She believed that "the more the entrance to the medical profession is widened the more chance of its being reformed."[3] Although eminently qualified, she did not choose to be a physician, for she preferred the role and function of nurse.

She regretted the fact that women lacked political power: "I am convinced that political power is the greatest power it is possible to wield for human happiness, and until women have their part in it in an open, direct manner, the evils of the world can never be satisfactorily dealt with."

She was drawn to philanthropic endeavors, always analyzing and planning programs of care for the welfare of others. She applied theoretical concepts to practical ends. When she began a systematic study of the "ameliorative treatment of physical and moral distress," she gathered her data by observation while visiting and observing at many institutions. She observed at the Trinita del Monti and Santo Spirito hospitals before enrolling in the program for nursing under the direction of Pastor Fliedner at Kaiserswerth. Although she did not become a Lutheran Deaconess, she finished the three-months' program. She then went to Paris to study and learn in the historic institution Maison de la Providence under the guidance of the Sisters of Charity of St. Vincent de Paul. She was determined to replace the ill-prepared, sadistic nurses of the period, who were so well depicted in Charles Dickens' *Martin Chuzzlewit,* with intelligent, kind, well-prepared nurses.

After her brief experience in nursing care, Miss Nightingale assumed an administrative role as superintendent of the *Establishment for Gentlewomen During Illness.* Within a short time she was asked to become superintendent of nurses at King's College Hospital. She had begun to plan her work there when the call came to go to the *Crimea.*

THE CRIMEAN WAR

Russia's desire for Constantinople, dating from the time of Peter the Great, culminated in the outbreak of the Crimean War in 1854. England and France came to the defense of endangered Turkey in March of that year. For the first time in modern warfare, a civilian correspondent, William Howard Russell of *The London Times,* reported on events; prior to this War, generals gave out the reports of success or failure. Now a vivid picture of the conditions of the soldier was presented to the public. It was an appalling presentation of the British Army's marked inefficiency and hopelessly outmoded bureaucracy. In addition to the astronomically high death rate from wounds and infections, cholera broke out among the troops and spread with frightening rapidity. One thousand cholera victims were received at the General Hospital even before the famous battle of Alma, in which England's casualties were 2,860 wounded and 619 dead. The next report received in London was of the famous battle of Balaclava, immortalized by "The Charge of the Light Brigade." The battle of

[2]Bishop, William J.: "Florence Nightingale's Message for Today," *Nursing Outlook, 8*:246–247, 1960.

[3]Correspondence with John Stuart Mill. Courtesy of Dr. Alfred Meyer.

Inkerman later resulted in 2,612 British soldiers killed and wounded.

It is recorded that "between the battle of the Alma and the battle of Inkerman something had happened to the conscience of the British nation. . . ."

Londoners were horrified by the gruesome accounts of the war, of the unbelievable neglect of the wounded and dying, as well as of the lack of relief of the excruciating pain and suffering of the English and Irish soldiers. Russell described the plight of the soldiers in Crimea to England and the world in an article in *The London Times:* "It is impossible . . . to see the melancholy sights . . . without feelings of surprise and indignation at the deficiences of our medical system. The manner in which the sick and wounded are treated is worthy only of savages. . . . Here the French are greatly our superiors. Their medical arrangements are extremely good, their surgeons more numerous, and they have also the help of Sisters of Charity who have accompanied the expedition in incredible numbers. These devoted women make excellent nurses." The following day, October 13, 1854, a letter published in *The London Times* inquired: "Why have we no Sisters of Charity?"[4] Immediately, the Army issued an appeal for nurses. Thus, at long last, female nurses were accepted into the English Army.

A memorable letter of Sir Sidney Herbert, the Secretary of State for War, contained a plea, for Florence Nightingale to supervise the military hospitals in Turkey.

> There is but one person in England that I know of who would be capable of organizing and superintending such a scheme. . . . My question simply is, would you listen to the request to go out and supervise the whole thing? You would, of course, have plenary authority over all the nurses, and I think I could secure you the fullest assistance and cooperation from the medical staff, and you would also have an unlimited power of drawing on the Government for whatever you think requisite for the success of your mission. . . . I must not conceal from you that upon your decision will depend the ultimate success or failure of the plan. Your own personal qualities, your knowledge and your power of administration, and among greater things, your rank and position in society, give you advantage in such a work which no other person possesses.[5]

Florence Nightingale was appointed Superintendent of the Female Nursing Establishment of the English General Hospitals in Turkey. It was decided that the number of Miss Nightingale's group of nurses should not exceed 40. Tremendous response by nurses to join the group was expected, but few applied, and only 14 of these were considered suitable. After Anglican sisterhoods were approached, however, six members joined Miss Nightingale's group. Eight sisters from the Sellonite order also answered the call. Catholic orders offered their services, and the government decided to attempt 10 Sisters of Mercy from Bermondsey. Mr. and Mrs. Bracebridge (friends of Miss Nightingale) accompanied the group, bringing the total number of participants, excluding Miss Nightingale, to 40. Before leaving England, each nurse had to sign an agreement that placed her totally under the rule of the Lady Superintendent. Florence Nightingale insisted that the authority vested in her should be absolute—supreme and not to be questioned.

Many of the medical officers of the army opposed the idea of women nurses. They felt that the nursing care given by untrained orderlies was as good as could be expected in war and that the presence of women would be burdensome.

Miss Nightingale and her band were assigned to the base hospital at *Scutari,* across the strait from Constantinople (now Istanbul). It was to Scutari that thousands of cholera victims and hundreds of battle casualties were taken by way of an agonizing journey across the Black Sea in "hospital ships." Once at Scutari there were no beds or blankets for the feverish cholera victims or for the wounded, many of whom were suffering the painful aftermath of surgery and amputations with subsequent infection.

Since hospital accommodations were nonexistent in Scutari, it was necessary to convert the artillery barracks into a hospital (Fig. 9–4)—an almost insurmountable task

---

[4] Cook, Sir Edward: *The Life of Florence Nightingale.* Vol. I. London, Macmillan, 1914, p. 147.

[5] Bishop, William J.: "Florence Nightingale's Message for Today," *Nursing Outlook, 8*:246–249, 1960.

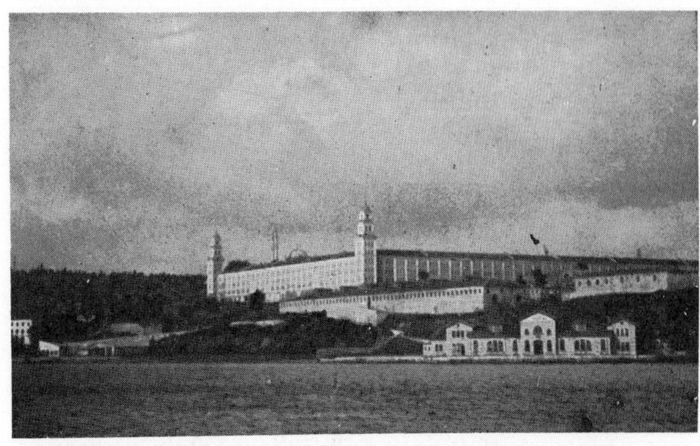

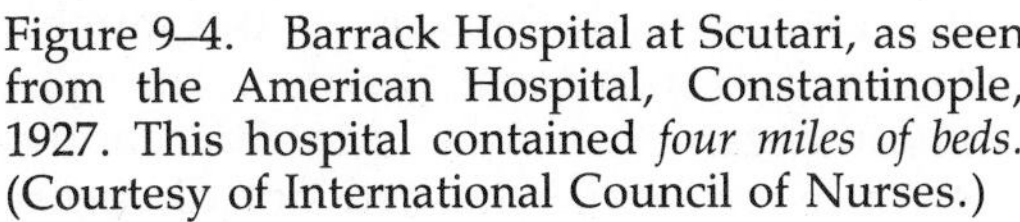

Figure 9–4. Barrack Hospital at Scutari, as seen from the American Hospital, Constantinople, 1927. This hospital contained *four miles of beds.* (Courtesy of International Council of Nurses.)

even under normal conditions. The huge, barnlike building that was to serve as the hospital was filthy and dilapidated. The barracks resembled a hollow square with a tower at each corner. It was a bleak setting and the building was in a state of decay. Underneath the building were large sewers that attracted rats and other vermin, which inhabited the premises. The odor was most offensive. It is little wonder that Florence Nightingale wrote, "I have been well acquainted with dwellings of the worst parts of most of the great cities in Europe but have never been in any atmosphere which I could compare with that of the Barrack Hospital at night."

When the sick and wounded arrived, they were confronted with a barren structure without hospital, medical, dietary or laundry equipment of any kind. They were placed on the floor in their vermin-ridden and blood-encrusted coverings. There were no basins, few utensils of any sort, no soap and no towels. There were no knives or forks, so the men ate with their fingers. It took four hours to serve a meal, and most of it was not edible. There was practically nothing in the barracks hospital that a very sick man could eat. There was no night nursing; the men, left alone in the dark, spoke of the terror of it. Under these conditions, the death rate was *42 per cent.*

This was the scene confronting Florence Nightingale and the team of nurses on their arrival. They faced resentment from the medical group as well as a seemingly impossible assignment. They had to transform this place of horror into a haven where patients could truly convalesce, and that required a miracle. The change that occurred at Scutari, however, was nothing short of miraculous (Fig. 9–5). After obtaining the obvious necessities, Miss Nightingale began by setting up five diet kitchens and a laundry. At the Barrack Hospital in Scutari, a missionary from New England, *Reverend Cyrus Hamlin* (the founder of Robert College in Istanbul), contributed his

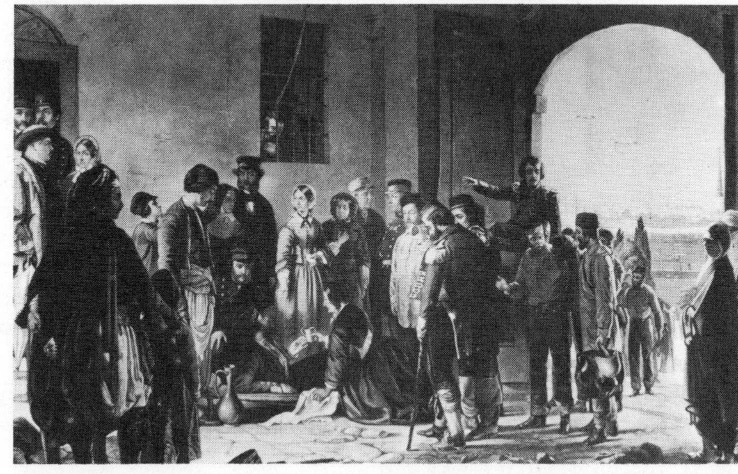

Figure 9–5. Florence Nightingale at Scutari, assessing patient needs and giving directions for care. (Nursing Mirror Photograph.)

services by baking bread and washing clothes for Miss Nightingale.[6] She had been told that the barracks had plenty of supplies, but they could not be found; some had been sent to the wrong ports and some were buried under munitions. She used her own funds for emergencies and asked friends at home to provide more. "Calamity unparalleled" was her evaluation of this unbelievable and unnecessary situation.

Reverend Hamlin presents an interesting picture of Florence Nightingale's personality in action. "She was a quiet, self-possessed, interesting, intelligent lady, evidently wholly absorbed in her work. She had the faculty of command." He recorded an encounter between Miss Nightingale and Dr. Menzies, a physician at the barracks. She asked him to kindly open a certain storehouse so that she might obtain supplies.

> Menzies replied: "No such articles are there, Miss Nightingale. They all went up to the front . . . ." Miss Nightingale replied: "Well I would like to have the door opened, or I shall send men to break it down."[7]

Dr. Menzies in shock and alarm opened the door, and Florence Nightingale found what she wanted. Soon afterward, Dr. Menzies was recalled to London and was replaced by another physician. This human dynamo had achieved her objective. Reverend Hamlin depicts her as "a person in perfect health . . . graceful and agile in form and movement . . . firm, determined."[8]

During the Crimean War Florence Nightingale made contributions to the field of dietetics. She believed that prescribing the diet for the patient was the function of the physician but that the science and art of feeding the sick was an essential part of nursing.[9]

There was another side to Florence Nightingale's personality. Smith describes her insatiable thirst for power as well as her derogatory response to those who opposed her.[10] These personality traits were evident in her reaction to the second group of nurses that came to Turkey.

In the course of the war, as the number of casualties increased, the need for more nurses became obvious. Mr. Bracebridge sent a letter (which he had not discussed with Miss Nightingale) to Secretary of State for War, Sidney Herbert, requesting additional nursing assistance. Mr. Herbert proceeded to comply with this request in spite of the promise made to Florence Nightingale prior to her departure for the Crimea that no nurses were to be sent to military hospitals except at her request and subject to her recommendation. Sidney Herbert cajoled another friend of his, Mary Stanley, a very able leader, to supervise the selection of this next group of nurses. England had requested the services of Irish Sisters of Mercy to join this second group. They responded enthusiastically. Eleven sisters from that order plus three sisters from Liverpool and one from Chelsea volunteered. Mother Mary Francis Bridgeman was unanimously selected to be the superior of these sisters. Mother Bridgeman came from a wealthy family, of Norman extraction, which possessed vast estates in the counties of Limerick and Clare.[11] Mother Bridgeman had sound administrative skills and extensive nursing care experience. She was respected for her leadership as a superior of her own order. While the sisters were preparing for their journey, Sidney Herbert informed Mother Bridgeman in writing that the Lady Superintendent would communicate with the second group of sisters only through Mother Bridgeman as their superior. She was to be in charge "in all matters outside the wards of the hospital"—a clear delineation of spiritual versus professional power. This policy was to prevent the predicament of the Sisters from Bermondsey—who had no official status, no autonomy as a religious community and no rights as individuals—from befalling this second group of sisters. As the time for departure drew near, Sidney Herbert reneged on this promise to the sisters. He

---

[6]Widmer, Carolyn L.: "Grandfather and Florence Nightingale," *American Journal of Nursing, 55*:569–571, 1955.

[7]Hamlin, Rev. Cyrus: *My Life and Times.* Boston, Congregational Sunday School and Publishing Society, 1893, p. 335.

[8]*Ibid.*, p. 337.

[9]Cooper, Lenna F.: "Florence Nightingale's contribution to dietetics," *Journal of the American Dietetic Association, 30*:121–127, 1954.

[10]Smith, Barry: "New Light on the Lady with the Lamp." Read at Yale University, November 6, 1981.

[11]Bolster, Evelyn. *The Sisters of Mercy in the Crimean War.* Cork, The Mercier Press, p. 40.

insisted that each nurse sign the agreement that required all allegiance to Florence Nightingale. This would negate the spiritual aspects of the religious community. This request was anathema to the sisters and therefore unacceptable. It should be noted that the sisters differed from the secular nurses in that they were not reimbursed for their services. Also, while the secular nurses were placed in first class on board ship, the sisters were quartered in steerage.

Meantime, news of the upcoming arrival of the second group of nurses reached Miss Nightingale. In her thinking their coming was a ghastly mistake of monumental proportions. Because she did not request them, much less select them, she viewed them with suspicion and contempt and maligned them and their efforts. She especially spoke ill of Mother Bridgeman. Documents reveal derogatory names that she used when referring to those she disliked or whose skills she envied.

After their arrival the sisters were ignored until a devastating epidemic of cholera broke out. The sisters were well prepared to care for patients with this affliction because they had developed great nursing skill during previous epidemics at home. Patients, physicians and orderlies praised the sisters for their superb care. Ultimately, the War Office assigned Mother Bridgeman the responsibility for the hospitals at Koulali and Balaclava. Here the sisters' nursing care received high commendation.

Florence Nightingale is also remembered for her correspondence with friends and families of soldiers and the special messages she wrote to soldiers' wives and children. She recognized the need for organized occupation and wholesome recreation for soldiers in hospitals and encouraged the establishment of coffee-houses that provided music and recreation. Teachers were assigned to give courses to those interested in increasing their schooling. Miss Nightingale was unsurpassed as a hospital administrator and hospital reformer. A choice comment made by Miss Nightingale illustrates her gift for identifying incomplete instructions: "We have gone over your draft very carefully and find that although it includes almost everything necessary, it does not define with sufficient precision the manner in which the meat is to get from the commissariat into the soldier's kettle."

In two months the hospital at Scutari had been transformed into an efficiently managed institution. As a result of sanitary improvements and the provision of good nursing care, in six months the death rate was reduced to two *per cent* (from 427 per 1000 in February 1855, to 22 per 1000 in June 1855), and nurses had won the respect of most of the surgeons (Fig. 9–6).

Florence Nightingale utilized the scientific method of gathering data and was skilled as a statistician, presenting factual evidence in a most graphic way. Dr. C. E. A. Winslow[12] referred to her as the "Lady with the Slide Rule," as well as a lady with the lamp of compassion and the broom of

[12]Winslow, Charles-Edward A.: "Florence Nightingale and Public Health Nursing," *Public Health Nursing, 46*:331, 1946.

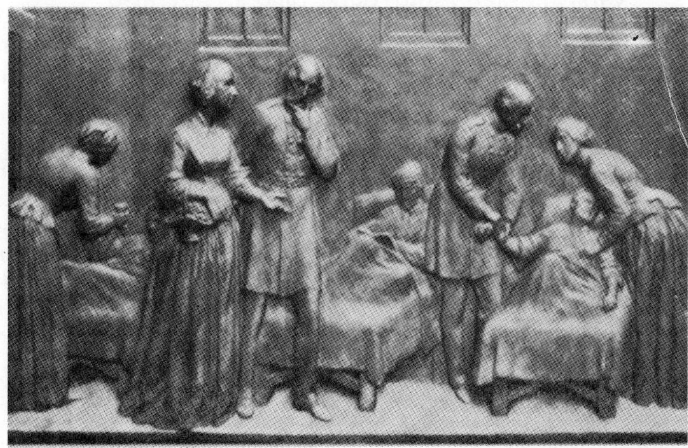

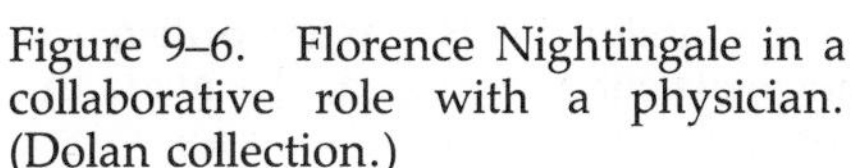

Figure 9–6. Florence Nightingale in a collaborative role with a physician. (Dolan collection.)

efficiency. She made rounds with her famous lantern, whose wind shield prevented the candle in the candlestick within the lantern from being extinguished (see illustration, p. 155.)

A War Office report said of the Irish Sisters of Mercy, "The superiority of an ordered system is beautifully illustrated in the Sisters of Mercy. Their intelligence, delicacy and conscientiousness invest them with a halo of extreme confidence. One can safely consign his most critical cases to their hands."

Early in 1856, peace was made; the military hospitals were closed and the nurses went back to England, Miss Nightingale last of all, returning in July 1856. By now she had become a popular heroine.

Florence Nightingale's war work encompassed far more than reorganizing nursing and saving lives. She had broken through the age-old prejudice against women in the army, leading to a new attitude toward nursing and the establishment of a new occupation for educated women. Smith has said that it was to Florence Nightingale's credit that she established in the mind of the public "the sanctification of nursing as a service."[13]

Before departing from the Crimean theater of operations, Miss Nightingale visited the cemetery where so many of the soldiers had been buried. She would never forget or forgive that so many lives had been lost needlessly by carelessness and ignorance. In her diary she noted, "I stand at the altar of those murdered men and while *I* live I fight their cause."

It has been said not only that Florence Nightingale was "The Lady with the Lamp" carrying light into dark places, but also that she was a sort of galvanic battery, stirring and frequently shocking the apathetic public into action. Because of her prodding, Parliament, through the actions of Sir Sidney Herbert, reformed the whole army medical system. Her *Notes on Matters Affecting the Health Efficiency and Hospital Administration of the British Army* formed the basis for these reforms. It took five years of hard, bitter fighting to carry the reforms through, but the pledge she had made to the dead soldiers to fight for their cause had been fulfilled. Army hospitals and barracks were entirely reconstructed on a sanitary basis, a new code of sanitary regulations was adopted, an army medical college was founded and recreation clubs were established.

The health of the soldiers in India also received her attention, and vast sanitary and irrigation projects as well as economic reforms were carried out by the government on her recommendations. Two of her reports, *Observations on the Sanitary State of the Army in India* (1863) and *Life or Death in India?* (1873), were forceful weapons in this campaign.

In 1883, she wrote a letter describing the proper method of analyzing the problems of sanitation and disease prevention in India, and she suggested 12 questions that should be addressed to gather the appropriate data for solution of the problem. Among them were:

What is the Sanitary Inspector (the Vaccination Officer) doing as executive? and what will be his power in the Villages?

Is an Enabling Act wanted, empowering local Governments to frame sanitary rules?

Miss Nightingale even inquired about the crucial issues of "unwholesome trades fouling the water."

The revolution that she initiated in military hospitals was carried over into civilian hospitals. Dr. Schrimpton[14] comments on her book *Notes on Hospitals* (1859): "This is the most practical, scientific work on the construction, management and administration of Hospitals." This book presented the most exhaustive study that had ever been made on hospital planning and administration. It contained clear, practical wisdom on every phase of hospital work.

Dr. Cope, in *Florence Nightingale and the Doctors,* comments:

Few of Miss Nightingale's contemporaries knew so much about hospitals as she did. When she was asked by the members of the Sanitary Commission in 1857 what British and foreign hospitals she had visited, she made this astonishing answer:

I have visited all the hospitals in London, Dublin, Edinburgh, and many county hospitals, some of the naval and military hospitals in England; all of the hospitals in Paris and studied

[13]Smith, Barry: "New Light on the Lady with the Lamp." Read at Yale University, November 6, 1981.

[14]Schrimpton, C.: *The British Army and Miss Nightingale.* Paris, A. and W. Galignani, 1864, pp. 30–34.

> with the Sisters of Charity; the Institute of protestant deaconesses at Kaiserswerth on the Rhine where I was twice in training as a nurse; the hospitals in Berlin and many others in Germany, at Lyons, Rome, Alexandria, Constantinople, Brussels; also the war hospitals of the French and Sardinia.[15]

Dr. Cope further has commented that to Miss Nightingale a visit to a hospital was not merely a formality but rather a time of concentrated observation. He commented on her skilled observational techniques and her "interest in the general layout of a hospital, as well as in the details of ward construction, sanitation and general administration" in addition to the importance of nursing care. "It is no wonder that she was consulted about the plans for new hospitals. Doctors everywhere recognized her as an authority, and she obtained an unrivalled acquaintance with the plans of hospitals" in England, Canada, Australia and the United States. The plans for the Johns Hopkins Hospital in Baltimore were taken to England for her criticism before the first buildings were built.

A BOOK ON NURSING

In December 1859, a modest black volume containing 77 pages and entitled *Notes on Nursing: What It Is and What It Is Not* was published. The fame of the author made it, in the vernacular of our day, a "best seller." Within a month of publication 15,000 copies had been sold, and by the time of Florence Nightingale's death well over 100,000 had been purchased. In 1860, Miss Nightingale rewrote the book and enlarged it. It was then published in New York and translated into Italian, German and French. In 1946, concern over the scarcity of copies of this priceless book prompted a reprinting for modern-day appreciation. Dean Emeritus Annie W. Goodrich of Yale University School of Nursing wrote in the foreword:

> The timeliness of the revival of *Notes on Nursing,* the plan and purpose of which is so clearly stated in Miss Nightingale's preface, cannot be questioned.
>
> Nearly a century has passed since this woman of great vision and wide experience, as her last contribution to humanity, epitomized in terse, sometimes caustic, but always convincing language, a message to the womanhood of the world.
>
> It is a book which should be owned not only by every member of the nursing profession, but which should find its place in every home, not to replace the ever-increasing body of knowledge relating to the development of that priceless possession of every nation, its child-life, but because it interprets in simple terms the age-old principle of healthy living.
>
> It should be noted that Florence Nightingale makes very clear the distinction between persons professionally qualified for the practice of nursing and the knowledge essential for every woman to whom may come at any time a call to render nursing service in some form.
>
> Though the message of this little book is for all, to none should its appeal be stronger than to the American nurses of the twentieth century who, as teachers, as citizens, and oft-times as mothers, have, through their acquired knowledge, the responsibilities that citizenship in a democracy implies. It is a tragic fact that, despite almost phenomenal advances in the art and science of living, ignorance, poverty and disease still obtain in great degree. Let us hope that this little book will, in this present edition, continue its career of usefulness.

Students today marvel at the continuing pertinence of Florence Nightingale's basic principles of good nursing care and the clarity with which she delineated the role identification for nurses:

> A good nursing staff will perform their duties, more or less satisfactorily, under every disadvantage. But while doing so, their head will always try to improve their surroundings in such a way as to liberate them from subsidiary work and to enable them to devote their time exclusively to the care of the sick. This is, after all, the real purpose of their being there at all, not to act as lifts, water carriers, beasts of burden or steam engines—articles whose labour can be had at vastly less cost than that of educated human beings.[16]

HEALTH AND A HOLISTIC APPROACH IN NURSING

Miss Nightingale stressed the importance of primary prevention as well as health maintenance. Her definition of health

[15] Cope, Zachary, M.D.: *Florence Nightingale and The Doctors.* Philadelphia, J. B. Lippincott Company, 1958. pp. 18–19.

[16] Report of the Committee on the Cubic Space of Metropolitan Workhouses with Papers Submitted to the Committee, 1867, p. 72.

was "not only to be well, but to be able to use well every power we have."

She taught that there were two major components of nursing—*health nursing* and *sick nursing*. Health nursing was "to keep or put the constitution of a healthy person in such a state as to have no disease"; that is, attaining and/or retaining the person's health. Sick nursing was described as "to help the person suffering from disease to live"; that is, to help him not merely to survive but to live as full and satisfying a life as possible, thus regaining a state of wellness. She stated, "Both kinds of nursing are to put a person in the best possible condition for nature to restore or to preserve health, to prevent or to cure disease or injury."

She was appalled at the wastefulness caused by inadequate preventive and restorative practices as well as at the lack of emphasis on health in nursing practice. In maintaining that the whole person should be understood and treated, she advocated a *holistic* approach. She insisted that prevention was better than cure. This philosophy predated the theories of microbiologists and psychologists. Bishop put Florence Nightingale in proper perspective with today's world when he commented:

> Miss Nightingale had always seen to the heart of things that the sick person must be treated and not the disease, that prevention is infinitely better than cure, and that nursing must hold to its ideal but must change some of its methods. And now after a hundred years the ministers of health, the global epidemiologists and the psychosomatic experts are just beginning to catch up with her.

Even now her ideas and ideals for nursing are not completely understood or realized.

THE NIGHTINGALE SCHOOL FOR NURSES

The remarkable achievements in the Crimea first showed the world that thousands of lives that were being wasted could be saved by good, intelligent nursing care and that skilled nurses were essential in military hospitals. The nurses' accomplishments indicated that the most intelligent and competent women were required for such work and that they must be especially prepared for it. It is no wonder, then, that when the Duke of Cambridge presided over a meeting to organize a plan for presenting a testimonial to Miss Nightingale after the Crimean War the resolutions were:

> That the noble exertions of Miss Nightingale and her associates in the hospitals of the East, and the invaluable services rendered by them to the sick and wounded of the British forces, demand the grateful recognition of the British people;
>
> that it is desirable to perpetuate the memory of Miss Nightingale's signal devotion, and to record the gratitude of the nation, by a testimonial of a substantial character;
>
> and that, as she expressed her unwillingness to accept any tribute designed for her own personal advantage, funds be raised to enable her to establish an institution for the training, sustenance, and protection of nurses.

The nation's testimonial of fifty thousand pounds, obtained by compulsory subscription from the soldiers of the Crimea as well as donations from the public, was channeled into the Nightingale Fund for a training school for nurses.

A council of distinguished persons was appointed to administer this Nightingale Fund, and they negotiated for the establishment of the Nightingale Training School. This council was important because Miss Nightingale needed the members' support to change the existing system of nursing service administration. The influence of the council coupled with the financial independence of her school from any other institution permitted the school's emergence as a totally autonomous entity. With cost factors not a restriction, Miss Nightingale could design the theoretical as well as the practical and clinical portions of her program.

Miss Nightingale's unique gift for enlisting and securing the wholehearted support of interested and influential people was propitious. Through the efforts of her supporters a milieu was provided that could nurture the kind of program, faculty and students Florence Nightingale insisted upon in order to achieve her objectives.

The Nightingale Fund Council sponsored the training school, provided a special building for it, authorized the curriculum, paid the instructors, entered into contracts with hospitals and handled business affairs.

The draft agreement defined the services to be provided by the hospital, such as allowing the use of requested areas for learning experiences and, conversely, specified the financial reimbursement to be made to the hospital from the Nightingale Fund. Included in the contractual arrangements with the hospital were the following stipulations: it must always have a staff of experienced nurses responsible for the care of patients; there must be a well-qualified charge nurse to direct and teach those assigned to her (ongoing in-service education); there must be labor-saving devices; and it must accept and respect the director of the program and the clinical instructor.

The Nightingale Training School for Nurses opened in 1860 as a completely independent educational institution. St. Thomas' Hospital was selected for the clinical learning experience: "A hospital alone was not to be the center for the education and practice of nursing." Because there was an emphasis on teaching patients and families about the preservation of health, the students were *also* to go into homes. In 1865, Florence Nightingale contributed to two books on nursing in a community setting. She is purported to have written an eloquent appeal for the use of community nursing in London. Miss Nightingale helped found the first Community Nursing Association in Liverpool and outlined the whole basis of our modern public health nursing movement.

The school of nursing that Florence Nightingale founded prospered. Because she was a highly educated woman, she exemplified vividly what higher education could do for a person preparing for public service. She was probably better educated than many men of her period, even most doctors. She was a champion of educational opportunities for other occupational groups. In the army she founded schools for soldiers and courses for the orderlies and cooks and even fostered the founding of a medical school for officers.

The aims of the *Nightingale School* were to train hospital nurses; to train nurses to train others; and to train district nurses for the sick poor. Thus, she endeavored to prepare nurses for: maintenance of health, prevention of disease, detection of illness, caring for the sick and providing nursing education. The length of the program was one year. The classes were small, permitting a high degree of selectivity—between 1000 to 2000 applications were received, but only about 30 students were admitted. There were two categories of students. One was educated probationers who paid a tuition fee. The other group of students was not required to pay a fee; their expenses were taken care of by the Nightingale Fund.

The expected behavior of the students was enunciated and shared with each student. It was important for the instructor and students to identify and use in their practice a body of nursing knowledge.

FLORENCE NIGHTINGALE AND THE "NURSING PROCESS"

Miss Nightingale was the originator of the concept of the nursing process. She insisted that *prepared and educated persons* were necessary to function properly in the nurse's role. She included in this role assessment and intervention according to a plan of care, followed by *evaluation.* She wrote, "Merely looking at the sick is not always observing. To look is not always to see. It needs a high degree of training. . . . It is most important to observe the symptoms of illness; it is, if possible, more important . . . to observe the symptoms of nursing: of what is the fault not of illness, but of nursing. Observation tells how the patient is; reflection tells what is to be done" (Fig. 9–7).

She defined nursing as that care that "put a person in the best possible condition for nature to restore or to preserve health, to prevent or to cure disease or injury." Miss Nightingale stressed that the sick person must be treated and not the disease; she espoused the philosophy of nursing the sick not the sickness many years before Dr. Osler made his famous statement: "It is better to know the patient who has the disease than the disease the patient has."

It was Miss Nightingale's opinion that "the very elements of what constitutes good nursing are as little understood for the well as for the sick." She felt strongly that nursing involved a separate body of knowledge and role function from that of medicine. She envisioned the nurse as a

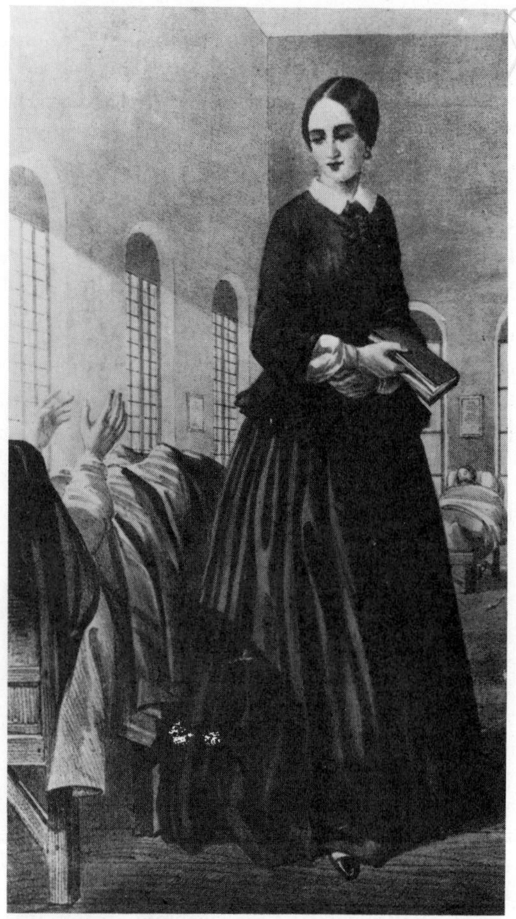

Figure 9–7. Florence Nightingale carrying out the "nursing process." (Nursing Mirror Photograph.)

colleague of the physician, working with him but having a distinct sphere of duty. She believed that it was the nurse who carried the main responsibility for the health, comfort and welfare of patients and society. She said, "It is the surgeon who saves a person's life—it is the nurse who helps this person to live."

Miss Nightingale insisted that it was essential for nurses to teach and control nursing. She selected with care the director and faculty of her school to guide the learning process in nursing. *Mrs. Wardroper* was chosen to direct the school and was referred to as "Matron." It is to Mrs. Wardroper that much of the success of the school (curriculum and teaching) should be credited. She inspired faculty, students and colleagues during the 27 years of her leadership. In *Notes on Nursing,* Miss Nightingale stressed, "The Matron [director of nurses] should be one whose desire is that students shall learn—a rarer thing than is usually supposed."

In 1875, a home sister, or clinical instructor, was appointed. She was *Mary Crossland,* who appears to have done a creditable piece of work in planning a program of clinical instruction (Fig. 9–8). Her efforts have been recorded in her letters to Miss Nightingale relating her progress. Her enthusiasm inspired several physicians to join in taking the students on clinical rounds. Seymer cites a letter written on November 8, 1879:

> Mr. Croft gave us rather a new style of clinical lecture this morning—some had expressed a desire to understand about aneurisms—so instead of beginning to tell, Mr. Croft asked questions: asked Miss G. if she had ever come across a case in the wards. She had, in a Medical ward. He then asked her to state what she had observed about the case, such as symptoms of pain, difficulty of breathing—cough—position

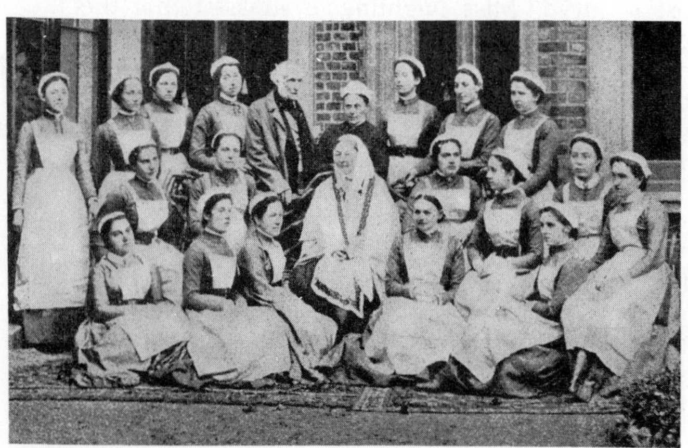

Figure 9–8. Miss Nightingale *(center)* and students at St. Thomas' Hospital, London, 1887. Lord Verney and Miss Crossland appear behind her. (Dolan collection.)

of patient—diet—treatment, to all of which she gave good answers. Then Mr. Croft explained the cause of the different symptoms—the effect of diet and treatment and what share a nurse had in seeing the treatment was carefully carried out.[17]

As early as 1867, Miss Nightingale's contractual agreements provided that in addition to the salary received from the hospital, the ward sister (head nurse) was to receive a salary from the Nightingale Fund for assisting in the training of students. Ward sisters were chosen for their teaching abilities and were responsible for instructing students on the wards. The medical instructors were to be paid in a similar fashion. The head nurses were to keep weekly summary records of the work of each student; the matron recorded monthly summaries. Students were to keep diaries of the day's activities and interactions as well as "nursing case papers," which were probably the forerunners of "process recordings." The students were to be taught to detect symptoms and the reasons for these symptoms and were to be given sufficient time to understand the reasons. Proper guidance for the student was stressed. For many years, Miss Nightingale selected the students and advised on details. Students were required to read and write well. People who saw the early Nightingale nurses were impressed with "the bright, kindly and pleasant spirit which seemed to pervade them." The students in the program were encouraged to ask questions and to use the resources of their well-equipped library and practice laboratory. In this well-rounded program the students were prepared for living as well as for earning a living.

Miss Nightingale, in *Suggestions for the Improvement of the Nursing Service of Hospitals,* inveighed against using nurses for cleaning and scrubbing. Her words were: "A nurse should do nothing but nurse. If you want a charwoman, hire one. Nursing is a specialty." Florence Nightingale was successful in her demands. The hospital provided a staff that included 16 head nurses, 54 staff nurses, three nurses' aides, 23 ward maids for cleaning and 14 scrubbers for the heavy cleaning work. Her forceful order—"If you want a cleaning woman—hire one, my nurses are to nurse"—was obeyed.

She also cautioned that premature responsibility and overwork for students endangered sound growth, caused frustration and disinterest in nursing and prevented full contribution to good nursing care. She insisted that arrangements be worked out with hospital administrations so that the person in charge of nursing service could improve the work environment in order to liberate nurses from subsidiary work so that they could devote their full efforts to the nursing care of clients. She anticipated the current emphasis on accountability to clients. She encouraged step-savers such as having hot water piped up to the patient's floor, a lift or elevator to bring up the patient's food, a system of bells with valves that flew open and remained open until the nurse could detect which patient needed her, a nursing environment that kept pace with progress and an attitude of willingness on the part of the matron (director of nursing service) to see that nothing prevented the students from nursing.

Florence Nightingale pleaded for nurses' education to become an ongoing endeavor. She was an ardent proponent of *continuing education.* She emphasized that "no system can endure that does not march" (in essence, move ahead intellectually). Miss Nightingale did not approve of graduation or registration: "Nursing is a progressive art in which to stand still is to have gone back." To have the idea that one had mastered a field of learning was abhorrent to one who said, "Progress can never end but with a nurse's life." For these reasons it is not surprising that the Nightingale Plan involved a continuing relationship between her school and its graduates. Each year there was recognition of satisfactory nursing service through a "gratuity paper," which was a type of certification.

Miss Nightingale's plans for the reorganization of nursing met with opposition, chiefly from physicians. Of a hundred physicians whose opinions were asked, only four favored her ideas. The other physicians previously had given the nurses at St. Thomas' their training and believed it was very good. One said, "Nurses are in

---

[17]Seymer, Lucy R.: "Mary Crossland of the Nightingale Training School," *American Journal of Nursing,* *61*:86, 1961.

much the same position as housemaids, and need little teaching beyond poultice-making and the enforcement of cleanliness and attention to the patient's wants." Another doctor said publicly, "A nurse is a confidential servant, but still only a servant. . . . She should be middle-aged when she begins nursing; and if somewhat tamed by marriage and the troubles of a family, so much the better." A few doctors did understand what the movement might mean. One said, "A trained and educated nurse would soon become most popular and trusted. She would cooperate with the physician, her presence would inspire confidence in the patient, and she would restore peace and order to a distracted household."

Miss Nightingale envisioned a collaboration between the nurse with the physician. The English physician, Dr. Saleeby, reflected, "If Lister was the father, then Florence Nightingale was the mother of modern surgery." Certainly without the reforms in nursing and hospital work the triumphs of modern medicine and surgery would have been impossible.

Despite its founder's prestige, the school faced many difficulties in its first 10 years. However, one by one the physicians began to accept Florence Nightingale's teachings, and slowly the public came to appreciate the skills of an educated nurse.

Miss Nightingale was personally acquainted not only with the Queen and her cabinet but also with every prime minister of her time and many royalty of other nations.

Florence Nightingale died in August 1910, at the age of 90. Her family was asked to allow her to be buried in Westminster Abbey, but they knew her wishes and refused. Her grave is in the family plot at East Wellow, near Romney, in Hampshire, and its only mark is a small cross with her initials and dates. (There are monuments to her in London, Derby, Milbank, Florence and Calcutta, and beautiful memorials in St. Paul's Cathedral, London, St. Thomas' Hospital, the Royal Infirmary, Glasgow, Scotland, and the Episcopal Cathedral in Washington, D.C.)

Florence Nightingale raised the status of nursing to a dignified occupation, improved the quality of nursing care and founded modern nursing education. John Greenleaf Whittier wrote a poem entitled "Florence Nightingale of England" in May of 1882.

> Where pity, love and tenderness
> Are found, (there) Christ must be;
> So wheresoe'er thy footsteps press
> His presence walks with thee.

SUMMARY

The Crimean War served as a catalyst to bring members of religious orders and lay nurses together for the benefit of those who needed nursing service. In the stressful environment of the war crisis, the gifts of the leaders, which might not otherwise have been known, shone forth for all to see and remember. Outstanding contributors to nursing included Mother Bridgeman and the Sisters of Mercy, the Anglican Sisters, and such individuals as Mary Stanley and Fanny Taylor, whose two-volume work of her experiences in the hospitals of Scutari and Koulali provide well-documented source material on this historic epoch.[18]

In retrospect, Florence Nightingale was intellectually and academically, as well as financially, wealthy. She was probably better educated than most men of her period, including most physicians. Miss Nightingale knew how to analyze situations, to present facts and to direct others and she had leadership qualities. Her students of nursing received a better preparation than most students of medicine. Miss Nightingale had an indomitable spirit with an attractive and gracious exterior. She was not a submissive, sweet, smiling, quiet person but a gifted, brilliant, dynamic, forceful leader whose thoughts and desires produced results. She had two aspects to her nature: a tremendous will that wilted those who opposed her and a fantastic compassion for all who suffered. She was admired the world over.

Florence Nightingale foretold the transition of nursing as it moved from the prescientific era to the scientifically oriented era in which it now functions. How different might nursing education and nursing service have been if Florence Nightingale's

[18]Taylor, Fanny: *Eastern Hospitals and English Nurses: The Narrative of Twelve Months' Experience in the Hospitals of Koulali and Scutari by a Lady Volunteer.* London, Hurst and Blackett, 1856.

philosophy had really been understood and practiced by all nurses; her ideas and plans have not yet been fully realized. Florence Nightingale's vision set into motion a most creative social force that exemplified man's concern for his fellow man. She became a legend in her own time and a living memorial to the fact that nursing has a vital independent, as well as a collaborative, role.

THE HERITAGE OF NURSING

Florence Nightingale—The Image of the Nurse as a Gifted Scholar, An Able Administrator and a Persuasive Leader

1. Florence Nightingale wielded political influence because:
   a. she was respected, admired and recognized as an extremely intelligent and well-educated person by some of the world's most brilliant men.
   b. she was admired for her humanitarian endeavors.
   c. she shared documented evidence from her research with the public.
2. Miss Nightingale's notable personal attributes included:
   a. graciousness and attractiveness.
   b. an indomitable spirit.
   c. warm human sympathies, which incited her to action for the welfare of others.
   d. exceptional intellectual gifts and a broad liberal education coupled with insatiable intellectual curiosity.
   e. logical reasoning powers, which led her to a scientific method of problem-solving.
   f. a vindictive response to those who opposed her.
3. Her nursing practice was:
   a. built on a body of nursing knowledge.
   b. based on a carefully delineated philosophy of nursing.
   c. defined and published in her book *Notes on Nursing—What It Is and What It Is Not.*
   d. client-oriented—"Nurse the sick one—not the sickness."
   e. based on the nurse's role in primary prevention.
   f. attuned to a modern definition of health, using a holistic approach.
   g. based on the nurse's functioning in a collaborative role with physicians.
   h. proven successful by the accomplishments in the Crimean War, which made the public aware of the need for properly designed programs of nursing education.
4. The Nightingale School for Nurses was:
   a. autonomous and financially independent.
   b. supported by influential leaders.
   c. sustained by carefully devised contractual agreement between the school and the institutions used for practical learning experience.
   d. planned to provide a milieu for learning and giving good care.
   e. staffed by nurse-faculty and controlled by nurses.
   f. opposed to preparing "physician's assistants."

5. Her *faculty and students* were:
   a. selected with great care.
   b. admonished to identify and use a body of nursing knowledge.
   c. encouraged to use "modern" teaching methods and learning skills.
   d. encouraged to use a "nursing process" method.
   e. aware of the call for practice-oriented research.
   f. cautioned to realize that nursing is a separate entity from medicine.
   g. required to participate in continuing education.
   h. forbidden to overwork.
   i. indoctrinated with the concept of accountability to clients.

The world and nursing were enriched by the image of the nurse as a gifted scholar, a creative thinker, a persuasive leader and an outstanding independent practitioner. Florence Nightingale was a genius whose ideas of and goals for nursing have not yet been realized.

REFERENCE READINGS

Bolister, Evelyn: *The Sisters of Mercy in the Crimean War.* Cork, The Mercier Press.
Cook, Sir Edward: *The Life of Florence Nightingale.* Vols. I and II. London, Macmillan, 1914.
Cope, Zachary: *Florence Nightingale and the Doctors.* Philadelphia, J. B. Lippincott Co., 1958.
Dolan, Josphine A.: *The Grace of the Great Lady.* Chicago, Medical Heritage Society, 1971.
Dolan, Josephine A.: "Florence Nightingale, Rebel With a Cause," *R. N. Magazine,* May 1970.
Hamlin, Cyrus: *My Life and Times.* Boston, Congregational Sunday School and Publishing Society, 1893.
Hobson, W.: *World Health and History.* Bristol, John Wright & Sons, 1963.
Nightingale, Florence: *Notes on Hospitals,* 3rd ed. London, Longmans, 1867.
Nightingale, Florence: *Notes on Nursing.* London, Harrison & Sons, 1859. (Philadelphia, J. B. Lippincott Co., 1946.)
Nutting, M. Adelaide and Dock, Lavinia L.: *A History of Nursing.* New York, G. P. Putnam's Sons, 1935, Vol. II.
O'Malley, I. B.: *Florence Nightingale, 1820–1856.* London, Thornton Butterworth, 1931.
Parton, James, et al.: *Eminent Women of the Age.* Hartford, Conn., S. M. Betts Co., 1868.
Seymer, Lucy R.: *Florence Nightingale.* London, Faber & Faber, 1940.
Seymer, Lucy R.: *Florence Nightingale.* New York, The Macmillan Co., 1954.
Seymer, Lucy R.: *Florence Nightingale's Nurses. The Nightingale Training School 1860–1960.* London, Pitman, 1960.
Seymer, Lucy R.: *Selected Writings of Florence Nightingale.* New York, The Macmillan Co., 1954.
Smith, F. B.: *Florence Nightingale: Reputation and Power.* London, Croom Helm, 1982.
Stewart, Isabel M.: *The Education of Nurses.* New York, The Macmillan Co., 1943.
Strachey, Ray: *The Cause, A Short History of the Women's Movement in Great Britain.* London, G. Bell and Sons, 1928.
The Nightingale Training School; St. Thomas' Hospital, 1860–1960. London, Nightingale Training School for Nurses, 1960.

The United States issued a commemorative stamp in honor of Mrs. Harriet Tubman, a courageous abolitionist and compassionate nurse during the Civil War.

10 Social Forces Affecting the Emergence of Educational Programs in Nursing

THE STATUS OF WOMEN

The midpoint of the nineteenth century was marked by the blossoming of Victorian society and the demand for emancipation of women, whose lives were devoid of educational and career opportunities.

The wealthy young woman frittered away her time with sewing, painting or musical activities. Life was very difficult, however, for the poor woman, who suffered daily from sheer exhaustion, poor nutrition and exposure to disease. Winslow Homer portrays her situation as well as those of all workers in one of his etchings (Fig. 10–1). Thomas Hood describes the working woman in his famous poem "The Song of the Shirt." The last verse of the poem epitomizes the pathos of her life.

With fingers weary and worn,
With eyelids heavy and red,
A woman sat in unwomanly rags,
Plying her needle and thread–
Stitch! stitch! stitch!
In poverty, hunger, and dirt,
And still with a voice of dolorous pitch
She sang the "Song of the Shirt!"

. . . .

"Work–work–work
Till the brain begins to swim;
Work–work–work
Till the eyes are heavy and dim!
Seam, and gusset, and band,
Band, and gusset, and seam,
Till over the buttons I fall asleep,
And sew them on in a dream!

"Oh, men, with sisters dear!
Oh, men, with mothers and wives!
It is not linen you're wearing out,
But human creatures' lives!
Stitch–stitch–stitch,
In poverty, hunger, and dirt,
Sewing at once, with a double thread,
A shroud as well as a shirt.

In London in 1840, women were refused admission to the first world convention to abolish slavery. The issue of segregation of

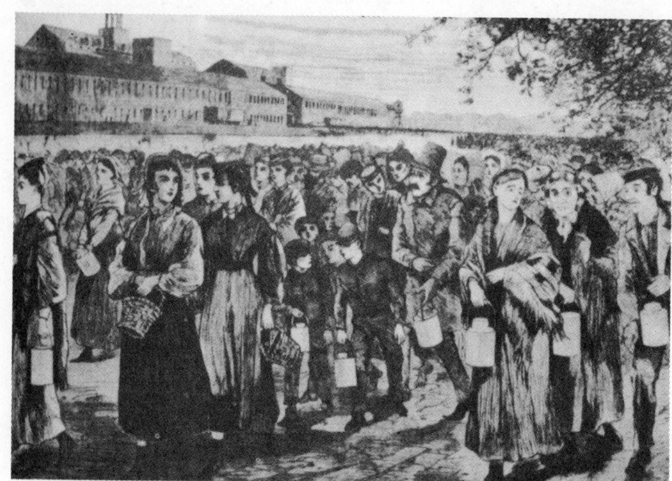

Figure 10–1. Workers of all ages facing a long day of labor with no creature comforts. An etching by Winslow Homer. (Dolan collection.)

women was not recognized. In 1848 in Seneca Falls, New York, there was a convention for women's rights. The crusade for women's rights was of monumental proportions and great historical significance. Susan B. Anthony and many others fought for the rights of women as human beings—for suffrage, an opportunity for higher education and an opportunity to practice the professions, including law and medicine.

Throughout the course of history women had been the midwives; now men were also midwives (in the role of obstetrician). There was no question in Victorian society of the indelicacy of men's delivering women in labor, but it was unthinkable for a woman to practice medicine or to study anatomy or physiology.

A milestone was reached when women were readmitted into the medical field. The pioneer was *Elizabeth Blackwell* (1821–1910), whose struggles to gain admission to medical school are well known. She was informed that she might as well lead a revolution as try to be a physician. Geneva Medical College in Geneva, New York, however, consented to admit her in 1847. After much tribulation, she received her degree of doctor of medicine. Her troubles were just beginning because she was unable to secure a hospital staff appointment, and patients seemed averse to having a woman physician, even though women midwives had been accepted for years.

In 1853, Dr. Blackwell set up a dispensary, and in 1857, she established the New York Infirmary for Women and Children. The infirmary was to provide a clinical setting for practical experience for women students of medicine. In 1865, she was responsible for founding the *Women's Medical College of the New York Infirmary for Women and Children.*

The die had been cast; the readmission of women into the field of medicine, even in small numbers, was now assured. The Women's Medical College of Pennsylvania was opened in 1850. There were eight candidates for the degree of doctor of medicine in the first class. The course consisted of two college semesters of three months each, or one academic year.

Lucretia Mott announced in her *Discourse on Women,* "A new generation of women is upon the stage." Florence Nightingale had demonstrated the societal benefits of well-educated women.

THE WAR BETWEEN THE STATES (1861–1865)

On April 14, 1861, when *President Lincoln* summoned 75,000 volunteers for the Union Army, the Union had no army nurse corps, organized medical corps, or ambulance or field hospital service. Members of many religious orders promptly volunteered and gave superior care to soldiers in their own hospitals, in army hospitals and on the battlefield (Fig. 10–2). One form of recognition of their outstanding contribution to both the Union and Confederate troops was the erection of the memorial monument, "Nuns of the Battlefield," in Washington, D.C. This remains a tribute to the nearly 600 sis-

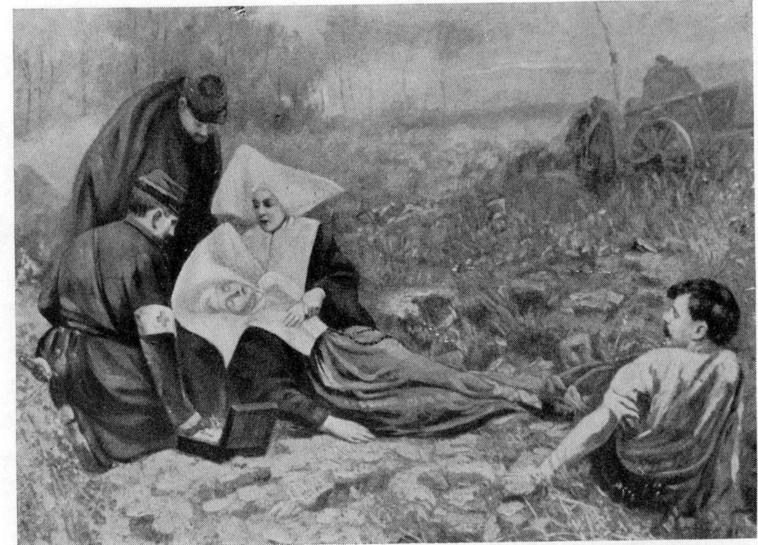

Figure 10–2. The Innocent Victim. A Sister of Charity killed on a Civil War battlefield while ministering to the wounded. (Dolan collection.)

ters of 12 religious orders who served so heroically during this crucial period. The nursing duties in some of the largest government hospitals was assigned to them. "There was an immense enthusiasm among the laity, but a total lack of experience and efficient organization. . . . The first hospitals were mostly empty barns or warehouses . . . but in the hands of the Sisters they became finally a model of European military sanitation."

All the Catholic nursing sisters received many compliments from the government because of their efficiency. Jefferson Davis paid them highest tribute and Abraham Lincoln gave them permission to purchase all supplies needed for their work. The sisters neither asked for nor received any compensation for their labors. These hundreds of devoted sisters, however, were not enough to care for so many wounded and sick. Hundreds of lay nurses were needed to supplement them. Outside the religious orders, there were almost no nurses with any real preparation. Nevertheless, women did request permission to be of assistance, and two such women were Clara Barton and Mother Bickerdyke.

Clara Barton (1821–1912) (Fig. 10–3) of North Oxford, Massachusetts, was born Clarissa Harlowe, but later changed her name to the simpler one by which she is known and remembered. When the Sixth Massachusetts Regiment arrived in Washington on April 19, 1861, she was there to feed them and dress their wounds. Another project she undertook was supervising the shipment of field supplies that had been sent down for the soldiers by wagon train. It is recorded that on one of her journeys with the wagon train, a herd of cattle to be used for food for the army was being driven ahead of the train. As the wagon train passed a Confederate hospital, the surgeon begged for assistance for his patients who were starving. The officer in charge of the cattle asked Miss Barton,

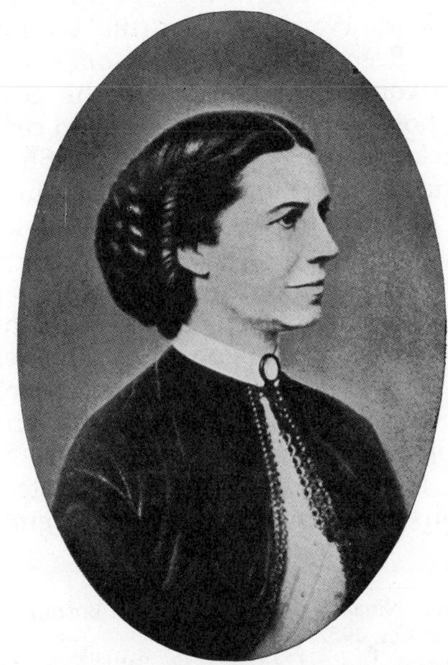

Figure 10–3. Clara Barton. (From a photograph taken during the Civil War.) (Dolan collection.)

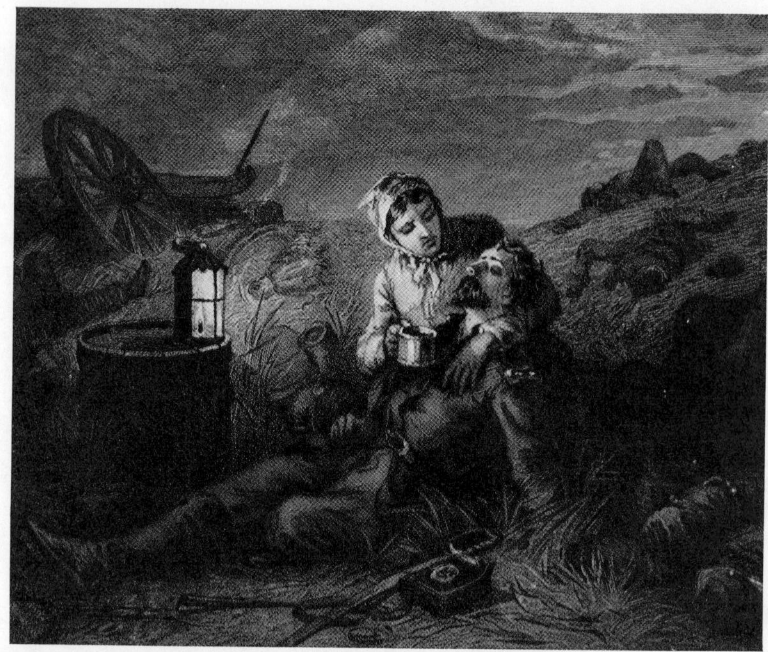

Figure 10–4. Mother Bickerdyke searching the battlefield at midnight in order to find and comfort the neglected or forgotten patient. (Dolan collection.)

"What can I do? I am a bonded officer and responsible for the property in my charge." "You can do nothing," she replied, "but ride on ahead. I am neither bonded nor responsible." Soon an ox was extricated from the herd and given to the grateful surgeon of the Confederate army.

Mary Ann Bickerdyke (1817–1901), affectionately called *Mother Bickerdyke,* responded to an urgent plea from her minister, Henry Ward Beecher (the brother of Harriet Beecher Stowe), for some women in his congregation to go to the government hospitals and battlefields and care for the sick and wounded (Fig. 10–4). She was a dynamic and kind-hearted woman who gave the soldiers very good care. Mother Bickerdyke was a widow of humble origin and moderate education, with two little sons. She had taken Dr. Hahnemann's short course in homeopathy and received a degree of Doctor of Botanic Medicine.[1] This training was useful in her nursing care of the wounded.

Dr. Brockett[2] described the devoted attention she showered upon the enlisted men who received a private's pay, private's fare and private's dangers. She stressed that these boys were dear to somebody, and she would be a mother to them and fight for their rights and comfort. She is remembered as the "Soldier's Friend." The soldiers idolized her. Indeed, Dr. Brockett stated, "Woe to the surgeon, the commissary or quartermaster, whose neglect of his men and selfish disregard for their interests and needs came under her cognizance."

Her efforts were memorialized by the

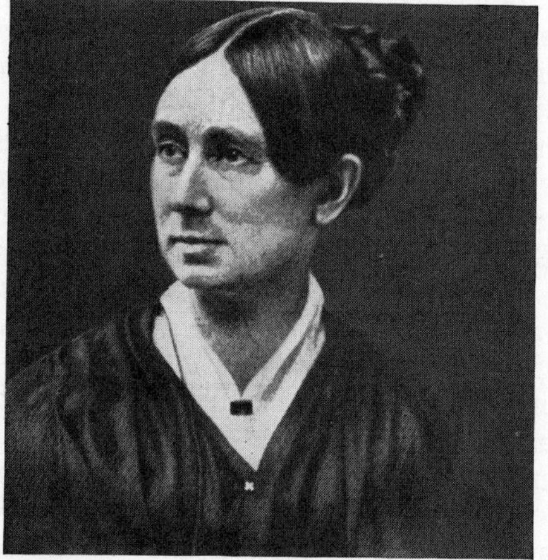

Figure 10–5. Dorothea Lynde Dix. (Dolan collection.)

[1]Baker, Nina B.: *Cyclone in Calico.* Boston, Little, Brown & Co., 1952, pp. 18–20.

[2]Brockett, L. P.: *The Camp, the Battle Field, and the Hospital; or Lights and Shadows of the Great Rebellion.* Philadelphia, National Publishing Company, 1866.

government when the hospital ship, the *S. S. Mary A. Bickerdyke,* was launched at Richmond, California, in 1943.

Although there were women such as Clara Barton and Mary Bickerdyke, the need for more nurses was still great. The public had been troubled by newspaper accounts of the medical treatment at some military camps, the lack of care for sick soldiers at these centers, the insufficiency of supplies and the inadequacy of transportation that resulted in a lack of surgical dressings and drugs.

On June 10, 1861, *Dorothea Lynde Dix* (Fig. 10–5) was appointed *Superintendent of the Female Nurses of the Union Army.* The Secretary of War gave her the responsibility and authority to recruit and equip a corps of army nurses.

Document 213
To Volunteer Nurses
War Department, Military Hospital

Be it known to all whom it may concern that the free services of Miss D. L. Dix are accepted by the War Department, and that she will give at all times all necessary aid in organizing military hospitals for the care of all sick and wounded soldiers, aiding the chief surgeons by supplying nurses and substantial means for the comfort and relief of the suffering; also, that she is fully authorized to receive, control and disburse special supplies bestowed by individuals or associations for the comfort of their friends or the citizen soldiers from all parts of the United States.

Given under the seal of the War Department this twenty-third day of April, in the year of our Lord one thousand eight hundred and sixty-one, and of the independence of the United States the eighty-fifth.

S/Simon Cameron
Secretary of War

Military rank, so very important, was not given to Miss Dix or the members of her corps. She did not have a background of preparation in nursing as Florence Nightingale did, but she had developed organizational skills as a result of her previous humanitarian efforts.

The qualifications of the army nurses were that the women who were recruited be over 30, plain-looking, dressed in brown or black with no ornamentation—no bows, no curls, no jewelry and no hoop skirts. Women from all parts of the country offered their services. Miss Dix soon had 2000 capable, enthusiastic women ready to serve the armed forces.

The mansion of *Robert E. Lee* was converted into a hospital, and here the wounded from the Civil War's first important battle, Bull Run, were brought. Now the mansion's beautiful estate is known as *Arlington National Cemetery*.[3]

Temporary hospitals were organized in any available buildings. Other structures were hastily erected or tents were pitched. Public buildings were commandeered. At one time the Union Army converted the Capitol in Washington into a hospital; 400 wounded were nursed in the Senate and House and 300 in the rotunda.

In many hospitals there were ward masters and orderlies who did as much of the nursing as they could. The women nurses dressed wounds, gave medicines and attended to diets (Fig. 10–6). The hours of

[3]In 1938 a statue of a nurse, designed and sculptured by Frances Rich, was erected in the nurses' section of Arlington National Cemetery. It was rededicated in 1971 "to commemorate devoted service to country and humanity by the Army, Navy and Air Force Nurses."

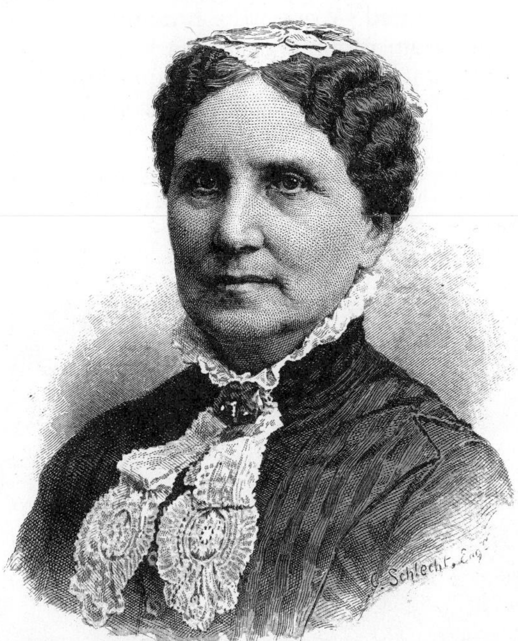

Figure 10–6. Mary A. Livermore (1820–1905), a devout advocate of suffrage and education for women, served with the United States Sanitary Commission during the Civil War. (Dolan collection.)

duty were long. There were many medical cases, fevers, dysentery and even smallpox, and many nurses died of disease contracted in the line of duty.

Despite all efforts, many soldiers had insufficient care and many died from neglect. After some battles hundreds of wounded were laid in open sheds or temporary shelters without bedding and with only a few surgeons to look after them. The so-called "ambulances" were often only springless wagons.

During the Civil War, many of the medicines made from herbs were obtained from the *Shakers*, or the *United Society of Believers in Christ's Second Coming*. They were the first group in the United States to grow herbs for the pharmaceutical market.[4] Their main industrial enterprise was the cultivation of herbs; they collected them, dried them or extracted the medicinal ingredients and packed and shipped them.

The Shakers were meticulously clean and had an efficient system of preparing the medicines. In addition to having beautifully cared-for gardens, they had an herb house where the herbs were dried and packaged; and another building, the extract house, where presses and boilers were located. Water was brought by clay pipes from mountain springs to provide a pure water supply. Raffinesque, the famous French-American botanist, said, "The best medical gardens in the United States are those established by the communities of Shakers or Modern Essenes."[5]

UNITED STATES SANITARY COMMISSION

In the late spring of 1861, handbills were distributed in New York City signed by more than 90 respected ladies announcing a mass meeting at Cooper Union. More than 4000 determined women attended. They organized *The Women's Central Association for Relief*. This group and others of similar interest and organization banded together, and their leaders cajoled a Unitarian clergyman, Henry W. Bellows, D.D., of New England, a physician, Elisha Harris, and three other physicians into going to Washington to plead for the establishment of a sanitary commission to investigate health conditions in the Union Army. As a result, the *United States Sanitary Commission* was established by order of President Lincoln on June 3, 1861. (See Figure 10–7.)

One of the reports of the Sanitary Commission revealed that 15 per cent of the physicians in the Northern regiments were either poorly qualified or totally incompetent. Needless to say, the medical officers of the Army resented the interference of the commission in attempting to improve

[4]Andrews, Edward D., and Andrews, Faith: *Shaker Herbs and Herbalists*. Stockbridge, Mass., Berkshire Garden Center, 1959, p. 3.

[5]Andrews, Edward D., and Andrews, Faith: *Shaker Herbs and Herbalists*. Stockbridge, Mass., Bershire Garden Center, 1959, p. 4.

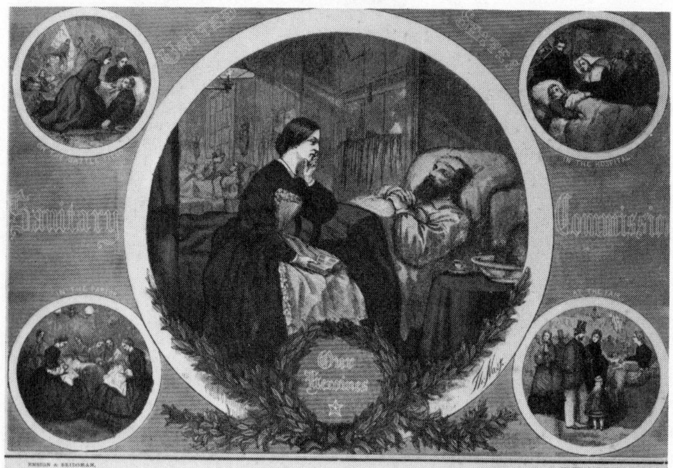

Figure 10–7. Thomas Nast's representation of the diversified yet unified activities of the United States Sanitary Commission—providing nurses on the battlefield and in the hospital; making supplies in the home; and raising money at the fair while arousing public interest and support for health care. (Dolan collection.)

the medical care of the soldiers. Much is now known that might not have been disclosed but for the commission's constant vigilance, and much was prevented that might have been disastrous for the welfare of mankind. The results of their endeavors included the establishment of pavilion hospitals that could be dismantled and moved and standards for camp water supply systems, latrines and garbage disposal.

After the first battles of the war, the wounded received practically no care. "Common soldiers, untrained, lazy, and indifferent or brutal, were cooks and nurses for the war hospitals, the largest of which had forty beds. There were no medicines, no stores, nor ambulances. The camps were dirty and unsanitary." Those who knew of these conditions were filled with shame and resolved to do something about it. When the Sanitary Commission first offered supplies and service, the Government Medical Bureau looked upon the proposal with suspicion, but dire need soon forced the Bureau to accept the commission's offer. The commission collected and distributed supplies of all sorts, planned camps and attended to their sanitation and tended the wounded on the field and in hospitals; in short, the commission undertook a large share of the health work for the army (Fig. 10–7). It provided such things as green vegetables, given by the farmers for the soldiers; thus, the commission prevented scurvy, the great army scourge. (Dehydrated vegetables were used to feed the soldiers, at the suggestion of a Harvard professor, in 1864.) In 1862, the commission equipped a hospital train, which was an entirely new practice (Fig. 10–8). Providing "the largest army charity the world has ever seen," the commission collected and spent over $5,000,000 in cash and $15,000,000 worth of supplies, an unprecedented amount for those days.

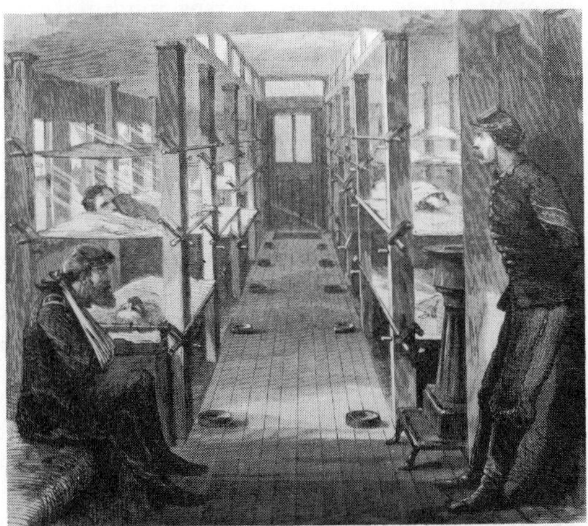

Figure 10–8. The interior of a hospital train. (Dolan collection.)

The Women's Central Association for Relief eventually became a branch of the U.S. Sanitary Commission and assumed the important activity of sending nurses to war areas where the need seemed most crucial. Preparatory to the nurses' departure, programs were planned for them at New York Hospital and Bellevue Hospital, as well as at several Boston hospitals, which provided one month's observation and work.

NURSE VOLUNTEERS

Many members of the *Woolsey* family participated in nursing. Austin[6] presents a fascinating account of a well-to-do family's involvement in the Civil War as well as in the development of a new approach to nursing education. Mrs. Woolsey and her daughters Abby, Jane, Carry, Hatty, Georgy and Eliza contributed their talents either in nursing care or in making hospital supplies.

Georgeanna (Georgy) Woolsey was one of the first young ladies to be admitted to New York Hospital for brief instruction and to "walk the wards." She then requested to join the ranks of Dorothea Dix. Georgy and her sister *Eliza Woolsey Howland* went to Washington to care for the army of the sick, who were housed in every available building. After a conference with Miss Dix, the sisters commenced their volunteer nursing activities at Georgetown Hospital. While they were carrying out their nursing duties it became obvious to them that chaplains were needed. Thereupon Georgy wrote to President Lincoln requesting the appointment of chaplains to hospitals. She even delivered the letter to the back door of the White House. The President responded by appointing seven chaplains.

[6]Austin, Anne L.: *The Woolsey Sisters of New York—1860–1900.* Philadelphia, American Philosophical Society, 1971.

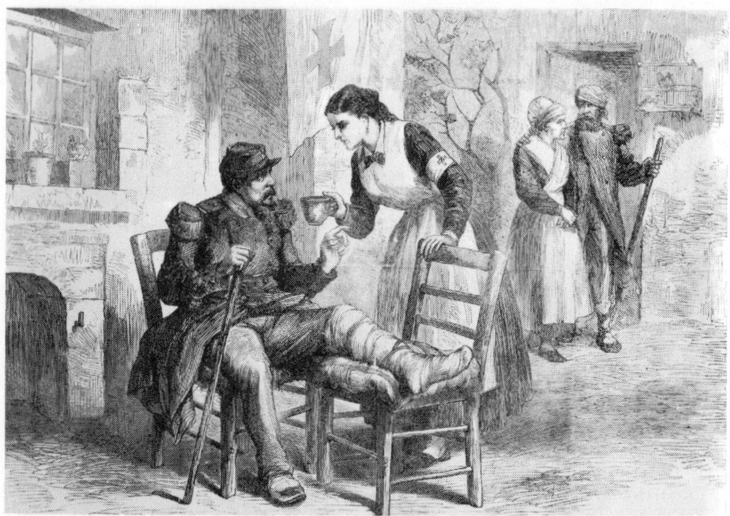

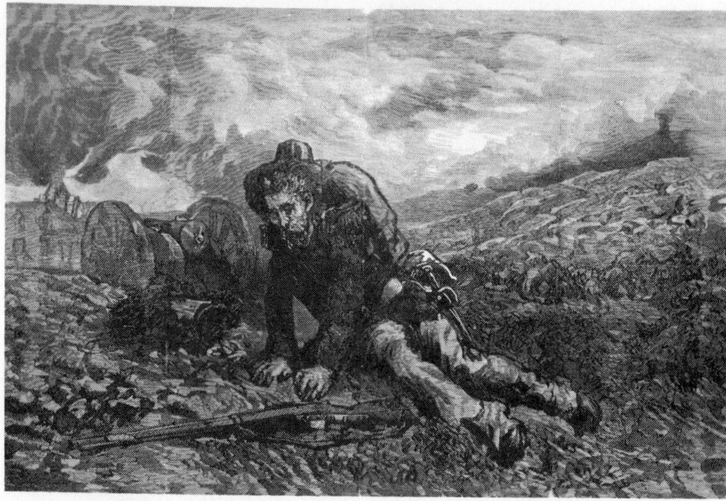

Figure 10–9. These pictures appeared in *Harper's Weekly* in 1871 and were titled "Cared For" and "Uncared For." They depict the importance of the nurse in helping people to live. (Dolan collection.)

The opposition of physicians to women nurses and the lengths to which they went to encourage the women to return home are well documented by many of the volunteer nurses, including Georgeanna Woolsey.[7] The almost insurmountable task faced by Miss Dix of providing nursing care despite the opposition of physicians can thus be understood. In 1864 Georgeanna Woolsey wrote:[8]

> No one knows, who did not watch the thing from the beginning, how much opposition, how much ill-will, how much unfeeling want of thought these women nurses endured. . . . Government had decided that women should be employed, and the army surgeons . . . determined to make their lives so unbearable that they would be forced in self-defense to leave. . . .
>
> Some of the bravest women I have ever known were among the first company of army nurses. They saw at once the position of affairs, the attitude assumed by the surgeons and the wall against which they were expected to break and scatter; and they set themselves to undermine the whole thing.
>
> None of them were "strong-minded." Some of them were women of the truest refinement and culture; and day after day they quietly and patiently worked, doing, by order of the surgeon, things which not one of those gentlemen would have dared to ask of a woman whose male relative stood able and ready to defend her

[7]Austin, Anne L.: *The Woolsey Sisters of New York—1860—1900*. Philadelphia, American Philosophical Society, 1971, pp. 50, 112.

[8]*Ibid.*, p. 112.

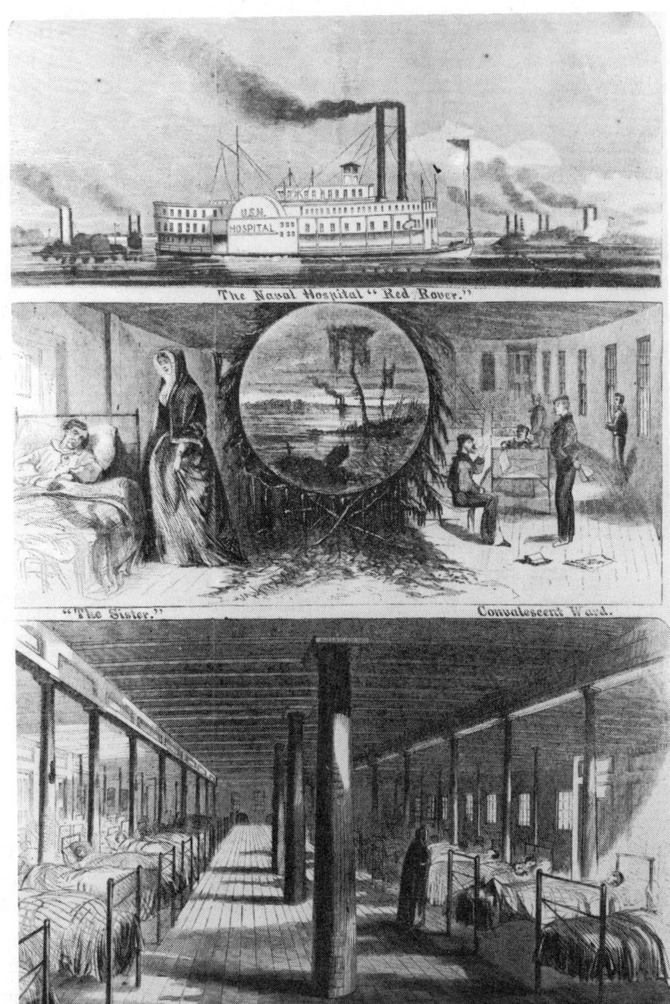
U.S.N.
HOSPITAL
The Naval Hospital "Red Rover."
"The Sister."
Convalescent Ward.
The Ward.
THE FLOATING HOSPITAL ON THE MISSISSIPPI.—Drawn by Mr. Theodore R. Davis.—[See Page 801.]

Figure 10–10. Hospital steamers—floating hospitals—transported many soldiers from the war theater. Nurses were in charge of providing care. (Dolan collection.)

and report him. I have seen small white hands scrubbing floors, washing windows and performing all menial offices. I have known women, delicately cared for at home, half fed in hospitals, hard worked day and night, and given, when sleep must be had, a wretched closet just large enough for a camp bed to stand in. I have known surgeons who purposely and ingeniously arranged these inconveniences with the avowed intention of driving away all women from their hospitals.

As the casualties increased, transport steamers, in effect, *floating hospitals,* were used to convey soldiers to hospitals for care (Fig. 10–10). Four nurses were assigned the duty of caring for patients on each transport—Georgeanna Woolsey, her sister Eliza Howland, *Katherine Wormeley* and *Christine Griffin.*

Jane Stuart Woolsey, after receiving nursing experience in hospitals in New York City, commenced her activities in the theater of war. Her refreshing reflections of this experience are presented in *Hospital Days.*[9] She praises the thoughtful inclusion in the wards in the theatre of war operations of game-boxes and books for patients who might enjoy them; the green shades that were lowered to protect the eyes of feverish patients; the prints on the wall for di-

[9]Woolsey, Jane Stuart: *Hospital Days.* New York, Van Nostrand, 1868, p. 47.

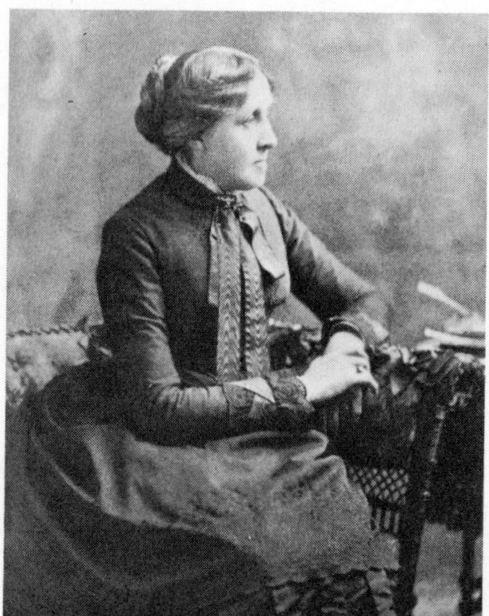

Figure 10–11. Louisa May Alcott in 1887. (Dolan collection.)

version; and the rocking chairs with their swinging motion to relieve nervous tension. Soft, light slippers were provided for the male nurses in the ward because it was understood that the heavy thud of a boot is "almost as intolerable to a patient as a 'sympathizer' sitting on the edge of his bed."

Indeed she comments:

> No one can count up the value of these things, not only in the flannels for discharged, broken-down men, and woolen socks and mittens for convalescents going on guard in puddles of snow-water, but the distraction from pain in wounded men, the occupation and interest furnished to wretched, bored, half sick, half well, wholly demoralized men who huddle in a hopeless way round the red-hot sheet-iron stoves.

Her concepts of nursing permeate her book. She describes her plan for learning about patients' fancies and home habits; noting changes in their physical and mental condition; talking with them, listening to them, and writing for them; helping them invent occupations and amusements to while away the hours; remembering that "many sad wives and poor children depend on my promptness"; and analyzing each patient's need and carrying out the best possible regimen to hasten his return to health.

Jane Woolsey relates an incident in which her sister Georgy collaborated with the physician for a better approach to patient care.[10]

> On one of these nights a nurse came hurriedly up with the word, "There's a man dying in Ward ——; we can't do anything for him."—"Has he taken anything since he came in?"—"No'm, can't eat nothin', doctor says mustn't give him no stimulants, stomach's too weak." "I'll have a look at him," says G (Georgy)—and after the nurse goes out—"the surgeon doesn't know a bronchitis from a broken leg. There's not a man in that ward who ought to die.—*If* he is dying, he is dying of starvation." She hunts up the doctor and asks if wine-whey, the lightest of stimulants, may be tried. Doctor didn't know what it was, but had no objection; "man couldn't live anyhow." The man took the cup full eagerly, was "out of danger" in the morning, got well,—the doctor directing the nurse to be very particular to "give him his wine-whey 'reg'lar' "—went back to the field and helped to take Richmond.

Jane Woolsey stressed that she followed "those who were assigned to carry trays," served those patients who were unable to serve themselves and checked to see that every person had enough food or obtained more suitable food. While she watched patients, she would make notes in a memorandum book that she carried: "Mr. M—— has expressed a longing for some Boston brown bread. Memo: try and get him some. For a patient whose appetite was on the wane and who didn't feel the effort to eat was worthwhile. Memo: try champagne in a long-spouted cup."

This most remarkable family received much gratitude from nurses and patients and their families for their devotion and superior nursing care.

Louisa May Alcott (1832–1888) (Fig. 10–11) was the daughter of Bronson Alcott, whose influence prompted the rise of the Transcendental Movement. Miss Alcott cooled feverish brows, soothed the fears of 12-year-old drummer boys and recorded her efforts in letters that she signed "Nurse Periwinkle." Later, her letters appeared in *Hospital Sketches,* published in 1863. Reflecting on her daily routine, she wrote:

[10] Woolsey, Jane Stuart: *Hospital Days.* New York, Van Nostrand, 1868, p. 121.

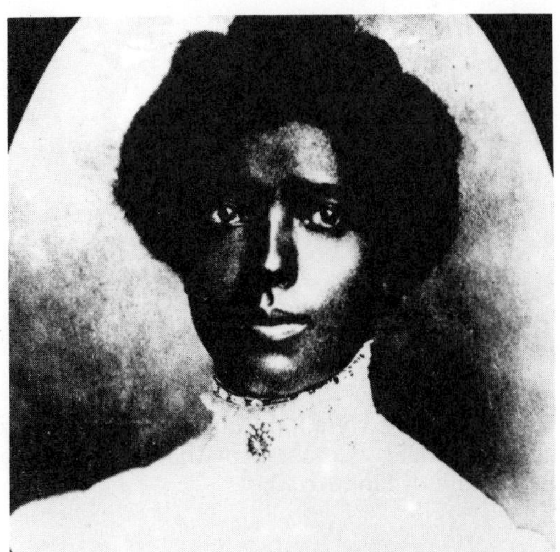

Figure 10–12. Sojourner Truth, a nurse in the Civil War. (Courtesy of Joyce A. Elmore.)

Up at six, dress by gaslight, run through my ward and throw up the windows, though the men grumble and shiver. But the air is bad enough to breed a pestilence . . . till noon I trot, trot, trot, giving out rations, cutting up food for helpless 'boys,' washing faces, teaching my attendants how beds are made or floors are swept, dressing wounds. . . . At twelve comes dinner for patients and afterward letter writing for them or reading aloud. . . . Supper at five sets everyone running who can run. . . . Evening amusements. . . . Then, for such as need them, the final doses for the night.

She reported that she "ministered to their minds by writing letters" to their families for them. She noted that many boys wore bags of camphor around their neck for protection against disease.

Her common sense and ability to protest against lack of organization in nursing service were displayed when she registered disapproval of the use of convalescents as attendants. She deplored not having enough help of the right kind.[11]

If any hospital director fancies this a good and economical arrangement allow one used up nurse to tell him it isn't, and beg him to spare the sisterhood who sometimes in their sympathy, forget that they are mortal, and run the risk of being made immortal, sooner than is agreeable to their partial friends.

[11]Alcott, Louisa M.: *Hospital Sketches.* Boston, James Redpath, 1863, p. 74.

Dr. Brockett's book *The Camp, the Battle Field, and the Hospital*[12] presents many nursing care studies of these heroic and able nurses of the Civil War era. Several case studies describe the activities of Louisa May Alcott. Of Georgeanna Woolsey, Dr. Brockett states in *Woman's Work in the Civil War*[13] that she was one of the most efficient ladies. Her constant cheerfulness, her ready wit and her never-failing resources of contrivance and management in any emergency made the severe labor seem light and, by keeping up the spirits of the entire party, prevented the ever-present scenes of suffering from rendering her co-workers morbid and depressed.

Harriet Tubman (1820–1913) was a fearless, courageous nurse who worked diligently to relieve the sufferings of those who needed her ministrations. In addition, as an abolitionist, she was a staunch worker in assisting her fellow blacks to gain freedom. Bradford has called her the "Moses of her people."[14] She had escaped to the north and had been active with the underground railroad movement before joining the Union Army in the Civil War. Miller has provided an annotated list of many books that deal with the contributions of this remarkable woman, who is purported to have made 19 trips to the South and to have assisted three hundred slaves in achieving freedom.[15]

Henry K. Durant, acting assistant surgeon in charge of the "Contraband Hospital," attested to Mrs. Tubman's "kindness and attention to the sick and suffering of her own race" in May of 1864. He further stated that he took "much pleasure in testifying to the esteem" in which she was held. This testimonial was countersigned by R. Saxton, the brigadier general, who penned, "I concur fully in the above."

[12]Brockett, L. P.: *The Camp, the Battle Field, and the Hospital; or Lights and Shadows of the Great Rebellion.* Philadelphia, National Publishing Company, 1866, pp. 293–454.

[13]Brockett, L. P.: *Woman's Work in the Civil War: A Record of Heroism, Patriotism and Patience.* Boston, R. H. Curran Co., 1867, p. 327.

[14]Bradford, Sarah: *Harriet Tubman—The Moses of Her People.* New York, Corinth Books, 1961, pp. 139–140.

[15]Miller, Helen Sullivan: *The History of Chi Eta Phi Sorority, Inc., 1932–1967.* Washington, D.C., Negro Life and History, Inc., 1968, pp. 169–172.

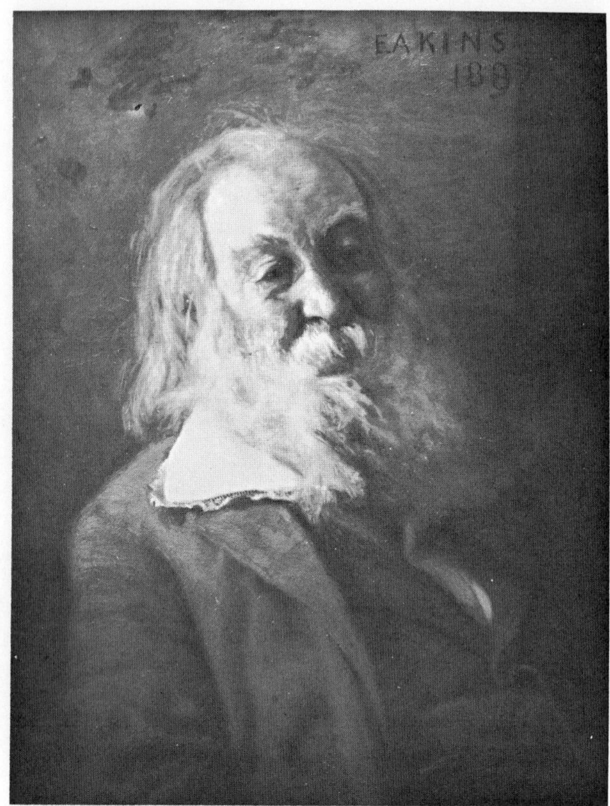

Figure 10–13. Walt Whitman, by Thomas Eakins (1887). (Courtesy of the Pennsylvania Academy of Fine Arts.)

Mrs. Tubman is recorded as holding the position of "nurse or matron" at the Colored Hospital in Fort Monroe, Virginia.[16]

Other black women made significant contributions to Civil War nursing. *Sojourner Truth* (Fig. 10–12) worked diligently for the women's movement and cared very competently for wounded soldiers in the Union Army. *Susie King,* wife of Sergeant Edward King of the 33rd W.S. Colored Infantry, served in the capacity of volunteer nurse for a little over four years. Elmore[17] stated that "physicians and hospitalized soldiers welcomed her" and that "she frequently accompanied Clara Barton on rounds." Her compassion and intelligence have been noted. She often brought solace to the soldiers by reading letters to those unable to read and worked to teach some of them to read and write.

Walt Whitman (1819–1892) (Fig. 10–13) has left a monumental record of the care of the sick during the Civil War in his collection of poems, *Drum-Taps,* and in his diary, *Specimen Days,* which contains vivid descriptions of his experiences as a hospital nurse in Washington. His younger brother George enlisted in the Thirteenth Regiment. When news reached Walt Whitman that his brother had been wounded, he rushed to Fredericksburg, Virginia, to be of assistance. His sensitive nature was so moved by the sick and wounded soldiers that he was unable to leave them. His major role was not so much to meet the physical needs of the casualties but to meet the psychological ones. The emotional trauma suffered by these heroic soldiers could be understood and appreciated only by those who witnessed it.

He was a familiar figure wandering from ward to ward, passing out books and other comforts, listening to the boys and writing letters for them. He used his literary talents to expose the inefficiency and negligence that he noted as he observed the military procedures. His objective in his articles was to move the indifferent public.

[16]Bradford, Sarah: Harriet Tubman—*The Moses of Her People.* New York, Corinth Books, 1961, p. 142.

[17]Elmore, Joyce Ann: "Black Nurses: Their Service and Their Struggle," *American Journal of Nursing,* 76:435, 1976.

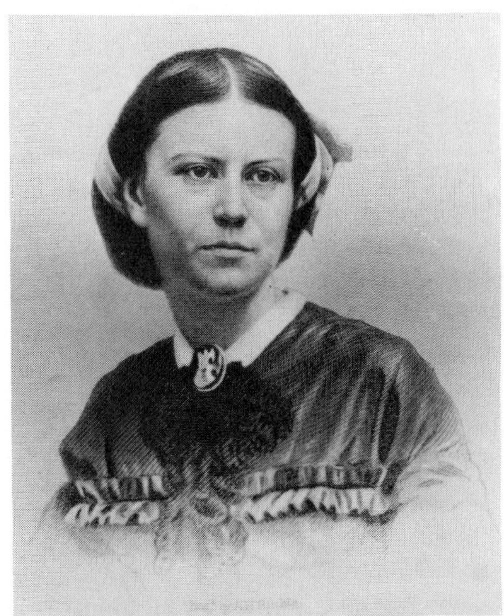

Figure 10–14. Margaret Breckinridge, a distinguished Civil War nurse. (Dolan collection.)

He played a dual role of war correspondent and nurse. His perceptions of the sufferings of the men and his efforts in their behalf are set forth in "The Dresser":

> Bearing the bandages, water and sponge,
> Straight and swift to my wounded I go,
> Where they lie on the ground after the battle brought in,
> Where their priceless blood reddens the grass, the ground,
> Or to the rows of the hospital tent, or under the roof'd hospital,
> To the long rows of cots up and down each side I return,
> To each and all one after another I draw near, not one do I miss,
> I onward go, I stop,
> With hinged knees and steady hands to dress wounds,
> I am firm with each, the pangs are sharp yet unavoidable,
> One turns to me his appealing eyes—poor boy! I never knew you,
> Yet I think I could not refuse this moment to die for you, if that would save you.

Austin records Walt Whitman's disdain for "lady nurses." He believed that older nurses were the "true nurses."[18] Conversely, it is interesting that the correspondence of Harriet Foote Hawley reveals the aversion that she felt whenever Walt Whitman appeared in the hospital units. She indicated that his presence had a disruptive influence.[19]

Many of the women who went to the Civil War in the nurse role, including the Woolsey sisters, Louise Lee Schuyler and Margaret Breckinridge, were women of sound educational backgrounds, strong political beliefs and socially prestigious families.

Margaret Breckinridge (Fig. 10–14), the granddaughter of a member of the U.S. Senate who later became Attorney General of the United States, was the daughter of John Breckinridge, D.D., an ardent churchman. The patriotic and humanitarian milieu in which she was raised prepared her for the outstanding contributions that she was to make as a nurse in the Civil War.

Harriet Foote Hawley and *Ella Louise Wolcott* describe the ghastly medical care and the need for delivery of higher quality health care.

Harriet Foote Hawley was the wife of Colonel Hawley, who later became editor of the *Hartford Courant* and eventually governor of Connecticut. In her correspondence, *Ella Louise Wolcott* left extensive documentation of the role and plight of the nurse in this war and of the encouragement she received from Dorothea Dix.[20]

On the Confederate side, religious sisters and lay women also gave heroic service. The Confederate Army did not appoint a director of nursing, but President Jefferson Davis bestowed the rank of captain on a most deserving candidate, *Miss Sally Tompkins.* Miss Tompkins was a well-to-do young Southern woman who was active in the charitable works of her church. After the battle of Bull Run when Judge Robertson offered the use of his home as a hospital, she was placed in charge of it because she had taken care of many sick persons. When private hospitals were ordered closed, she begged President Davis to intercede for the soldiers and her hospital, and the Robertson hospital was not closed. She refused the customary remu-

[18]Austin, Anne L.: "Nurses in American History—Wartime Volunteers," *American Journal of Nursing,* 75:816–818, 1975.

[19]Unpublished biographical records. Courtesy of Edward J. Foote.

[20]Dolan collection of Wolcott and Dix letters.

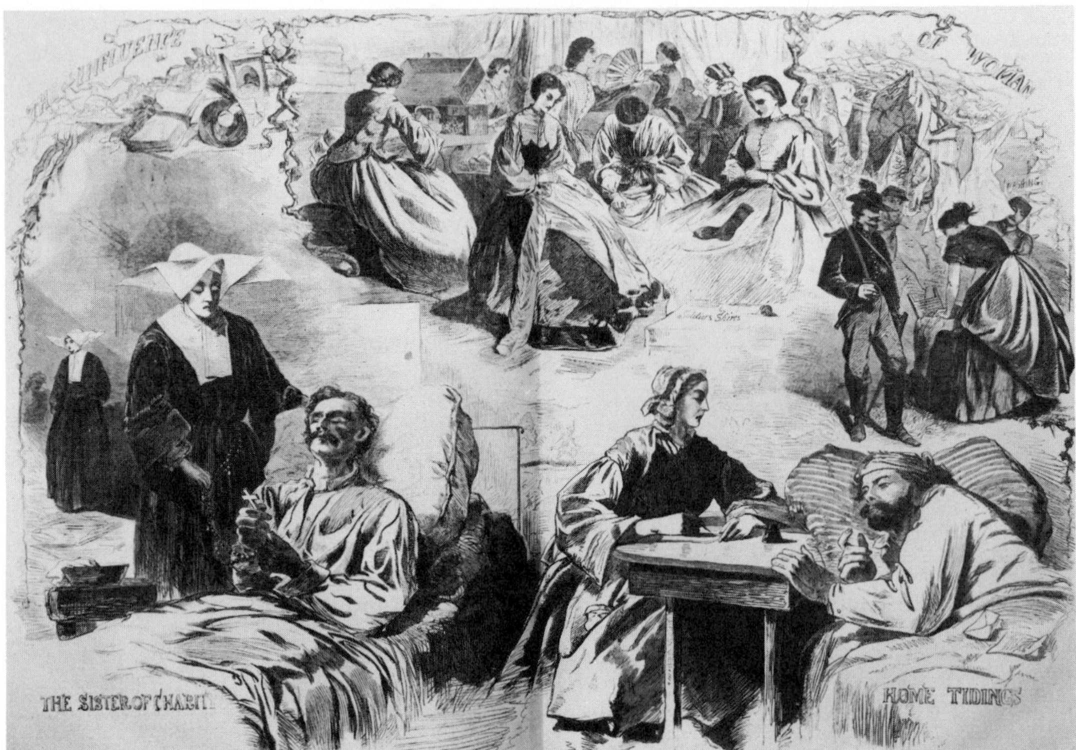

Figure 10–15. A montage of the activities and the influence of women during the Civil War. An etching by Winslow Homer. (Dolan collection.)

neration but accepted food, medicines and other supplies in lieu of a salary.

The nursing care given by Miss Tompkins must have been of a superior quality, because by the end of the war, her records indicate that only 73 patients died out of 1333 who had received care in the Robertson hospital.

Many refined, self-sacrificing women nursed the wounded of the Confederate Army day and night. Among these were Miss Kate Cumming, Mrs. Ella Newsom and Mrs. Gilmer. Their heroic benevolence inspired others to join them. Hospitals were named in honor of Mrs. Newsom and Mrs. Gilmer.

Kate Cumming's diary of her activities as a volunteer nurse with the Confederate Army has been preserved as an important primary historical source for this epoch.[21] It was first published in 1865. She states, "I had never been inside of a hospital and was wholly ignorant of what I should be called upon to do, but I knew that what one woman (Florence Nightingale) had done, another could." Impressive are her accounts of the sick and wounded, and of their care, or lack of it, on battlefields and in hospitals. She relates problems concerning the quartermaster, transportation, food, shelter, fuel, lighting, clothing and communications. She describes amputations, hospital gangrene, contagion, smallpox and typhoid fever. With deep humility she bemoans the fact that she "failed to be more useful." Many of these cultured, dedicated women recognized the need for well-educated nurses.

THE RED CROSS SOCIETY

One of the significant movements of the nineteenth century was the development of the Red Cross Society. It was originally an association of citizens who undertook to render effective help in time of war or calamity. In the beginning, help was ex-

[21]Cumming, Kate: *Kate: The Journal of a Confederate Nurse.* Richard Barksdale Harwell, Ed. Baton Rouge, Louisiana State University Press, 1959.

tended only in time of war, but soon aid was given in all calamities that involved a considerable number of people.

For centuries there had been societies for helping the wounded in time of war, many of which had done efficient work. The Red Cross idea was far greater than anything that went before it, in that it placed the work on an *international* basis and suggested teamwork among nations, a thing almost unheard of before the mid-nineteenth century. The plan originated in the mind of *Jean Henri Dunant,* a Swiss, and it owes its effectiveness to his ingenuity.

In 1859, while traveling in Italy, Dunant saw the field of Solférino on the day after the battle, in which 300,000 were engaged, had taken place. He helped care for the wounded and was horrified by the needless suffering that he saw. He wrote a vivid description of it, and began interviewing kings, princes, generals and church officials and lecturing on the subject. It was his vision and persistence that brought about this work of such incalculable value.

In 1863, Dunant formulated a plan in which he proposed to organize in every country an association for war relief. Each association was to be an independent society, with a strong international bond of affiliation and a guaranteed neutrality of supplies and personnel. The result was that in October 1863, an international conference was held at Geneva, Switzerland, where representatives of 16 nations agreed to a provisional program. This led to the formation of an international Red Cross society. The United States, then in the midst of the Civil War, sent no official delegate.

In August 1864, a formal diplomatic congress was held, in which participants signed the *Geneva Convention.* This agreement stipulated that each nation that ratified the convention should have a national committee or society, civil in character and function, which alone would have the right to send a surgical corps to a war. Such organizations were at that time under way in 28 countries. The well-known emblem of the society, the red cross, was also adopted.[22]

[22]During the Serbian War of 1876 the Turkish Government notified the powers that it would use the red crescent instead of the red cross as the insignia of its relief societies. Moslem countries participating in the Red Cross use the crescent to differentiate them from Christian countries.

The convention was ratified at that time by 12 nations; by 1925 there were 52 national Red Cross organizations. Additions have been made to its program from time to time, and its provisions are now recognized as a part of international law.

In some countries similar societies that were already in existence were affiliated with or absorbed by the Red Cross, keeping the original idea of cooperation. Soon after its organization, the Red Cross began extending its relief efforts to victims of natural disasters, such as, earthquakes, extensive floods, forest fires, famines and all catastrophes for which more than local help was needed. The present emphasis of the Red Cross is on improvement of health, prevention of disease and relief of suffering.

In every country the society makes preparation beforehand for war or disaster, they have at various centers great storehouses containing such things as tents, portable houses, furniture, tools, clothing and medical and surgical supplies. The Red Cross personnel are men and women who can temporarily leave their regular occupations; its organization provides means of getting a group of previously instructed workers together on an hour's notice. The efficiency of its organization has repeatedly been shown in times when governments were helpless because of official "red tape."

The First World War caused an unprecedented development in the Red Cross. In 1919 the health authorities of the world formed a league that is a federation of the various national Red Cross societies. This league has expanded its program to include public health and has become interested in the control of tuberculosis and venereal diseases and in child welfare.

Because their endeavors involved the education of nurses, the *Division of Nursing* was promptly created by the society. Its directors have included Alice Fitzgerald and Katherine Olmsted of the United States, Mrs. Maynard Carter of England and Yvonne Hentsch of Switzerland.

The *Florence Nightingale Medal* (Fig. 10–16) was established in 1912 by the International Red Cross Committee to be given in alternate years to nurses "who have distinguished themselves in an exceptional manner by great devotion to their patients in time of war or peace." This medal has been given to organizations, graduate nurses,

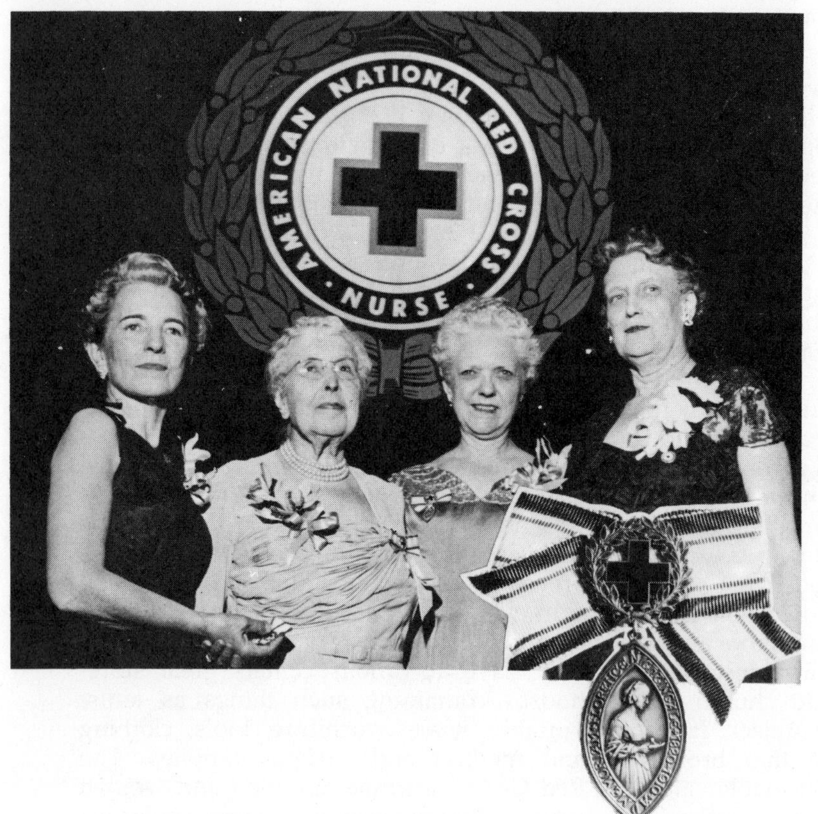

Figure 10–16. Ann C. Magnussen *(far right)* presenting the Florence Nightingale Medals at the National League for Nursing Convention in 1959 to *(left to right)* Lucile Petry Leone, Effie Jane Taylor, and Ruth Sleeper. (Dolan collection.)

nurses' aides and posthumously, to nurses who died in war.

In some European countries, the Red Cross has its own hospitals and educates its own nurses. Educational courses vary greatly in length and content. Some courses last three months, some three years in an accredited school of nursing. Some consist of lectures to laymen and schoolchildren, or instruction in first aid. Red Cross hospitals sometimes care for the sick poor or the members of the armed forces in peacetime.

The United States, the thirty-second country to enter the Red Cross, formed the *American Red Cross Society,* largely as a result of the tireless efforts of *Clara Barton.* She was a nurse who served during the Civil War and who, in 1870, undertook the work of the Red Cross in the Franco-Prussian War. In 1881, she organized in Washington a Red Cross Committee and in 1882, persuaded the government to ratify the Geneva Convention and give the committee official standing.

PUBLIC HEALTH—A COMMUNITY ENDEAVOR

In the 1860s, New York City was filled with filth and debris; sicknesses ravaged the inhabitants. Garbage and refuse were thrown in the streets, and the air was polluted by the slaughterhouses and leather tanneries. Communicable diseases, such as tuberculosis, smallpox, diphtheria, scarlet fever, yellow fever, cholera and dysentery, were rampant in the congested tenement house districts.

It took a group of concerned public-spirited citizens, who banded together into the Citizens' Association, to fight for sanitary and health reform. The health picture viewed by the Citizens' Association was discouraging, but persistence, plus the added impetus caused by the reappearance of dreaded cholera, assisted in the passage of the necessary legislation. After years of having submitted health bills into the legislature without success, in 1866, the association's the Metropolitan Health Bill was passed and the Board of Health came into being. An interesting highlight that prompted the bill's passage was reported as follows:

> "Why I believe I have got smallpox for I begin to itch all over," cried a New York State legislator as he listened to Dr. Stephen S. Smith explain the sanitary requirements of the Citizens' Association's metropolitan health bill. The date was February 13, 1865, and Smith described how wholesale clothing dealers had goods manufactured in tenement houses. City inspectors

often found the clothing thrown over the beds of children with scarlet fever, measles, or smallpox—a condition which helped make the city vulnerable to epidemics.[23]

One of the first acts of the new Board of Health was to establish a bureau of records and vital statistics and an office of sanitary superintendence. When the United States faced another outbreak of cholera in 1866, isolation of the victims was enforced, and disinfectants were used to cleanse their homes and surroundings. A central depot for distributing disinfectants was established and a special disinfecting corps was organized (Fig. 10–17). This was a successful project, and the new Board of Health was credited with preventing a more devastating outbreak of cholera.

A vigorous program aimed at a general clean-up of New York City then ensued. Unsanitary conditions of every nature became the target of the Board of Health. Establishments that were considered to be health menaces were required to relocate. Inspections of garbage and refuse disposal systems were enforced and cellars were cleaned out by the members of the Board of Health. Cellar apartments were ordered to be drained, renovated or vacated.

Food markets were inspected as part of the initial plan for regulating and controlling the quality of produce. Finally, in 1869, a chemical laboratory was set up to analyze the water supply of the city; well water was found to be contaminated with the drainage from privies. Typhoid fever was discovered to be transmitted in this way. The results of an analysis of cosmetics revealed that they contained injurious quantities of lead. Kerosene, which was used in the lamps of this period, was mixed with naphtha, causing many explosions that resulted in fires and serious burns. The Board of Health made the use of naphtha as an ingredient illegal. The Board of Health had achieved phenomenal success in their initial efforts at consumer protection.

Practicing physicians were required to register cases of infectious disease with the Bureau of Records and Vital Statistics. Birth, stillbirth, marriage and death certificates were examined with great care. The incredibly high infant mortality rate, particularly in the tenement districts, became apparent. Deaths of children under five years of age accounted for 48 per cent of the total mortality; deaths of children under two years amounted to approximately 40 per cent of the total mortality.

A "summer corps" of physicians visited the tenement districts during July and August to treat the sick and distribute to mothers a pamphlet on infant care. The absence of, and urgent need for, nurses was

[23]McMahon, Margaret, and Erhardt, Carl: "Highlights of the First 100 Years," *Public Health Reports,* U.S. Department of Health, Education and Welfare, No. 1, *81*:87, 1966.

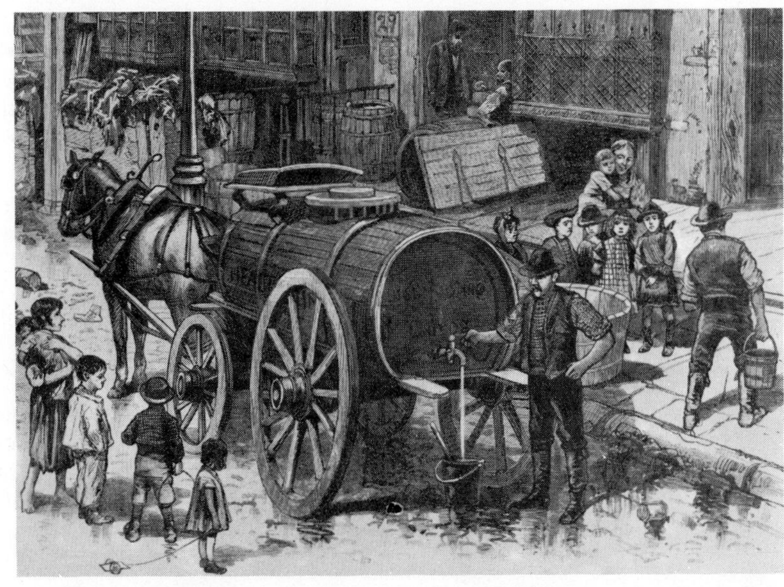

Figure 10–17. The disinfecting corps of the Health Department distributing disinfectants. (Courtesy of New York Academy of Medicine and New York City Department of Health.)

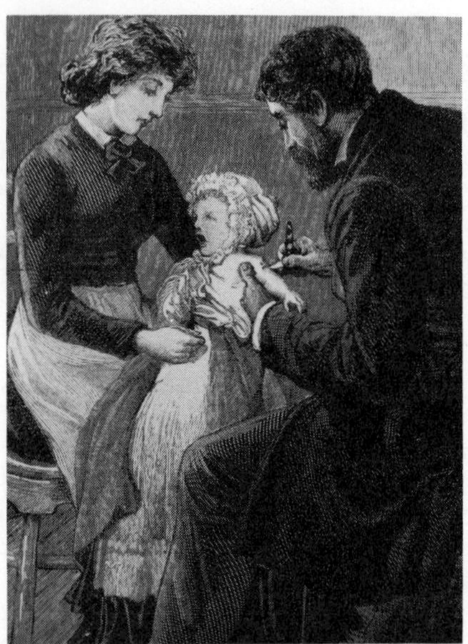

Figure 10–18. This 1871 newspaper drawing shows an early vaccination clinic where mothers brought their small children for smallpox vaccinations. (Courtesy of New York Academy of Medicine and New York City Department of Health.)

obvious! In 1867, Elisha Harris, counsel to the Board of Health, predicted that nurses would become our "missionaries of health," advising the public on health and sanitation.

Tuberculosis, called consumption or phthisis, was purported to be responsible for one-fifth to one-sixth of all deaths and seemed to afflict the underprivileged and minority groups most severely. Poor food and unsanitary living conditions were considered to be the cause of tuberculosis.

An epidemic of smallpox, which resulted in a high death rate, struck New York City in the winter of 1874–75. It was the duty of the Health Department to provide a special corps of physicians to vaccinate the public (Fig. 10–18). Efforts were devised to prepare vaccine.

The smallpox epidemic prompted legislation to transfer the Smallpox Hospital on Blackwell's Island, under the control of the Commissioners of Charities and Corrections, to the control of the Health Department. It was renamed Riverside Hospital. Buildings were renovated, and the nursing services of the Sisters of Charity were secured. The Board of Health eventually purchased a steamboat called the *Psyche* to transport patients to Riverside Hospital. Toward the end of the nineteenth century this hospital became too small for the demands made upon it, and a new and larger isolation hospital was constructed on North Brother Island. A larger steamboat was also required, and the *Mayor Franklin Edson* was procured for hospital service. It was reported that the after-cabin of the boat was divided in two parts to permit transportation of two types of contagious diseases without danger of mixed infection.

The Health Department recognized opportunities to provide health education, and pamphlets on child care, food handling, ventilation and prevention of disease were made available for distribution. Families were instructed in the need for cleanliness, disinfection and isolation of sick persons from other members of the family.

SUMMARY

At a time of critical need in the history of the country many dedicated and gifted persons responded to the call for nurses. The proper scientific and social ingredients had been added to the culture medium for the growth of nursing.

THE HERITAGE OF NURSING

The Image of Capable Leadership in the Civil War

In this period of crisis (1861–1865), many dynamic leaders emerged to increase public awareness of the urgent need for schools of nursing and programs of health maintenance and community health leadership in the United States. In the Civil War, the proven ability of the nurse leadership demonstrated that competent independent nurse practitioners existed.

The public was aware of:

1. the need for hospitals.
2. the necessity for better-prepared persons to accept the role of nurse and to provide good care for patients.
3. the existence of a potential nurse leadership force, which was seen during the Civil War.
4. the desire of these leaders to "change the system" and develop schools of nursing.
5. the need for community health programs and trained health care personnel at the termination of the war.

Most wars have been followed by health care reforms. The Crimean War showed Great Britain and the world what good nursing was, what must be done to improve nursing and how proper nursing education could provide quality nursing care. During the Civil War, socially, politically and intellectually endowed leaders emerged who struggled to upgrade health care by encouraging the establishment of schools of nursing. An enormous debt of gratitude is owed to these courageous, gifted, politically experienced, influential and visionary leaders.

REFERENCE READINGS

Adams, G. W.: *Doctors in Blue: The Medical History of the Union Army in the Civil War.* New York, Collier Books, 1961.

Alcott, Louisa May: *Hospital Sketches.* Boston, James Redpath, 1863. (New York, Sagamore Press, 1957.)

Alcott, Louisa M.: *Life, Letters and Journals.* Ednah D. Cheney, Ed. Boston, Roberts Brothers, 1889.

Austin, Anne L.: *History of Nursing Source Book.* New York, G. P. Putnam's Sons, 1957.

Austin, Anne L.: "Nurses in American History: Wartime Volunteers—1861–1865," *American Journal of Nursing, 75*:816–818, 1975.

Austin, Anne L.: *The Woolsey Sisters of New York—1860–1900.* Philadelphia, American Philosophical Society, 1971.

Baker, Nina B.: *Cyclone in Calico.* Boston, Little, Brown & Co., 1952.

Barton, W. E.: *Life of Clara Barton.* Boston, Houghton-Mifflin Co., 1922.

Blackwell, Elizabeth: *Pioneer Work in Opening the Medical Profession to Women.* London, Longmans, Green and Co., 1895.

Boyden, Anna L.: *Echoes from Hospital and White House.* Boston, D. Lothrop and Company, 1884.

Bradford, Sarah: *Harriet Tubman—The Moses of Her People.* New York, Corinth Books, 1961.

Brockett, L. P.: *The Camp, the Battle Field and the Hospital; or Lights and Shadows of the Great Rebellion.* Philadelphia, National Publishing Company, 1866.

Cumming, Kate: *Kate: The Journal of a Confederate Nurse.* Richard Barksdale Harwell, Ed. Baton Rouge, Louisiana State University Press, 1959.

Elmore, Joyce Ann: "Black Nurses: Their Service and Their Struggle," *American Journal of Nursing, 76*:435, 1976.

Holland, Mary A.: *Our Army Nurses.* Boston, B. Wilkins & Co., 1895.

Jolly, Ellen R.: *Nuns of the Battlefield.* Providence, R.I., Providence Visitor Press, 1927.

Leech, Margaret: *Reveille in Washington, 1860–1865.* New York, Harper & Brothers, 1941.

Livermore, Mary A.: *My Story of the War.* Hartford, Conn., A. D. Worthington & Co., 1890.

Lowenfels, Walter: *Walt Whitman's Civil War.* New York, Alfred A. Knopf, 1961.

Marshall, Helen E.: *Dorothea Dix: Forgotten Samaritan.* Chapel Hill, University of North Carolina Press, 1937.

Phelps, E. S.: *Our Famous Women.* Hartford, Conn., A. D. Worthington & Co., 1884.

Rathbone, William: *Sketch of the History and Progress of District Nursing from Its Commencement in the Year 1859 to the Present Date.* New York, Macmillan Co., 1890.

Reed, William H.: *Hospital Life in the Army of the Potomac.* Boston, William V. Spencer, 1866.

Wilson, Forrest: *Crusader in Crinoline: The Life of Harriet Beecher Stowe.* Philadelphia, J. B. Lippincott Co., 1941.

Woolsey, Jane Stuart: *Hospital Days.* New York, Van Nostrand, 1868.

Wormeley, Katharine P.: *The Other Side of the War with the Army of the Potomac.* Boston, Ticknor, 1889.

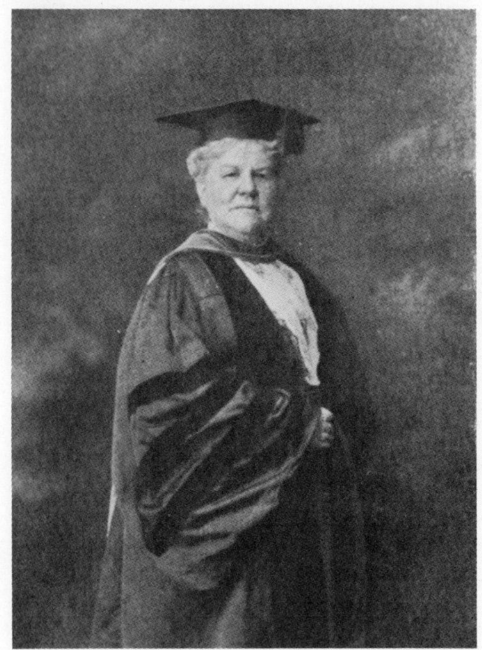

Louisa Lee Schuyler in her doctoral robes after receiving an L.L.D. from Columbia University in 1915 for starting the first nursing school in the United States. (Dolan collection.)

11 Nursing Leaders' Responses to the Establishment and Promotion of Educational Programs

THE NEED FOR NURSING EDUCATION

Florence Nightingale's work in the founding of her school in England was well known in America. It was not long before others began to share her vision that better nursing could be undertaken by educated women.

The first attempt to train nurses on this continent was made by the Ursuline Sisters of Quebec, who, about 1640, taught Indian women to care for their sick.

The family of Dr. Valentine Seaman, of New York, claims that he was the first person in the United States to found a school for nurses. His son says, "In 1798 Dr. Seaman introduced the first regular school for trained nurses, from which other schools have since been established." He enrolled about 24 pupils and gave them a course of lectures in anatomy, physiology, care of children and midwifery.

The Crimean War, the educational endeavors of Florence Nightingale and the Civil War had focussed attention on the necessity for nurses and on the importance of an educational system in which to prepare them. Interest, stimulated by physicians as well as enlightened citizens, led to efforts to inaugurate a program for the preparation of nurses.

In 1869 at a meeting of the *American Medical Association*, Dr. S. D. Gross as chairman presented a report of the *Committee on the Training of Nurses*, which recommended that nursing be placed under the control of the medical profession. The committee proposed that there should be a school for the training of nurses in every large hospital, not only to meet the demands of that hospital but also to train nurses to care for families in their homes. The nurses were to be trained by the medical staff, as the medical students were. The county medical societies were to take the responsibility for the schools in their districts. Fortunately, the recommendations of the committee were not adopted.

The most popular woman's magazine of the late nineteenth century was *Godey's Lady's Book and Magazine*. Mrs. Sarah Hale, its editor, wrote a significant editorial entitled "Lady Nurses," which appeared in the February 1871 issue:[1]

> Much has been lately said of the benefits that would follow if the calling of sick nurse were elevated to a profession which an educated lady might adopt without a sense of degradation, either on her own part or in the estimation of others. . . .
>
> There can be no doubt that the duties of sick nurse, to be properly performed, require an education and training little, if at all, inferior to those possessed by members of the medical profession. . . . The manner in which a reform may be effected is easily pointed out. Every medical college should have a course of study and training especially adapted for ladies who desire to qualify themselves for the profession of nurse; and those who had gone through the course, and passed the requisite examination, should receive a degree and a diploma, which would at once establish their position in society. The graduate nurse would in general estimation be as much above the ordinary nurse of the present day as the professional surgeon of our times is above the barber-surgeon of the last century.

Mrs. Hale, in this brief, thought-provoking editorial, identified the need for *professional nurses* who had completed a well-planned educational program with a specific body of knowledge that was different from, but taught in as great a depth as, that required of members of the medical profession. This knowledge was to be obtained in an educational rather than a service-centered institution. Completion of training was to be marked by the granting of an academic degree in addition to professional certification. Her words fell on deaf ears, and in 1873 a Dr. Aeneas Munro in *The Science and Art of Nursing the Sick*, stressed the need for requiring that nurses be able to read and write and bemoaned the fact that so many could not do either.

In both England and America, the need for trained nurses was so great that schools of nursing inevitably took root and grew. As in England, the pioneer nurses in America were unusual women who had vision, force, great courage and persistence. These few women laid the solid foundations on which nurses now stand.

At the time of the Civil War, there were said to be only 68 hospitals in the country; in 1872, a survey found 178. From that time on, the number of hospitals increased rapidly, largely because of the improvement in nursing and the fact that physicians and patients found that better care and more convenient service could be provided in the hospital than in the average home. The process seemed slow, but by 1900 there were about 2000 hospitals in the United States. From that time on they multiplied at an incredible rate, and those already in existence expanded their facilities.

THE INCEPTION OF SCHOOLS OF NURSING

The New England Hospital for Women and Children, staffed by women physicians, took its first step toward founding a school of nursing when Dr. Marie Zakrzewska arrived in 1859. She suggested practical instruction in the hospital for women medical students and the establishment of a school of nursing. The hospital charter was issued in 1863 and included a nursing school.

In the 1864 Annual Report of the New England Hospital for Women and Children, the adoption of the first bylaws on June 5, 1863 was recorded:

> The object of the Institution shall be
>
> 1st. To provide for women medical aid of competent physicians of their own sex.
>
> 2nd. To assist educated women in the practical study of medicine.
>
> 3rd. To train nurses for the care of the sick.[2]

In the early 1870s a committee was appointed to develop a plan for instituting a

[1]Hale, Sarah: "Lady Nurses," *Godey's Lady's Book and Magazine*, *82*:188–189, 1871.

[2]Munson, Helen, W.: "Linda Richards," *American Journal of Nursing*, *48*:552, 1948.

training school for nurses. The plan was described as:

Education of Nurses

In order more fully to carry out our purpose of fitting women thoroughly for the profession of nursing, we have made the following arrangements:

Young women of suitable requirements and character will be admitted to the Hospital as school nurses, for one year. This year will be divided into four periods; three months will be given respectively to the practical study of nursing in the Medical, Surgical, and Maternity Wards, and night nursing. Here the pupil will aid the head nurse in all the care and work of the wards under the direction of the Attending and Resident Physicians and Medical Students.

In order to enable women entirely dependent upon their work for support to obtain a thorough training, the nurses will be paid for their work from one to four dollars per week after the first fortnight, according to the actual value of their service to the hospital.

A course of lectures will be given to nurses at the Hospital by the physicians connected with the Institution beginning January 21. . . . Certificates will be given to such nurses as have satisfactorily passed a year in practical training in the Hospital.[3]

The thrust of this program was to prepare competent assistants for the physicians and to service the hospital. Nurses received a small fee for their services rather than a planned program of education and were considered employees rather than students. They were taught by physicians, many of whom did not know what nursing could or should be. Such a program of nursing education in hospitals provided the nurses with practical experience obtained within the hospital, such as in the medical and surgical wards, as well as provided the hospital with services on a round-the-clock basis.

On September 1, 1872, the *New England Hospital in Boston* (later transferred to Roxbury, Massachusetts) admitted a class of five students to its newly formed *Training School.* This school was administered under the direction of Susan Dimock, M.D. She had finished her medical education in Switzerland and had been to Kaiserswerth and knew its methods. Dr. Zakrzewska, who had suggested the establishment of a school of nursing, taught bedside nursing. The course was one year in length. No classwork was required, although lectures were given during the winter months. Books were not available to give a background in nursing, so lectures without demonstrations composed the educational aspects of the curriculum. How different from the program of Florence Nightingale!

The course was a rigorous one. The hours of duty extended from 5:30 A.M. to 9:00 P.M. Students lived in rooms among the hospital wards because they had to be available to take care of the patients night and day. Days off for illness had to be made up. At the end of the year on October 1, 1873, one student graduated.

When the second year began, a nurse was hired as a head nurse and instructor of the students of nursing, and a more structured program was started. The length of the program was expanded to 16 months, and by the time the school celebrated its fifth anniversary, the length of the program had increased to 18 months. To enrich the course of study, one month in the diet kitchen at the hospital and one month of district nursing in the community were provided. There were now two head nurses and a superintendent of the training school. In 1893, the program was lengthened to two years and in 1901, to three years.

Melinda Ann (Linda) Richards (1841–1930) was the one student who graduated on October 1, 1873, and she has been called "America's first trained nurse" (Fig. 11–1). Miss Richards had been a nurse in the Boston City Hospital. Going there with the idea of learning nursing, she had been greatly disappointed to find that the nurse's work and position were little more than that of a maid. She had been offered a position as head nurse there, but had refused it, claiming that she did not know enough and wanted more training. She was then directed to the New England Hospital.

Miss Richards recorded her experiences, in which she mentions that students did not have uniforms but instead wore dark washable dresses.[4] She relates that "every second week" the students had a free

[3] *Ibid.*, p. 552.

[4] Richards, Linda: *Reminiscences of Linda Richards.* Boston, Whitcomb and Barrows, 1911.

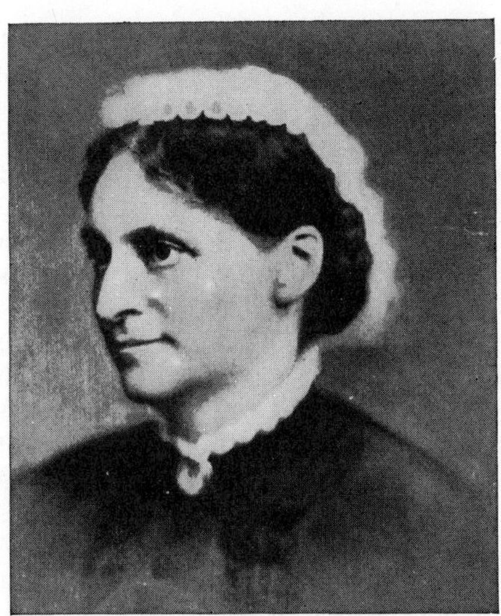

Figure 11–1. Linda Richards. (From a painting given to the New England Hospital for Women by its alumnae.) (Dolan collection.)

afternoon from two to five o'clock. They had no evenings out, no hours for study or recreation and no regular leave on Sunday. During the year's program only twelve lectures were given by the visiting staff of physicians, and the only clinical instruction was given by the women interns when the physician ordered a treatment and the intern and student nurse together figured out the procedure. Medicines were kept in bottles that were numbered, not labeled, and consequently the students learned nothing of the medicines, their actions or untoward effects to be observed. In addition to the absence of textbooks, there were no entrance requirements and no final examinations.

Miss Richards has given an account of the high maternal mortality rates due to epidemics of puerperal fever and of the astonishing duty of the patients in labor to make shrouds for the hospital. Many a patient must have wondered if she were making her own!

Linda Richards' first assignment as a graduate was as night superintendent at Bellevue Hospital in New York City. After a year there, she went to the Boston Training School as the new superintendent of the school. In addition to performing the administrative duties for which she was hired, she insisted upon giving actual patient care herself. She often worked day and night. She even requested a room in the hospital, in place of the comfortable room provided her outside the hospital, in order to watch the patients at night so that she could be called at any hour.

In 1877, Linda Richards visited England, where she met Florence Nightingale and studied the methods of teaching nurses at St. Thomas' Hospital. Between 1885 and 1889, she was a medical missionary in Japan, establishing and directing the first training school for nurses there. In the following years, she assumed the position of superintendent of nurses at the New England Hospital for Women and Children, Brooklyn Homeopathic Hospital, Hartford Hospital and University of Pennsylvania Hospital. Her efforts were later directed to establishing schools in hospitals for the mentally ill. She died on April 16, 1930.

On August 1, 1879, *Mary Eliza Mahoney* (1845–1926) (Fig. 11–2) completed her 16-month course at the training school of the New England Hospital for Women and Children and thus became America's first black nurse to graduate from a school of nursing. In addition to the previously described course of 12 months of nursing experience in medical, surgical and maternal nursing and night duty, training school students were sent into the homes in the community for private duty under the direction of the school in order "to prove

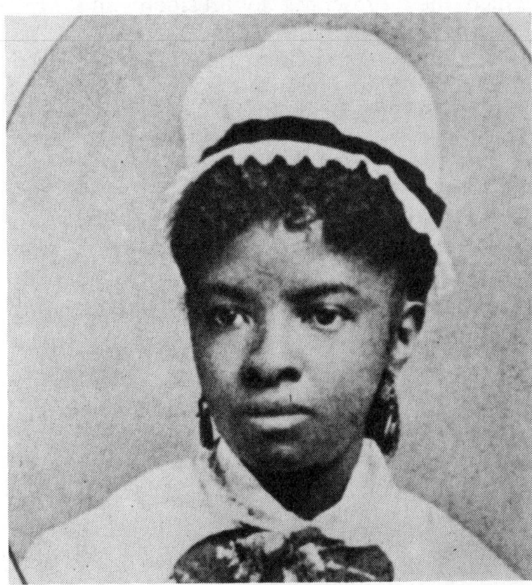

Figure 11–2. Mary Eliza Mahoney (1845–1926). (Dolan collection.)

[their] competency in all of these clinical areas." Out of the class of 40, 22 students were dropped by the school, and only four students, including Mary Mahoney, graduated. In *Pathfinders,* Thoms gives a description of Mary Mahoney, when she gave the address of welcome at the first convention of the National Association of Colored Graduate Nurses:

> Miss Mahoney was small of stature, about five feet in height and weighed less than one hundred pounds . . . she was most interesting and possessed an unusual personality and a great deal of charm. . . . Although at this meeting Miss Mahoney seemed pleased to see and to know of the upward trend of the nursing profession, to hear her make comparisons between the years 1879 and 1909 would almost lead one to believe that the training of today was rather a hit-or-miss proposition. However, she was an inspiration to the entire group of nurses present. At the close of the convention she was made a life member of the Association, exempt from dues, and was elected chaplain. . . . Through her efforts on this occasion a demonstration for nurses was held at the New England Hospital. . . .
>
> Miss Mahoney was a remarkable person. . . . She seldom missed a national nurses' meeting. Her last attendance was in Washington, when the Association met in August, 1921, as a guest of the Freedmen's Hospital Alumnae Association. This circumstance made it possible for the nurses to be received at the White House by President Warren G. Harding. The nurses carried a large basket of American Beauty roses which they presented to President and Mrs. Harding with the request that the National Association of Colored Graduate Nurses be placed on record as an organized body of two thousand trained women ready when needed for world service.[5]

In her honor, the *Mary Mahoney Medal* was initiated in 1936 by the National Association of Colored Graduate Nurses. This medal is symbolic of the opportunities in nursing for those of all races, creeds and national origins.

U.S. SCHOOLS ON THE NIGHTINGALE PLAN

Largely because of the vision, competent planning and political influence of the well-educated and highly esteemed nurse leaders of the Civil War, schools of nursing on the Nightingale Plan were started in the United States. The influence of many of these gifted and productive individuals has been recognized and acknowledged. One such person, Louisa Lee Schuyler, was awarded an honorary Doctor of Laws (L.L.D.) in 1915, by Columbia University for her unusually significant accomplishments. It was the second time in the history of Columbia University's 161 commencements that a woman was granted this honor, and the university applauded her success as the "originator of the first American training school for nurses." Annie Goodrich recorded the event and the response of appreciative nurse leaders.

> In conferring the degree upon Miss Schuyler, President Butler said:
>
> "Louisa Lee Schuyler: A pioneer in the service of noble women to the state; founder of the State Charities Aid Association and of the system of visitation of state institutions by volunteer committees of citizens; originator of the first American Training School for Nurses; initiating and successfully advocating legislation for the state care of the insane; powerfully aiding the first public movement for the prevention of blindness in little children; worthy representative of a splendid line of ancestors, distinguished through two centuries for manifold services to city, state and nation; great granddaughter of General Philip Schuyler of the American Revolution, great granddaughter of Alexander Hamilton of the class of 1777, I gladly admit you to the degree of Doctor of Laws."[6]

It was eminently fitting that when convening in San Francisco, three national organizations representing over 30,000 professional nurses sent a message of congratulation to Miss Schuyler. The telegram read as follows:

> "The American Nurses Association, the National League of Education and the National Organization for Public Health Nursing, assembled at the Greek theatre of California send greetings of veneration, gratitude and congratulation to their friend, the originator of the first school for nurses in America, and whose life of service has been so deservedly recognized by Columbia University."

[5]Thoms, Adah B.: *Pathfinders.* New York, Kay Printing House, 1929.

[6]Goodrich, Annie W.: "Louisa Lee Schuyler—An Appreciation," *American Journal of Nursing,* 15:1079, 1915.

Austin[7] has presented a detailed and scholarly account of the Woolsey sisters whose service during the Civil War was discussed in Chapter 10. Of Abby Howland Woolsey and her sister Jane, in particular, Stewart has written: "Armed with practical hospital experience and having not only intelligence but education, stamina, and good social position, these women were formidable opponents. Without such supporters it is doubtful whether the early Nightingale schools could have survived."[8]

"In 1873, the famous trio of schools evolved, Bellevue Training School in New York City, the Connecticut Training School in New Haven and the Boston Training School. These three schools were purported to be patterned after the Nightingale Plan, but all three differed significantly from that model."[9] To appreciate the similarities as well as the differences, the ingredients of the Nightingale Plan should be recalled (see Chapter 9).

Bellevue Hospital Training School

In 1872, Louisa Lee Schuyler, who organized the New York State Charities Aid Association, enlisted the aid of certain of its members, including Miss Abby H. Woolsey, to inspect Bellevue Hospital. They found a deplorable state of affairs. Women who were ex-convicts did most of the nursing and collected fees from the patients for the crude and inefficient services that they rendered them; drunkenness and foul language were common; the patients' food was poor and they slept on bundles of straw. The physicians of the house staff took temperatures, gave treatments and recorded the condition of patients. It was a repetition of the worst days in the hospitals of Old England. Dr. W. Gill Wylie, who was an intern there, said, "The nurses had the impossible task of attending to from twenty to thirty patients each. The night watchman was expected to assist in the care of patients. The wards looked fine on the surface, but sepsis followed slight operations or injuries, and about 50 per cent of the amputations were fatal. One out of every eleven maternity cases died."

It was reported that in Bellevue Hospital there were 900 patients, "most of them in want, many in positive distress." The crowded conditions required that three patients sleep on two beds, which were presumably strapped together, and five patients occupy three beds. There were no night nurses and only three night watchmen.

The report of these conditions stirred the women's nursing committee, which had asked in 1871 for a nurses' training school; the matter had been referred to the medical board, which did nothing about it. The committee felt that nursing *must* be improved, but most of the medical board disapproved of the women's interest in the matter. General James Bowen was the only commissioner who supported them. A clergyman said publicly that it was not proper for ladies to visit a hospital of this sort.

Opposing the proposed training school were the medical staff, who feared exposure of their poor medical techniques; the hospital administration, who feared their jobs would be threatened; and the politicians, who feared publicity about their gross abuse of their offices.

However, there were physicians who supported the plans for the new project and Dr. W. Gill Wylie, who became a house surgeon at Bellevue, was prominent among them. In 1872, he went to England hoping to have an individual conference with Florence Nightingale. This young man waited until he arrived in Paris to send her a letter requesting an interview. Because of postal delays and the death and burial of her niece, Florence Nightingale did not receive the note until after Dr. Wylie had left England. Perhaps this was fortunate, because an individual conference might not have been recorded, but Miss Nightingale's reply exists for critical perusal. Some of the highlights are as follows:

> You say "the great difficulty will be to define through instruction the duties of the nurse as distinguished from those of medical men" and you are anxious to get "my views relative to the subject."

[7]Austin, Anne L.: *The Woolsey Sisters of New York, 1860–1900*. Philadelphia, American Philosophical Society, 1971, Chap. IX.

[8]Stewart, Isabel: *The Education of Nurses*. New York, The Macmillan Co., 1943, p. 89.

[9]Dolan, Josephine A.: "Nurses in American History: Three Schools—1873," *American Journal of Nursing*, 75:989, 1975.

Is this a difficulty?

Most carefully do we in our training avoid the confusion both practically and theoretically of letting women [nurses] suppose that nursing duties and medical duties run into or overlap each other—so much so that though we have often been asked to allow ladies intending to be "Doctors" to come in as nurses to St. Thomas's Hospital in order to "pick up" . . . as they phrased professional medical knowledge. We have never consented even to admit such applicants—in order to avoid even the semblance of encouraging such gross ignorance and dabbling in matters of life and death as this implies.

You who are a "medical man" who knows the difference between the professional studies of the medical student . . . and the nurse will readily see this.

A nurse is not a "medical man" nor is she a "medical woman."

This letter reiterated Miss Nightingale's feeling that the nurse and physician have different spheres of duty, deliver different kinds of care and need different educational preparation for their respective professional role. More specifically, Miss Nightingale desired to encourage the new schools in the United States to be organized to prepare nurses rather than physicians' assistants.

Meantime the women's committee, under the leadership of Miss Schuyler,[10] had reached an agreement with hospital authorities, and six wards were set apart for use in an experimental nurses' "training class." Funds were raised by subscription, and a house was rented for the nurses' home.

The objective of Bellevue's program was "to train nurses for the care of the sick in order that women shall find a school for their education and the public shall reap the advantage of skilled and educated labor."[11]

There was confusion from the beginning about whether the emphasis should be on charitable service or education for nursing. In 1893, Miss Louise Darche, in addressing the International Congress on Hospitals, Dispensaries and Nursing, stated, "When the ladies who inaugurated the first training school in America formed a committee for the purpose of starting a school for nurses . . . it was not because of a need for a school as a school for nurses; nor was it for the purpose of creating a new field of labor for women, a profession; but simply and solely because of the great need of one of the great charity hospitals for better nursing.[12]"

The hospital administration agreed to place the school under the control of nurses but required that the school pay all expenses incurred beyond the cost of the old system. Thus, the students had to carry out the scouring and scrubbing that had previously been done by the maids.

Abby Woolsey prodded nursing schools to appeal for funds as educational institutions, as college did, rather than on the basis of charity. She encouraged nursing schools to be more like normal schools, the predecessors of state teachers' colleges.

In May 1873, the *Bellevue Training School for Nurses* was founded. Sister Helen of the Sisterhood of All Saints, who was in the United States to set up a branch of the sisterhood in Baltimore, was selected to direct the training program. Miss Euphemia Van Rensselaer succeeded Sister Helen as the superintendent.

Five students enrolled in the first class. The length of the course was one year, but the nurses were bound by contract for an additional year of service. The students learned by imitation and by trial and error. The classroom instruction consisted of one evening class weekly in the parlor of the nurses' home.

Bellevue attempted to use Nightingale methods and attracted educated applicants. The school report of 1879 recorded that well-educated women were leaving the teaching field to enter nursing. In 1882 in *Century Magazine,* North noted progress in an article entitled "A New Profession for Women."[13] The accompanying illustrations were intended to show that educated women were enrolling in the Bellevue Training School (Fig. 11–3). In this same article, North discussed the nurses who

[10]The National Institute of Sciences also recognized Miss Schuyler as the founder of Bellevue's training school.

[11]Dock, Lavinia L.: "History of the Reform in Nursing in Bellevue Hospital," *American Journal of Nursing,* 2:90, 1901.

[12]Darche, Louise.: "Proper Organization of Training Schools in America," In *Hospitals, Dispensaries and Nursing,* Sec. III. Report of International Congress of Charities, Correction and Philanthropy, Chicago, Illinois, 1893, pp. 513–523.

[13]North, Franklin: "A New Profession for Women," *Century Magazine,* pp. 38–47, July 1882.

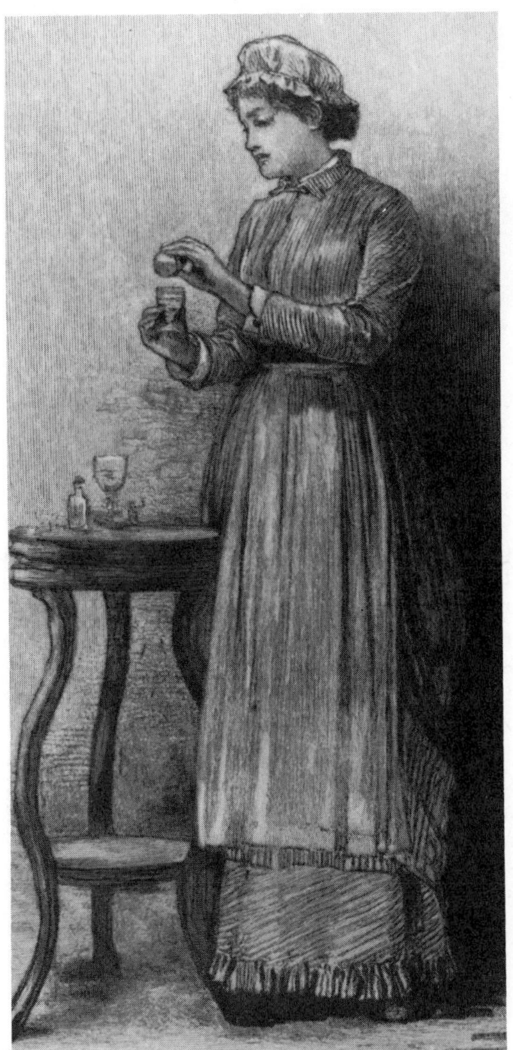

Figure 11–3. "The Nurse—A New Profession for Women." The nurse who posed for this picture was Isabel Hampton, a well-educated member of the student body of the Bellevue training school. (Dolan collection.)

joined in community work projects with the Women's Branch of the City Missions (Fig. 11–4).

It is interesting to note that this group of educated students of nursing was well accepted by the medical staff. An interdisciplinary team approach was taken in conducting clinical case conferences. Sometimes the chief of staff discussed the medical aspects and then asked the well-prepared head nurse to present the nursing assessment and plan of care for the enlightenment of both students of nursing and students of medicine (Fig. 11–5).

Linda Richards became night superintendent in October 1874 and started the practice of keeping records and writing orders.

Bellevue Training School provided a pin for each graduate to distinguish its graduates from those of other schools. The pin was designed by Tiffany and Company in 1880. The seal was a crane against a circle of blue surrounded by a wreath of poppy leaves and poppy blossoms. The crane was chosen as a symbol of vigilance, and the pin represented a trinity of purposes: to be vigilant, to be constant and to be merciful.[14]

There was a very high mortality rate at Bellevue Hospital because of blood poisoning, or septicemia. The medical house staff dressed the wounds, going from patient to patient and spreading infection. Sponges for cleaning wounds were pieces of real sponge, and a single one was often used to cleanse the wounds of many patients.

The incredibly high mortality rate caused by puerperal fever (two deaths in every

[14]Giles, Dorothy: *A Candle in Her Hand*. New York, G. P. Putnam's Sons, 1949, p. 155.

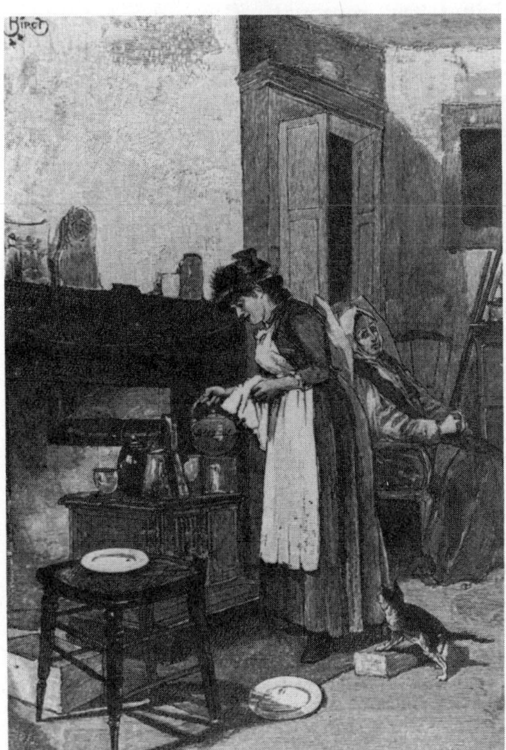

Figure 11–4. Caring for a sick person in a tenement house. (Dolan collection.)

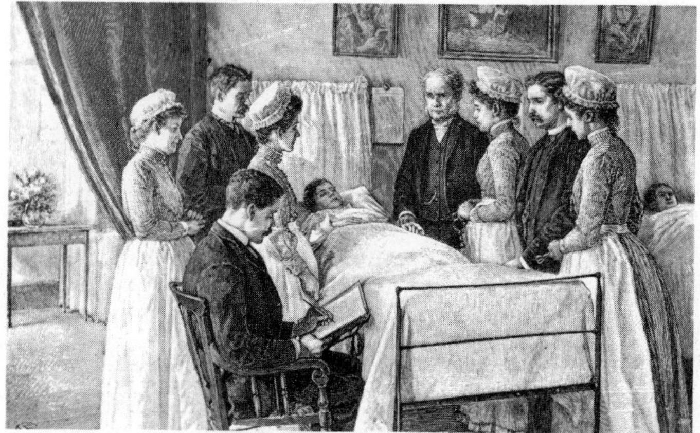

Figure 11–5. A bedside consultation using an interdisciplinary approach. The chief of staff and instructor or head nurse discuss with students of medicine and nursing the appropriate means for ascertaining and satisfying the needs of the patient. (Dolan collection.)

five deliveries) prompted the training school to offer to take charge of the entire maternity ward. The students of nursing had reported the unbelievable plight of the maternity patients. The obstetricians were violently opposed to the training school's offer. The training School then made a request for assistance to the State Charities Aid Association, which resulted in the assignment of the three maternity wards to the Bellevue Training School in May 1874. Linda Richards was asked to direct this project. Strong community backing was solicited for removal of pregnant women from Bellevue's wards, and the Advisory Committee of the State Charities Aid Association presented the following ultimatum to the medical board of the hospital: "Gentlemen, we have learned the cause of mortality in the Lying-in wards of this hospital. We give you forty-eight hours to remove these women. If they are here at the end of this time, the whole story will be published in the Evening Post." The president of the New York Board of Charity ordered the immediate removal, to the Charity Hospital on Blackwell's Island, of the 25 women who were waiting to be delivered. Every patient survived. The maternity wards of Bellevue were closed. The theory of Dr. Semmelweis (see pp. 151–153) had been proved once again: the medical students and medical house staff had been guilty of transferring puerperal sepsis.

Connecticut Training School

In 1872, the New Haven Hospital appointed a committee of three physicians and a layman to report on the practicability of training nurses. Dr. Gill Wylie's report on European schools of nursing aided them in their investigation. The committee reported in April 1873 that it was not expedient for the hospital itself to undertake such a work, but recommended the establishment of a school as a separate organization with the hospital as its field.

Another of the famous Woolsey sisters, Georgeanna Woolsey Bacon (Fig. 11–6), and her husband, Dr. Francis Bacon, joined a wealthy philanthropist, Charles Thompson, in establishing the *Connecticut Training School* in New Haven.

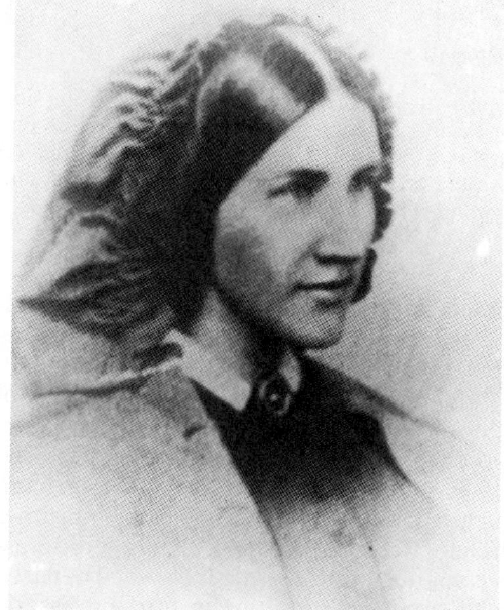

Figure 11–6. Mrs. Georgeanna Woolsey Bacon. (Courtesy of Anne L. Austin and the American Philosophical Society.)

Agreement of the Hospital Directors with the Officers of the Training School.

At a meeting of the Directors of the General Hospital Society of Connecticut, held, respectively, on the 18th and 24th of April, 1873, the following Resolutions, as amended, were adopted.

1. That the office of Superintendent of Nursing, or Head nurse, be created by the Directors of this Hospital.
2. That the office be declared distinct from that of the Steward or Matron, concerning itself only with the direct personal care of the sick or wounded *in the wards* for men and women and with the supervision of the pupil nurses.
3. That the Head nurse be responsible to the resident and attending physicians for such care, *reporting to them,* and that she be assisted by the proposed class of pupil nurses whom she shall instruct, and who *report to her.*
4. That the pupil nurses be allowed to assist in the preparation of special diet, furnished on the order of physicians only.
5. *That the rough work of the wards be done,* as heretofore, *by the convalescents, or such other persons as the Steward shall appoint.*
6. That quarters and a comfortable table (such as is now furnished for private patients and the one woman nurse at present employed) be supplied to these nurses.
7. That the officers and committee of the Training School shall have the selection, dismissal, and general supervision of the Head nurse, and pupil nurses; it being understood that the number of pupil nurses shall be limited to six, this number to be increased as the needs of the Hospital, in the opinion of the Prudential Committee, may require. It is further to be distinctly understood, that the officers and committee of the "Training School," are in no way to interfere with the responsibility of these nurses for the care of the patients, to the attending Physicians and Surgeons; nor with such regulations of the Hospital as are established and ordered by the Directors. That a standing committee of three of the officers of the Training School shall be annually appointed by the Training School, to act in connection with the President and the Prudential Committee of the Hospital, in investigating any complaint that may be preferred by any of the Hospital authorities, against any Head or pupil nurse, and such joint head may, by a major vote dismiss any head or pupil nurse, for reasonable cause.
8. That the committee of the Training School shall direct and superintend such instruction of the nurses outside the wards of the Hospital, as may, in their judgment best conduce to the end for which the school is established, provided that the patients of the Hospital are not neglected.
9. That the pupil nurses not on duty in the wards may accompany the attending and consulting physicians, with their consent, on their daily rounds, for the purpose of obtaining such bedside instruction as these gentlemen may consent to furnish.
10. That the resident physicians be asked to give such facilities for instruction as it may be in their power to afford; and generally to cooperate with the committee in their effort to prepare the nurses for valuable work.
11. That the connection of the Training School with the Hospital may take effect whenever, in the opinion of the Prudential Committee, the new Hospital Building is ready for occupation.
12. That the Secretary be instructed to communicate the above action of the Directors of the Hospital to the officers of the Training School.

The above is a true copy of the record.

Attest,

C. A. Lindsley,
Secretary.

May 16th, 1873.

Figure 11–7. One of the earliest training school contracts. (Dolan collection.)

As a result of productive strategy meetings, an acceptable agreement was reached between the director of the General Hospital Society of Connecticut and the officers of the Connecticut Training School (Fig. 11–7). The school was founded, but there were no pupils, so it advertised for "probationers" in country newspapers, through ladies' missionary societies and in notices at railway stations and in post offices. All the early schools of nursing found it hard to convince young women that it was necessary to spend even six months' in learning nursing. The Civil War, however, had done much to call attention to the need for proper education for nursing.

In October of 1873, the Connecticut Training School at the New Haven Hospital was established, with four pupils. Miss Bayard, a graduate of the school of the Woman's Hospital of Philadelphia, was in charge (Fig. 11–8).

Many serious and frustrating obstacles became apparent when the hospital steward and his wife exhibited animosity toward the new director and her students. The couple were terrified of losing their jobs, and, therefore, fought the new system. Miss Bayard resigned when incorrect and adverse newspaper publicity about the new school was printed.

A new director, Mrs. Allen, arrived and the distraught steward continued to cause conflict whenever he could. She resigned May 13, 1874; however, there were courageous women who were willing and able to direct the school who guided it successfully. The desire of the teachers and students to save the lives of their patients prompted them to work longer hours than were expected and to request a ward for teaching purposes. The school contracted with the hospital to provide nursing services in exchange for educational services because it was critical for the students to see good patient care. This contract meant that instructors and students covered the wards day and night. (Sleeping arrangements had been provided on the top floor of the hospital.) The school tapped its meager budget to purchase food and milk to supplement the patients' diets. From the beginning, the aims of the nursing schools seemed to emphasize charitable service, with education incidental to this service.

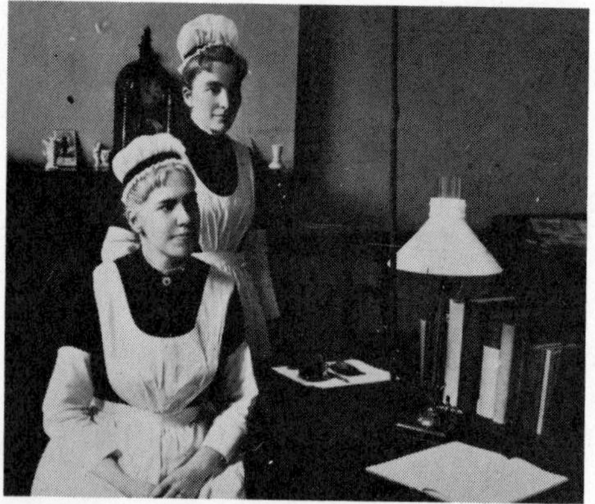

Figure 11–8. The Superintendent and Assistant Superintendent of Nursing in the office of the Connecticut Training School. (Courtesy of Yale Medical Library.)

The physicians liked the work of the nurses and were, from the first, enthusiastic about the school (Figs. 11–9 and 11–10). Mrs. Georgeanna Woolsey Bacon wrote:

> Our first four pupils arrived late in the evening, and in a dreary storm. . . . They and their superintendent found themselves at once plunged into hard work. The north ward was full of typhoid fever, ten cases, six men and four women, and wards 1 and 2 East and West were opened and filled during the first week. The committee's journal reads: 'Our nurses for the first five weeks did very hard work. The fever cases were severe, some of the patients entirely delirious. . . . The four nurses in turn sat up night after night and did duty during the day in the other wards, or diet kitchen, where the special diet for thirty was cooked and distributed to all parts of the hospital by the nurses who cooked it. . . . No class of nurses has ever had such demand made upon its endurance as this pioneer class of pupils met and struggled through. All the typhoid fever cases recovered. . . . Everything was in a transition state. The nurses were crowded, as their numbers increased, into the three small rooms in the top floor, four in a room,—the clothes horse screens which divided their beds one from another were the first screens of the kind used in the hospital. . . . By the end of our second year we were able to send out our first graduates to private families.

Shortly after its founding, the school was allowed to take eight students. At the end of its second year the student nurses were sent into private nursing. The payment for their services went to the training school. Fortunately, this practice was discontinued in 1905, and by discontinuing it, the Connecticut Training School became eligible to

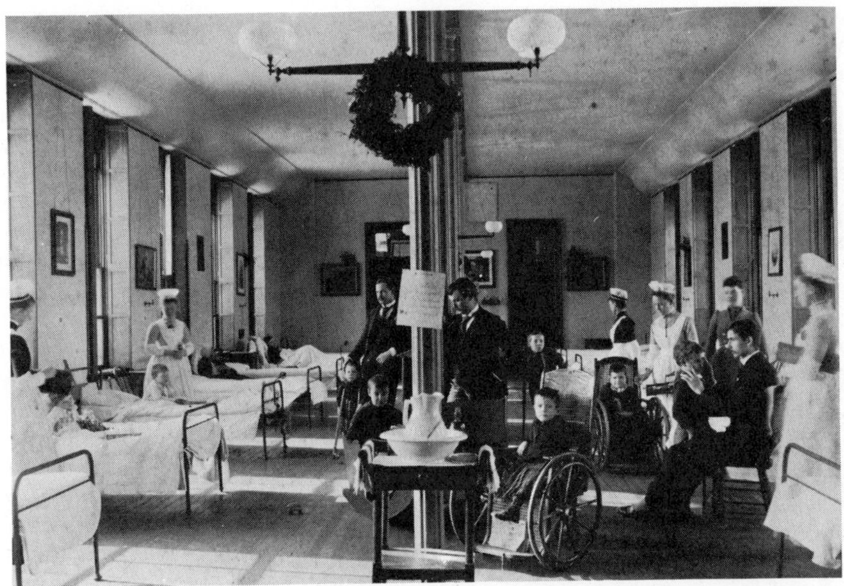

Figure 11–9. A pediatric unit under the aegis of the Connecticut Training School (ca. 1878). Note that there are two faculty members supervising three students. (Courtesy of Yale Medical Library.)

register with the Regents in New York State.

In 1877, the school published the *New Haven Manual of Nursing*, a textbook created by a committee consisting of both nurses and physicians; it was a comprehensive text and soon found wide acceptance among the nursing schools, which by then were being organized throughout the country.

An 1881 report on the Connecticut Training School says:

> The work was so hard many nurses broke down and were obliged to give up their profession. The members of the Training School Committee went on the wards and helped at this time. The Board of Managers feel the Hospital cannot go on successfully without the school, and the community cannot dispense with the

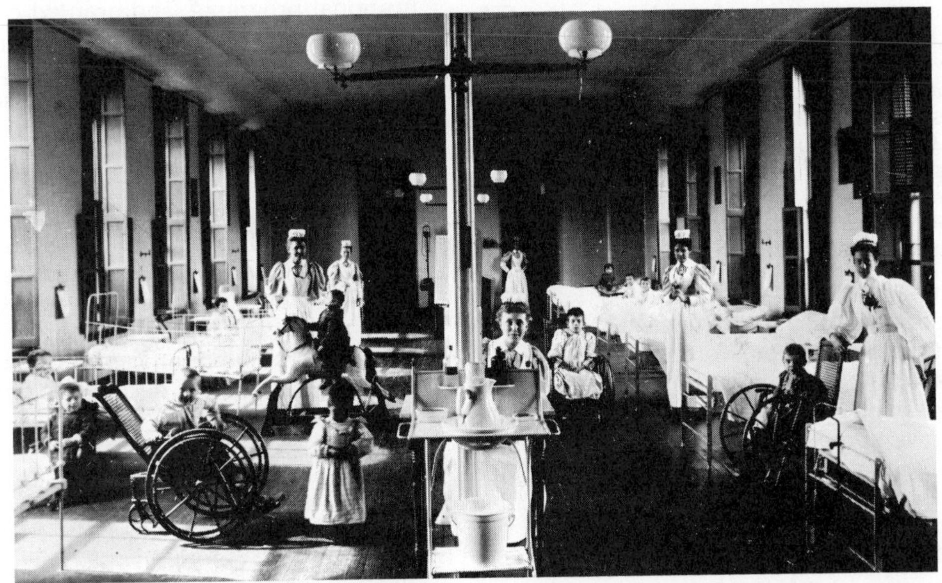

Figure 11–10. The same pediatric unit shown in Figure 11–9, about the turn of the century. Note one instructor at the right and five students. (Courtesy of Yale Medical Library.)

services of the nurses here trained. If there were no school we should have to hire nurses and the lowest rate for which they could be engaged for this harassing work would be $15 monthly.

An interesting comment appears in the 1881 yearly report on the school:

It is perhaps well to state once for all, the school is thankful they are able to relieve suffering in the hospital, but the school does not exist primarily for this purpose but for the training of nurses for the public; [it is] the only school in this country or in Europe which is not supported by the hospital which it serves.

Margaret Stack notes: "The Board of Directors were able for thirty-three years to direct and finance the Training School without assistance from the Hospital."[15]

The public took kindly to the nurses, and there was an immediate demand for their services.

Boston Training School

In 1807, the *Massachusetts General Hospital* was founded by a group of prominent physicians. It was a private enterprise, though designed for nonpaying patients, and a model hospital, noted for its cleanliness and good nursing. Mrs. G. L. Sturtevant, who was nurse there in 1862, described the working conditions:

The nurses were paid $7.50 a month, head nurses $12. There were no maids; the nurses washed the dishes and did the cleaning. The night watchers left the ward at 5 A.M., making a verbal report to the head nurse. The day nurses went on duty at that hour, had breakfast at six, and remained on until 9:30 P.M., taking an occasional hour off if they could get it. They slept in small rooms between the wards, two nurses in a folding bed. In the daytime the room was used for doctors' consultations or for dressings and minor operations.

In April 1873, the Women's Education Association of Boston suggested the organization of a school for nurses to offer a desirable occupation for self-supporting women as well as to meet the obvious need for well-prepared private duty nurses in the community. This association consisted of enterprising people who were identified with many welfare movements in Boston, especially educational and philanthropic ones.

An agreement was worked out between the trustees of the Massachusetts General Hospital and the directors of the training school. At first the suggestions from trustees of the hospital implied that they wanted control, but by skillful negotiation, the directors of the developing school retained control of the program.[16]

It was finally agreed that the hospital should allow the school to open as an experiment. Subscriptions were secured for the expenses of the school, and pupils were sought. Six young women were accepted, and on November 1, 1873, the *Boston Training School* was opened.

Mrs. Billings was engaged as superintendent and spent three months observing Bellevue's program in preparation for her new position. Two head nurses and four students joined Mrs. Billings and took charge of the assigned clinical wards. The two wards in "The Brick" building of the hospital were given over to the school because "it [the building] stands by itself; represents both medical and surgical departments; and offers the hard labor desirable for the training of nurses."[17]

Once the program started, the Women's Education Association severed connections with the school (its function was the initiation rather than the administration of educational programs) and granted control of the training program to the board of directors of the school. The hospitals paid the school of nursing for the nursing service it provided.

The school grafted its new system onto the hospital's system of nursing and depended on voluntary contributions for maintenance. Three months after the school opened Mrs. Billings resigned (she was succeeded by Baroness Mary von Oluhansen), and by that time the pupils had acquired such a body of knowledge that one of the head nurses decided to enter the school as a student.

[15]Stack, Margaret K.: "Resume of the History of the Connecticut Training School for Nurses," *The American Journal of Nursing*, 23:829, 1923.

[16]Curtis and Denny: "Early History of the Boston Training School," *The American Journal of Nursing*, 2:333, 1902.

[17]Parsons, Sara E.: *History of the Massachusetts General Hospital Training School for Nurses*. Boston, Whitcomb and Barrows, 1922, p. 21.

Linda Richards became the next director. She found the school still on trial and rather discredited by the staff. She saw that the nurses were working much as their untrained predecessors had done; there were no maids, and therefore, nurses were occupied doing dish-washing and dining-room work, washing poultice cloths and taking turns at doing night duty and acting as head nurse. Cotton was expensive, so all soiled dressings and poultice cloths, of which there were many, had to be washed (in the patients' bathtub) and ironed by the nurses.

Miss Richards reorganized the work, got classes under way and developed the school. "Her major job was to prove to the staff that trained nurses were better than untrained ones. One means she sometimes used to demonstrate this was to care for the sickest patients herself. Gradually the staff realized their value and began to refer to 'our school' with pride." By the end of her first year, Miss Richards had convinced the physicians that the new regime was a success, and the school was accepted by the trustees. Later Miss Richards was told by the superintendent of the hospital that the trustees had voted another ward to be given to the school. He assured her: "The School is safe. Before another year comes round you will have the nursing of the entire hospital in charge." Parsons states: "By the end of 1876 Miss Richards had charge of all the nursing in the Hospital and her pupils were employed in eight wards."[18]

Miss Richards remained for two and one-half years, and when she left to study training school work in England, the school was operating on a permanent basis. For some decades *training school for nurses* was the accepted term for nursing schools and students of nursing were called *pupils.*

In the development of the new program at Massachusetts General Hospital,[19] it is noted that in 1874, a thermometer was requested for the use of nurses in taking care of patients and a month of night watching was added to the program; in 1875, cooking became an essential addition to the training program, there being no cooks in hospitals; in 1876, pupils were permitted in the operating room; in 1889, a class on "insanity" and one on "bacteriology" were added to the course; in 1891, pupils were responsible for cleaning and sterilizing instruments for Saturday operations; and by 1896, pupils were required to assist with operations on Saturday. (The reason for permitting students in the operating room only on Saturday is not given.) Gradually, a graduate nurse was placed in charge of the operating amphitheater, and pupil nurses assisted at operations and, finally, assumed the responsibility of administering the ether. In 1895, *Miss Annabella McCrae* became a full-time instructor in the teaching of nursing procedures. In 1896, pupil nurses received instruction in the administration of hypodermic injections.

In 1896, The Boston Training School ceased to be an independent school and was made an integral part of the Massachusetts General Hospital.

Hartford Hospital Training School

Hartford Hospital Training School in Hartford, Connecticut, was established in 1877 and patterned somewhat on Nightingale lines. In a review of the first two years of its existence, however, one reads:

> The compensation for services of the pupil-nurses is board, washing, care when sick, instruction in nursing, lectures, etc., with $10 per month the first year, and $14 per month the second year. The nurses spend one hour each day in recitation from the textbook used in the school. Two days in the week they receive instruction in the diet-kitchen. Lectures are given by the house physician two days in the week and occasionally by the visiting physicians and others."[20]

The pattern of service to the hospital and compensation on an employee basis is again evident. The "doctor's lectures" became the vogue.

[18]Parsons, Sara E.: *History of the Massachusetts General Hospital Training School for Nurses.* Boston, Whitcomb and Barrows, 1922, p. 40.

[19]Sleeper, Ruth: "The Two Inseparables—Nursing Service and Nursing Education," *The American Journal of Nursing, 48*:678–681, 1948.

[20]*Nineteenth Annual Report of the Executive Committee of the Hartford Hospital.* Presented to the Corporation at their Annual Meeting, December 10, 1879. Hartford, Conn., Press of the Case, Lockwood and Brainard Company, 1880, pp. 10–11.

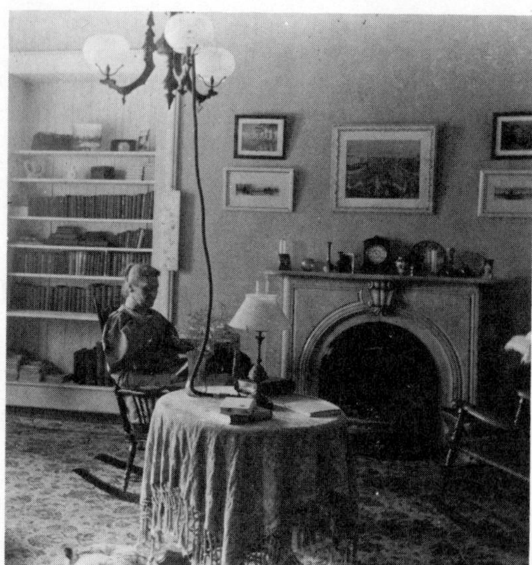

Figure 11–11. Miss Linda Richards, Matron of Hartford Hospital Training School, 1895–1897, in the living room of her apartment, probably preparing for the next day's classes. (Dolan collection.)

In 1895, when Linda Richards (Figs. 11–11 and 11–12) became the fourth matron and superintendent of nurses of the Hartford Hospital Training School, she said, "This is one of the pioneer schools of the country, having been the fourth school organized." Miss Richards introduced a system of ward maids who relieved the nurses of cleaning and dining-room work. She urged the hospital administration to build a nurses' home apart from the hospital where the students could rest properly, and she insisted on trained nurses as head nurses on the wards.

CANADIAN SCHOOLS ON THE NIGHTINGALE PLAN

In 1874, nursing education in Canada was initiated when the St. Catharine's Training School and Nurses' Home came into being. The name was changed later to the *Mack Training School for Nurses* in connection with St. Catharine's General Hospital in honor of the founder, Dr. Theophilus Mack.

Excerpts from the correspondence between Miss Lavinia Dock and Dr. Howard Dittrick of Cleveland appear in the history of the Mack Training School for Nurses.[21]

> Miss Nightingale's new plan of training was begun in St. Thomas's Hospital in 1860, and only four or five years after that, Dr. Mack, having comprehended her work and its meaning—determined to have a hospital with a home for nurses on Miss Nightingale's plan, with a trained nurse at its head. Thus he outdistanced all others on the American continent.
>
> Today, when this system is universal, we do not realize its immensely revolutionary character in Miss Nightingale's day. It was unknown in English hospitals, although British matrons held dignified and respected positions. It heralded in fact, a phase of the "woman movement.". . .

[21]*Seventy-fifth Anniversary (1874–1949) of the Mack Training School for Nurses.* St. Catharine's General Hospital, p. 3.

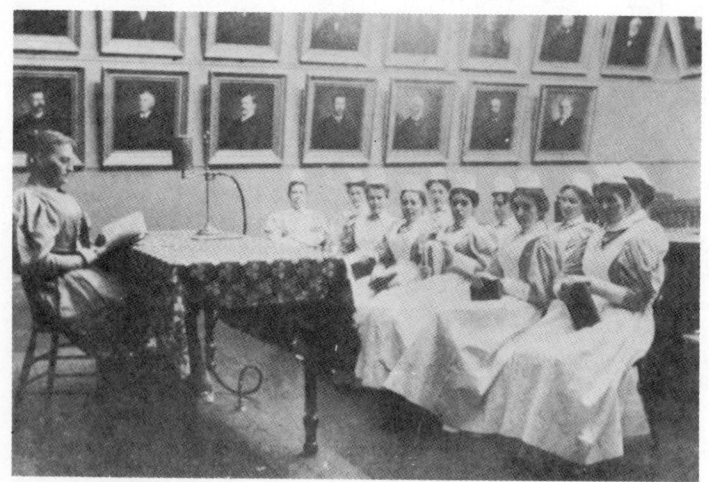

Figure 11–12. Miss Linda Richards teaching a class of students at Hartford Hospital Training School. (Dolan collection.)

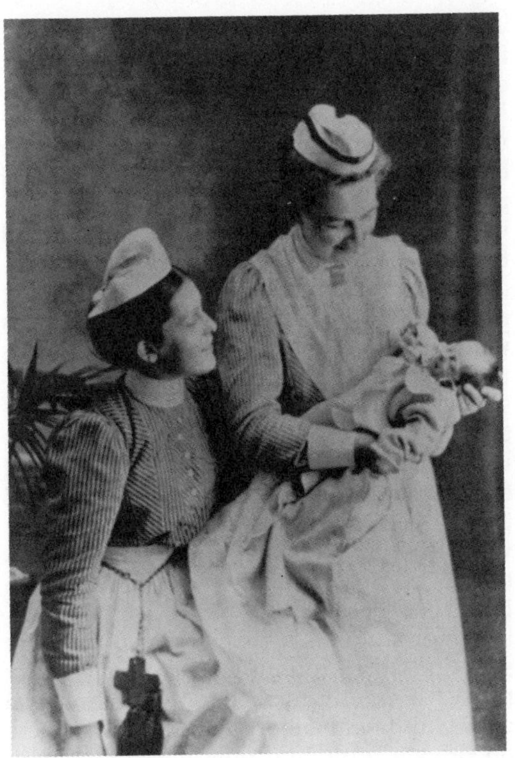

Figure 11–13. A student and graduate nurse conferring at St. Catharine's General Hospital in Ontario. (Dolan collection.)

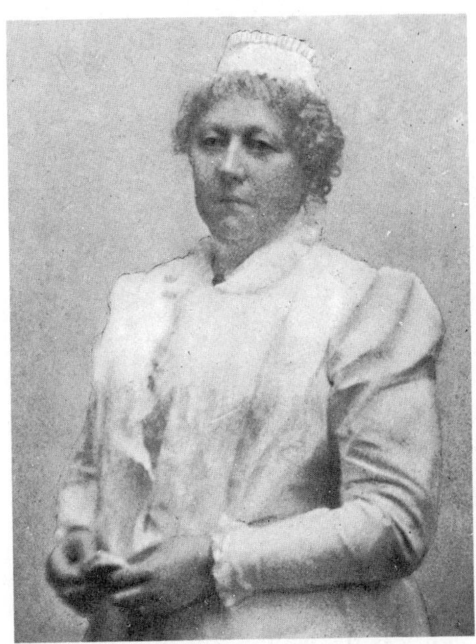

Figure 11–14. Nora Gertrude Livingston. (Dolan collection.)

Dr. Mack and his intelligent community, familiar with Miss Nightingale's work . . . in the English hospital world, adhered to her principles, and determined as early as 1864 to establish and follow them loyally. Beginning in a small way, in that year—they developed their purpose so well that in 1873 they sent Miss Money to England to bring out a staff of nurses trained in the "Nightingale System," and she returned with three from Guy's Hospital, and several probationers.

The final success of the training school was the result of the efforts of Dr. Mack, who had sent to England for nurses and founded a school that has always been worthy of the name and has produced many able nurses (Fig. 11–13). Its establishment made the emergence of trained nursing in Canada practically simultaneous with that in the United States.

The *Montreal General Hospital* was founded in 1821, and in 1875, the hospital board applied to Florence Nightingale for help in establishing a school. She sent them five nurses, but they were not successful. Finally, under the direction of *Nora Gertrude Livingston* (Fig. 11–14), a graduate of New York Hospital, a superior school was established, which gave the first preliminary course and was the first three-year nursing school in North America. *Flora M. Shaw* (Fig. 11–15), one of its graduates, established the University School at McGill University in 1920.

The nursing school of the *Toronto General Hospital* has a similar history to that of the

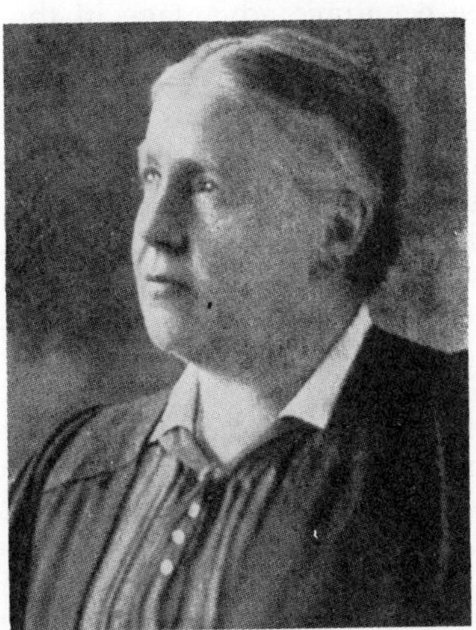

Figure 11–15. Flora Madeline Shaw. (Dolan collection.)

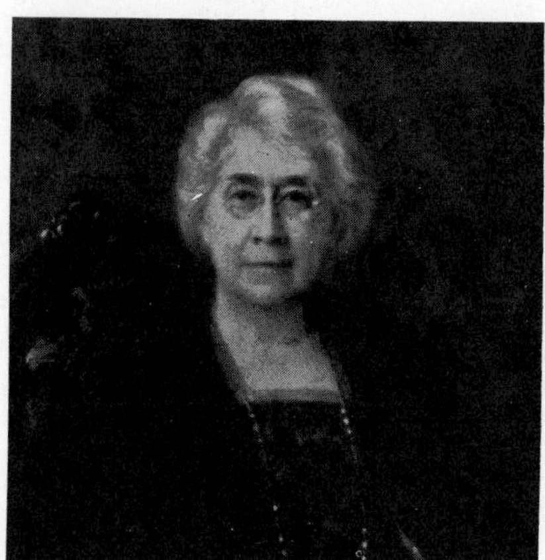

Figure 11–16. Mary Agnes Snively. (Dolan collection.)

Montreal General Hospital. In 1877 an attempt was made to establish a nursing school, but the school did not really flourish until 1884 when it was taken over by *Mary Agnes Snively* (Fig. 11–16), one of the founders of the Canadian Nurses' Association and a graduate of Bellevue Training School. During her 26 years of service, Miss Snively elevated the standards of the Toronto General Hospital school.

Good nursing education had been established in Canada and the United States, and with the early schools of nursing came the dawn of modern nursing.

PROBLEMS OF EARLY SCHOOLS

It was most unfortunate that hospitals saw an economic advantage in the establishment of schools of nursing. A few recognized the duty of providing skilled nurses for the community, but most hospitals stated frankly that their schools were organized "to provide better nursing *for the hospital*." Also it was promptly discovered that students in training were not only more easily disciplined and controlled than hired nurses but also cheaper and more satisfactory.

In consequence, during the 1880s and even more so in the 1890s, many schools were started in small private and special hospitals, where it was impossible to give adequate training or experience. The independent schools disappeared as hospitals began to control the "training" of nurses. Serious problems developed because of the sudden emergence of so many new schools. The number of schools increased from four in 1873 to four hundred by the turn of the century.

Society had accepted the social and financial obligation to educate teachers for elementary and secondary schools but did not recognize the obligation or benefit of financing programs to prepare nurses and thereby upgrade patient care.

The early schools of nursing faced many problems; one of the most difficult was whether to supply nursing service or to educate students of nursing. This led to a fusion of the two aims. The necessity of obtaining financial aid was a serious problem. Drives to encourage wealthy residents of the community to donate funds stimulated the schools to promise in return that they would permit students to care for members of the donors' families in their homes in times of illness.

Senior students were the ones who were sent into the community as private duty nurses. Sometimes in periods of financial crises, all members of the senior class were on private duty, and only the least experi-

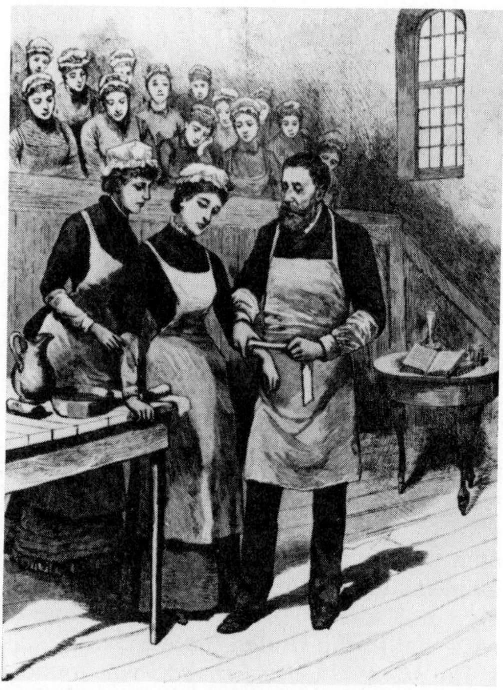

Figure 11–17. A demonstration on bandaging in 1886. This is an example of those classes taught by physicians that many training schools referred to as "Doctors Classes." (Dolan collection.)

enced students were available to give nursing care to the hospitalized patients. The fees obtained from caring for these wealthy patients in their homes went into the school treasury.

An interesting handwritten note from the office of the Editor-in-Chief of the *American Journal of Nursing* signed by Miss Sophia F. Palmer on August 12, 1904, was sent to the superintendent of nurses of the Connecticut Training School. It read, in part: "The objection to sending nurses out [into homes] is that it deprives the nurse of a part of her legitimate education whether the money is used for the hospital or the training school. . . . Either the hospital or the community should carry the burden of the cost of the schools." Miss Palmer sarcastically stated that this use of nursing students "is a great reflection upon the city and the members of the Board of Directors of the hospital."

In many schools, students upon admission were immediately assigned to the wards as workers (employees) and, when placed on the hospital payroll, were paid a stipend. Students were not sustained by the kind of self-respect that is accorded members of a profession. It has been stated that "heavy demands on the wards made it impossible for all students to attend their weekly lecture [class]." Certain students were assigned to take complete notes and later to read them to those who were unable to attend the class.

The first year of the two-year program provided experience in patient care, and the second year included ward administration and responsibility for the instruction of new students. The roles of the second-year students therefore, included comforters of patients, housekeepers, providers of financial aid (private duty), trainers of themselves and teachers of younger students. This type of "training" was not comparable to good apprenticeship training whereby one learned one's skill by working with a "master." Their experience was considered learning "by doing"—at the patient's expense.

DIVISIONS OF NURSING

Three divisions of nursing, hospital work, private duty and visiting or district nursing, were open to the new graduate.

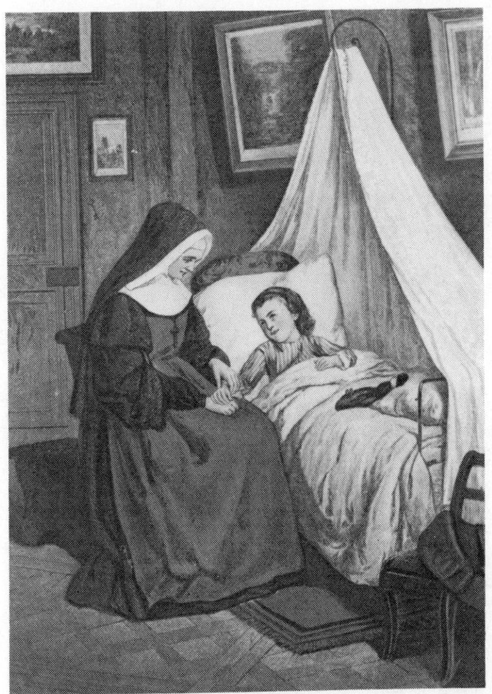

Figure 11–18. A Sister of Mercy cares for a sick child in her home. (Dolan collection.)

The only *hospital nursing* positions employing training school graduates at first were those of superintendent of nurses, perhaps an assistant, and operating-room and night supervisors. Usually the head nurses were students. Physicians gave lectures, and the superintendent of nurses gave most of the classes, in both sciences and nursing arts. Gradually the better schools added instructors, graduate head nurses and graduates for general duty.

As the increasing number of schools produced a body of trained nurses, there was a marked demand for them to do *private duty* in homes (Fig. 11–18). People did not go to hospitals for medical illnesses, rarely for obstetrics and not always for surgery. Even major operations were often done in private homes. The vast majority of graduate nurses did private duty. People began to understand what a trained nurse was and to have confidence in her abilities; 24-hour nursing duty was the rule for years.

DUTIES OF NURSES

An item of equipment that has become commonplace is the clinical thermometer,

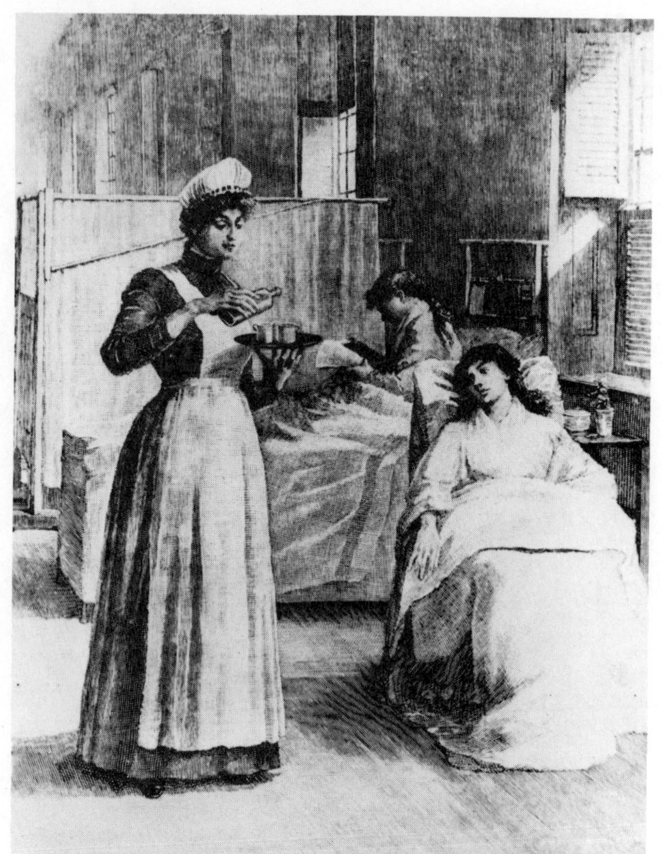

Figure 11–19. The nurse role no longer encompassed the timeless teaching aspects of nursing care once nurses were forced to reply, to a patient's questions, "I don't know, ask your doctor." (Dolan collection.)

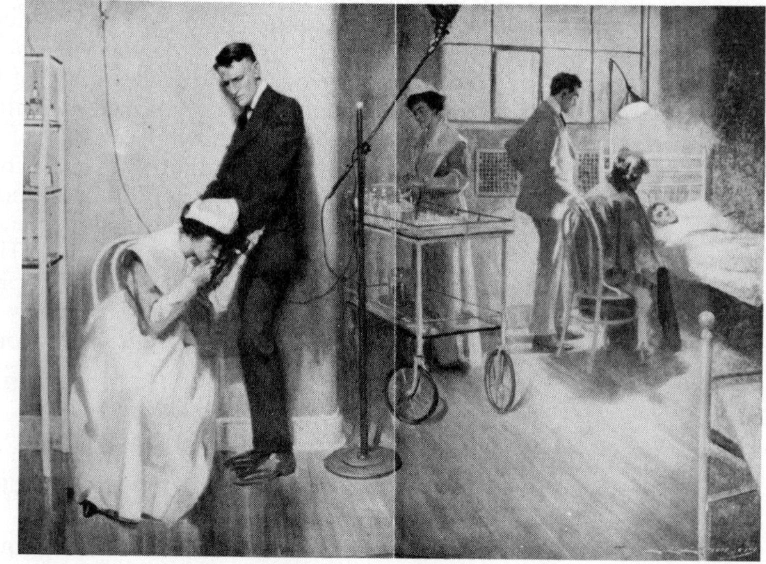

Figure 11–20. A scene from Mary Roberts Reinhart's book *K* in which the student nurse cries, "They say I poisoned him. . ." (Dolan collection.)

and yet it was scarce and not readily available to nurses in the latter part of the nineteenth century. The physician carried the thermometer and on occasion he, not the nurse, took a patient's temperature. A nurse's assignment involved making and applying turpentine stupes to relieve abdominal distention and to encourage peristaltic action. She applied mustard plasters and poultices made of ginger or onions or flaxseed, which assisted in drawing out the "laudable pus" from an infection. She gave carbolic acid gargles to patients, and of course, prepared and gave numerous enemas, cleansing as well as nutritive, which occupied much of her time and effort. Since intravenous infusions were unknown during this period, nutritional supplementation was achieved by the rectal administration of egg nog with brandy or chicken broth. Cupping and the application of leeches were also duties of the nurse.

Answering a patient's questions about his condition or planning a program of teaching him about his health needs was not permitted. Nurses were instructed to answer very briskly, "I don't know—ask your doctor" (Fig. 11–19). The physician's demanding that the nurse not answer any questions but refer them to him lowered the status of the nurse and prevented health teaching. Since the contents of medicines were not identified at first, nurses often were not able to answer questions about medication. Some nurses were blamed for causing severe reactions in patients. A famous nurse, *Mary Roberts Rinehart*, whose novels became popular at the turn of the century, reflected on the plight of the nurse in such a predicament (Fig. 11–20).

Because of ignorance of the causes of many diseases, of the effects of surgical intervention and of the ways in which disease was spread, as well as the lack of important pharmaceutical preparations such as antibiotics, many patients were hospitalized for long periods. The physical, emotional, spiritual, recreational and nutritional aspects of nursing care were crucial to the patient's comfort and well-being. It is a well-known fact that many patients came to the hospital for nursing care only because their chances of being cured were thought to be slim. Many patients, families and doctors have recorded that it was nursing care alone that brought patients back to health. Many interesting beds were designed and even an invalid lift to assist in making the long hours more comfortable for the patient (Figs. 11–21, 11–22 and 11–23).

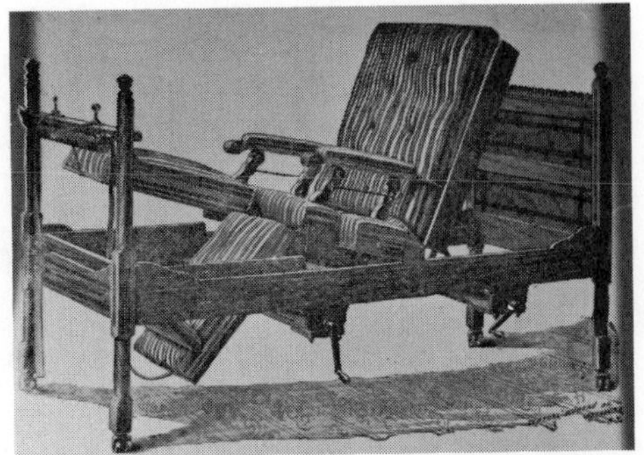

Figure 11–22. An adjustable chair bed (ca. 1880). (Dolan collection.)

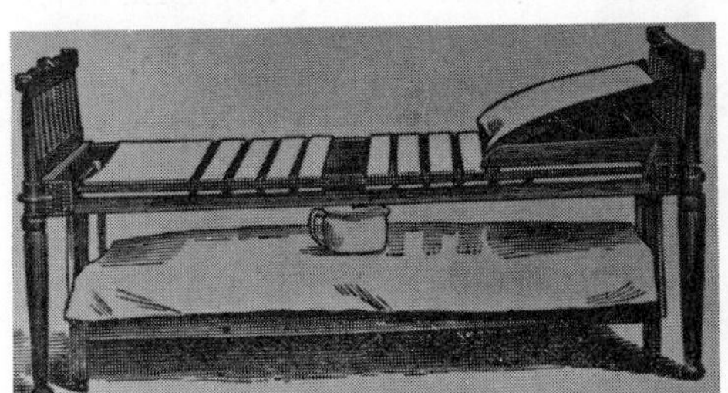

Figure 11–21. The Crosby invalid bed (ca. 1877). (Dolan collection.)

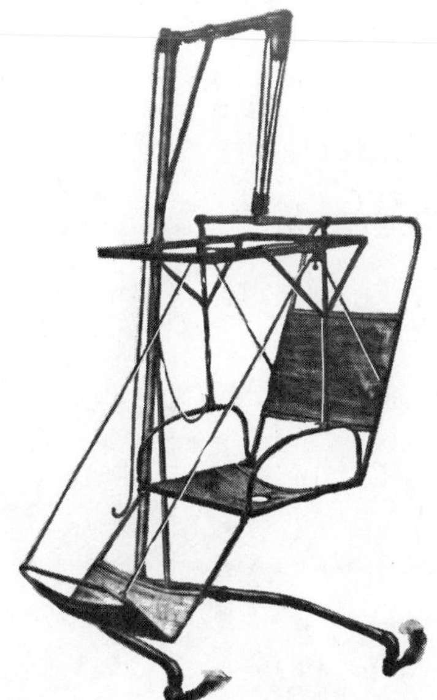

Figure 11–23. An invalid lift (ca. 1880). (Dolan collection.)

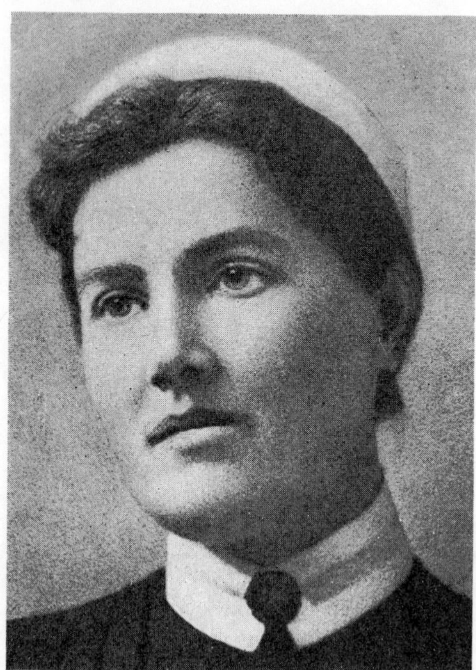

Figure 11–24. Isabel Hampton Robb. (Dolan collection.)

NURSING LEADERSHIP

In *A Century of Nursing,* written in 1876, Abby Woolsey stressed the desirability of elevating nursing to an educated and honorable profession. She pleaded for quality in educational programs, expressing the belief that nursing schools should be equal to teachers' colleges. A committee of the Bellevue Training School mapped plans for a "College of Nursing," but this college did not become a reality.

John Eaton, federal commissioner of education, in a public address implied that the training of nurses should be an educational endeavor and must be planned on educational lines. His address was published under the title, "Training Schools for Nurses," by the Bureau of Education, Washington, D.C., in 1879.

In addition to the founding of these early schools of nursing in the last quarter of the century, there were some dynamic leaders in nursing education, and teaching tools, such as textbooks, were made available.

Isabel Hampton Robb (1860–1910) was an outstanding leader in nursing and in nursing education (Fig. 11–24). Born in Welland, Ontario, Canada, she attended St. Catherine's Collegiate Institute for several years, and then accepted a teaching position there. She decided to enter the field of nursing and in 1881 was admitted to Bellevue Training School as a student nurse (Fig. 11–25) and graduated in 1883. She was a remarkably constructive thinker and had the rare ability both to create and to apply new ideas.

In 1886, Isabel Hampton became *Superintendent of Nurses at Illinois Training School in Chicago.* The school contracted with Cook County Hospital for clinical experience for the students. The ability of Miss Isabel Hampton as an organizer began to

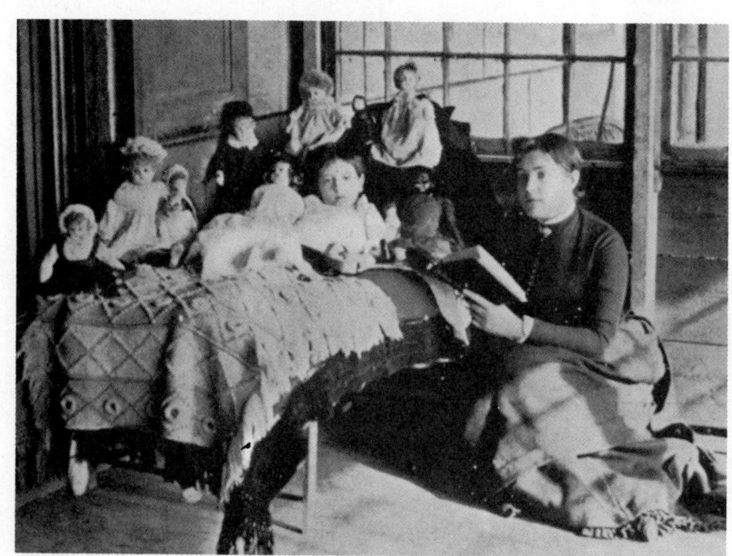

Figure 11–25. Isabel Hampton as a student nurse caring for a little girl surrounded by her dolls. (Dolan collection.)

be noted in this position. She put into practice a graded system of theory. She terminated the practice of students' doing private duty as part of their education.

In 1889, Miss Hampton journeyed to Baltimore to organize a new school at *Johns Hopkins Hospital*. Here her fertile mind gave birth to new ideas, and many innovations were attempted. She became "Principal" instead of "Superintendent"; she established policies for a 12-hour day, which included time allowance for meals, definite recreation, rest and study periods and a limit on the day's work. Her aim, which she had the ability and persistence to achieve, was quality nursing care that combined a happy balance of intellectual and manual skills. Of her leadership qualities, Nutting commented:

> Planning, initiating, directing, and controlling,—such activities provided for her an element in which she lived and moved with the greatest ease and freedom. She was in every sense of the word a leader, by nature, by capacity, by personal attributes and qualities, by choice, and probably to some extent by inheritance and training; a follower she never was.[22]

Recognizing the need for nursing textbooks, Miss Hampton wrote *Nursing—Its Principles and Practice for Hospital and Private Use*.

The International Congress of Charities, Correction and Philanthropy was to be held, during the World's Fair in Chicago in 1893, and Miss Hampton was asked to organize a section for nursing. For help with this project she sought the thinking and advice of Florence Nightingale as well as nurse educators in this country. Miss Nightingale shared her thoughts generously through correspondence, and a firm friendship blossomed between these two dynamic leaders. During the congress, the nurse educators were called together by Miss Hampton, and the *Society of Superintendents of Training Schools for Nurses* evolved. She became the first president.

Miss Hampton's attractiveness, combined with her poise and charming manner, have been recorded by many admirers. Dr. Hunter Robb became her chief admirer and in June of 1894 they were married. She retired from active nursing but remained an ardent supporter in the fight for better preparation for nurses, especially nurse educators, and a better quality of care for patients.

Her revolutionary but sound ideas were presented in 1895 at the annual convention of the American Society of Superintendents of Training Schools for Nurses. She advocated a *three-year course* and an *eight-hour day* at a time when many students were working twice that number of hours. She also suggested terminating the practice of giving stipends each month and, with the money thus saved, establish libraries. This would change the status of the nurse in school from employee to student.

Mrs. Robb felt that an organization was needed for *all nurses*, not just for nursing school administrators. In 1896, she became the first president of the newly formed *Nurses Associated Alumnae of the United States and Canada*, which was a nationwide union of nurse training school alumnae associations. In unity there could be strength.

Unlike Florence Nightingale, Isabel Hampton Robb believed that the status as well as the preparation of practitioners of nursing would benefit by licensing examinations and registration. Such forms of legal control would improve nursing as they had improved medicine and law. Legal control would protect patients from incompetent nurses as well as elevate the standards of nursing. Her efforts played a large part in the development of the courses established in 1898 at Teachers' College of Columbia University.

Isabel Hampton Robb's brilliant career ended abruptly in 1910 when she was killed in a tragic accident. A trust fund was established to perpetuate the memory of this brilliant leader. The *Isabel Hampton Robb Scholarships* have permitted many nurses to receive a more enriching educational background; let us hope that this fund has helped to elevate the quality of nursing care as well as that of nursing education.

Mary Adelaide Nutting (1858–1948) (Fig. 11–26) was born in Quebec and later attended private schools in Montreal, Boston and Ottawa, receiving special instruction in music and art. She was a member of the first class to graduate from the training

[22]Nutting, M. A. "Isabel Hampton Robb—Her Work in Organization and Education," *American Journal of Nursing*, 10:19, 1910.

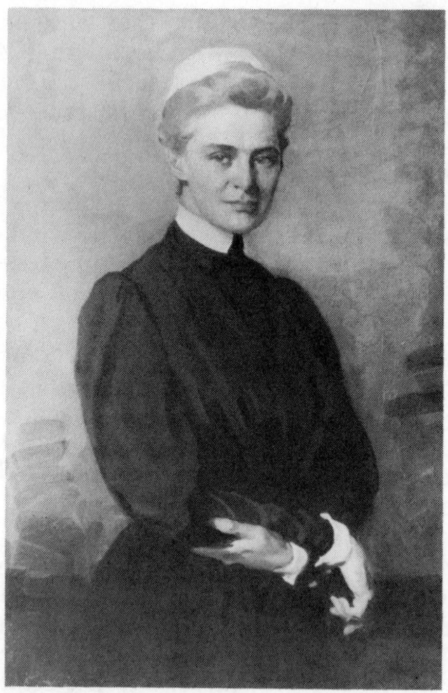

Figure 11–26. Mary Adelaide Nutting. (Dolan collection.)

school at Johns Hopkins and became principal of this school when Isabel Hampton Robb resigned. Her concepts of nursing education seemed to parallel those of Mrs. Robb, and Miss Nutting carried out many of the reforms Mrs. Robb had initiated.

In 1907, Miss Nutting was appointed to the faculty of Teachers' College of Columbia University and became the *first professor of nursing in the world,* a position that she held until her retirement in 1925. Out of gratitude for her outstanding leadership, the *Adelaide Nutting Historical Nursing Collection* was dedicated to her memory and has been exhibited at Teachers' College.

Among her many achievements were: raising the standards of basic nursing education; assisting in the establishment of nursing organizations; preserving the profession's history in the four-volume *History of Nursing,* written in collaboration with Lavinia Dock; encouraging provision for financial support for schools of nursing and, thus, permitting separation of schools of nursing from hospital ownership and control; developing programs at Teachers' College for nurses in teaching, public health, supervision and administration; and coordinating nursing services during World War I. She also wrote a brochure entitled *A Sound Economic Basis for Schools of Nursing,*[23] and *The Educational Status of Nursing.*[24]

Miss Nutting received an honorary Master of Arts degree from Yale in 1921. The Liberty Service Medal was awarded to her for her humanitarian and patriotic services. The National League of Nursing Education designed the *Adelaide Nutting Medal for Leadership in Nursing Education,* presenting the first medal to Miss Nutting in 1944.

UNIFORMS

Nurses' uniforms were not designed or worn by lay nurses until the latter part of the nineteenth century. *Euphemia Van Rensselaer* (Fig. 11–27) has been credited with recognizing the need for a uniform and designing one. Miss Van Rensselaer was born in 1840 of an illustrious family. Her mother was Elizabeth King, the daughter of Governor King of New York and the niece of Charles King, president of Columbia University; Euphemia's grandfather, Rufus King, was an early American statesman

[23]Nutting, M. A.: *A Sound Economic Basis for Schools of Nursing.* New York, G. P. Putnam's Sons, 1926.

[24]Nutting, M. A.: *Educational Status of Nursing,* Bulletin No. 7, U.S. Bureau of Education, 1912.

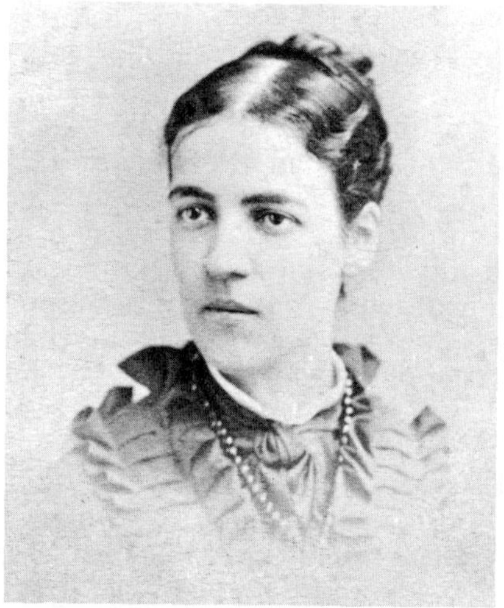

Figure 11–27. Euphemia Van Rensselaer (Sister Marie Dolores) in 1878. (Courtesy of Mrs. Christopher Wyatt.)

and served as ambassador to Great Britain on two occasions. Miss Van Rensselaer's father was Brigadier-General Van Rensselaer; his death from typhoid fever prompted her to become a trained nurse.

According to her niece, Miss Van Rensselaer initiated the practice of wearing a uniform while serving as a nurse at Bellevue Hospital.

> The story I heard from my Mother was that Euphemia Van Rensselaer volunteered for service at Bellevue when the two Miss Schuylers—granddaughters of the General—organized the States Charities Aid Association. Up to that time the only nurses were the old women collected by the Hospital. The Misses Schuyler, inspired by Florence Nightingale, were determined to relieve this impossible situation and procured volunteers. In 1876 it was determined to have uniforms but this did not suit the volunteers. It was then that my Aunt set the example by taking home some material and having a uniform made for herself. When Miss Van Rensselaer was seen duly clad the others decided to follow suit. She later became an Anglican nun in Clewer, England and then when her brother, who was a clergyman in the Episcopalian Church came over to Rome, she followed him and joined the Sisters of Charity. She was sent to Nassau to found a Mission and on her return organized Seton Hospital for tuberculosis which was taken over later by the City. She then organized the Grace Institute—a trade school for women—and ended her life in a Day Nursery in her brother's parish—St. Francis Xavier's—the Jesuit Church at 16th Street and Sixth Avenue. She died about 1912 in the New York Foundling Asylum.[25]

Euphemia Van Rensselaer designed the blue and white uniform, apron and cap of the Bellevue Training School.

The nurse's cap has always been and still is distinctive. It probably originated when all women wore caps indoors; this would account for the lace frills on the cap that Florence Nightingale designed for her school in 1860. At one time the cap that entirely covered the hair was thought correct, and the "dusting cap" pattern was much used. Since these were ugly, the style gave way to one which covered the knot of hair that was at that time worn on top of the head. Caps either were un-washable (book muslin or organdy) or had elaborate frills that required special laundering. About 1910, simply made, easily laundered caps began to be used. The use of black bands on the sleeves of the uniform for graduates or seniors shows the military influence, an attempt to indicate rank. The present customs involving stripes are so varied, however, that they are meaningless.

NURSE AUTHORS

In the early years of nursing, practically all textbooks used by nurses were written by physicians. Miss Nightingale's *Notes on Nursing* (1859) probably did much to make nurses feel that they were capable of writing their own textbooks and knew best how to present the art of nursing.

With the exception of the Bellevue Training School's *Handbook of Nursing* (1878) and the Connecticut Training School's *Handbook on Nursing* (1879), the first American nursing textbook was written by Mrs. Clara Weeks-Shaw, a graduate of the New York Hospital. This text, *A Textbook of Nursing* (1885), made the distinction between true nursing care and the mere execution of the physician's orders.

Diana C. Kimber has been credited with writing the *first textbook on anatomy for nurses* in 1893. She was born in Oxfordshire, England. After receiving an excellent liberal education in both England and Germany, she came to New York and entered Bellevue Training School in 1884. The teaching field attracted her, and feeling the need for a textbook on anatomy, she undertook to write one. It was the *first scientific book written by a nurse for nurses.* She returned to England in 1898 and entered an Anglican nursing sisterhood. From this spiritual environment, she went forth to care for the sick poor in their homes, carrying out her high ideals of service.

Minnie Goodnow (Fig. 11–28), well-known author, educator, war nurse and administrator, was one of the pioneers in the field of textbook writing. She wrote the first textbook on chemistry for nurses in the United States in 1911, the well-known *Nursing History* in 1916 and the first *Physics for Nurses* in 1919. Miss Goodnow saw ac-

[25]Personal correspondence with Mrs. Christopher Wyatt (Euphemia Van Rensselaer Wyatt).

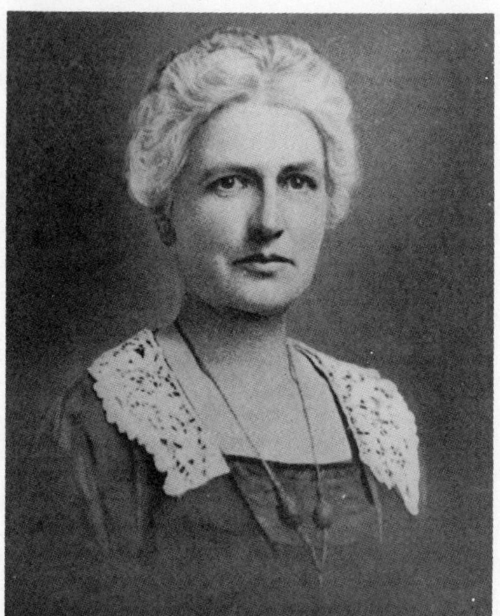

Figure 11–28. Minnie Goodnow was the author of *Nursing History,* the predecessor of *Nursing in Society*. (Dolan collection.)

tive service overseas during World War I and had a colorful career as an administrator for over 40 years. She died in 1952.

Bertha Harmer was a graduate of Toronto General Hospital. She received the degrees of B.S. and M.A. from Columbia University and was an instructor at St. Luke's Hospital, New York City. Assisting in organizing the Yale School of Nursing, Miss Harmer became one of its professors. For some years she was in charge of the Graduate School of Nursing at McGill University, Montreal. She wrote a textbook entitled *Principles and Practice of Nursing*. She died in 1934.

Lavinia L. Dock (1858–1956), one of the great women in nursing history, contributed to the improvement of the status of women and was active in many social welfare movements. Miss Dock graduated from Bellevue Hospital in 1886. She held executive positions in Bellevue, Johns Hopkins and the Illinois Training School and worked at the Henry Street Settlement. She held the position of Secretary of the International Council of Nurses and was one of its chief promoters. Her *Textbook on Materia Medica for Nurses* was published in 1890.

The first general history of nursing, with the exception of two pamphlets, was written by M. Adelaide Nutting and Lavinia L. Dock. Its four volumes constitute a standard reference. The school at Johns Hopkins University, Baltimore, was the first to put the history of nursing into its curriculum.

THE HERITAGE OF NURSING

The Image of the Early Schools

Schools on the Nightingale Plan were established:

1. as a result of the vision, competent planning and political influence of the highly esteemed nursing leaders of the Civil War.
2. despite opposition from medical staff, hospital administration and politicians.

The early schools on the Nightingale Plan differed from the true Nightingale program in that:

1. the educational objectives were more restrictive.
2. the ability to select learning experiences on the basis of educational needs of the learners was lacking.
3. the control of the program was far less centralized.
4. the environment was less conducive to learning.
5. the programs were inferior in faculty, philosophy, content and teaching strategies.

6. the preventive, social and psychological components of nursing were not stressed.
7. the focus of the programs was "sick nursing"; there were no health components or community-based learning experiences.
8. the students were not free from non-nursing duties.
9. the nursing service demands superseded the learning needs. (Students were utilized as head nurses instead of the stable experienced staff required by the Nightingale School.)
10. the confusion in aims—nursing education versus nursing service—had brought about a fusion of both at the expense of the educational program.
11. the recognition of responsibility for continuing education of graduates was nonexistent.
12. the lack of financial backing was a crucial handicap.

The principal similarities between early American training schools and the Nightingale school were that nurses were in charge of the programs, the teaching and the students. The advantage of utilizing even this small aspect of the Nightingale Plan was that nursing retained its identity and became recognized as a distinct department within the hospital organization.

Great nurse educators emerged to guide the strengthening of programs of nurse education, provide teaching and learning aids, and chart the course for improving the educational preparation of nurses for delivery of care.

REFERENCE READINGS

Bacon, Francis: "History of the Connecticut Training School," *The Trained Nurse*, pp. 187–193, October 1895.

Bernheim, Bertram: *The Story of Johns Hopkins*. Surrey, England, Windmill Press, 1949.

Christy, Teresa E.: *Cornerstone for Nursing Education*. New York, Teachers' College Press, 1969.

Colvin, Sarah T.: *A Rebel in Thought*. New York, Island Press, 1944.

Cooper, Page: *The Bellevue Story*. New York, Thomas Y. Crowell, 1948.

Curtis, and Denny: "Early History of the Boston Training School." *American Journal of Nursing*, 2:331–335, 1902.

Dock, Lavinia L.: "History of the Reform in Nursing in Bellevue Hospital," *American Journal of Nursing*, 1:90, 1901.

Giles, Dorothy: *A Candle in Her Hand*. New York, G. P. Putnam's Sons, 1950.

Goodrich, Annie W.: "Louisa Lee Schuyler—An Appreciation," *American Journal of Nursing*, *15*:1079–1082, 1915.

Hampton, Isabel A., et al.: *Nursing of the Sick—1893*. New York, McGraw-Hill Book Co., 1949.

Hanaford, Phoebe: *Daughters of America, or Women of the Century*. Augusta, Me., True & Co., 1882.

Hobson, Elizabeth C.: "Founding of the Bellevue Training School." In *A Century of Nursing*. New York, G. P. Putnam's Sons, 1950.

Marshall, Helen E.: *Mary Adelaide Nutting*. Baltimore, Johns Hopkins University Press, 1972.

North, Franklin H.: "A New Profession for Women," *Century Magazine*, pp. 38–47, July 1882.

Parsons, Sara E.: *History of the Massachusetts General Hospital Training School for Nurses*. Boston, M. Barrows, 1922.

Pugh, Garrett F., and Fisher, A. J. B.: *Ethics and Health in Late Victorian Society*. London, Arundel, 1970.

Richards, Linda A.: *Reminiscences of Linda Richards*. Boston, M. Barrows, 1911.

Seelye, Rev. L. Clark: *The Need of a Collegiate Education for Women*. North Adams, Massachusetts, American Institute of Instruction, 1874.

Stack, Margaret K.: "Resume of the History of the Connecticut Training School for Nurses," *American Journal of Nursing*, *23*:825–829, 1923.

Staupers, Mabel K.: *No Time for Prejudice*. New York, Macmillan Co., 1961.

Stewart, Isabel M.: *The Education of Nurses*. New York, The Macmillan Co., 1943.

Thoms, Adah B.: *Pathfinders*. New York, Kay Printing House, 1929.

Weeks-Shaw, Clara S.: *A Textbook of Nursing*. New York, D. Appleton & Co., 1897.

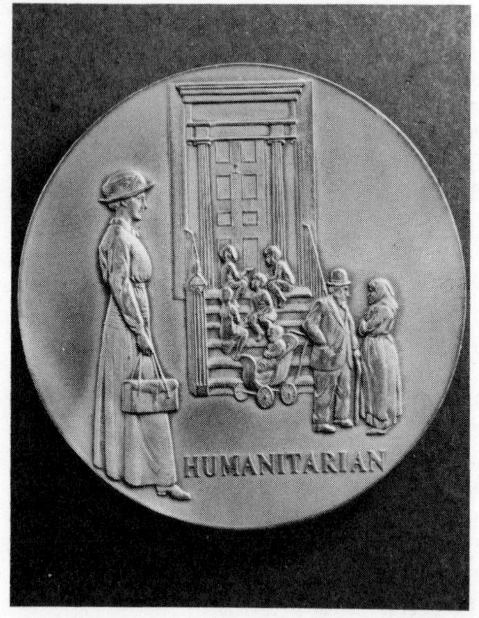

Lillian Wald Commemorative Medallion honoring her induction into New York University "Hall of Fame for Great Americans." (Fitzpatrick collection.)

12 Relationship of Nursing to Welfare Services and Society in the Late Nineteenth Century

SOCIAL WELFARE

The closing years of the nineteenth century saw a resurgence of *humanitarianism*. Many individuals and groups endeavored to relieve the physical and social sufferings of others.

Leprosy continued to plague many people, and devoted care for its victims was still needed. In 1873, *Father Damien* de Veuster (1840–1889), a young Belgian priest, requested to be sent as a missionary to Molokai in the Hawaiian Islands. There he singlehandedly cheered his heartsick patients, built homes for them, nursed them and buried them. His magnificent story of courage, devotion and sacrifice inspired his patients and followers.

In 1894, the State of Louisiana recognized the need for a place to care for the many victims of leprosy. Money was raised to buy an abandoned sugar plantation in the town of Carville to house the lepers, and a physician, Dr. L. A. Wailes, volunteered to take care of them. Soon afterwards, when he realized that more assistance was needed, he resigned his task. In 1896, the Sisters of Charity of St. Vincent de Paul received a petition for help from the board of directors of the "Louisiana Leper Home," and the nuns offered to send some members of their community. Sister Beatrice, a trained nurse from Boston, joined four other nurse nuns and took over the settlement. The Sisters worked for many years under incredible hardships to make the institution a suitable place in which to live and work. Patients received a home and nursing care. In 1917, Congress passed a law authorizing the purchase of this institution by the United States Government and named it the *National Leprosarium*. Because of World War I, the transfer of ownership was not completed until 1921. Since then, the U.S. Public Health Service has been responsible for this institution. The Sisters of Charity have remained an integral part of the staff.

A journal article, "Nurses at Carville," identifies three primary objectives in the care of the patient with leprosy (Hansen's disease)—the importance of a strong nurse-patient relationship, the accurate recording of observations, assessments and facts, and the "nurse's role as an educator on health problems related to leprosy."[1]

In 1971, *Sister Mary Anne Hain,* director of nursing at the Carville, Louisiana, Public Health Service Hospital, was the recipient of the Federal Nursing Service Award given annually by the Association of Military Surgeons of the United States to a nurse member for outstanding accomplishments in the advancement of professional nursing.

William Booth (1829–1912) was an ardent religious leader fired with enthusiasm to rescue poor souls who were living in the slums of London. He knew that hunger, dirt and misery had to be relieved before spiritual assistance could be rendered. In 1878, he organized and became the first general of the *Salvation Army.* He taught Christian principles and practiced Christian living by giving food, clothing and shelter to the poor as well as aiding them in finding suitable, useful work. His labors extended to other lands. The gracious assistance given by his army to the United States' soldiers during World Wars I and II can never be forgotten. William Booth's book, *In Darkest England and the Way Out* (1890), reflects his belief that to restore a man to humanity is to restore him to God.

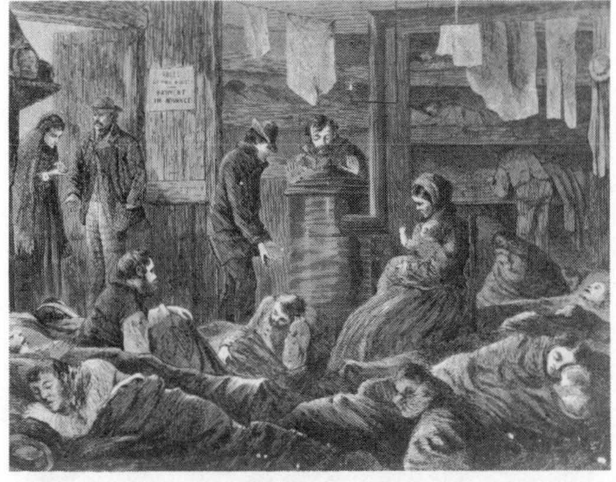

Figure 12–1. Underground lodging for the poor in New York. (Dolan collection.)

The *Settlement House Movement* was started at Toynbee Hall in London by Oxford University students who studied community problems and wanted to alleviate them.

Jane Addams (1860–1935) graduated from college in 1881. One night two years later, she wandered through London's East End and for the first time saw the slums of a big city. She was determined to do what she could to relieve the problems of the slums. In Chicago in 1889, she and Ellen Gates Starr purchased a big old house and opened its doors to the neighborhood; this was the beginning of *Hull House.* Help of any sort was available to neighbors. This was the spirit of social service. Jane Addams was also a leader in the fight for suffrage for

[1]Hughes, Sister Ann Elizabeth, Bertonneau, Sister Dorothea and Enna, Carl D.: "Nurses at Carville," *The American Journal of Nursing, 68*:2564–2569, 1968.

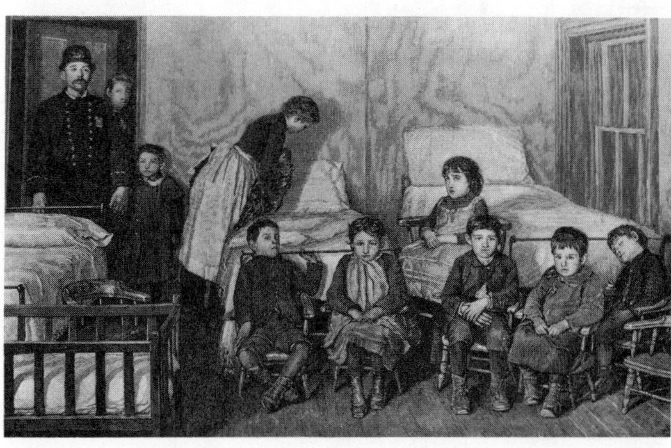

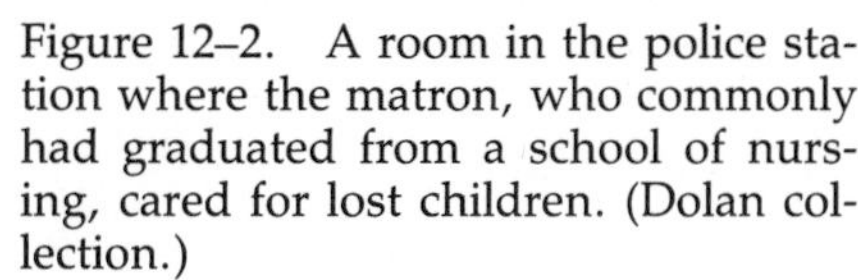

Figure 12–2. A room in the police station where the matron, who commonly had graduated from a school of nursing, cared for lost children. (Dolan collection.)

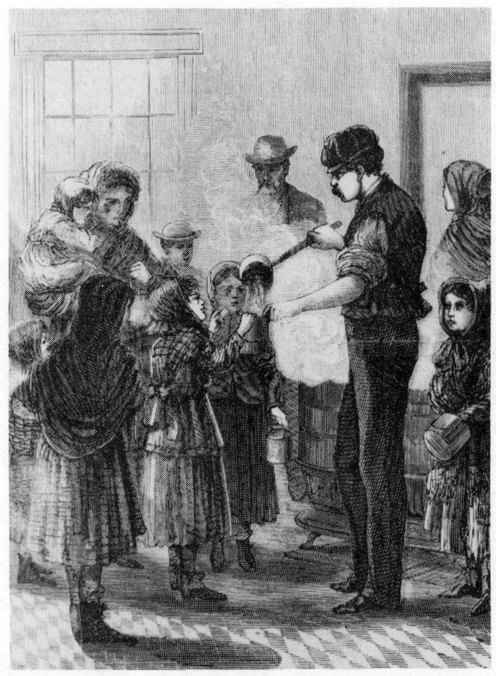

Figure 12–3. The New York YMCA's soup kitchen for the relief of the poor. (Dolan collection.)

women. She, with Nicholas Murray Butler, was the recipient of the 1931 Nobel Peace Prize.

The Young Men's Christian Association (YMCA) was started to develop the spiritual, social, physical and intellectual well-being of men (Fig. 12–3). It was organized in 1844 in London and in 1851 in the United States. Physical training has become an important part of the program.

During the Civil War, several branches of the YMCA joined to form the United States Christian Commission to work for the welfare of soldiers in camps and hospitals. In the First World War, the commission cared for prisoners and provided recreation for the soldiers. In the Second World War, it cooperated with other agencies to form the United Service Organization (USO), which planned recreational programs for the members of the armed forces.

In 1885 in London, Lady Kinnaird encouraged a group of women to provide homes for women workers. That same year in the south of England, Emma Roberts started a prayer union. In 1887, the two groups united to form the Young Women's Christian Association (YWCA) to assist women and girls spiritually, socially, intellectually and physically.

In 1866, there was a YWCA in Boston. Local associations spread until the YWCA became the vast organization it is today. The YWCA units in this country have been a source of housing for women in every large city.

Another humanitarian project was the establishment of the *Grenfell Mission. Sir Wilfred Grenfell* (1865–1940) was an English medical missionary who went to Labrador in 1892 (Fig. 12–4). There he built a chain

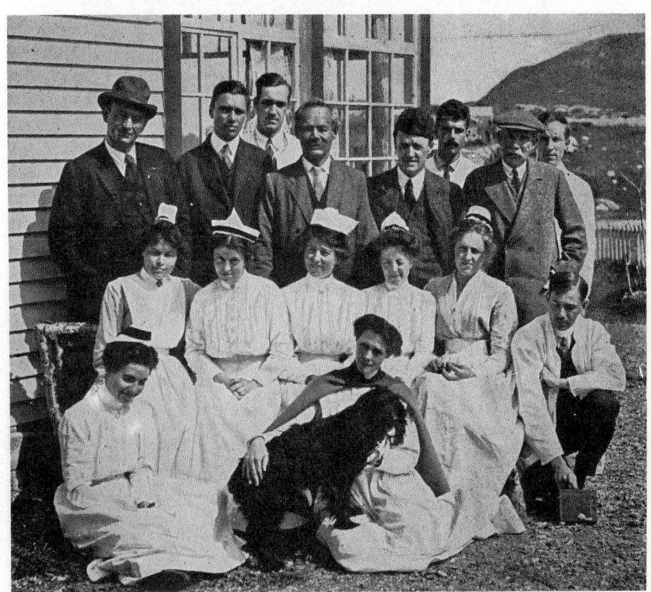

Figure 12–4. Dr. Grenfell *(center)* and his staff at St. Anthony's Hospital, Labrador, 1914. (Dolan collection.)

of hospital centers and nursing stations, established cooperative stores and built schools, libraries and orphanages. In 1912, the International Grenfell Association consolidated the work of the American, Canadian and English branches that supported his mission. Sir Wilfred supervised the work of his staff and cruised along the eastern Canadian coast in the hospital steamer, *Strathcona II,* giving assistance to those in need. Patients were reached by dogsled in the winter and by boat in the summer. Thus, another amazing project had been developed for the welfare of mankind.

NURSING IN THE SPANISH-AMERICAN WAR

The year was 1898, and American patriotism was being fanned to fever pitch by the slogan "Remember the 'Maine.' " The United States battleship *Maine* had been sunk mysteriously on the fifteenth of February in Havana harbor. This was one of the many incidents that finally caused President McKinley to ask Congress for authority to intervene in Cuba's struggle to be free from Spanish control and domination. He was authorized to permit enlistment of volunteers.

There was no organized army nurse corps at the time, although training schools were in existence and trained nurses were available; furthermore, there was no system by which nurses could be provided for war service. To remedy this situation, Congress appropriated the necessary funds and gave the surgeon general the authority to employ nurses under contract.

Although the Nurses Associated Alumnae of the United States and Canada (now the American Nurses' Association) represented the trained nurses of both countries, it had been in existence for such a short time that it was not recognized as the spokesman for nurses nor was it prepared to undertake the task of listing qualifications or recruiting nurses for this war service. Consequently, a physician, *Dr. Anita Newcomb McGee,* assumed the task. The surgeon general believed that nurses would not be useful because military surgeons were opposed to their presence in military hospitals. Through Dr. McGee's prompting, however, the surgeon general asked the Daughters of the American Revolution to carry out the procurement of nurses. Because Dr. McGee was vice president of the Daughters of the American Revolution, the group accepted the surgeon general's request to recruit nurses. Dr. McGee established standards of admission to the service as well as a valuable system of keeping records. Credentials were evaluated, statements being obtained from schools from which the applicant graduated along with the required certificate of good reputation.

Nurses were recruited; they were needed desperately, not so much because of war casualties but because of the typhoid fever that afflicted many of the soldiers in camp. Other communicable diseases that threatened the troops in Cuba were yellow fever, malaria and dysentery.

When Dr. McGee was appointed acting assistant surgeon general, she was responsible for the Army Nurse Division. At this time she terminated the assistance of the Daughters of the American Revolution. The efforts of Dr. McGee and the excellence of the work of the nurses in this war led to the establishment of a permanent Army Nurse Corps. Commenting on the achievements of the nurses in general, an officer said, "When you were coming, we did not know what we would do with you. Now we do not know what we would have done without you."

Many members of the Nurses Associated Alumnae of the United States and Canada and many women prominent in the nursing world served in the war, among them Mary Gladwin, Eugenie Hibbard, Esther Hasson and Anna Maxwell. A total of nearly 1600 graduate nurses served.

These army nurses won the esteem and recognition of the officers and men (Fig. 12–5). Their supporters included the surgeons who had been most prejudiced against them. The continued employment of women as army nurses is due to the skill and devotion that female army nurses showed at the time of the Spanish-American War.

During the Spanish-American War, a military physician, *Major Walter Reed,* was appointed chief of a committee to study the cause and spread of typhoid fever in the army camps. After much searching, the commission determined that flies, in addi-

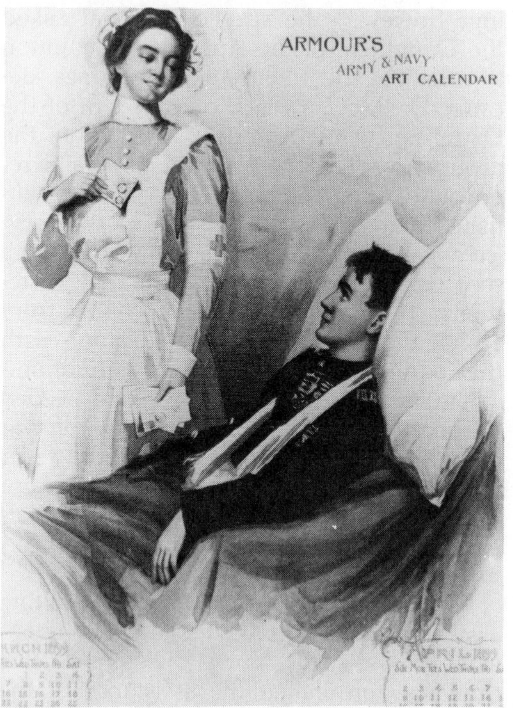

Figure 12–5. A calendar portrayal of the image of the "Angel of Mercy" prominent in the minds of the military and public. (Dolan collection.)

tion to unclean practices in general, were the most obvious source of the illness.

At the end of the war, it was apparent that disease had taken a heavier toll of lives than the bullets of the enemy. Yellow fever had been a particularly virulent and fatal enemy. Burning sulfur candles as a means of preventing this disease did not appear to be successful. When a person died, all his personal effects, including even his home, called "fomites," were burned. These actions were still no solution to the problem. The United States government sent physicians to Cuba with the assigment of finding some method to control this malady, which had been endemic in Havana for more than 200 years. The physicians were *Drs. James Carroll, Aristides Agramonte, Jesse W. Lazear and Walter Reed.*

Dr. Carlos Finlay, a Havana physician, had been striving for 19 years to convince his medical colleagues that yellow fever was caused by a common house mosquito. Major Walter Reed and Dr. Agramonte consulted Dr. Finlay, who shared his theories about yellow fever and even gave them a supply of mosquito larvae of the suspected species. Human volunteers were needed. Heroic Americans volunteered. The first ones were physicians. Some survived, but others died, martyrs to the cause of science. The experiments proved that yellow fever was transmitted by the bite of the mosquito now called *Aëdes aegypti.*

One of the heroines of this scientific project was a nurse, *Clara Louise Maass* (1876–1901).

Miss Maass attended the Christina Trefz Training School for Nurses of the Newark German Hospital—now called *Clara Maass Memorial Hospital.* She enrolled at age seventeen and was one of the first five students to graduate from the two-year program in 1895. She was a member of the hospital staff for the next three years, becoming head nurse in 1898. With a spirit of patriotism, Miss Maass was one of the first to sign up as a contract nurse during the Spanish-American War. She commenced working in Army field hospitals in the South and in Cuba until she completed her service in February 1899. She rejoined the U.S. Army the following November and was sent to the Philippines, where an attack of dengue—more popularly known as "breakbone fever"—shortened her term of service, causing her to return home to recuperate.

In October of 1900, Miss Maass received a cablegram from Dr. William Gorgas urging her to return to Cuba, where he and Dr. Walter Reed were conducting research efforts to identify the cause of yellow fever. She volunteered for this civilian nursing assignment and served in Havana through the spring of 1901, nursing the victims of the fever.

To validate a theory that mosquitoes were the carriers of yellow fever, Clara Maass offered to be bitten. She suffered a mild attack of the fever in June 1901, but offered to be bitten again on August 14. This time the fever proved fatal, and she died at Las Animas Hospital in Cuba on August 24, 1901.

Clara Louise Maass was the only woman to volunteer and, therefore, the only woman to die in these experiments. Her death proved without a doubt that mosquitoes alone are the cause of yellow fever. The experiments ceased, and ultimately, the disease was conquered. Miss Maass died in

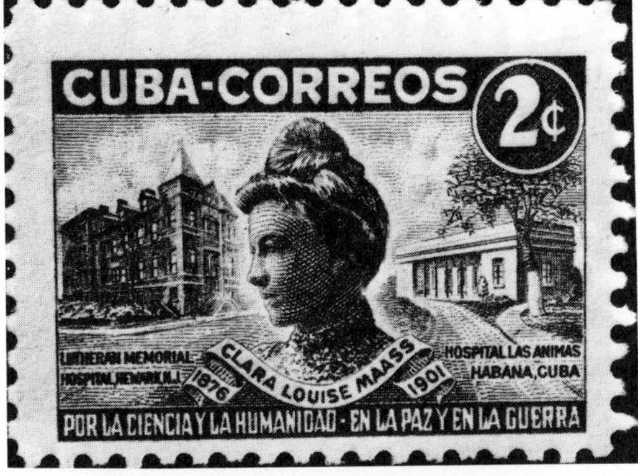

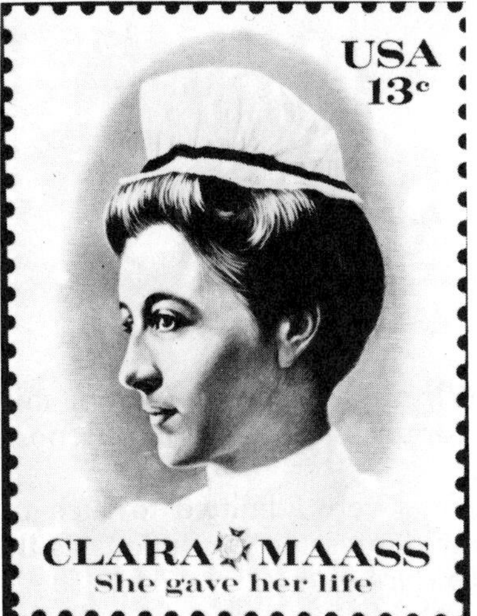

Figure 12–6. Clara Maass, a nurse heroine honored by two countries, Cuba and the United States. (Dolan collection.)

Havana but her body was later sent to Fairmount Cemetery in Newark for burial with full military honors.

It has been recorded that "Clara Maass was a gallant, courageous woman . . . a highly skilled nurse . . . a warm, compassionate human being who was deeply committed to humanity. She lived to serve those who needed her." She died for the same reason.

In 1951, Cuba issued a commemorative stamp praising her heroic sacrifice. In 1976, the United States honored her contribution to humanity and the nursing profession with the issuance of a commemorative postage stamp. She is the first individual American nurse to be so honored (Fig. 12–6).

The significance of Miss Maass' courageous act became even more evident when a devastating epidemic of yellow fever occurred in the southern United States. Some people, including health care providers, packed their families and possessions and attempted to flee to safety. The lack of physicians added to the devastation of the population. Many nurses, such as the Sisters of Charity, aided the sick to the best of their ability (Fig. 12–7).

PUBLIC HEALTH PROBLEMS

Two community problems of vital importance were those of controlling contagious

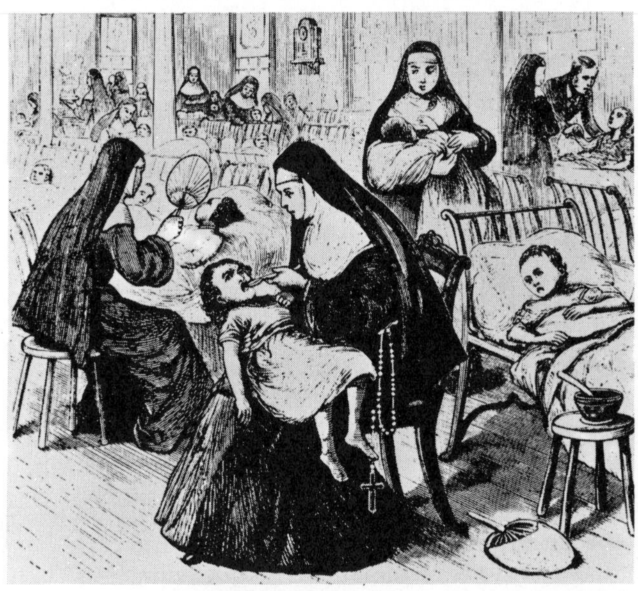

Figure 12–7. The Sisters of Charity caring for victims of yellow fever, at St. Vincent's Infant Asylum in New Orleans. (Dolan collection.)

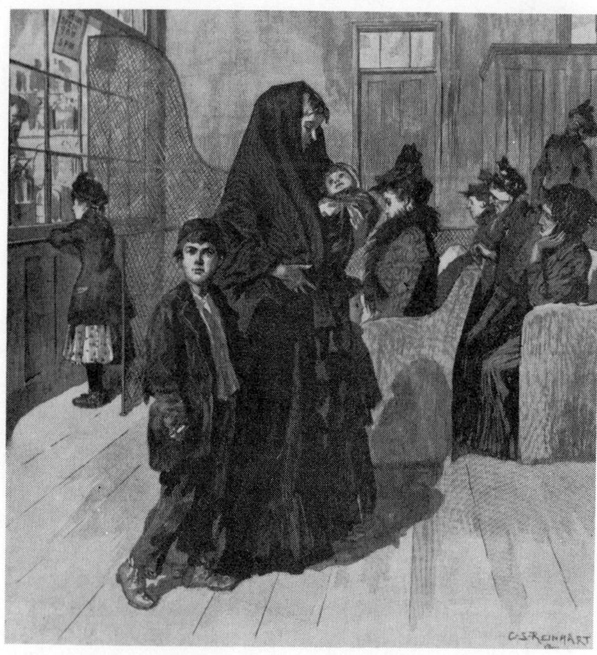

Figure 12–8. A public dispensary in the 1890s. (Dolan collection.)

disease and improving environmental sanitation. Many civic improvement groups attempted to solve these problems. *The Association for Improving the Condition of the Poor,* as well as the *State Charities Aid Association,* emphasized the dangers in tenement dwellings of overcrowding, poor ventilation, inadequate water supply and absence of decent privies. As a result of their efforts, the sanitary police force was increased, and by 1887, the New York Health Department was required by law to inspect tenement dwellings twice a year.

Public dispensaries were available for medical care of the poor (Fig. 12–8). The need for well-prepared nurses to teach and care for people in homes, outpatient facilities and clinics, as well as assist in a dynamic program of prevention of disease, was obvious.

The microorganism, the tubercle bacillus, that caused the disease was identified about 1882 by Dr. Robert Koch. In the 1870s and again in the early 1900s, *tuberculosis* was among the leading causes of death. It was determined that this infection was transmissible through contact with an infected person, as well as through drinking milk from diseased cattle. A tuberculosis control program was initiated; it included hospital facilities to isolate and care for victims of this disease, tuberculin tests for cattle, regular inspections of milk and meat supplies and mandatory reporting of cases.

Patients were admitted to such psychologically depressing institutions as the *Hospital for Incurables* (Fig. 12–9). The importance of healthful surroundings was pointed

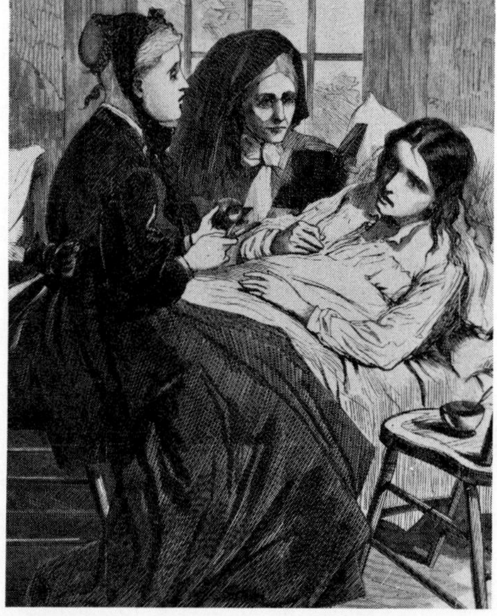

Figure 12–9. A patient and her visitors at the Hospital for Incurables on Blackwell's Island. (Dolan collection.)

out by Dr. Edward L. Trudeau, who was stricken with tuberculosis in 1872 while nursing his brother. He had been taught as a medical student that tuberculosis "was a noncontagious, generally incurable and inherited disease, due to inherited constitutional peculiarities, perverted humours and various types of inflammation." Opium and opium derivatives were often taken to soothe the effects of the disease. Trudeau, fearing an early death, retired to the Adirondack Mountains where many with tuberculosis went. He was surprised to discover a lack of suitable living arrangements for patients of moderate means. In 1885, he established the Adirondack Cottage Sanatorium, later known as the *Trudeau Sanatorium,* in which the importance of rest, sunshine, fresh air and nutrition was emphasized.

The widespread acceptance of the inevitability of tuberculosis, often referred to as the white plague or galloping consumption, is reflected in several operas of the period, such as Verdi's *La Traviata* and Puccini's *La Bohème.* The association of this disease with celebrities of the century is discussed in Waksman's book,[2] in which a special chapter is devoted to the victims of tuberculosis in literature and the arts. Among the victims of tuberculosis were Keats, Shelley, Robert Louis Stevenson, Goethe, Schiller, Washington Irving, Elizabeth Barrett Browning, Chopin and Chekhov. Edgar Allen Poe described the effects of tuberculosis, which he had observed firsthand in his family. Ralph Waldo Emerson and the Brontës also described the disease.[3] There are presentations of the disease in *Nicholas Nickleby, David Copperfield* and *Wuthering Heights.*

There was clearly a need for good nursing care for tuberculosis patients and their families.

PUBLIC HEALTH NURSING

In Liverpool, England, in 1859, after a lengthy illness, the wife of *William Rathbone* died. Mrs. Rathbone had had all the comforts that wealth and affection could provide. In his grief, Mr. Rathbone pondered the predicament of the poor families bereft of money and comfortable surroundings who might be faced with long-term sickness. He asked Mrs. Mary Robinson, the nurse who had been such a comfort to his wife and family, to try an experiment for three months. Supplied with the necessary appliances for usual bedside care as well as medicines and nourishing foods, she was to give nursing care and comfort to poor patients. Included in her assignment was the responsibility to teach families to improve their standard of living. The conditions Mrs. Robinson found in the homes of

[2]Waksman, Selman A.: *The Conquest of Tuberculosis.* Berkeley and Los Angeles, University of California Press, 1964.

[3]Hobson, W.: *World Health and History.* Bristol, John Wright & Sons, 1963, Chapter X.

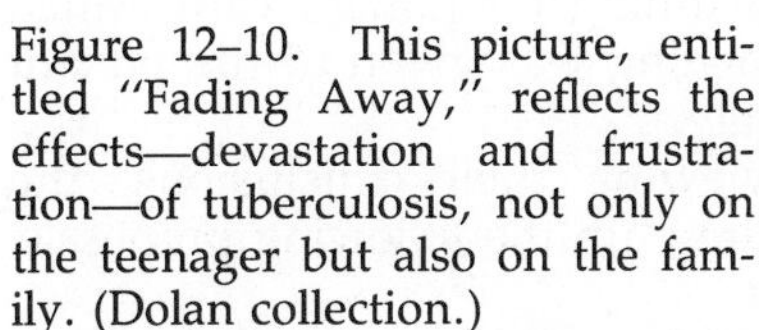

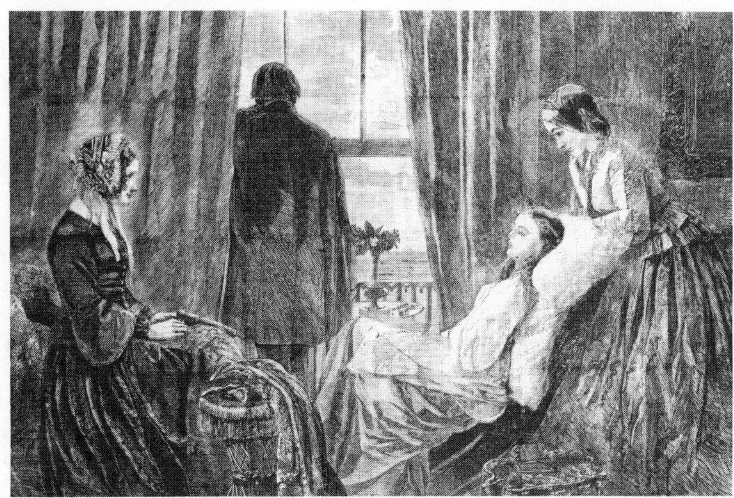

Figure 12–10. This picture, entitled "Fading Away," reflects the effects—devastation and frustration—of tuberculosis, not only on the teenager but also on the family. (Dolan collection.)

the poor were worse than anything she could have imagined, and in despair she returned after one month to Mr. Rathbone to resign from her assigment. After much persuasion on his part, she returned to the poor families to continue her project.

Mr. Rathbone believed in the value of personal service in relieving the needs of the poor. He convinced the Liverpool Relief Society to adopt a system of dividing towns into districts and districts into sections. To each district a committee of "Friendly Visitors" was assigned. Initial inquiries were conducted with tact and kindness by paid agents and then the case was turned over to the care of the friendly visitor of that section.

Mr. Rathbone's book, *Social Organization of Effort in Works of Benevolence and Public Charity by a Man of Business,* presented his beliefs and suggestions for social welfare. He was convinced of the need and value of district nursing. He believed that many persons with long-term illnesses would not be admitted to a general hospital, that many patients preferred to stay at home with their loved ones, that there were not enough hospitals available to meet the demands made upon them and that the cost of patient care was far less when the patient stayed at home. These were urgent reasons for developing district nursing.

Mr. Rathbone consulted Florence Nightingale, who encouraged him to organize a training school for nurses in the Liverpool Royal Infirmary. This training school would have the dual benefits of improving the nursing care within the hospital and of providing nurses for the sick of the community. Mr. Rathbone had a home constructed for nurses, which he presented to the Royal Infirmary; this gift solved a housing problem. In 1862, the *Training School and Home for Nurses of the Royal Infirmary* began a program to provide hospital nurses, private duty nurses and district nurses.

In 1865, in the town of Derby in England, a trained nurse was made Lady Superintendent in charge of all district nursing units to supervise the quality of the nursing care they gave.

An interesting project developed in relation to *Mrs. Ranyard's Bible and Domestic Mission,* which Mrs. Ranyard had organized in 1857. The Bible women visited the poor to read to them and pray with them. These eager women recognized the requirement of being prepared to minister to ever-present physical as well as spiritual needs. Finally, in 1868, the nurses' branch of the mission was established in London. Proper preparation as a Bible woman was followed by three months' training in the medical and surgical wards of the hospital, plus a month's training in obstetrics. No classes seem to have been given; mere presence in the hospital setting seemed all the preparation that was available. Caring for patients with contagious diseases was not permitted because of the danger of spreading infection.

In 1874, a committee was established in London called *The National Association for Providing Trained Nurses for the Sick Poor.* The objectives of this group were to increase the quantity and improve the quality of nursing care. The committee developed a logical plan for obtaining these objectives by determining what nurses were available, what preparation was needed and how other groups had handled these problems. *Miss Lees,* a pupil of Florence Nightingale, was placed in charge of the investigation. Seven hundred to 800 letters were sent to clergymen and medical officers in London. Data revealed a great need for nurses, but personal interviews showed that district nurses had poor preparation, if any. The data also showed the ways in which nurses carried infection from one house to another.

The conclusions of this committee were: There was need for more district nurses. Hospital nurses' training schools should provide preparation for care of the sick in their homes. Under the prevailing system there was too much emphasis on distribution of alms and too little on giving nursing care. Nurses needed to be given guidance, direction and supervision. There was too little consultation between nurses and physicians in planning for patient care. Much too little teaching was given to the patient and his family.

After reviewing their conclusions, the committee drew up the following proposals:

1. An independent training school should be established in close proximity to a hospital, as Miss Nightingale's school was to St. Thomas' Hospital. The school should be under the control of its own trustees of the school.
2. Close to the hospital should be a dis-

trict home where four to six nurses could live with a superintendent (supervisor). After the year's training in the hospital, a three months' apprenticeship should be given in district nursing.

3. Payment should be obtained for the nursing service, but only if the patient could afford to pay. This would permit many patients to receive care who were in need of as well as deserving of this service.

4. In case the previous suggestions were not acceptable or feasible, a superintendent could be appointed to manage a less elaborate but essentially identical program without developing the special training school.

This remarkable report was published in 1875 and received favorable attention from the public. The fourth suggestion was adopted, and Miss Lees was appointed superintendent. Many gentlewomen were recruited to provide nursing for the sick poor because it was Miss Lees' belief that this type of nursing required the highest caliber of women, who were well educated, to provide the actual nursing care and to teach health care to the patients. This organized effort was called *the Metropolitan and National Nursing Association for Providing Trained Nurses for the Sick Poor.*

The uniform adopted and worn by the Metropolitan Nurses was a dress of brown trimmed with dark blue linen, with a large apron and oversleeves of the same material to be worn when on duty. The outdoor uniform consisted of a dark blue cloak or blue alpaca in summer. A black straw bonnet, trimmed with black silk and piped with pale blue silk, lined with white muslin with a stiffly crimped muslin border and wide white muslin strings, completed the uniform. At that time, bonnets were worn when the nurses were on duty. A leather bag pinned to the uniform contained pin cushion, scissors and dressing forceps. Each nurse carried a small leather handbag, containing disinfectants, hand towel, soap and surgical dressings.

The training of these nurses was the important function of this association. Miss Lees selected applicants with care, and they remained in the central office for one month under observation as they accompanied a more experienced nurse on calls. If these applicants were considered suitable, they went into the hospital to serve for one year and then returned to the central office for a six months' course in district nursing under the guidance of the superintendent (supervisor), who went with the trainees on each new case, teaching them how to care for each patient. This appears to have been a good use of the apprenticeship system. Special classes were given in anatomy, physiology, hygiene, diseases of women and ways of peptonizing foods. Applicants had to pass examinations after the completion of the classes.

This experiment proved successful. The benefits of better educational methods, along with greater individual intellectual capacity, were pointed out by Miss Lees (then Mrs. Dacre Craven) in her address given at the World's Fair in Chicago:

> District nurses should feel themselves beyond and before all things, the servants of the sick poor. They instruct—but practically and by example. District nursing means, the care of the sick poor in their own homes, where there are no proper appliances, and where the nurse can rarely see the doctor,—in some cases, not at all. She must know how to put the room of each patient into such good sanitary condition that the patient may have a fair chance of recovery, and how to extemporize hospital appliances where these are required. She must be so well trained in nursing duties as not only to know how to observe and report correctly on every case under her charge, but to allow no change to pass unnoticed; and to be able to apply, provisionally, suitable treatment, until the medical man shall have arrived. She must know how to purify the foul air of the room without making a draught; to dust without making a dust; to ice drinks without ice; to filter water without a filter; to bake without an oven. . . . She must be content to be servant and teacher by turns. . . . A district nurse must have a real love for the poor and a real desire to lessen the misery she may see among them; and such tact as well as skill that she will do what is best for her patients even against their will. No district nurse should ever give alms or relief of any kind, beyond the highest of all—that of nursing service. . . . A nurse's business is to nurse—but she has also to teach the poor those sanitary laws which are household words with the well-to-do.[4]

Thus, important groundwork for the development of community nursing had been laid. Another opportunity for community nursing was presented when *Queen Victoria*

[4]Proceedings of the International Congress of Nurses, 1893.

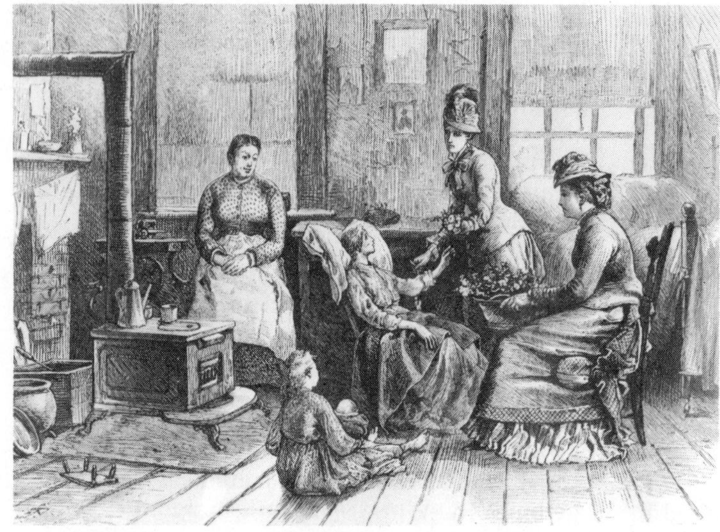

Figure 12–11. Members of the Flower Mission visiting the sick. (Dolan collection.)

celebrated the fiftieth anniversary of her reign as Queen. Of the 76,000 pounds raised by the women of England, 70,000 pounds were used to establish the *Institute for the Training and Supervising of District Nurses.* Properly qualified nursing associations already in existence were given an opportunity to affiliate with this institute, and a form for affiliation was devised. This consolidation was proposed to upgrade and standardize the community nursing service.

In 1889, the *Queen Victoria Jubilee Institute for Nurses* was founded by royal charter. This institute was connected with the historically famous St. Katherine's Hospital, founded by Queen Matilda in 1148. This group of nurses was called "Jubilee Institute Nurses" but became known as the *"Queen's Nurses."*

The plan for preparation of these nurses resembled the one developed by Miss Lees. The program ranged from four to 18 months in length, according to the background of the individual, and was given at the Maternity Charity and District Nurses' Home. This type of preparation provided trained nurses and midwives. In addition to this plan, there was special training available for those who would work in rural areas.

In the United States, after the War of 1812 left wives and children without many breadwinners and after the devastation and death wrought by the epidemics of yellow fever, a *Ladies' Benevolent Society* was organized for the relief of persons suffering from anguish, sickness and poverty. Cases were investigated, and relief was given in proportion to needs. Work was provided for the unemployed.

By 1832, Dr. Joseph Warrington had organized the society of *Lying-in Charity for Attending Indigent Women in Their Homes.* This group instructed prudent women to be nurses.

By 1877, the *Woman's Board of the New York City Mission* recognized that the need was as great for nurses to go into the homes of the poor to care for physical needs as it was for their missionary members to care for spiritual needs. These nurses received their training at Bellevue.

In 1886, *Visiting Nurse Society of Philadelphia* employed nurses to care for the sick in their homes. The service was extended to persons of moderate means who paid the society, as well as to the poor to whom the care was given free. A uniform was adopted in 1887, and in 1891, Miss Linda Richards assumed charge of the Visiting Nurse Society of Philadelphia.

In 1886, the *Instructive District Nursing Association* was founded in Boston, Massachusetts. Teaching was an important aspect of the home care of the sick, and the principles of hygiene and sanitation as well as health subjects and aspects of illness were taught. The Instructive District Nursing Association was the first to recognize the educational opportunities in visiting nursing. Brainard writes:

It was a fortunate thing that the first District Nursing Association in America should have laid such stress on the educational side of the work, and as proof that their attitude was accepted by America as the right and proper one, we may cite the words of Isabel Hampton (the late Mrs. Robb) who five years later in an address to the International Congress of Nurses (1893) said: "In District Nursing we are confronted with conditions which require the highest order of work, but the actual nursing of the patient is the least part of what her work and influence should be among the class which the nurse will meet with. To this branch of nursing no more appropriate name can be given than 'Instructive Nursing,' for educational in the best sense of the word it should be."[5]

The *Chicago Visiting Nursing Association,* established in 1889, was another early agency. A white Maltese cross was sewn on the sleeve of the uniform of each nurse member of this agency. Miss Edna Foley, a graduate of Hartford Hospital, was one of the early superintendents of this public health nursing agency. She was the author of the *Visiting Nurse Manual* and president of the National Organization for Public Health Nursing from 1920 to 1921.

Another pioneering endeavor was the course in public health nursing given by the *University of Michigan* to provide instruction for students who were engaged in field work with the Detroit Department of Health as well as for those with the Visiting Nurse Service.

Lillian D. Wald (1867–1940), who graduated from the New York Hospital Training School for Nurses in 1891, was shocked by the neglect of a critically ill woman who lived in a tenement. Miss Wald conceived the idea of establishing a neighborhood nursing service for the sick poor of the lower East Side in New York City (Fig. 12–12). She was fortunate in interesting two prominent and wealthy lay persons, Mrs. Solomon Loeb and Jacob H. Schiff, in her plan, and she had the encouragement and support of a nursing classmate, *Mary Brewster.*

Duffus[6] entitled his biography of Lillian

[5]Brainard, Annie M.: *The Evolution of Public Health Nursing.* Philadelphia, W. B. Saunders Co., 1922, p. 208.

[6]Duffus, R. L.: *Lillian Wald, Neighbor and Crusader.* New York, The Macmillan Co., 1938.

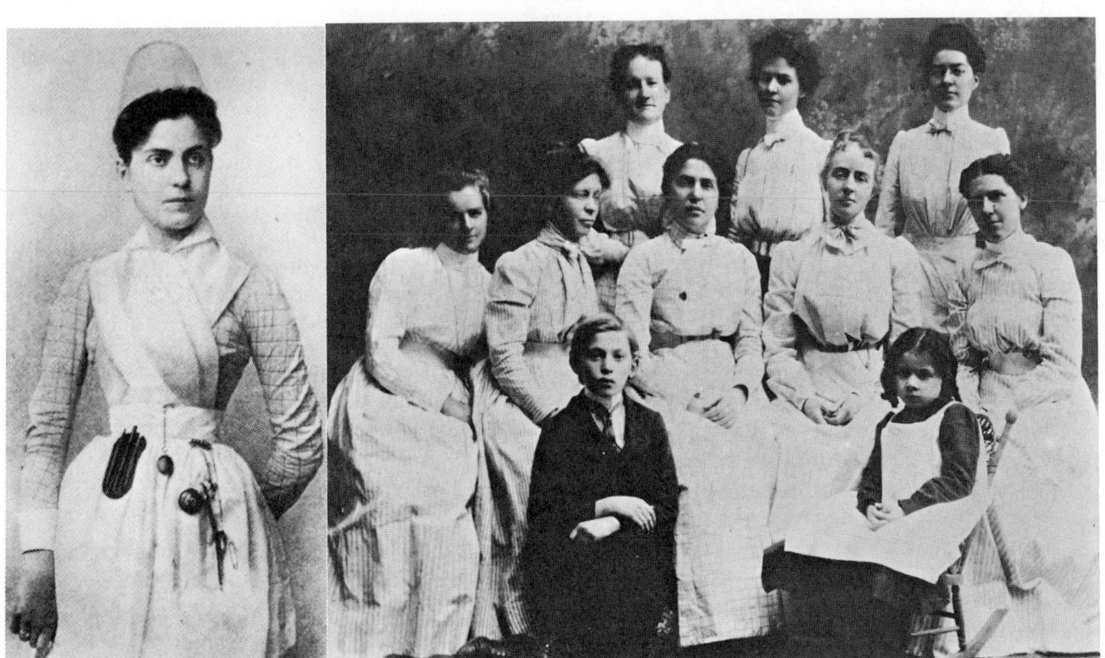

Figure 12–12. *Left,* Lillian Wald in her student uniform. In the early years of the Visiting Nurse Service, the nurses wore the uniform of the school from which they were graduated. *Right,* Lillian Wald and her staff. She is seated in the middle of the second row with Lavinia Dock to her right. (Courtesy of the Visiting Nurse Service of New York.)

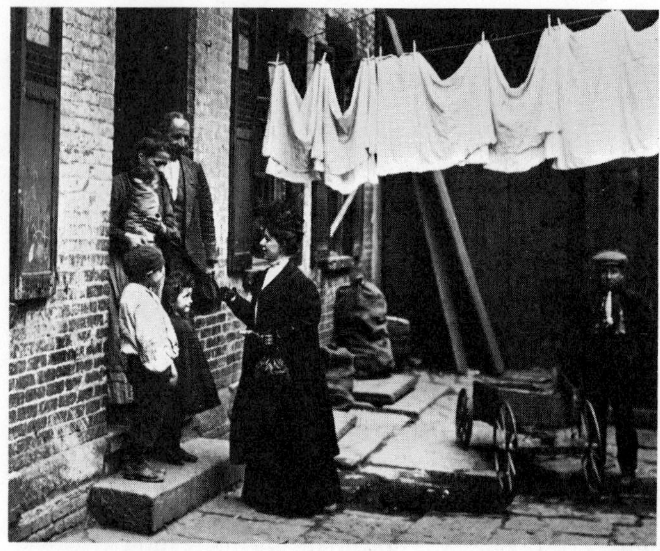

Figure 12–13. A nurse from the New York City Department of Health instructing tenement dwellers about health and sanitation in 1895. (Courtesy of New York City Department of Health.)

Wald *Neighbor and Crusader*, and this title was apt, for neighborliness was her motivating thought and approach as she carried on her intensive crusade of assistance to the less fortunate. Her concept was that the nurse's visit should be like that of a very interested friend rather than that of an impersonal, paid visitor. The experiment was a success, and the world-famous *Henry Street Settlement* was opened in 1893 on the top floor of a house purchased by Mr. Schiff. Here both nurses and social workers were added to the staff. In due time, in addition to the nursing service, there was an organized program of social and educational activities. It became a *generalized social settlement project*.

As nursing in general, and community nursing in particular, enlarged its range of duties and opportunities, more nurses with special assignments and preparation were needed. Nurses were specializing in maternity care, in infant welfare and in tuberculosis work. Gradually, there came to be an overlapping of functions, with several nurses working in the same household at the same time; this was a most disturbing situation for everyone, including the perplexed family. Eventually, a plan was developed for all nursing to be of a general nature with special instruction in the care of patients to be given by supervisors who had specialized preparation and who acted as resource persons.

There have been *public health nurses* in Canada from about 1885. Their work became highly developed under the *Victorian Order of Nurses for Canada* and was for some years considered superior to almost any other in the world. The Victorian Order was founded in 1897 by Lady Aberdeen. It was named in honor of Queen Victoria, who celebrated her Diamond Jubilee in that year.

> The Victorian Order nurses go into the simple homes in the little fishing villages in Nova Scotia and Cape Breton; into the workingman's cottages in the larger towns; into the tenements in the cruel slums of our larger cities; into the schools, the milk stations, the homes where tuberculosis holds its victims; into the little hospitals, away up in the mining towns or out on the beautiful prairies; out into the ranches in the ever lovely foothill region, where they become the country nurses; or into the tiny hospitals in the mountains, and away out to the Pacific coast branches. The Victorian Order nurse seems to fit into her particular corner as if she had been there all her life and it was good to be there. The committees, with hardly an exception, work as though their existence depended on the results, throwing all their energies into the service and loving their work.

The Victorian Order has worked mainly in three areas: public health nursing, chiefly in cities; hospital nursing for small hospitals in outlying and thinly populated districts; for the Lady Minto Cottage Hospital Fund; and visiting nursing in Canada's many sparsely settled places, including work among the Indians, for the Lady

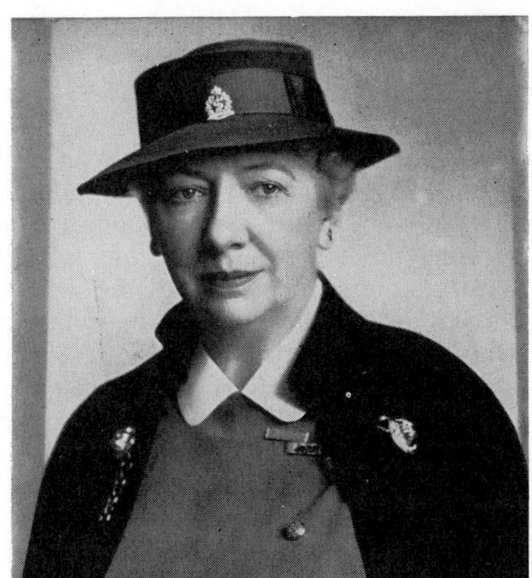

Figure 12–14. Lieut. Col. E. L. Smellie, formerly Matron-in-Chief, Royal Canadian Army Medical Corps. (Courtesy of *The Canadian Nurse.*)

Grey Country District Nursing Scheme. The order has always had much lay interest and support.

Elizabeth Smellie (Fig. 12–14), member of the original Victoria Order of Nurses' committee, was head of the order for many years and organized the Canadian Women's Army Corps during World War II.

INFANT WELFARE

Marked progress had been noted in interest in the welfare of infants and contributions toward their care (Fig. 12–15). The *Crèche,* a type of day nursery for the care of poor babies, was established through the efforts of the Mayor of Paris in 1844.

During the later years of the nineteenth century, it was realized that one of the major causes of the high infant mortality rate was the milk used in the feeding of infants. It was essential to obtain a supply of pure cow's milk. In 1889, two milk distribution centers were constructed, one in New York City and one in Germany. The objective was to provide clean milk for poor sick babies. This project was of relatively little value because once the child became well impure milk was again used, and sickness returned.

BACTERIOLOGY, PREVENTIVE MEDICINE AND ASEPTIC SURGERY

It was *Louis Pasteur* (1822–1895), the great French chemist, who finally disposed of the long-accepted theory of spontaneous

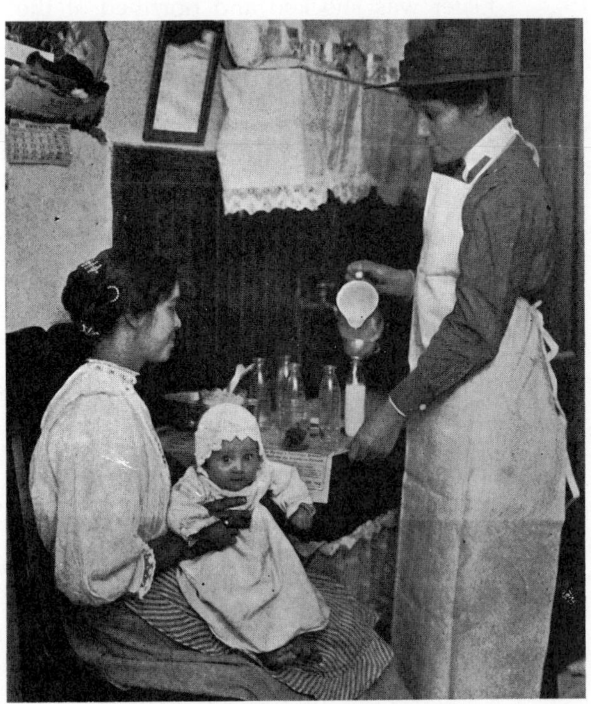

Figure 12–15. The baby welfare nurse. (From Brainard, Annie M.: *The Evolution of Public Health Nursing.* Philadelphia, W. B. Saunders Co., 1922.)

generation, or abiogenesis. In 1860, Pasteur confirmed the presence of airborne bacteria. He found that living ferments abounded on many objects and in water. He experimented with heating flasks of broth, expelling the air in the process, and demonstrated that no growths of bacteria appeared. Thus, his experiments proved that bacteria could be killed by heat. Pasteur also discovered that *anthrax* was caused by bacteria. He devised a vaccine that, when inoculated into animals, protected them against the disease. Pasteur's last and perhaps greatest accomplishment was his study of *rabies* in 1880. His efforts resulted in the development of a method of vaccinating dogs[7] and, thus, immunizing them against rabies. The fact that the cause of the disease had not been established was a serious disadvantage; nevertheless, he produced the well-known *Pasteur treatment for rabies*.

Joseph Lister (1827–1912) was the first to apply Pasteur's discoveries to the field of surgery. The conditions existing in the hospitals at this time were terrible. Surgical patients and those admitted with injuries, as well as obstetric patients, were exposed to severe infections, such as blood poisoning (septicemia), erysipelas, puerperal fever, tetanus and "hospital gangrene."

Lister was shocked and horrified at the contagious nature of infection associated with open wounds and with the appallingly high death rate that followed such infection. He dedicated himself to the duty of investigating and then correcting methods of surgery, as well as dissipating the obnoxious odor of the wards, which was partly due to poor ventilation.

He observed the swiftness of the surgeon, who operated amid the screams of his unanesthetized patient; then he watched for the inevitable signs of infection, which seemed localized in the hospital wards. With the availability of anesthesia, many more surgical operations were performed and the amount of infection increased. The surgeons talked freely about the formation of "laudable pus." Lister believed that infection must be due to the surgeon, his instruments, his assistants and his methods of carrying out technique. He had studied the work of Pasteur and immediately applied the germ theory of disease to his surgical procedures. He looked for some method of keeping germs out of wounds and decided upon the use of carbolic acid. In 1865, Lister used carbolic acid (phenol) successfully in treating a compound fracture. He disinfected his instruments with it, saturated the surgical dressing with it and sprayed the solution into the air above the incision during the operation. His success in preventing infection increased as his methods and techniques improved. Lister's contributions added chemicals to the armamentarium against bacteria. Aseptic surgical technique has now replaced Lister's technique, and hospitals are no longer places of stench, horror and death.

Robert Koch (1843–1910) was the brilliant German physician who proved that every infectious disease was caused by a specific microorganism. Thus was laid the foundation for the science of bacteriology. Koch proposed four "postulates" by which a specific organism could be proved to cause a certain disease:

1. Obtain a specific organism from blood or tissue of a diseased person.
2. Make a pure culture of this organism.
3. Produce the disease condition in another person or animal by inoculation with material from the pure culture.
4. Procure the same specific organism from the now-diseased second person or animal.

His contributions included a method for growing or culturing microorganisms; a system of staining microbes with different colored dyes so that they could be seen and photographed with the microscope; and the detection and identification of the specific causative organisms of several diseases, such as the anthrax bacillus and the tubercle bacillus. In addition to identifying the bacillus of Asiatic cholera, Koch proved that this disease spreads by way of water, food and clothing.

Now the solution to the perplexing and mysterious problem of what causes disease (formerly thought to be such things as evil influences, dėmons, the night air) was found to be the existence of these invisible causative organisms called microbes.

As spontaneously as fire spreads through

[7]It has since been realized that many other animals can transmit rabies.

dry timber, one scientific investigation of bacteria led to another. Many specific organisms were identified, and there was hope that vaccines or medications for treatment and prevention of disease would be forthcoming.

In 1872, *Ferdinand Cohn,* who first classified bacteria as plants, published the first modern classification of bacteria.

In 1874, *Armauer Hansen,* of Bergen, Norway, isolated the lepra bacillus. Leprosy is now called *Hansen's disease* after him.

The discoveries of bacteria continued in rapid succession throughout the rest of the nineteenth century.

Ernst von Behring (1854–1917) was a Prussion doctor who, in the later part of the nineteenth century, spent some time at Koch's Institute for Infectious Diseases. His studies there resulted in the introduction of a new method of disease prevention—that of using serum from immunized animals. In 1892, he produced diphtheria antitoxin, and later that year he prepared tetanus antitoxin.

On Christmas night in 1891, von Behring successfully treated a child suffering from diphtheria, using diphtheria antitoxin.

Another theory that needed to be exploded was the still popular humoral theory. It was examined scientifically by the great German pathologist *Rudolf Virchow* (1821–1902). He proposed in 1855 that the basic unit of life was the cell, that cells change in response to internal as well as external stimulus or irritation and that changes in cellular structure result in pathological conditions.

The field of *psychiatry* benefited from the efforts of members of several generations of the Tuke family of England; the field seems to have been a family undertaking. William Tuke was a devout member of the Society of Friends, more commonly known as Quakers. He was opposed to brutality in any form. After he visited several hospitals, including Bedlam, and observed the inhumane treatment given to these unfortunate creatures (Fig. 12–16), his abhorrence extended to the cruel methods used in the care of the mentally ill.

Through the efforts of William Tuke and his son and daughter-in-law, money was raised to establish a home where these patients could be treated as human beings. The home, called *The Retreat,* seemed well named because it was a place of security, a haven during a stormy period of life. An additional advantage of the home was that good care was provided inexpensively. The construction of the building was unique because in place of barred windows, it had window frames made of steel that looked like wood. The building itself had a homey, comfortable appearance, in a setting of trees. The interior atmosphere was as conducive to convalescence as the exterior.

William's grandson Samuel continued

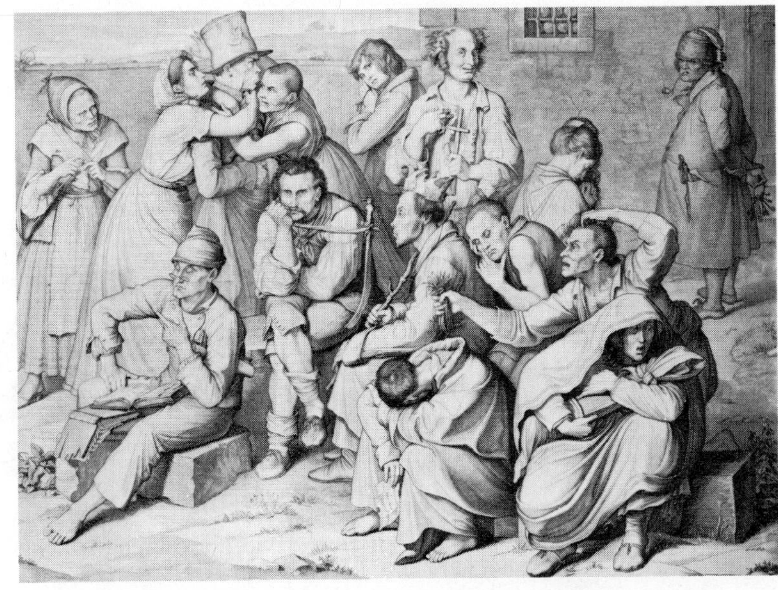

Figure 12–16. The Madhouse, by Wilhelm Kaulbach. (Courtesy of Philadelphia Museum of Art.)

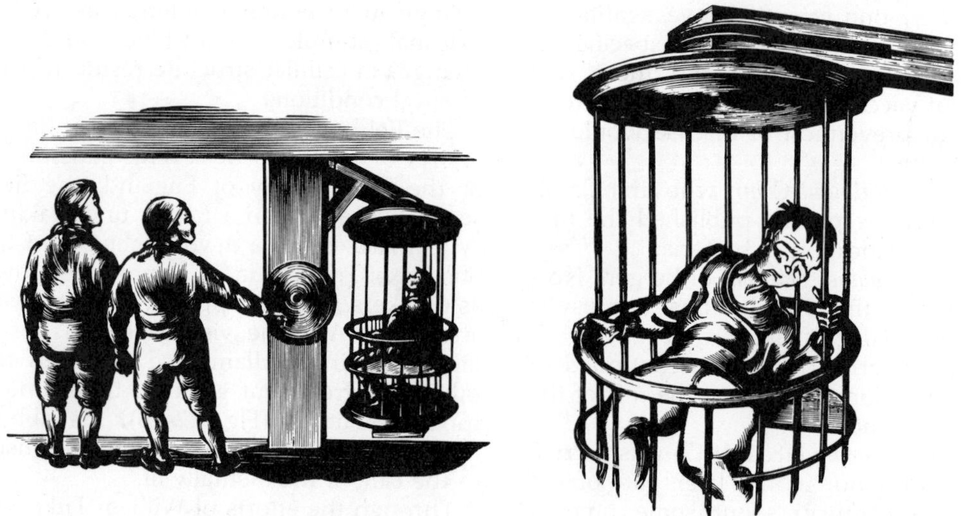

Figure 12–17. A whirling cage—an early device for calming psychiatric patients. (Courtesy of Smith Kline & French Laboratories.)

the fight for better care of the mentally ill. In 1854, he described the disgraceful conditions of the York Insane Asylum and Bedlam. The directors seem to have labored under the impression that these patients were devoid of feelings, because some of the patients were chained in a sitting position; others were placed in a squatting position; many of them were nude; and all of them were cold, even to the point of freezing; and the lack of sanitary facilities made the total environment unbearable. Solitary confinement of the patient in a chamber of horrors and occasional floggings were used as disciplinary measures along with other fear techniques, (Figs. 12–17 to 12–20).

William Tuke's great-grandson Daniel also continued the fight for the better treatment of the mentally ill. He became a physician and eventually one of England's most celebrated psychiatrists. He gave courses in psychology, maintained a private practice and was chief psychiatrist at the York Retreat. Tuberculosis interrupted his work, and he had to seek a climate

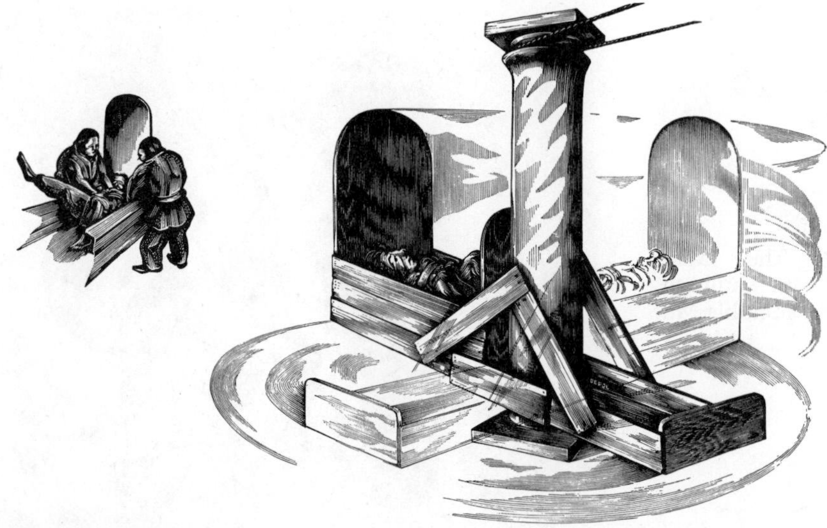

Figure 12–18. The revolving bed—an early device for calming patients with mental illness. (Courtesy of Smith Kline & French Laboratories.)

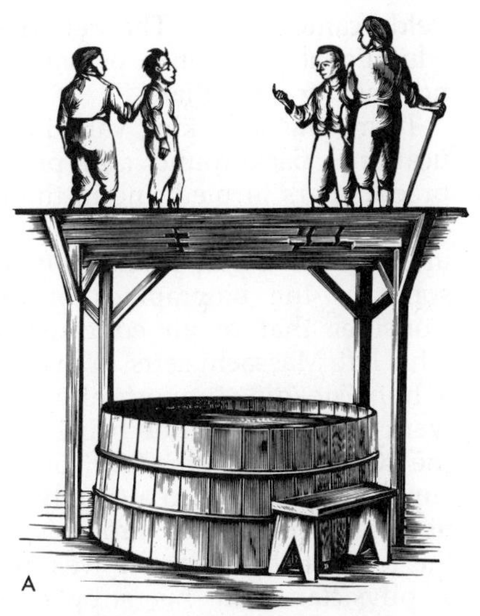

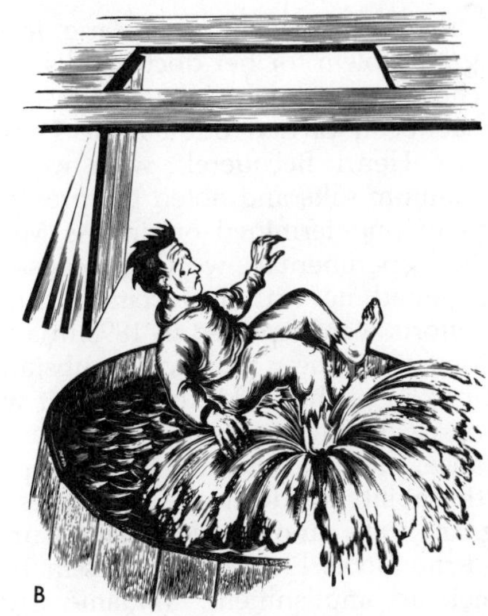

Figure 12–19. *(A)* Enticing the patient to an early form of shock therapy. *(B)* The resulting shock therapy. (Courtesy of Smith Kline & French Laboratories.)

more conducive to cure. Among his writings are *A Manual of Psychological Medicine, History of the Insane in the British Isles, The Influence of the Mind upon the Body in Health and Disease* and his famous compilation *Dictionary of Psychological Medicine.*

DISCOVERY OF RADIUM AND X-RAYS

Two discoveries occurred at the close of the nineteenth century that were of tremendous significance to many aspects of society including the medical field.

The first was the discovery of the X-ray in 1895 by the German physicist *Wilhelm Roentgen* (1845–1922). In his capacity as a professor of physics and mathematics, he had been fascinated by the studies on radiation. He discovered the x-ray, this great gift to society, when in his laboratory. He found that these rays penetrate many things, including human flesh, but bones remain opaque. The photograph he took, which revealed the rays' powers, was scarcely believable even to him.

His news was eagerly received, and honors, including the Nobel Prize in Physics in 1901 and an honorary degree of Doctor of Medicine, were accorded Roentgen.

The application of x-rays to the field of medicine was at first only for diagnostic purposes. Later, however, its therapeutic uses were realized.

The second discovery, that of *radium* by *Pierre* and *Marie Sklodowska Curie,* came

Figure 12–20. Placing a disturbed patient in a revolving cage. (Courtesy of Smith Kline & French Laboratories.)

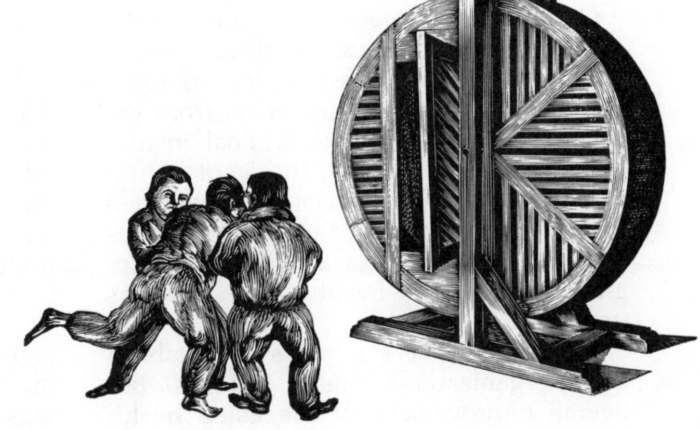

about in a most unusual way. Marie, in selecting a problem for her doctoral dissertation, chose to pursue further some research that had been carried out by the French physicist Henri Becquerel, who worked with uranium salts and noted the presence of rays of undetermined origin. As Marie Curie's experimental work progressed, Pierre joined her in this exciting study. Their efforts were reported in 1898 in a paper discussing a new radioactive substance contained in pitchblende, the ore that was the source of the uranium. The extracted substance, radium, has been found to possess the ability to destroy some types of malignant cells and tissues. The Curies shared the Nobel Prize for physics in 1903 for their accomplishment. Madame Curie received it again for chemistry in 1911; in 1906, her husband had been struck and killed by a motorist. They both made monumental contributions to society.

PROGRESS IN MEDICAL EDUCATION

There was an obvious need for a unifying force to weld the members of the allied health groups. The needs to discuss common problems, to share evidence of progress, to set standards for acceptable practice, to upgrade the educational background of the practitioner all played a part in the establishment of local and then national organizations.

In 1832, the British Medical Association was formed; in 1841, the Pharmaceutical Society of Great Britain was established; in 1847, the American Medical Association was founded; and in 1852, the American Pharmaceutical Association was created.

One of the first items of business of the newly formed American Medical Association was a resolution asking for the separation of the licensing functions from the teaching functions of educational institutions. Beginning in 1883, the *Journal of the American Medical Association* was published for the dissemination of information to its members. The process of intellectual upgrading in the health sciences was underway.

The fruition of the plans to establish these organizations was a triumph, but overall improvement of the allied health fields came slowly. The betterment of the educational preparation of practitioners was not easy or immediate.

There was a striking variation in the educational background and preparation of practitioners in medicine in the nineteenth century. Examples of the lack of uniformity in educational preparation can be found in some of the biographies of the period. Consider that of an educated gentleman who left Massachusetts to avail himself of a homesteading opportunity. In 1871, he went to Kansas, after being wounded in the Civil War. Needing pharmaceutical supplies, he wrote to a supply firm for the necessary medicines. Probably because of the tone of the letter, he was mistaken for a physician and his supplies were addressed to "Dr. Waugh." When they arrived at the small town railway office, the clerk noticed the address, paying particular attention to the gentleman's title. Immediately "Dr. Waugh" began to practice medicine, although under marked and voluble protest. When Kansas required doctors to be licensed, this gentleman, without instruction, formal or otherwise, was reputed to have been the only one to pass the medical examination in three counties.

The amount of medical education practitioners received ranged from no preparation in basic education or medicine to good preparation. The profession was going through a period of trial and error in determining what constituted adequate training. Students learned by becoming apprentices to physicians, by attending proprietary schools and, at last, by receiving instruction in the first schools under the sponsorship of universities. As early as 1848 the need for practical demonstration as well as clinical teaching for students of medicine was recognized.

In reviewing the accomplishments of the *Association of American Medical Colleges,* which was organized in 1890, one notes a recommendation of a minimum standard of high school graduation as the only prerequisite for the study of medicine! Conversely, Johns Hopkins University in 1893 made a bachelor's degree a prerequisite for admission to its medical school. This wide diversity in the background of physicians compelled the leaders in medicine to consider the establishment of some required standards for preliminary education.

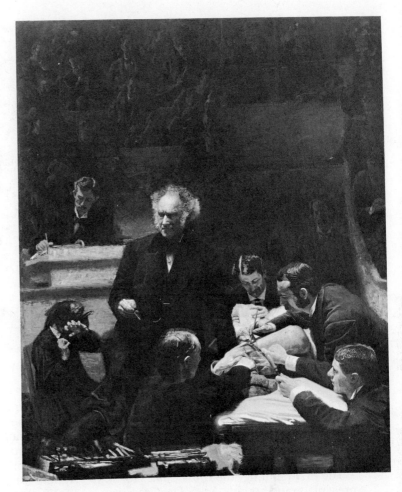

Figure 12–21. The Gross Clinic, by Thomas Eakins (1875). (Courtesy of Jefferson Medical College, Philadelphia.)

An outstanding *medical center* came into existence in Baltimore when Johns Hopkins University opened in 1876. Johns Hopkins Hospital was founded in 1889, and Johns Hopkins School of Medicine was established in 1893. The new school of medicine was a graduate school; the faculty felt that a sound liberal education was essential before the student attempted professional study.

In 1883, Rochester, Minnesota, became famous with the founding of Saint Mary's Hospital, the Mayo Clinic and Saint Mary's School of Nursing.

CONTRIBUTIONS IN HEALTH CARE

In this century many devices, including the hypodermic syringe, the cystoscope, the laryngoscope and the bronchoscope, were invented. These instruments were useful for diagnostic as well as therapeutic purposes. Many bacteria had been identified, and three ways of destroying bacteria—by heat, chemicals and vaccines—were determined. The closing years of the nineteenth century were filled with important discoveries and developments in bacteriology and parasitology. Among the most outstanding events were the demonstrations of the malarial parasite in the mosquito by Sir Ronald Ross, the use of serum against snake venom by Albert Calmette, the explanation of the side-chain theory by Paul Ehrlich, the use of ultraviolet light by Niels Finsen and the discovery that the mosquito transmits yellow fever by Walter Reed, James Carroll, Jesse Lazera, Aristides Agramonte and Carlos Finlay.

Thomas Eakins (1844–1916), a famous American painter, has left two paintings that show the remarkable progress made in

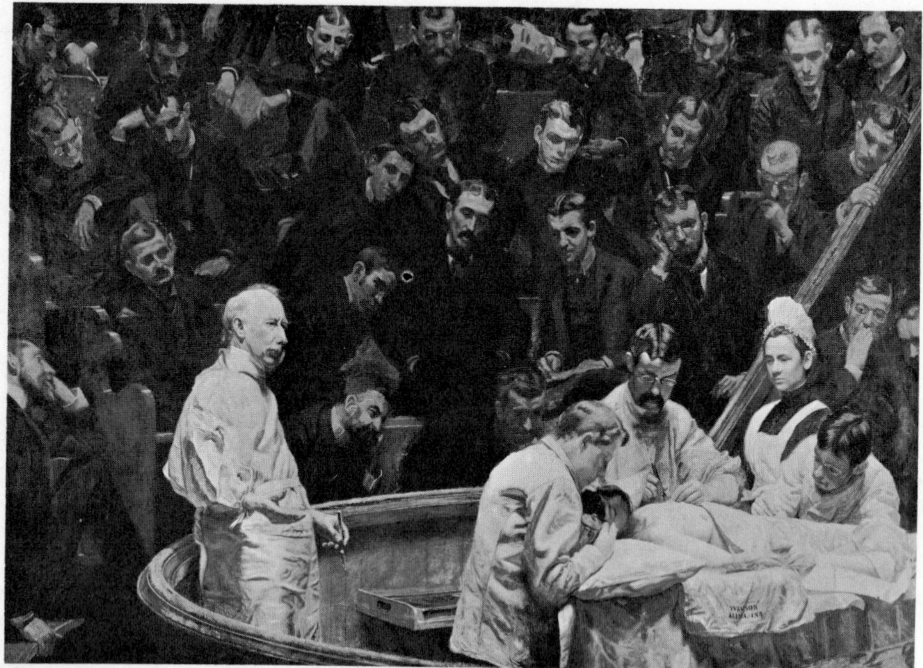

Figure 12–22. The Agnew Clinic, by Thomas Eakins (1898). (Courtesy of Philadelphia Museum of Art.)

the scientific basis of patient care in the last quarter of the nineteenth century. Creating a most unusual "before-and-after" effect, Eakins used the same amphitheater for the setting of each picture.

The first painting, the *Gross Clinic* (1875), presents grand rounds, with Dr. Gross explaining to medical students the surgical operation that is being performed (Fig. 12–21). He appears to be completely oblivious to the feelings of the patient and to the agonizing horror of the patient's mother, who sits to the doctor's right. The second picture, the *Agnew Clinic* (1898), shows Dr. Agnew presiding at grand rounds (Fig. 12–22). The setting for both pictures is presumably a surgical clinical amphitheater, the audience presumably medical students,

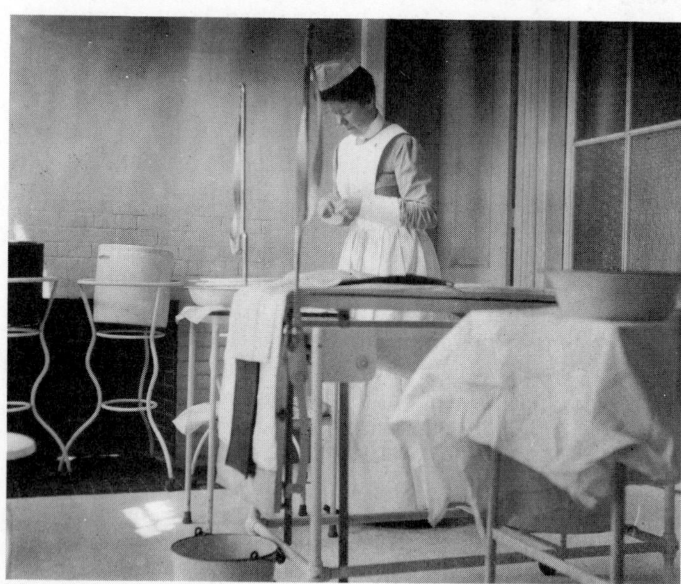

Figure 12–23. A student of nursing preparing an operating room for a surgical procedure.

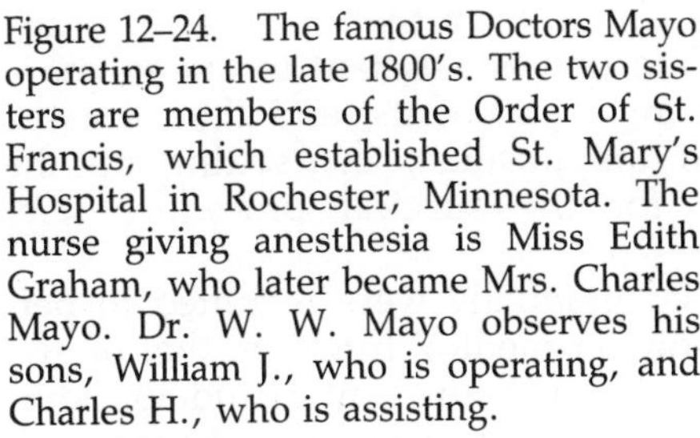

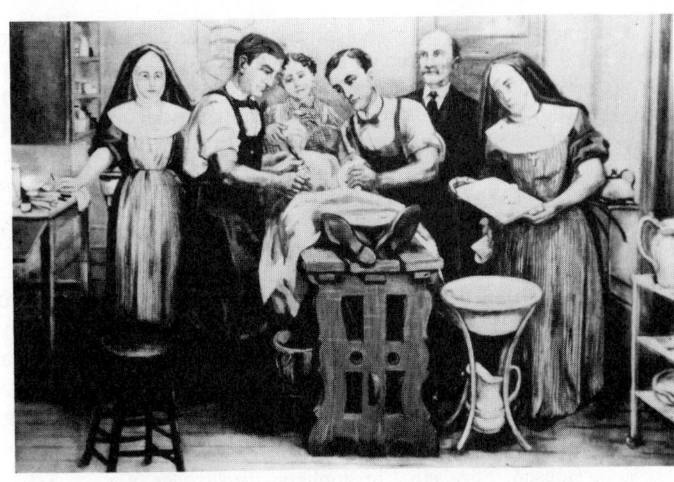

Figure 12–24. The famous Doctors Mayo operating in the late 1800's. The two sisters are members of the Order of St. Francis, which established St. Mary's Hospital in Rochester, Minnesota. The nurse giving anesthesia is Miss Edith Graham, who later became Mrs. Charles Mayo. Dr. W. W. Mayo observes his sons, William J., who is operating, and Charles H., who is assisting.

but the scene has definitely changed in the years from 1875 to 1898. The scientific investigations of Pasteur, Koch and Lister have resulted in many changes: the surgeons are aware of the necessity of shedding their street clothes and replacing them with white operating gowns; the instruments have been bathed in carbolic acid solution; the patient is covered; the anesthetist is giving ether (note the can of ether in his hand and the ether cone over the patient's nose and mouth); thus, the advantageous use of ether by Dr. Morton has been noted; and since schools of nursing had been opened, a nurse appears in the operating room but as assistant to the patient, not to the surgeons. This nurse's name was *Mary V. Clymer* and her diary-type notebook was discovered in November of 1961. School records reveal that at her graduation in 1889 she was awarded the Nightingale medal. Her instruction included cooking, and her diary records her ability to concoct such things as jellied soups, beef tea and arrowroot biscuits. The ingredients for poultices and good liniments are also presented. "A good nurse," she relates, "must be kind, firm, gentle, and possessing a good deal of magnetism. Never be curious. Be watchful but not officious. Unnecessary noise with tongue or coal scuttle is to be avoided."

A Mrs. Hobson tells how nurses began to attend in the operating rooms:

> Miss Euphemia Van Rensselaer, belonging to the distinguished family of that name, who is described as "very handsome," and with an air of distinction in her bearing [is the heroine]. It is recorded that female patients were taken to the amphitheatre for operations before all the [medical] students, unassisted and unprotected by the presence of a nurse. We felt that this could not be allowed from our wards, and I consulted a friendly surgeon, Dr. Crosby. He said he should be delighted to have a nurse *attend his patients*, but, he added: "Medical students are a rough lot, and they may make it unpleasant for the nurses." . . . Miss Van Rensselaer stepped into the breach. "I will go with the patient and take Miss B______ with me; I am not afraid." The day came and I went to the hospital to await the result. I saw the patient carried out, followed by [the] two nurses. It was an anxious moment. To have had those

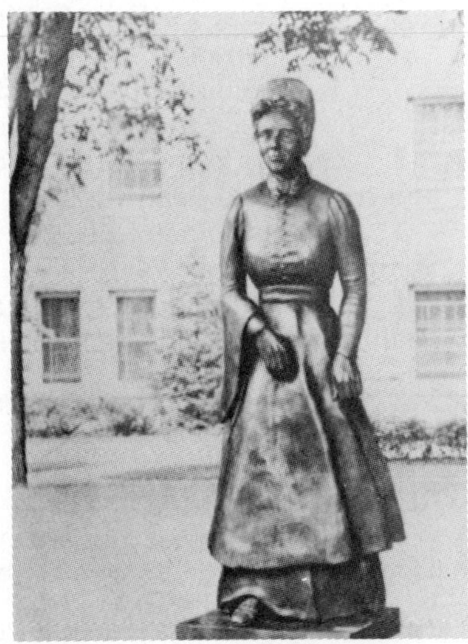

Figure 12–25. Statue of Edith Graham Mayo, Rochester's first trained nurse and Saint Mary's first nurse-teacher.

nurses insulted by jeers and howls, and perhaps forced to retire, would have been very serious, and it was quite possible. Nearly an hour passed; finally I heard the students thundering down the stairs. I waited anxiously until I could see Dr. Crosby, and rushed to meet him. His face beaming with smiles, he extended both hands: "Their presence was a benediction; I never had a more successful operation, and the students were as quiet as if they were in church," he exclaimed. Miss Van Rensselaer told me later that the theatre was crowded, and when they entered with the patient there was a faint murmur as if in surprise. It ceased and during the operation the order was absolute.[8]

[8]Hobson, Elizabeth Christophers: *Recollections of a Happy Life*. New York, G. P. Putnam's Sons, 1916.

Gradually the scene in the operating room changed. More operations were performed, and the role of the nurse in this setting shifted from that of assistant to the patient to that of assistant to the surgeon, in passing instruments, and that of assistant to the hospital, in "setting up the room" for the surgical procedure (Fig. 12–23).

Nurses gradually were recruited to perform another medical function, that of giving anesthesia. Many senior students, during operating room experience, began to be assigned the giving of ether to patients who were having their tonsils removed. This was the beginning of the role of nurse anesthetist (Fig. 12–24).

THE HERITAGE OF NURSING

The Influence of Social Welfare and Scientific Progress on the Image of the Nurse

Prepared nurses responded to the call for assistance in social crises and adapted to the changes in delivery of care resulting from the new scientific discoveries.

1. In times of social crisis, nurses responded to the acute needs of the poor.
    a. Clearly defined leadership was observed.
    b. Community Health nursing reemerged.
    c. A new role evolved for nurses in that the community health nurse participated in case-finding, health teaching and active cooperation with clients. Community nurses had much greater freedom of action. This role was in sharp contrast to that of the nurse in a hospital setting.
2. Leaders came forth to care for those with special health problems and to promote health-related legislation.
3. Nurses joined the war effort and won commendation during the Spanish-American War.
4. The foundation of the field of bacteriology had a significant effect on health care and laid the basis for procedure-centered delivery of care.

REFERENCE READINGS

Brace, Charles Loring: *Dangerous Classes of New York and Twenty Years' Work Among Them*. New York, Wynkoop, 1872.

Brainard, Anne W.: *The Evolution of Public Health Nursing*. Philadelphia, W. B. Saunders Co., 1922.

Burton, Katherine: *Sorrow Built a Bridge*. New York, Longmans, Green & Co., 1937.

Cunningham, John T.: *Clara Maass—A Nurse—A Hospital—A Spirit*. New Jersey, Rae Publishing Co., 1976.

Deutsch, Albert: *The Mentally Ill in America*, 2nd ed. New York, Columbia University Press, 1946.
Duffus, R. L.: *Lillian Wald, Neighbor and Crusader*. New York, The Macmillan Co., 1938.
Faxon, Nathaniel W.: *The Hospital in Contemporary Life*. Cambridge, Mass., Harvard University Press, 1949.
Hobson, W.: *World Health and History*. Bristol, John Wright & Sons, 1963.
Hughes, Sister Ann Elizabeth, Bertonneau, Sister Dorothea and Enna, Carl D.: "Nurses at Carville," *The American Journal of Nursing, 68*:(12) 1968.
Osler, Sir William: *Aequanimitas*. Philadelphia, Blakiston Co., 1932.
Pugh, Garrett F., and Fisher, A. J. B.: *Ethics and Health in Late Victorian Society*. London, Arundel, 1970.
Riis, Jacob: *How the Other Half Lives*. New York, The Macmillan Co., 1890.
Waksman, Selman A.: *The Conquest of Tuberculosis*. Berkeley and Los Angeles, University of California Press, 1964.
Wald, Lillian: *House on Henry Street*. New York, Henry Holt, 1915.
Wald, Lillian: *Windows on Henry Street*. Boston, Little, Brown & Co., 1934.

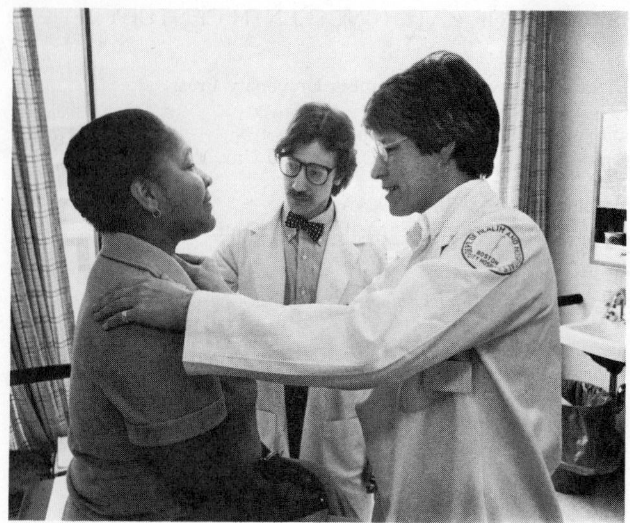

Jean Steel R.M.M.S., Assistant Professor of Nursing and Coordinator of Primary Care at Boston City Hospital, discussing a client's problem with internist Dr. Waltman, and thus functioning in an independent-interdependent role.

13 Scientific, Technological and Societal Movements of the Twentieth Century

Nursing has prospered in this century, which has seen the exploration of outer space, as well as the investigation of every area of the earth and of the human, the development of new sciences and the expansion of old ones and the fusion of many sciences—literally, an explosion of knowledge and technology. It has been said that much that was unknown has become known and much that was invisible has become visible.

The twentieth century has also witnessed a phenomenal improvement in the general standard of living, the lengthening of the span of life, the identification of the causes of many diseases, the ability to conquer most bacterial diseases and the provision for a scientific plan of care for the patient and his family. In the latter part of the century, social movements, such as the civil rights, student, consumer and women's movements, had a profound influence on the direction of health care. The preventive, rehabilitative as well as curative aspects of patient care have received increasing attention. The exigencies of wars, the marked progress in transportation and communication, the remarkable inventions and scientific achievements have had an influence on keeping individuals healthy, initiating changes in the care of the sick, expanding the health care field in general and refining nursing in particular. This century has encompassed the transition from candlelight to satellite, from the horse and buggy era to the space age. The struggle for freedom and independence of new nations, the trauma of international tensions and the threat to survival itself have all had a hand in writing current history.

PROGRESS IN TRANSPORTATION AND COMMUNICATION

The automobile and airplane and helicopter have created many occupational opportunities and have made it possible to bring medical assistance to a patient much

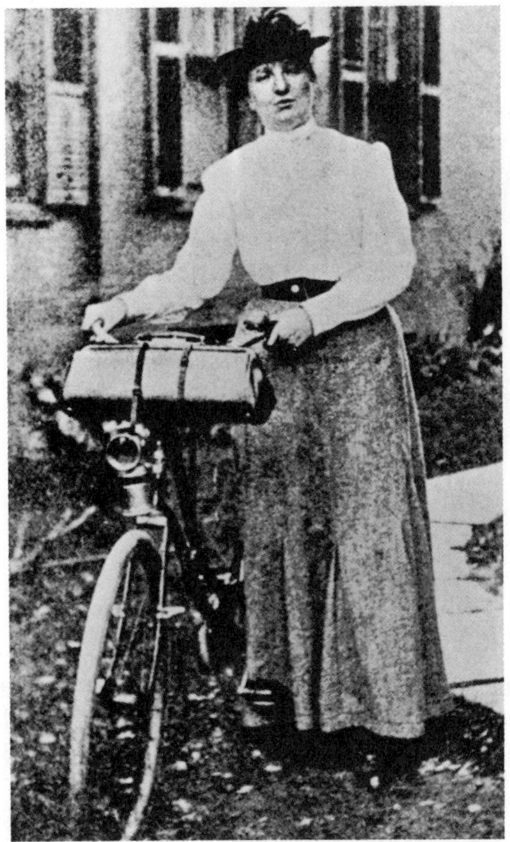

Figure 13–1. At the turn of the century, a public health nurse, Martha Wilkinson of Hartford, Connecticut, used the accepted mode of travel to make her rounds. The famous symbol of the public health nurse, the "black bag," contained broth and jellies in addition to health supplies. (Dolan collection.)

more quickly than ever before. The creation of different forms of travel has changed American life. Travel opportunities not only have broadened knowledge and provided recreational diversions but also have encouraged contact with new diseases and increased the accident rate.

Helicopters have proved of immeasurable value because of their high degree of maneuverability. Many patients whose lives might otherwise be lost because of improper care or delay are quickly flown great distances to medical centers. Additionally, the use of helicopers as miniature hospitals, serviced by professional teams, is an innovation in the delivery of care. Patient transport has changed dramatically since the nineteenth century (Figs. 13–3 and 13–4).

In the area of *communications,* the use of the computer has become widespread, as has that of the telephone, motion picture, radio and television. These technological advances have benefited the educational field and have helped to make the clients we serve more knowledgeable about health and illness than ever before.

PROGRESS IN SCIENCE RELATED TO HEALTH CARE

During the twentieth century there were many offshoots from the main stem of biological and physical sciences, and a marked growth in older, better-established ones occurred.

One of the most significant scientific advances occurred in 1905 when Albert Einstein proposed his theory of relativity. Also in physics, much evidence was accumulated about the electrical nature of living systems, and gradually the relationship of human beings with electrical fields was explored. Another advancement in physics has been the use of *ultrasound* in diagnosing and treating diseases.

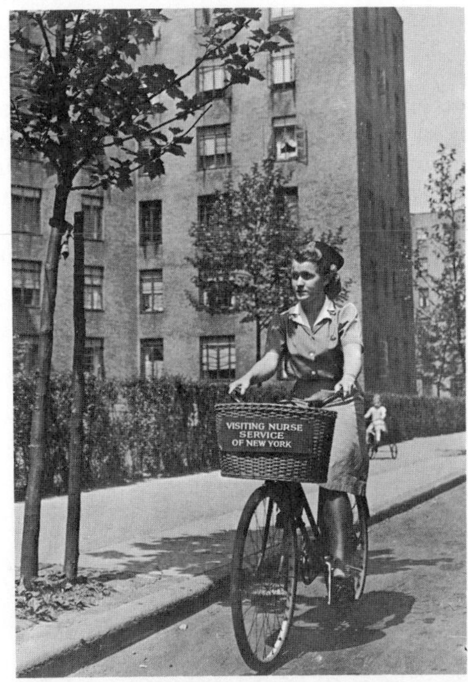

Figure 13–2. In 1944 during the gasoline shortage of World War II, nurses again rode bicycles in the Bronx and in Queens in New York. (Courtesy of the Visiting Nurse Service of New York.)

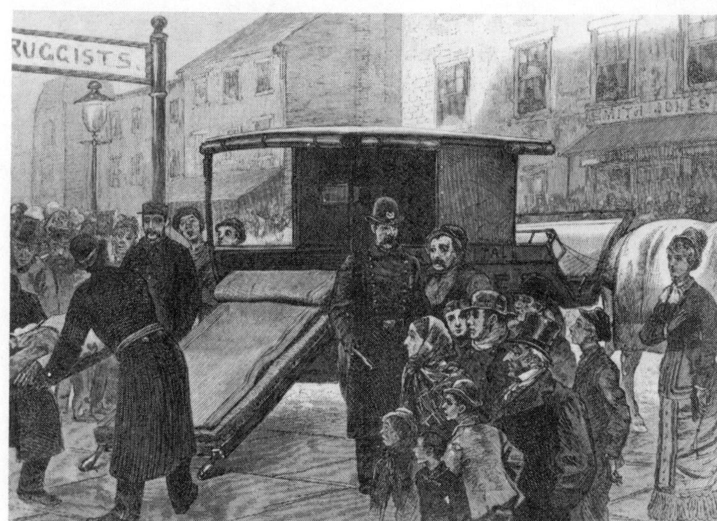

Figure 13–3. A New York City ambulance in 1879. (Dolan collection.)

The science of *bacteriology* has increased in scope and depth. The *electron microscope* has made it possible to study *viruses* and many other disease-causing organisms in greater detail than had previously been possible. Many valuable vaccines have been developed in this century. Associated sciences, such as *parasitology*, have evolved.

An examination of the structure of the cell has become as important to the biologist as the study of the atom has been to the physicist and chemist. Thus *cellular biology* and *cytology* developed. The application of the scientific bases of *pathology* in studying diseased tissues has resulted in more accurate diagnostic tests and has aided research for more efficient ways of treating patients. Developments in chemistry, including the introduction of biochemistry, make this science seem little related to the alchemy of centuries past.

When atoms were split or smashed artificially by means of a cyclotron, the *atomic age* was ushered in. There are many useful purposes for atomic energy, such as *radioactive isotopes* for medical research. Medicine now includes the use of nuclear reactors, cobalt machines, x-rays combined with motion pictures, CAT scanners and computers to plot programs for administration of lethal rays to diseased tissues. The atom in medicine has become a potent force in patient care. There is an atomic energy research center at Oak Ridge, Tennessee and medical atomic energy research centers at Brookhaven, Long Island and at

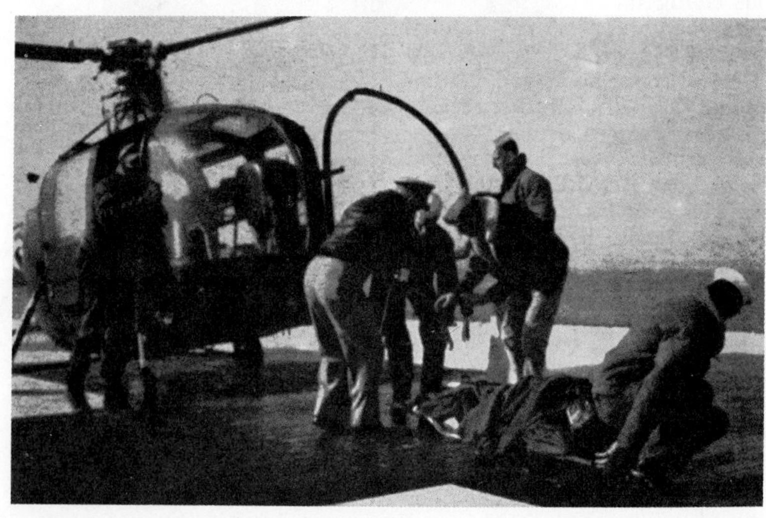

Figure 13–4. A helicopter awaiting a patient. (Dolan collection.)

the M.D. Anderson Hospital and Tumor Institute, Texas.

Chemical progress has benefitted society in many ways—in the pharmaceutical industry as well as in the areas of food and nutrition and cosmetics. *George Washington Carver* (*ca.* 1864–1943) employed his theories of "chemical gymnastics" to change the simple peanut into a multiplicity of useful preparations.

Biochemists have added much to our knowledge of the chemistry of digestion; studies in *nutrition* have advanced the knowledge of this subject in this century. By using a fluoroscopic screen, Dr. Walter B. Cannon studied the digestive organs of cats that had eaten radiopaque meals. In addition, he studied the effects of emotions on digestion and added to our knowledge of utilization of food, transmission of nerve impulses and actions of the endocrine glands.

Vitamins, those necessary ingredients discovered to exist in small amounts in certain foods, have been synthesized chemically, so that vitamin deficiency diseases are now being eliminated from the roster of illnesses.

In 1910 when *Dr. Paul Ehrlich* (1854–1915) and his Japanese assistant *Dr. Sahachiro Hata* proclaimed that Salvarsan (606) was the magic "chemical bullet" for the treatment of syphilis, *chemotherapy* became a vital factor in medical science.

Many drugs were synthesized in the chemical laboratories, and chemotherapy became a major form of patient care. In 1936, sulfanilamide, the first of the many sulfa "miracle" drugs, was used for the treatment of bacterial infections. *Sir Alexander Fleming* (1881–1955) of St. Mary's Hospital in London was responsible for the discovery of *penicillin* in 1939. The expansion and scientific progress in the field of pharmacology in the twentieth century has revolutionized health care.

Tuberculosis was a dreaded disease during the nineteenth century. The tubercle bacillus had been proved to cause destructive lesions in many parts of the body in addition to the lungs—in the brain (meningitis), skin (lupus), glands of the neck (scrofula), bones, joins and spine (Pott's disease), and kidneys and intestines. *Laennec* provided an instrument for listening to the chest; the combined efforts of many stressed that the disease was contagious; *Robert Koch* detected the causative organism; *Wilhelm Roentgen* discovered x-rays, which were used to detect evidence of tuberculosis in the body; and because of the development of tests, bovine tuberculosis could be controlled in cattle. In 1900, tuberculosis (all forms) was the second leading cause of death, causing 194.4 deaths per 100,000 people in that year, or 11.3 per cent of all deaths. Owing to new methods of treatment and prevention, by 1959 the death rate from this disease had fallen 98%, to 6.7 per 100,000 people, and death from this disease constituted only one per cent of all deaths.

MEDICAL, TECHNOLOGICAL AND SOCIAL ADVANCES

A second industrial revolution in the twentieth century brought new machinery and new methods of production into many agricultural as well as industrial areas. This revolution helped simplify work but more importantly it improved food purity. In the dairy industry, for example, in addition to testing the cattle, farmers now use milking machines that milk the cows under sanitary conditions, thus eliminating milk handlers. The milk is sent under proper refrigeration to plants where it is pasteurized.

In 1851, Dr. John Gorrie was granted the first patent for a cool-air machine. Dr. Gorrie firmly believed that if the room temperature could be lowered for patients who had high fevers, his treatments would have a greater degree of success. He relinquished his medical practice and devoted his full time to the problem of cooling air, and of freezing water artificially, or ice-making. The achievement of his objectives led to the development of air conditioning. In 1914, Dr. Gorrie's statue was placed in Statuary Hall of the Capital at Washington, D.C., in recognition of his pioneering efforts. He had laid the foundation for the ultimate development of *refrigeration,* which has been so essential in shipping and storing fruits, vegetables, meats and dairy products. Cleaner, more healthful produce is available, permitting a more varied and balanced diet for more people. Packaging of frozen foods has provided the opportunity for a well-balanced diet through all seasons of the year. Cryotherapy, cryosur-

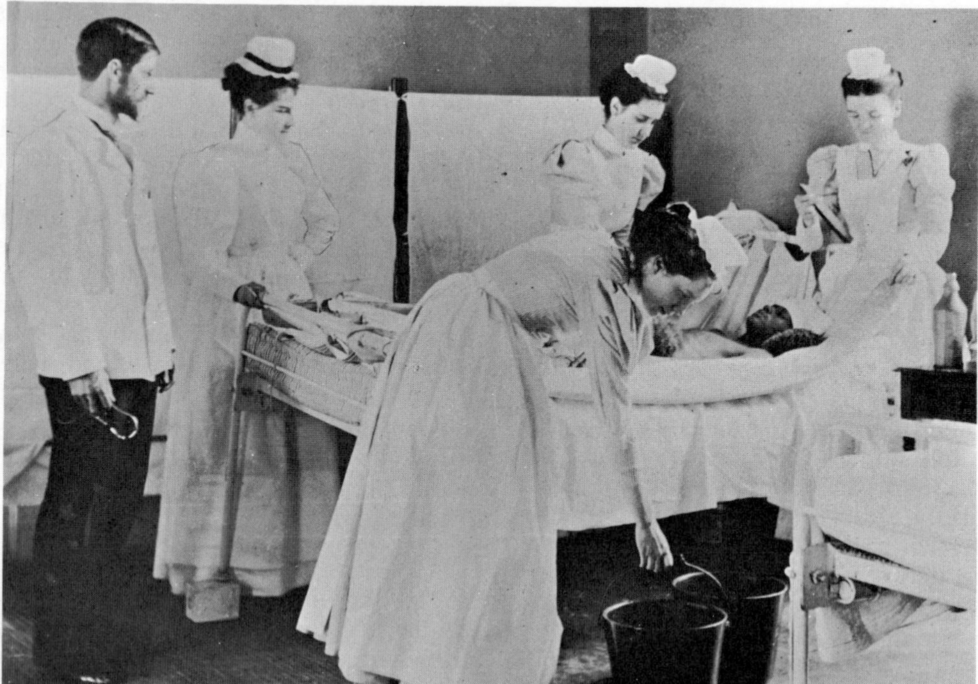

Figure 13–5. Three students of nursing prepare to give a patient who has typhoid fever a slush bath, using the ice water in the pails, to reduce his temperature (in 1905). The foot of the bed has been elevated with shock blocks. (Courtesy of Hartford Hospital School of Nursing.)

gery and hypothermic equipment have also been developed in this century (Fig. 13–5).

Cities have grown rapidly because of the increase in the numbers of factories, the mechanization of farming and the advancements in transportation. Improvements have been made in water supply purification, in meat inspection laws, in sanitary garbage collection and disposal, in sewerage systems, in street cleaning, in housing laws, in health supervision of an increasing number of public parks and recreation centers, in industrial hygiene and safety measures and in atmospheric sanitation.

Many major health problems have developed as a result of air pollution and the disposal of radioactive waste.

The feats of scientists and engineers have been phenomenal. The theoretical principles behind many of their inventions are being applied to techniques and equipment used in the care of the sick. The advancements of those scientific endeavors that have changed health care have been so great that a comprehensive account of them is impossible. The following are some highlights.

In 1901, *Karl Landsteiner* described his research in blood grouping, which led to a knowledge of blood testing and made blood transfusions possible (Figs. 13–6 to 13–8). In the same year, *Willem Einthoven* invented the string galvanometer, which provided the impetus needed to develop electrocardiography.

The year 1921 witnessed the announcement by Drs. Banting and Best of the isolation of *insulin* as the active ingredient in the pancreas needed for proper metabolic activity in diabetic patients. Endocrinology became an important and recognized field. Advances in surgery of the chest were also made. The victims of an incurable disease, *pernicious anemia,* were aided by the research of Drs. Minot and Murphy in Boston, who recommended that raw liver be included in the diet. Now pharmaceutical companies prepare liver for injection, and another once fatal illness can be controlled.

In the early 1930s an artificial respirator called an "iron lung" was invented that was instrumental in keeping many patients alive, especially those who were paralyzed by poliomyelitis. These respirators have been reduced in size and are now battery

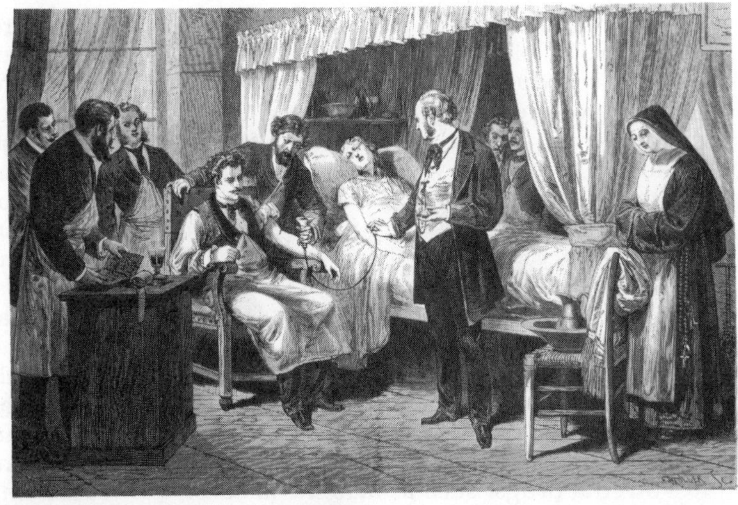

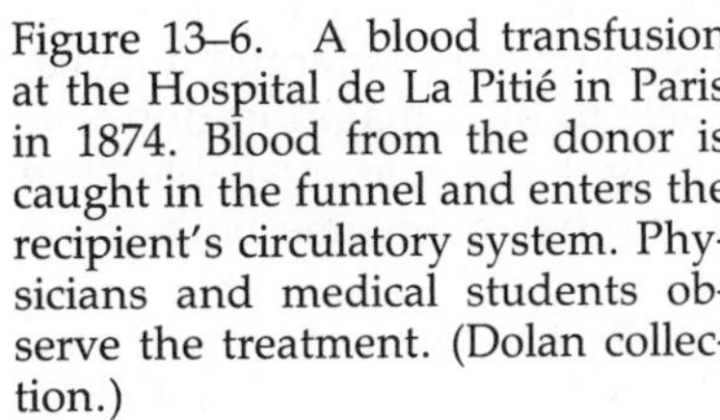

Figure 13–6. A blood transfusion at the Hospital de La Pitié in Paris in 1874. Blood from the donor is caught in the funnel and enters the recipient's circulatory system. Physicians and medical students observe the treatment. (Dolan collection.)

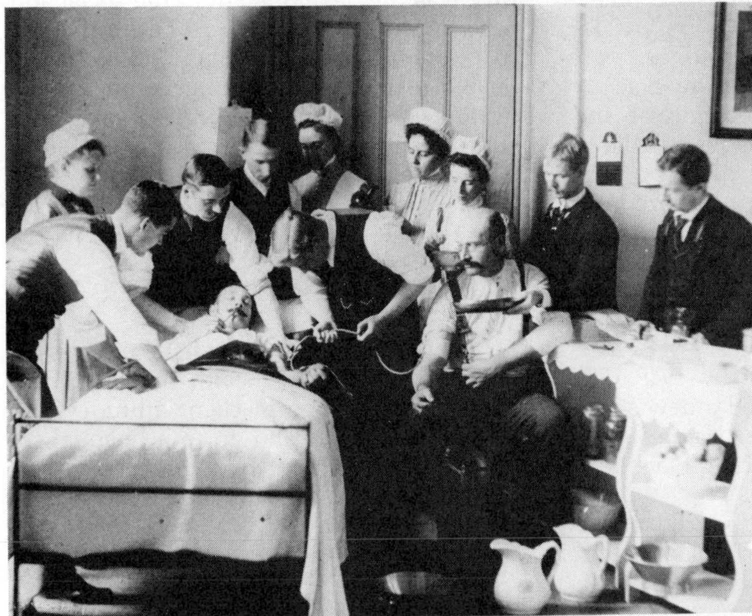

Figure 13–7. Blood transfusion, Bellevue Hospital 1888. (Dolan collection.)

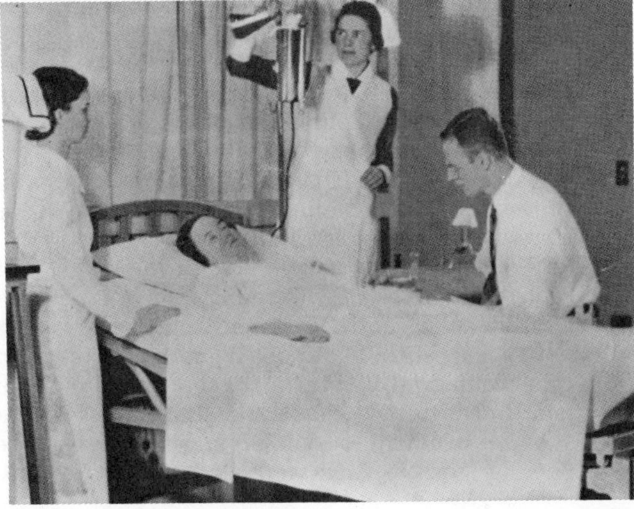

Figure 13–8. Blood transfusion, New Haven Hospital, 1938. (Dolan collection.)

powered. Methods of preserving the components of blood for therapeutic purposes were introduced. *Blood banks* were established for preserving human blood plasma and serum, which were used in transfusions. *Shock therapy* was used in psychiatry. The development of *corneal transplants* provided the miraculous gift of sight for recipients.

In the decade between 1940 and 1950, World War II presented many new problems to medicine that resulted in advancements in *atomic medicine, tropical medicine* and treatment of war injuries. In addition to blood banks, many other banks, such as those for bone and tissue, became a reality. Powerful drugs, such as atabrine (a substitute for quinine), antihistamines (for relieving allergic conditions), cortisone, ACTH and, of course, radioactive isotopes, were processed. Supersonic and ultrasonic vibrations were used in medicine at this time. In 1944, *Dr. Helen Taussig*, a pediatrician, carried out a research project on the plight of blue babies and emphasized the need for corrective surgery. Her efforts resulted in the development of a successful surgical technique by *Dr. Alfred Blalock*, of Johns Hopkins. Cancer detection tests, such as the vaginal smear test by *Dr. Papanicolaou*, became available by 1948. The field of rehabilitation received a new status because of the efforts of *Dr. Howard Rusk*, whose philosophy and teaching have been a boon to humanity.

In 1955, *Dr. Jonas Salk* produced a vaccine for the prevention of poliomyelitis. Mass inoculation of children and adults with Salk vaccine or Sabin oral vaccine has been responsible for the virtual disappearance of poliomyelitis.

During the years since 1950, *space medicine* has evolved as an offshoot of the growing field of astronautics. The use of electric monitoring, automatic thermometers, dialysis equipment, inhalation therapy and data processing and computers has become common in patient care. The lifesaving battery-operated pacemakers are now being replaced by nuclear-powered devices.

In the 1960s and 1970s many clinical innovations, such as open heart surgery, transplantation of human organs, implantation of artificial organs and artificial tissue, replacement of joints, genetic engineering and in vitro fertilizations, have been introduced. New scientific devices, such as ultrasound apparatus and lasers, have been utilized.

Until recently, the degree of magnification possible was restricted by the ability of the human eye to observe enlarged images. Another obstacle to high magnification was the amount of light that was available. The *electron microscope* has overcome both these limitations.

The span of life has been increased as a result of increased research in health science, public health and sanitation, improvements in the living conditions of the less fortunate and the elimination of contagious and infectious diseases.

Also important during the twentieth century was the development of the social and behavioral sciences, such as anthropology, psychology and sociology. These fields have had a profound influence on the education of health care professionals and subsequently on the methods developed to deliver health care.

IMPROVEMENTS IN HOSPITALS

In this century hospitals have progressed from pest houses to health centers. There has been a change in client attitude from dismay and refusal to go to a hospital for care to one of acceptance in recognition of the advantages of participating in a program of health care.

Three Works on the Status of Hospitals at the Turn of the Century

It is rewarding to contemplate the role of hospitals at the turn of the century and their influence, in conjunction with certain physicians and nurses, in shaping the health care system with which the profession of nursing has had to cope.

Hand Book for Hospitals. In 1883, the State Charities Aid Association of New York published a book entitled *Hand Book for Hospitals.* It had been prepared to assist public-spirited citizens in understanding proper organization and management of hospitals. The citizens were requested to consider the purpose for which hospitals were built and to remember that everyone needs good care. In addition, the book stressed that when the nurse is considering a plan of care, the importance of the family and family ties of patients should receive careful attention. According to the *Hand Book,* hospital administrators should exercise control in demanding that all things purchased for the welfare of patients and staff be of good quality. It was proposed that even the ice, which was purchased in a period before refrigeration, should not be cut from ponds or streams that received drainage or seepage from foul sources which would make it unfit for use. In discussing the details of hospitals, including its appliances, the advantages of *air beds,* which could be seen at the General Hospital in New Haven, and *water beds,* which were in use at Hartford Hospital, received attention from the association. Many step-saving techniques and devices were described. A dining room for every ward was recommended, with only the seriously ill and those patients who would be offensive to other patients being served in bed. The social and psychological contributions that a cheerful, attractive setting amid sociability and good food made toward achieving a patient's recovery were also noted.

The association's concerns extended to the nurses, and it requested suitable living arrangements for their physical and mental health: "The efficiency of the nurse is so important for her charge [the patient] that her health and comfort should be considered for this reason as well as for her own sake."[1]

Two types of patients received special attention, with an earnest plea for better care for both—maternity patients and the mentally ill. The plight of the pregnant woman, including the constant danger of puerperal fever, and the cruelty in the plan for care of the "insane" person were clearly delineated. The need for well-planned care, including diversional therapy, for the mentally ill patient was presented by Dr. Mary Putnam Jacob: "Rightly understood it means the creation around each patient of a new world, built up out of his own awakened and directed activities."[2]

In concluding the book, the State Charities Aid Association begged the reader to reflect again upon the objective "for which the hospital building, its corps of nurses, and its superintendence exist" and reiterated, "Let no one forget that this primary object is the curing of the sick. A hospital is not founded solely to provide a field of experiments and break in raw young medical men to practice."[3] The association believed that it was the moral obligation of citizens of communities to provide a healthful setting so that the sick poor could return home as well and as soon as possible. Readers were charged to become active in considering human rights.

This book produced a heated reaction on the part of many physicians, who believed rebuttal of the arguments should be published in the hope of stifling many of the proposals. The person who rose to rally physicians and their influential friends against the book's proposals was Dr. Charles Francis Withington.

The Relation of Hospitals to Medical Education. From their inception, hospitals had been designed to provide relief during times of sickness for those who were unable to provide for themselves. Many philanthropists had insured the delivery of such care for the poor through generous endowments with stipulations for use of these funds.

Dr. Withington pleaded the cause of medical leaders to permit hospitals to be used for clinical instruction for medical education. He acknowledged that money and instructions left in trust, with the lapse of time and change of circumstances, mandated a reconsideration with a modification, if not a redirection, of the use of such funds in a way that might not have been the intention of the donor.[4] He further stated that few endowed institutions are administrated precisely as their originators supposed they would be. It was his feeling that if these generous people were alive and apprised of all the facts in the case, they would exercise the same judgment and generosity that characterized their lives

[1]State Charities Aid Association: *Hand Book for Hospitals.* New York, G. P. Putnam's Sons, 1883, p. 88.

[2]State Charities Aid Association: *Hand Book for Hospitals.* New York, G. P. Putnam's Sons, 1883, p. 188.

[3]State Charities Aid Association: *Hand Book for Hospitals.* New York, G. P. Putnam's Sons, 1883, p. 235.

[4]Withington, Charles Francis: *The Relation of Hospitals to Medical Education.* Boston, Cupples, Upham, 1886.

and would endorse the actions made necessary by changed conditions.

Dr. Withington believed that intelligent and conscientious administrators of endowed institutions had a moral obligation to conform to the needs of medical students for clinical experience. He wrote *The Relation of Hospitals to Medical Education* to ease the conscience of the hospital administrators and placate the public, who might protest this trend of ignoring the obligation of providing for the comfort and well-being of individuals and of permitting patients to be used for the purpose of advancing medical science.

The first section of the book addressed itself to the "peculiar obligation" of hospitals in regard to medical education, especially the hospital's right to use its clinical material, i.e., its patients. He recognized the need of medical educators for patients and the impossibility of obtaining the consent of well-to-do persons who pay for their medical attention to allow themselves to be used for purposes of clinical instruction. It was his feeling that nonpaying patients, in consideration of the benefits they received, should give such compensation as they had it in their power to give, which was to provide the opportunity for clinical instruction.[5] He referred to the presence of "various appliances" that the hospitals could provide, such as postmortem examinations and opportunities to perform surgical operations.

The second section of Dr. Withington's book presented "the possible conflict between the interests of medical science and those of the individual patient and his indefeasible rights."[6] He agreed that occasionally it was "at the expense of the individual that truths of the greatest general utility have been learned." He assured the public that in this country this exchange is less likely to happen, but "even with us it may be well to draw up . . . a Bill of Rights which shall secure patients against any injustice from the votaries of science. The occupants of hospital wards are something more than merely so much clinical material during their lives and so much pathological material after their death."[7]

Dr. Withington inveighed against human experimentation for its own sake and without patient knowledge and encouraged the use of volunteers for such programs of experimentation. He did not discuss patient consent, although he said that physicians had no right to make any person the unwilling victim of an experiment. "A temptation kindred to the above is the recommendation of hopeless surgical operations," and he believed that surgeons "had no right to take advantage of the patient's extremity to recommend a procedure which can have no other advantage than to enhance the operator's reputation for boldness."[8]

Another source of tribulation for a poor patient was that of overfrequent physical examinations, which were often injurious. A patient who was critically ill with pneumonia was subjected to the frequent exposure of the chest and the auscultation and percussion by students who wanted to learn about the pneumonic process. Dr. Withington made no mention of the exhaustion of the patient and the interruption of his rest; these disturbances should have been objected to by the nurse in charge of the patient. And one wonders what Withington believed the proper role of the nurse to be, because he discussed the value of medical students' checking the exact amount of pleuritic effusion or the precise size of a hypertrophied heart without compromising the patient's safety and then commented, "It is our duty to learn them, for there is no conflict between the interests of science and the individual." Dr. Withington seems to have contradicted himself.

The only instance in which he mentioned the presence of a nurse was the statement that physicians should not examine a female patient without a nurse in the room. He admitted that the greatest objection women had to coming to a hospital was the unnecessary exposure to which they were subjected and the unnecessary

[5]Withington, Charles Francis: *The Relation of Hospitals to Medical Education*. Boston, Cupples, Upham, 1886, p. 9.

[6]Ibid., p. 14.

[7]Ibid., p. 15.

[8]Withington, Charles Francis: *The Relation of Hospitals to Medical Education*. Boston, Cupples, Upham, 1886, p. 17.

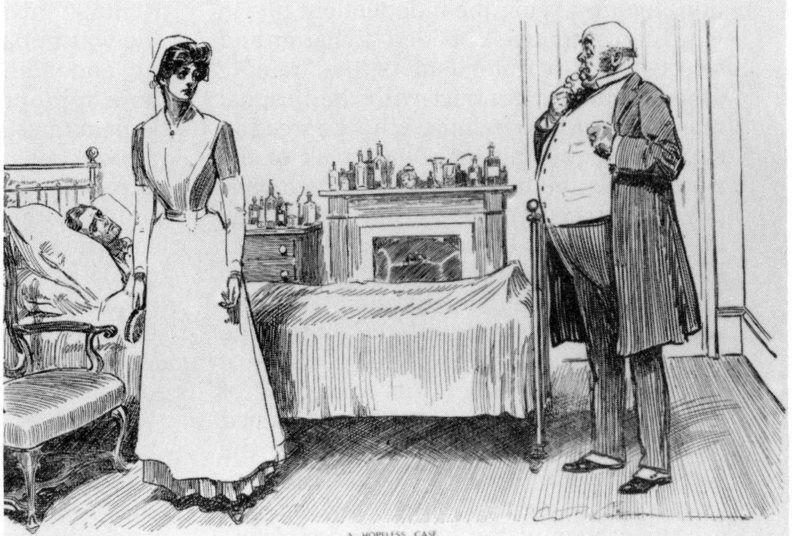

Figure 13–9. A Hopeless Case, by Charles Dana Gibson, depicts the limits of medicine and the profound importance of the role of skilled nursing care. (Dolan collection.)

pelvic examinations performed by students. He blithely stated, "There is no violation of modesty when there is no consciousness of exposure. An operation may be performed upon a woman before a whole amphitheatre of students and provided she is unconscious . . . of her surroundings and never learns . . . of the circumstances, there has been no violation of her modesty."[9]

The last section of the book referred to the factors that increased the educational value of hospitals, such as having a medical school affiliate with a hospital and attracting intelligent young medical men as house officers. The "preparation of young men, through the educational influence of hospitals, for the practice of their profession . . . by no means exhausts the educational capacity of the hospital." Dr. Withington made the disconcerting statement, "The most useful handmaid of medicine is nursing,"[10] adding that "in many cases, notably in the acute fevers, the labor of the nurse is undoubtedly more important than that of the physician. For the reduction of medicine from a science to an art good nursing is absolutely indispensable."

Dr. Withington reported that many well-known physicians who had experience in hospitals whose nurses had attended training schools as well as hospitals whose nurses had not, agreed that the character of the nursing care was vastly better where training schools existed. There were several reasons for favorable response on the part of physicians toward nurses who were as well prepared as training schools permitted them to be: The hospital stay was decreased for the patient, thereby enabling a greater number of patients to be treated in a year. The nurse who was doing private duty in the home provided "enormous relief to the practitioner [of medicine] who no longer is obliged to attend personally to pass a catheter, make a hypodermic injection or renew a surgical dressing. Much time thus saved from the drudgery of his profession can be devoted to scientific improvement."[11] He also recognized that significant information about the patient or symptoms or other phenomena of disease that might not be noted by the physician in the short time of his visit could be noted and recorded or reported by a well-prepared nurse.

Dr. Withington argued the benefits of training schools for the medical profession and for the hospitals. He indicated that there were two systems of nurse educa-

[9]*Ibid.*, p. 20.

[10]Withington, Charles Francis: *The Relation of Hospitals to Medical Education.* Boston, Cupples, Upham, 1886, p. 29.

[11]*Ibid.*, p. 30.

tion, the first being the independent one in which a committee obtained a charter and selected a superintendent of the training school. Under a contract with the hospital management, the training school agreed to supply the nursing for some or all of the wards while the hospital furnished a money payment for compensation for work done or maintenance of nurses or both. Dr. Withington made no mention of students of nursing securing an education. With the second method of nurse education, "the hospital management itself, for the sake of securing good nursing for its wards and of supplying the community with well-trained nurses," for private duty, "undertakes the same work, but of course there is no contract between the two parties, and the one executive head of the hospital administers also the training school."[12]

Dr. Withington then summed up his discussion on nursing by focusing on how nurses should be allocated and under whose control they should be placed: "Independent training school managers may in their zeal for the education of their pupils, make such a distribution of the latter, that the hospital administration shall suffer. The balance of advantage to all interests, therefore, seems to be with the method which makes the training school a department of the hospital and under its administrative control. Then the hospital staff at whose immediate disposal this most important instrument [nursing] lies, can in case of failure or incompetency look, as in all other cases of difficulty, to the one executive head to have the matter righted."[13] It is important to realize that he was not pleading that medical education become a department of the hospital and under its control nor in case of medical incompetency that the practitioner of this important "instrument" (medicine) be chastised by the hospital administrator.

The preceding material from what must have been a controversial book exemplifies some of the reasons for the trials that nursing has faced in this century.

Nurses and Nursing. *Nurses and Nursing* was purported to have been written by a "nurse" named Lisbeth D. Price in 1892. She was not a graduate of a school of nursing and admitted that "compiler" was a more appropriate term than "writer" of the book in question. An obstetrician wrote the introduction, stressing the need for the book and the capability of the author. According to him, the book's purpose was to "lay down the laws for the conduct and direction of nurses, and their responsibilities towards physicians, patients, and themselves." He indicated that capable, well-educated nurses are *almost* as essential as the educated physician.

Miss Price begins her preface with the opening remark that "a strong line of demarcation should be drawn between that which a nurse should know and that which she should not know, that the theoretical portion of her studies must of necessity be more or less superficial." Miss Price stated that the reason for her literary contribution was that the textbooks that she had seen, "though in the main seemed good, are prone to enter into certain subjects too deeply," and the practical side of nursing had been treated too superficially.

The initial chapter of her book bore the title "The Limitations of the Duties of the Nurse." She commenced:

"There are few professions—perhaps it may be said with truth, that there is *no* profession—which has its limitations marked with such rigid distinctions, as that of nursing. . . .

"There are many reasons . . . for these strong limitations. The chief one is this: the profession of nursing is dependent upon the medical profession; from it, in fact, it has emanated."[14] Her lack of knowledge of her heritage is obvious. She also made another incredible statement: "The 'doctor's duty to the nurse' is a perversion of fact that looks distorted, even in writing; no such relation exists. The nurse to the doctor should be a human automaton, that listens to him attentively, and obeys him implicitly, nothing more. . . . "

Thus the turn of the century saw the publication of three works that expressed varying points of view on the value and status of nurses: The first presented the ef-

[12]Withington, Charles Francis: *The Relation of Hospitals to Medical Education*. Boston, Cupples, Upham, 1886, p. 33.

[13]*Ibid.*, p. 34.

[14]Price, Lisbeth D.: *Nurses and Nursing*. Philadelphia, George W. Jacobs and Co., 1892, p. 1.

forts of a public-spirited group of citizens seriously interested in the welfare of all human beings, including nurses. The second was by a medical educator speaking for his colleagues and his students and trying subtly to mold the nurse's role and her educational program to the desires of medicine. In the third, a "nurse," who appears to have been flattered into permitting herself to assume the role of chastiser of her own colleagues, presented the role of the nurse as that of a passive and self-effacing servant to the physician.

Changes in this Century

Since the turn of the century, there has not been a great overall increase in the number of hospitals but in the size of hospitals. The total space of the modern hospital, which was once occupied only by patients' beds, is now shared with diagnostic testing areas and therapeutic equipment needed for patient service.

The architecture of the newer buildings has been planned with greater understanding of the needs of the patient as well as those who care for him. Still greater progress in this area is needed.

There were marked benefits in the older arrangement of patient units. In the open wards of older European hospitals, patients had both privacy and companionship along with ready access to nurses for care (Fig. 13–10). In the open wards of American and European hospitals in the early twentieth century, privacy was not so great, but nursing desks were part of the ward and nurses were readily accessible (Fig. 13–11). In newer units, clients complain of lack of communication with nurses, who perform clerical functions at a head nurse station, removed from the client. Communication is through an "intercommunication" system in the wall, which increases the feeling of depersonalization.

Many hospitals have progressive units, ranging from an *intensive care* unit for the patient who is critically ill, to a do-it-yourself unit in which a minimal amount of care is required. The ancient custom of relatives *"rooming-in"* with the sick loved one has been revived (Fig. 13–12). A motel system of patient care, designed to reduce expenses, is another innovation.

Color is used more effectively in hospitals today than it has been in the last two centuries, and utilized for its therapeutic value. Safety aspects are noted as is the use

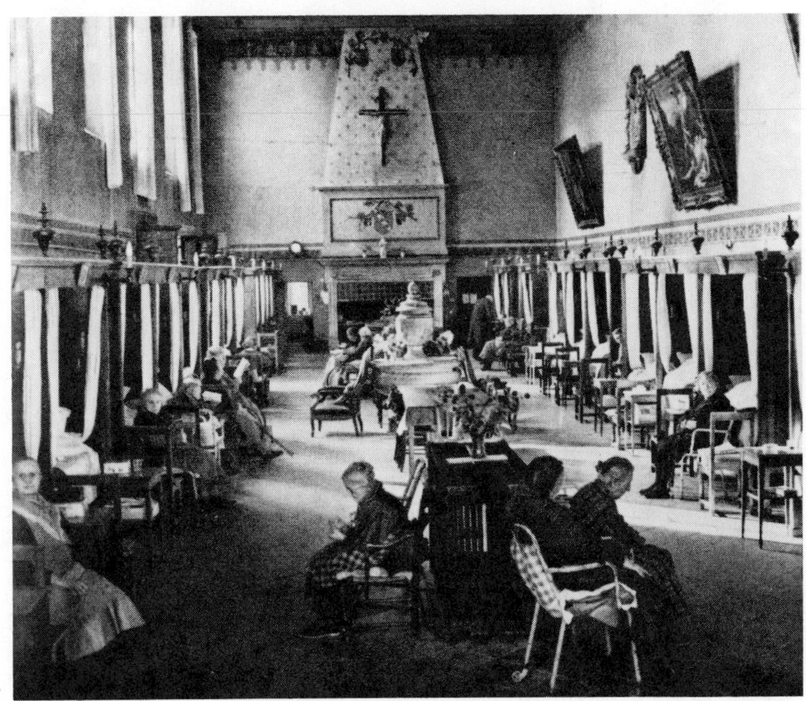

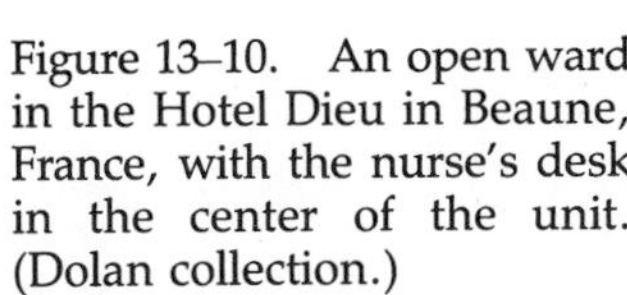

Figure 13–10. An open ward in the Hotel Dieu in Beaune, France, with the nurse's desk in the center of the unit. (Dolan collection.)

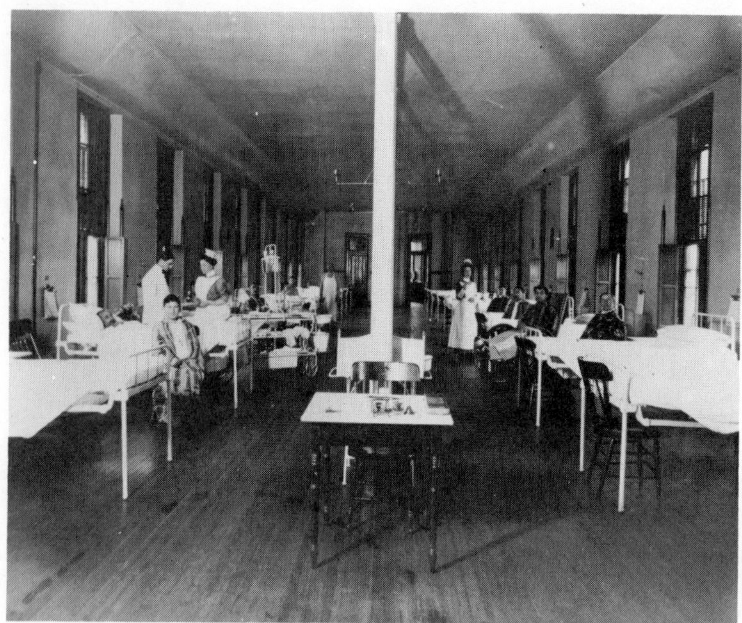

Figure 13–11. An open ward in an American hospital in the early part of this century. The ease with which a patient could communicate with a nurse is apparent. Note the iron beds. (Dolan collection.)

of many modern inventions to make care easier for both patients and nurses.

The construction of beds has been another area of marked change; iron beds that nurses had to lift in order to elevate the foot or head have been replaced by electric beds. Certain varieties of beds provide greater comfort and ease in assisting a patient or permitting him to do things for himself.

ADVANCES IN PUBLIC HEALTH

At the beginning of this century, the circumstances surrounding the transmission of such diseases as typhoid fever, cholera, summer diarrheas and food poisoning were beginning to be studied. The control of milk-borne, water-borne and food-borne diseases was demanding attention. Compounding these problems of disease were the overcrowded conditions in cities as a result of waves of immigrants from Europe. Eventually, adequate measures for obtaining sanitary water supplies and sewage disposal systems were put into practice.

A famous woman physician of this period was *S. Josephine Baker* (1873–1945).[15] The growing field of *public health* interested Dr. Baker, and in 1901 she joined the New

[15]Baker, S. Josephine: *Fighting for Life*. New York, The Macmillan Co., 1939.

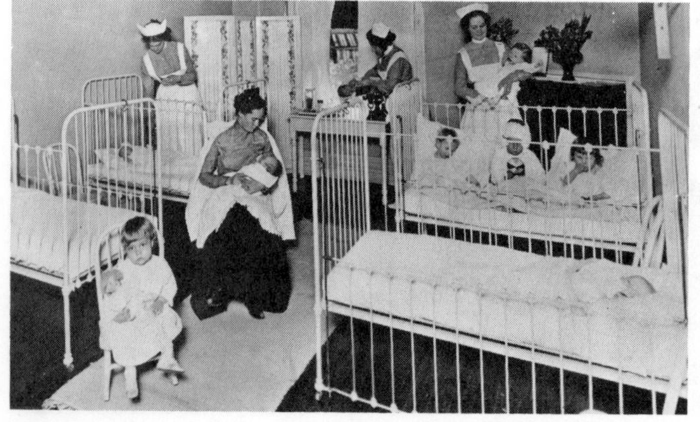

Figure 13–12. Mother permitted to "room-in" with her sick infant in the early twentieth century. (Courtesy of Northwestern Hospital.)

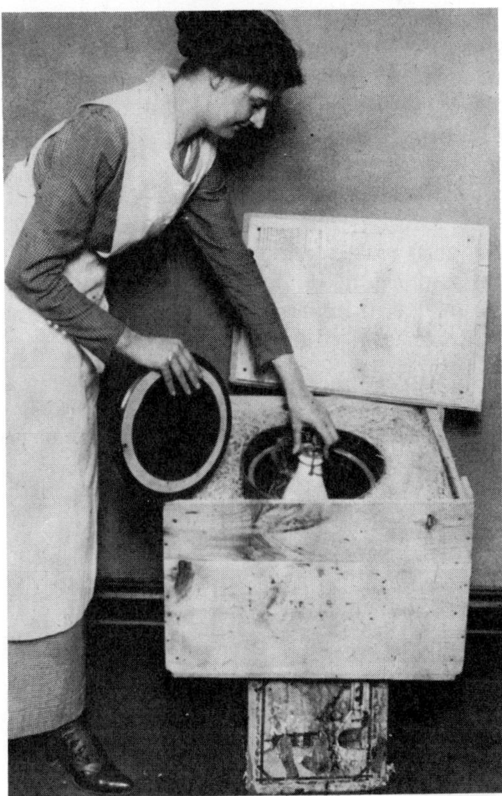

Figure 13–13. Nurses taught an improvised method of keeping milk cold to prevent it from becoming a culture medium for the growth of bacteria. (Dolan collection.)

York City Department of Health. She recognized the need for a program of health education to prevent needless suffering and misery. She became assistant commissioner of health and engaged in an expanding program dedicated to the health and welfare of children. She was responsible for the creation of the New York City Division of Child Hygiene and directed its program. Her goal in establishing this important section was "to prevent children from dying by preventing them from becoming ill." Educational programs absorbed her interest, and she emphasized the need for well-prepared nurses whose role in teaching would be recognized.

When she first started her crusade in the interest of infant welfare, she blamed much of the high infant mortality from gastrointestinal diseases on the city milk supply. She believed that the raw milk sold in the local grocery stores was a "diluted germ culture." She suggested the establishment of baby health stations where bottled pasteurized milk, sold more cheaply than the raw milk, would be accompanied by educational material on child care. The taxpayers did not approve this plan, but it won the financial support of a wealthy woman who maintained 30 of these baby stations. The success of the stations prompted the adoption of the station plan by the municipal authorities.

New laboratory techniques received impetus from the eager workers in departments of health. In 1907, an outbreak of typhoid fever in New York City was traced to a contaminated water supply. In the same year "Typhoid Mary" was located by Major George A. Soper of the U. S. Army and was taken into custody by the New York City Health Department. Laboratory tests allowed for the adoption of registration and supervision of typhoid carriers. By 1917 foodhandlers were being examined to detect possible typhoid carriers.

Bureaus for health education were established, followed by bureaus of infectious diseases, preventable diseases and industrial hygiene. The use of statistics provided significant data for determining solutions to public health problems.

The identification of the causative organisms of many communicable diseases, together with the knowledge of the vectors of disease and the institution of programs of immunization, led to civic action. If a person became ill with a contagious disease, his home and family members were quarantined, and the home was placarded to warn all neighbors and friends of the presence of a contagious disease.

The federal government attempted to control, inspect and supervise the quality of foods as early as 1879. At that time, a bill was submitted to Congress to prohibit the adulteration of substances to be used as food and drink. The bill did not pass.

American novelist and socialist *Upton Sinclair* (1878–1968) was instrumental in bringing about certain health reforms. His novel *The Jungle,* which described the shockingly filthy conditions in the Chicago slaughterhouses, evoked horror in the minds of the public and then incited the public to action. President Theodore Roosevelt received scores of letters demanding federal action to raise standards in the meat industry. *The Jungle* galvanized the consumer cause and put the federal government firmly into the consumer protection business.

In 1906, President Roosevelt signed the bill that enforced the proposal to prohibit the manufacture and sale of adulterated and misbranded foods. This law was to be administered by the Department of Agriculture. In 1931, the *Food and Drug Administration* was created, and in 1938, President Franklin D. Roosevelt signed a bill that created the *Federal Food, Drug, and Cosmetic Act*.

The influence of public-spirited citizens continued in the fight for better health. Newspaper journalists such as *Jacob Riiss* brought the social and health problems of immigrants to public awareness. The ecology movement was greatly influenced by Rachel Carson's *Silent Spring* (1962), as well as by the multifaceted activities of Ralph Nader, whose *Unsafe at Any Speed* (1965) roused Congress to study and take action against the automotive industry for manufacturing unsafe automobiles. In 1962, President John F. Kennedy wrote what has been called the consumer bill of rights: the right to be informed, the right to choose, the right to safety and the right to be heard.

White House Conferences

Several White House Conferences have been devoted to the interests of children and youth.

1909—The First White House Conference centered on the care of dependent children. As a result of this conference:

1912: Congress established the United States Children's Bureau.

1915–1919: The Children's Bureau helped states create divisions of Maternal and Child Health. All of the activities of the Children's Bureau have been directed toward three worthwhile objects: "(1) to insure to the children of the nation the right to be born as normal healthy babies and to develop into vigorous young persons ready to take their places in the adult world; (2) the remedying of conditions in our society which are obstacles to normal child health and development; and (3) the prevention of these harmful conditions."

The Children's Bureau has been concerned with employed children. The Congressional act establishing the bureau specified the need for investigation of "dangerous occupations, accidents, and diseases of children; employment and legislation affecting children in the several states and territories."

1919—The Second White House Conference emphasized child welfare standards. Concern was expressed for the high maternal and infant death rates due partially to too rapid industrialization. Results of this conference included the following:

1921: The Sheppard-Towner Act (Maternal Child Act) was passed.

1924: The Child Labor Law amendment was proposed.

1928–1931: The Committee on Cost of Medical Care was appointed.

1930—The Third White House Conference stressed child health and protection. This conference provided impetus for passage of the Social Security Act in 1935, and in addition resulted in the following:

1930: The Children's Charter was enacted.

1935–1936: The National Health Survey was attempted.

1940—The Fourth White House Conference selected as its theme "Children in a Democracy." Continued study of responsibility of federal, state and local government for maternity and child care was approved. Religion was emphasized. Grants-in-aid for research and for upgrading health professions were proposed. Results of this conference were as follows:

1942: The Emergency Maternity and Infant Care Act was passed.

1946–1947: The Hill-Burton Act (hospital construction) was adopted.

1948: "The Nation's Health"—a report to the President—was prepared.

1950—The Fifth White House Conference accepted the challenge of fostering mental and social health. This was the first of many conferences that encouraged all disciplines to work together on problems. Youth was also represented. Two major problems discussed were delinquency and mental retardation.

1960—The Sixth White House Conference for Children and Youth used the same techniques as had been used in 1950 for multidisciplinary conferences, but 7000 people attended and the results are not as easy to summarize. The problems of the "migrant minor," the American Indian child, the physically handicapped child, the illegitimate child and the black child were discussed. Results were:

1960: The President asked governors to set up physical fitness programs in each state.

A permanent White House Conference committee was established to improve implementation on local level of recommendations of the 1960 conference.

Eventually, well-child clinics were set up. In the 1950s babies were tested to detect phenylketonuria (PKU), and state laws required PKU testing for all newborns. In the 1960s legislation was enacted for reporting "the battered-child syndrome" in the hope of preventing child abuse. During the 1970s several White House conferences on children were held. Notable among them was one in which the children themselves determined the issues and made recommendations for actions and congresses in which specific topics, such as sudden infant death syndrome and child abuse, were focussed on.

During the 1970s and 1980s, White House conferences on aging were conducted. These conferences coincided with the increased emphasis on the social and health needs of older Americans and the development of the specialty field of gerontology. In 1980, special emphasis was given to the needs of disabled persons. This concern was related to the passage of federal legislation that protected the rights of handicapped individuals and paved the way for increased access of the handicapped to opportunities in employment and education.

Federal Health Services

In this century, federal government has assumed a progressively more active role in recognizing problems of health and enacting health legislation.

The Public Health Service was established by an act of 1798, which authorized marine hospitals for the care of American merchant seamen. In 1902, Congress renamed the Marine Hospital Service the Public Health and Marine Hospital Service and placed it under the direction of a surgeon-general. In 1912, this name was changed to the *United States Public Health Service* (USPHS). The duties of this branch of the federal service rapidly became more complex, and in 1918, it added the Division of Venereal Diseases. In 1929, the service acquired a narcotics division, renamed the Division of Mental Hygiene, which was responsible for hospital facilities at Lexington, Kentucky, and Forth Worth, Texas, that provide care and treatment for those addicted to narcotics.

The nurse leadership of the USPHS has provided strong nurse role models. The current Deputy Surgeon General and Chief Nurse Officer of the governmental service is the highly respected nurse leader and author, Dr. Faye G. Abdellah (Fig. 13–14).

In 1921, Congress established the United States Veterans' Bureau as a civilian agency of the federal government and, in the following year, assigned all Public Health Service hospitals to it. In 1930, to further coordinate government activities affecting war veterans, the Veterans' Bureau, the National Homes for Disabled Volunteer Soldiers and the Bureau of Pensions of the Interior Department were merged into a new agency called the *Veterans' Administration* (VA). The federal government organ-

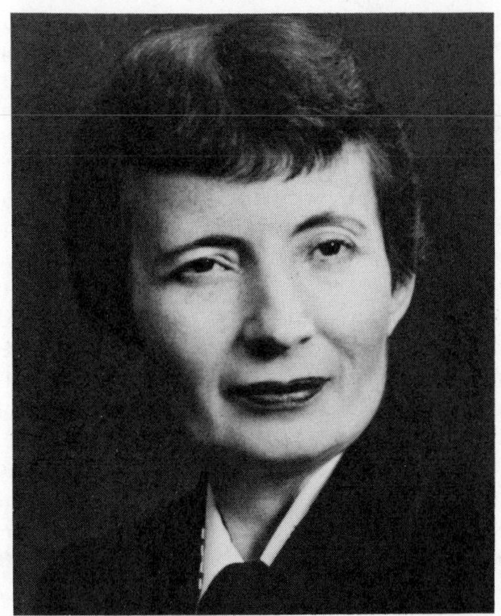

Figure 13–14. Faye G. Abdellah, Ed. D., LL. D., F. A. A. N. Deputy Surgeon General and Chief Nurse Officer, U. S. Public Health Service.

ized this agency to respond to the health needs of retiring servicemen and women. Mrs. Mary McCarthy Hickey, R.N., was the first Superintendent of Nurses. Since its inception, the nursing service of the VA has been the largest organized nursing service in the country. In 1980, the agency's nursing personnel, totalling about 60,000 individuals, worked in facilities located throughout the continental United States and its territories.[16] The VA, which administers the largest network of hospitals and health centers in the United States, continues to provide competent health care to U.S. veterans.

The passage of the *Federal Social Security Act* of 1935 had important, far-reaching effects. The *National Cancer Act* of 1937 brought into existence the *National Cancer Institute.* In 1946, the *Hospital Survey and Construction* (Hill-Burton) *Act* was passed, and in 1948, the *National Heart Institute* was founded. The *National Institute of Allergy and Infectious Diseases* and the *National Institute of Dental Research* were formed by reorganizing several existing units. *The National Institutes of Health* were developed. In 1952, the USPHS established, on the grounds of the National Institutes of Health in Bethesda, Maryland, a research hospital center called the *National Clinical Center.*

In the early 1960s, programs evolved for the training and education of health manpower and the construction of educational facilities. In 1963, attention was focused on mental health, and the *Mental Retardation Facilities and Mental Health Centers Construction Programs Act* was enacted.

The Federal Security Agency. In 1946, the Federal Security Agency was reorganized, which resulted in the transfer of several agencies to it: the Children's Bureau from the Department of Labor, the Food and Drug Administration from the Department of Agriculture, and the National Office of Vital Statistics from the Bureau of the Census of the Department of Commerce.

In 1953, an act of Congress changed the Federal Security Agency to the Department of Health, Education and Welfare. This department, now called the *U.S. Department of Health and Human Services,* is the nation's chief health coordinating agency. Division of Nursing, under the aegis of this agency, is responsible for administering student loans for nursing as well as funding programs of nursing education and nursing research.

Medicare. Former Secretary of Health, Education and Welfare John W. Gardner urged governors to take maximum advantage of expanded federal aid authorized for state health and welfare programs under the Social Security Amendments of 1965. In his letter, Secretary Gardner stated to the governors, "The new law lays the foundation for a medical care program for public assistance recipients and other low income persons that, within the next ten years, could go far to reduce one of the major causes of poverty and other social problems—the disabilities resulting from preventable or remediable health problems among persons in all age groups who cannot afford the medical care they need." Noting the American Nurses' Association's long-term backing of the extension of Social Security, President Lyndon Johnson asked the ANA's president and the director of the Washington office to join the official party of 200 who were to be present for the signing of the Medicare bill on July 30, 1965, at the Truman Library in Independence, Missouri.

The starting date for Medicare was July 1, 1966; services in extended care facilities were not covered until January 1, 1967. Additional provisions specifically designed to benefit future generations included: increased authorization for maternal and child health, crippled children and child welfare services; increased funds for grants to help colleges and universities train more professional personnel to work with crippled children, particularly the mentally retarded and those with multiple handicaps; and a five-year program of special project grants to provide comprehensive health care and services for preschool and school-age children, particularly in areas with concentrations of low-income families. Nursing organizations strongly supported the passage of this federally sponsored legislation.

Along with the passage of the Social Security Amendment, the program of *Medicaid* was also established to assist those

[16]Keough, Gertrude: *History and Heritage of the Veterans' Administration Nursing Service, 1930–1980.* New York, National League for Nursing, 1981, p. 2–3.

who were faced with the problems of poverty. As the costs of health care rise, national health insurance looms as a possibility. Third-party payments to nurses for the delivery of care have received attention and are being provided in some instances.

Voluntary Health Agencies

Many voluntary health agencies have exerted a tremendous influence on the preservation of health as well as prevention of disease throughout this century. Research efforts have been aided by their financial assistance. Some of the better-known voluntary agencies are the National Tuberculosis and Respiratory Disease Association, the American Cancer Society, the American Heart Association, the National Foundation for Infantile Paralysis and the National Association for Mental Health.

HEALTH SERVICES WORLDWIDE

World Health Organization

International health work has been carried on for many years. In 1902, the Pan-American Sanitary Bureau was established; in 1907, the International Office of Public Health came into being; and in 1921, the Health Organization of the League of Nations was developed. In 1923, a consolidation occurred, with the International Office of Public Health being absorbed into the Health Organization of the League of Nations.

In 1946, a constitution for a *World Health Organization* (WHO) was accepted by 61 nations. This new organization absorbed the duties of the Health Organization of the League of Nations and the United Nations Relief and Rehabilitation Administration (UNRRA). The Pan-American Sanitary Bureau became the regional headquarters for WHO for the Americas; its international headquarters are in Geneva, Switzerland. The organization's main objective has been to assist all peoples in the attainment of the highest possible level of health. The World Health Organization, as a specialized agency of the United Nations, has been the world's directing and coordinating authority in international public health. It acts as an educational channel whereby health workers may receive the latest scientific and medical information and get assistance in applying this knowledge in their own countries.

Unicef

Just as the children of the United States have the United States Children's Bureau, the children of the world have an agency specially dedicated to their interest and needs—the *United Nations International Children's Emergency Fund* (UNICEF). UNICEF has spent large sums of money on food, clothing and medicines for victims of catastrophic emergencies as well as for children in underdeveloped countries. Programs for the eradication of specific diseases have been instituted.

Project Hope

In 1958, Dr. William Walsh founded Project Hope. He stated, "Hope began not as a job but as a philosophy, not an idea but an ideal based on the premise that we in America did not have the obligation of taking care of the world but rather because of our blessings, to help the world take care of itself. The essence is teaching; the basis is partnership."[17] The name "Hope" signifies *Health Opportunities for People Everywhere.* The project was an attempt, using a personal approach, to bring about a healthier, happier and, it was hoped, a more peaceful world. Thus, in 1960 the first peacetime hospital ship, the S.S. Hope, sailed on its mission of mercy and education. This former naval hospital ship was rechristened and renovated and transformed into a floating, well-equipped, teaching health center. The well-qualified staff, representing the fields of nursing, medicine, dentistry and allied health education, shared their knowledge in a mutually beneficial relationship with their host country. For 14 years many countries received the benefits of this remarkable project and its participants served as the nation's foremost ambassadors of goodwill. This aspect of Hope's contributions to society terminated in 1974.

---

[17]*Around the World with HOPE.* Virginia, Project Hope, 1982.

Currently, Hope's activities are designed and directed from its international headquarters, *Project Hope Health Sciences Education Center*, in Virginia. This unique international learning center is the only one in the western world devoted exclusively to the *health sciences*. Within the structure of this center is the *International Nursing Interchange* (INI), which evolved from the recommendation of 21 world nursing leaders that an administrative and study center be established for nurses. In June 1981, the Inaugural Conference of the INI was convened with nurses representing 21 countries, the International Council of Nursing and WHO. This conference was followed in October 1981 by the first official meeting of the *Advisory Council of the INI* which included members from the United States, Colombia, Egypt, Holland, Japan and Jamaica. This council recommended:

1. convening an International Nurse Research Group.
2. designing an invitational conference to develop innovative approaches to meeting primary health care needs of the elderly through nursing.
3. developing courses in health policy formulation and evaluation for decision-makers in nursing, in the role of the nurse in primary health care, and in the nursing needs of the elderly.

The major thrust of the INI is to enhance the contribution of the nursing profession to the world's health and thereby advance nursing practice, education and research worldwide. The *Center for Health Sciences Information, Research and Analysis*, also part of Project Hope, offers a coordinated system for providing for professionals and the public accurate, factual information gleaned from research and analysis and methods of dissemination of reliable health-related findings and data.

The Peace Corps

In his Inaugural Address on January 20, 1961, President John F. Kennedy urged, "Ask not what your country can do for you—ask what you can do for your country." The Peace Corps has provided an opportunity for citizens to represent their country while working directly with peoples of other countries to provide economic, social and educational assistance and to stress the cause of peace through personal sharing and the encouragement of mutual understanding.

The Peace Corps was launched on March 1, 1961, when President Kennedy issued an executive order establishing the corps on a temporary basis. Through the corps, a pool of trained manpower helps other countries meet pressing problems. Teachers, nurses, doctors, librarians, social workers, laboratory technicians, community development workers, agricultural extension workers, sanitary engineers and workers in various other occupations have volunteered to work for the Peace Corps.

Contributions of Individuals to World Health

The remarkably unselfish and heroic efforts of many medical missionaries have been observed and their valiant work recorded. The contributions of *Dr. Albert Schweitzer* and *Dr. Tom Dooley*, in their efforts as ambassadors of good will, will not go unremembered.

FOUNDATIONS—PRIVATE SUPPORT

Historically the health fields have had opportunities for innovation because of financial support from such private organizations as the Rockefeller, Millbank, Commonwealth, Kellogg and Robert Wood Johnson foundations.

THE HEALTH PROFESSIONS

The health professions during the past century have evolved from having the status of a craft to having that of a profession. The developmental sequence in becoming a medical professional has gone from learning the field through trial and error, to taking an apprenticeship, to attending a proprietary school and finally to going to a specialized school in a university. This transition had a profound influence on the delivery of health service for society.

In 1848, a year after its organization, the

American Medical Association stressed the need for clinical teaching to include demonstrations in order to provide proper education of medical students. Physicians had been more interested in the practice of medicine than in the educational preparation of practitioners of medicine. When the *Association of American Medical Colleges* was organized in 1890, it recommended high school graduation as a minimum prerequisite for medicine. When *Johns Hopkins School of Medicine* opened in 1893, however, a bachelor's degree was required of applicants for admission to the medical school, which offered a four-year program. These two diametrically opposed courses of action prompted the need for a standard in order to establish uniformity in medical training.

The failure of schools of medicine to keep abreast of scientific progress led to the establishment of *state medical boards* during the closing years of the nineteenth and early years of the twentieth centuries. These boards were empowered to examine all candidates and to license those who were successful in meeting the standards set by the boards of examiners in medicine. For some years the boards were hampered by lack of financial backing and by too many political controls.

In 1904, the American Medical Association established a *Council on Medical Education* to investigate the problems of medical education, which had been identified as lack of educational standards, lack of prepared faculty and meager resources.

The Council on Medical Education asked the *Carnegie Foundation* to make a survey of medical education. This foundation was eminently qualified to do this because it had already completed similar studies of law and theology. A forceful scholar, *Abraham Flexner*, undertook the survey. His report, often referred to as "The Flexner Report," was published in 1910 in the book *Medical Education in the United States and Canada*. It was a highly explosive document that shocked and aroused the public to action. In summarizing his findings, Flexner made the following major points:

1. There were too many medical schools in the United States, most of them inadequate and unstable.
2. The bulk of the students were ill qualified. Their education was shoddy, and the majority arrived at medical schools without having completed high school. Moreover, admissions standards varied widely.
3. Teaching in the medical schools was mainly didactic, with insufficient time devoted to laboratory work.
4. Medical schools lacked adequate laboratory facilities to provide students with a learning experience essential for understanding disease, much less a scientific basis for practicing medicine.
5. Students were taught by ill-qualified professors, most of whom were actively engaged in private practice. These local practitioners were not paid by the institutions.
6. The teaching was carried out in an institution that had very nominal connections, if any, with a university.

The changes that were instituted because of the Flexner Report were remarkable. Devastating public criticism provoked an immediate revolution in medical education. The proprietary schools of medicine disappeared, and university medical schools were established. Many of the weaker schools closed, partly because of social pressures and inability to attract students. Many schools gained in strength through university affiliation, and nearly all schools were able to secure financial backing through private endowment or state support. The apprentice gave way to the university student of medical science. The faculty became university professors whose time was devoted entirely to instruction and research.

The admission requirements for medical schools changed and were enforced for all candidates for the profession of medicine. By 1914, high school graduation was required for medical school admission; by 1916 this changed to a requirement of one year of college, and by 1918 to two years of college. A base of broad liberal education was becoming essential for the professional superstructure of medicine.

Flexner's criticisms stimulated a more dynamic intellectual climate. There was a dramatic metamorphosis of the physician from an artisan to a scientist. The medical teaching was patient-centered rather than procedure-centered. The physician accepted newly discovered facts. The numbers of medical researchers and clinical investigators increased, and they contributed important scientific discoveries.

In 1962, medical educators engaged again

in systematic self-evaluation. The trend now seems to be a shortening of the total program of medical education with greater emphasis on humanities.

The Flexner beacon has lighted up over a half century of medical progress. It shines brightly today, for this study revolutionized the whole basis for the education of physicians in the U.S., and in the decades that followed, American medicine shot far ahead of medicine of the rest of the world.

CRITERIA FOR PROFESSIONS

While a Rhodes lecturer at Oxford University, Abraham Flexner delivered an electrifying and eloquent defense of the academic spirit. His famous *Flexner Criteria for a Profession*, which have been used as guidelines for changing subprofessional status to professional status, are as follows:

1. Professions involve essentially *intellectual operations* accompanied by significant individual responsibility.
2. They are *learned in nature*, and their members are constantly resorting to the laboratory and seminar for a fresh supply of facts.
3. They are not merely academic and theoretical, however, but are definitely *practical* in their aims.
4. They possess a *technique capable of communication* through a highly specialized educational discipline.
5. They are *self-organized*, with activities, duties and responsibilities that *completely engage their participants and develop group consciousness*.
6. They are likely to be more *responsive to public interest* than are unorganized and isolated individuals, and they tend to become increasingly concerned with the achievement of social ends.
7. They abide by a code of ethics whose ambiguities have been clarified and interpreted, rendering it completely understandable.
8. They receive a high level of compensation in terms of both money and satisfaction.[18]

This set of criteria was used as a basis for one designed by the Bixlers, which has achieved a wider acceptance among professionals.

1. A profession utilizes in its practice a well-defined and well-organized body of specialized knowledge which is on the intellectual level of higher learning.
2. A profession constantly enlarges the body of knowledge it uses and improves its techniques of education and service by the use of the scientific method.
3. A profession entrusts the education of its practitioners to institutions of higher education.
4. A profession applies its body of knowledge in practical services which are vital to human and social welfare.
5. A profession functions autonomously in the formulation of professional policy and in the control of professional activity thereby.
6. A profession attracts individuals of intellectual and personal qualities who exalt service above personal gain and who recognize their chosen occupation as a life work.
7. A profession strives to compensate its practitioners by providing freedom of action, opportunity for continuous professional growth and economic security.[19]

CONCEPTS OF HEALTH

As this century has progressed, the public's view of health has changed. At the turn of the century, when shortened life spans were further attenuated by constant exposure to uncontrollable infectious agents, freedom from disease was equated with being healthy. However, as environmental, scientific and technological advances were made during the first half of the century, a different concept of health evolved. This new concept is reflected in the 1960 statement by WHO that defined health as "a state of complete physical, mental and social well being and not merely the absence of disease or infirmity."

Ironically, subsequent attempts by individuals to broaden WHO's definition more closely parallelled Florence Nightingale's definition that health was "not only to be well, but to be able to use well every power we have." As if to further emphasize the value of Nightingale's definition, recent explanations of the concept of health have included such terms as "biopsychosocial balance," "adaptive capacity" and "individually perceived states of health." There are also scholars who prefer to avoid

[18] Flexner, Abraham: "Is Social Work a Profession?" *Proceedings of the National Conference of Charities and Correction, 1915, pp. 576–581.*

[19] Bixler, Genevieve K., and Bixler, Roy W.: "The Professional Status of Nursing," *American Journal of Nursing*, September, 1945.

the term "health" and instead use the phrase "high level wellness."

In spite of over two decades of increased interest in the concept of health, most attempts at measuring health have been directed toward negative indicators such as mortality, incidence and prevalence. An exception is Dunn's 1959 theory of levels of wellness, which is based on a hypothetical graduated health–illness continuum.[20] It remains a popular method for determining an individual's state of health, and has the advantage of identifying an individual's potential for attaining the elusive state of optimum health.

[20]Dunn, Halbert L.: "High Level Wellness for Man and Society," *American Journal of Public Health*, 49:786–792, 1959.

RESPONSES TO SOCIETAL IMPERATIVES

During the 1970s, federal government programs raised the American public's expectations for better employment, education and health care. Opportunities in each brought about the development of new skills and an awareness that citizens could both influence and control programs of health care delivery. As a result, new categories of health care personnel emerged, neighborhood health centers were established, and self-help groups came into being. The focus of health services began to shift to primary care. A consequence of the social movements was the blurring of traditional health care roles. This led to the need to reexamine the roles in light of their current value and acceptance.

THE HERITAGE OF NURSING

Events of the Twentieth Century

The early years of the twentieth century are noteworthy for their impressive number of scientific advances. From about 1950, however, we have witnessed an explosive growth in scientific knowledge and an improvement in technical skills as well as social and political development.

Amidst the strife of wars, of financial crises, and of social and health problems, there has been a profound improvement in the overall standard of living. Because of remarkable research efforts in all aspects of health, there has occurred a lengthening of the life span and an increased delivery of scientific health care. The Hospital has changed from pest house to health center and patients have gone from passive acceptance of medical opinion to greater self-direction and decision making.

In the past 20 years of this century the fantastic historical milestones of exploration of outer space and the penetration of the most minute internal structures of the human body have been realized. Workers in health professions have had to recognize that in order to perform their skills properly, they need an education that utilizes this vast scientific knowledge base.

It is against this background that the progress and plight of nursing are scrutinized in the succeeding chapters.

In retrospect, certain societal factors had a significant effect on the development of health care in the twentieth century. These included:

1. social movements, such as the civil rights, student, consumer and women's movements.
2. increased scientific advances.
3. advances in technology.

4. changes in the health care delivery system and the roles of providers and recipients of health care.
5. progress in public health.
6. development of voluntary and government health organizations.

REFERENCE READINGS

Abdellah, Faye G., Beland, Irene L, Martin, Almeda and Matheney, Ruth V.: *Patient-Centered Approaches to Nursing,* New York, The Macmillan Co., 1960.

Apple, Dorrian: "How Laymen Define Illness," *Journal of Health and Human Behavior, 1*:219–225, 1960.

Ashley, Jo Ann: *Hospitals, Paternalism, and the Role of the Nurse.* New York, Teachers' College, Columbia University, 1976.

Becker, Marshall H.: *The Health Belief Model and Personal Health Behavior.* New Jersey, Charles Slack, 1974.

Berthold, Jeanne S.: "Theoretical and Empirical Clarification of Concepts," *Nursing Science, 2*:406–422, 1964.

Besson, Gerald.: "The Health-Illness Spectrum," *American Journal of Public Health, 57*:1904, 1967.

Cannon, Ida M.: *Social Work in Hospitals: A Contribution to Progressive Medicine.* New York, Russell Sage Foundation, 1923.

Danto, A. Morgenbesser, S.: *Philosophy of Science.* New York, Meridian Books, 1960.

Dubos, Réné *The Dreams of Reason.* New York, Columbia University Press, 1961.

Dubos, Réné: *So Human an Animal.* New York, Charles Scribner's Sons, 1968.

Dubos, Réné: *Beast or Angel: Choices that Make Us Human.* New York, Charles Scribner's Sons, 1974.

Dubos, Réné: *The Professor, the Institute, and DNA.* New York, Rockefeller University Press, 1976.

Dunn, Halbert L.: "High Level Wellness for Man and Society," *American Journal of Public Health, 49*:786–792, 1959.

Dunn, Halbert: "Man, Energy and the Life Process," *Main Currents in Modern Thought, 15*:00, 1958.

Fischer, Roland: *Interdisciplinary Perspectives of Time.* New York, New York Academy of Science, 1967.

Hadley, Betty Jo: "Current Concepts of Wellness and Illness: Their Relevance for Nursing," *Image, 6*:21–27, 1974.

Keough, Gertrude: *History and Heritage of the Veterans' Administration Nursing Service, 1930–1980.* New York, National League for Nursing, 1981.

Mauksch, Ingeborg, and David, Miriam L.: "Prescription for Survival," *American Journal of Nursing, 72*:2189–2193, 1972.

McClure, Walter: "National Health Insurance and HMO's," *Nursing Outlook, 21*:44–48, 1973.

McGlothlin, W. J.: "The Place of Nursing Among the Professions," *Nursing Outlook, 9*:214–216, 1961.

Merton, Robert K.: *Issues on the Growth of a Profession.* New York, American Nurses' Association, 1958.

Merton, Robert K.: "The Search for Professional Status," *American Journal of Nursing, 60*:662–664, 1960.

Rogers, Martha E.: "Nursing: To Be or Not To Be?" *Nursing Outlook, 20*:42–46, 1972.

Rogers, Martha E.: *Educational Revolution in Nursing.* New York, The Macmillan Co., 1961.

Rogers, Martha E.: *Reveille in Nursing.* Philadelphia, F. A. Davis Co., 1964.

Selye, Hans: *The Stress of Life.* New York, McGraw Hill Book Co., 1976.

Stein, L. I.: "The Doctor-Nurse Game," *American Journal of Nursing, 68*:101–105, 1968.

Uprichard, Muriel: "Ferment in Nursing," *International Nursing Review, 16*:222–234, 1969.

A twentieth century calendar depicts the timeless significance of nurses' precious nurturing skills in the lives of people. (Dolan collection.)

14 The Emergence of Nursing as a Social Force in Health Care: Early Twentieth Century

Nursing and nursing education responded to the rapid changes in society and to the advances in science and technology ushered in during the twentieth century. The major social movements, especially the women's movements, influenced the development of nursing. The emerging nursing organizations provided a forum within which social, scientific and technological advances were deliberated and disseminated.

At the turn of the century, there was a marked expansion in the number of schools of nursing, and it seemed that this trend would continue. The high quality of many schools was due to the vision of leaders of nursing who were attuned to social progress as well as needs of society. Many schools, however, were of poor quality because the problems and obstacles to progress faced by the early schools had not been overcome. Students still were a source of cheap labor and were exploited by vested interests. The desire of various groups to control schools of nursing (including their students and faculty) as well as nursing itself has been a constant and frustrating issue. The role of the nurse had been molded by the social concept of woman's role in society. Nurse leaders were adamant for the rights of women (they had long been involved in human rights) and were found among the marchers in the suffragettes' pilgrimages (Fig. 14–1). An article in the *New York Herald Tribune*[1] describes an immortal triumvirate of suffragettes who led the march from New York City to Albany to demand the right of women to vote; one of these lead-

[1]Bugbee, Emma: "Suffragettes' 1912 Pilgrimage," *New York Herald Tribune*, Sunday, March 28, 1965.

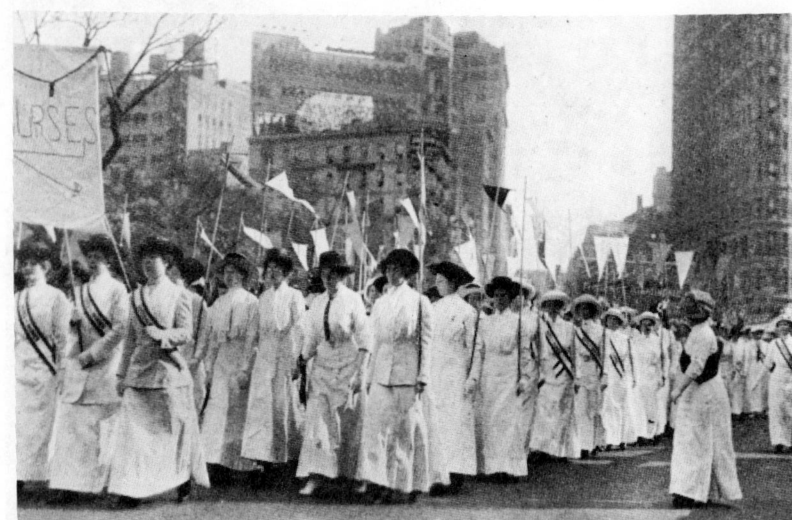

Figure 14–1. "Nurses in Suffrage Procession," from the *British Journal of Nursing,* July 1, 1913. (American Journal of Nursing Company Collection, Nursing Archives, Mugar Memorial Library, Boston University.)

ers was "Little Doc Dock" (Lavinia L. Dock), a member of the staff of the Henry Street Settlement. The nurse leaders fought the male-dominated society in which the status of the physician was superior and the role of the nurse was seen to be a subservient, dependent one.

ORGANIZATIONS FOR NURSES

During the nineteenth century, it was realized that in unity there was strength. This concept had been followed by industrial, social and political groups in forming unions and societies for workers. Members of other professional fields had associations for their members that brought individuals together for united action, such as the American Medical Association and the American Bar Association.

Group consciousness had permeated the professional boundaries of nursing, resulting in the formation of official organizations. In 1887, Mrs. Bedford Fenwick founded the first nurses' organization, the *Royal British Nurses' Association,* (Fig. 14–2). In North America, the first signs of union appeared in the organization of alumnae associations. These groups fostered the idea of cooperation but each focussed only on the schools and hospital of its alumnae group. Later, opportunities of a broader scope were recognized. There was need for the development of nurse influence. Nurse leadership in the ranks of educators recognized that there was an urgent need to work collectively to control and upgrade the nursing schools and to provide qualified faculty if the nursing care delivery system was to survive and improve.

American Society of Superintendents of Training Schools

In 1893 at the World's Fair in Chicago, eighteen superintendents of training schools gathered and held an important meeting. The person who initiated this meeting was Mrs. Bedford Fenwick of London; she encouraged the inclusion of nursing at the

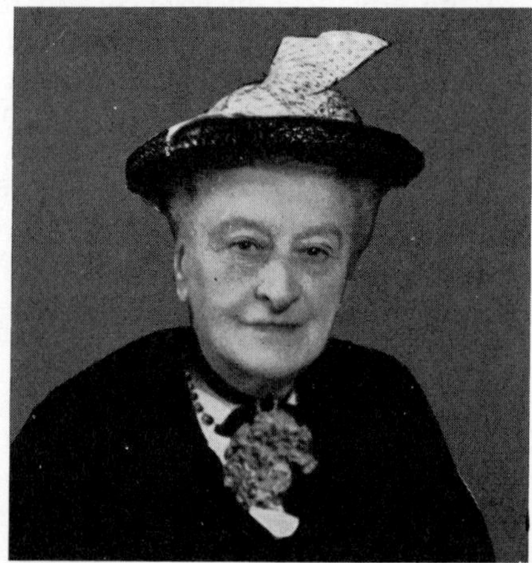

Figure 14–2. Mrs. Bedford Fenwick. During the Greco-Turkish war in 1897, she was in charge of a military hospital. (Dolan collection.)

Hospital and Medical Congress that was being held at this international gathering. Dr. John S. Billings, chairman of the Congress, agreed that nurses should be included, and a sub-section on nursing was provided. The chairman was Miss Isabel A. Hampton, Superintendent of Nurses at Johns Hopkins Hospital.

This meeting resulted in the formation of the *American Society of Superintendents of Training Schools,* (ASSTS), which aimed to improve training schools by establishing universal requirements for admission, a more thorough and extensive curriculum, a longer period of education, shorter hours of duty and better living quarters and working conditions as well as to maintain a universal standard of training and to further the best interests of the nursing profession. In order to qualify for membership of the association, the applicant had to be a graduate in good standing of a training school that was connected with a general hospital and gave not less than a two-year course of instruction and had to hold the position of superintendent of a training school connected with a recognized general hospital. These requirements were not waived for anyone, regardless of her prestige or position.[2]

This ASSTS banded together the educational leaders of nursing in this country and Canada. Because of their efforts, standards for the education of nurses were established and enforced. From the first meeting, which aimed for better education by enriching programs, many reforms were carried out and needed improvements were identified. The dynamic nursing leaders also decided to urge the alumnae association to unite. The ASSTS later became the *National League of Nursing Education* and subsequently the *National League for Nursing.*

Nurses' Associated Alumnae of the United States and Canada

Alumnae associations felt the need to expand their efforts, to keep abreast of progress and trends and to unite for greater control of the position of the nurse. As a result of the determination of delegates of 10 alumnae associations, a meeting was convened, and the outcome of this momentous conclave was the inception, in 1896, of the *Nurses' Associated Alumnae of the United States and Canada.* Isabel Hampton Robb was the first president and continued in this office until 1901. The chief objective of this organization was to secure legislation to differentiate the trained from the untrained nurse and thereby protect nurses, physicians, and the public.

In 1899, the group's name was changed to the *Nurses' Associated Alumnae of the United States* because New York law did not permit the incorporation of representatives of two nations. State nurses' associations were organized in 1901 to work toward state legislation to control nursing practice.

The American Federation of Nurses was formed in 1901 by the affiliation of the ASSTS and the Nurses' Associated Alumnae of the United States. The purpose of the affiliation was to take advantage of the opportunity it afforded for membership in the National Council of Women and participation in the proceedings of the International Council of Nurses (ICN). In 1905 the American Federation of Nurses withdrew from the National Council of Women and joined the International Council of Nurses.

American Nurses' Association

The *American Nurses' Association* (ANA) was established in 1911 as a successor to the Nurses' Associated Alumnae of the United States. It is the professional organization for registered nurses in the United States and holds membership in the ICN. State nurses' associations in all states are constituent units of the ANA.

The ANA is the largest professional organization in the world. It has the potential to mobilize tremendous nurse power for client advocacy and for upgrading health care. The overall purposes of the association are to foster high standards of nurse practice and to promote the welfare of nurses so that all people may have better nursing care. It represents registered nurses and serves as their spokesman with allied professional and governmental groups and with the public.

[2]*First and Second Annual Reports* [1894–1895] *of the American Society of Superintendents of Training Schools.* Harrisburg, Pa., Harrisburg Publishing Company, 1897, pp. 8–9.

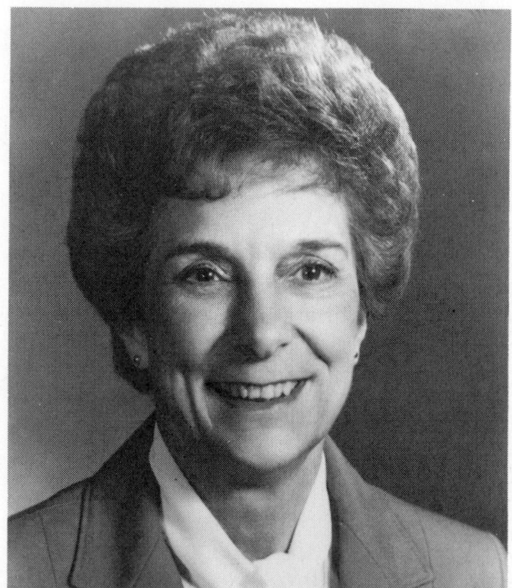

Figure 14–3. Dr. Helen Preston Glass, President of the Canadian Nurses' Association.

Canadian Nurses' Association

The *Canadian Nurses' Association* (CNA), which was founded in 1908, was in reality a consolidation of the Canadian Society of Superintendents of Training Schools for Nurses, established in 1907, and the Canadian National Association for Trained Nurses, formed in 1908. The present name was adopted in 1924. The Canadian Nurses' Association comprises 10 provincial associations and the Northwest Territories Nurses' Association. The CNA has been the official organization of registered nurses in Canada and is a member of the ICN.

International Council of Nurses

An opportunity for the union of all nurses throughout the world became a possibility with the founding of the *International Council of Nurses*. The ICN is the oldest international association of professional women. It was founded in 1899 by Mrs. Bedford Fenwick, assisted by nursing leaders from many countries. Its constitution was adopted in 1900. The first meeting of the council was held in Buffalo, New York, in 1901. Active membership was offered to self-governing national nurses' associations, and nurses in every country were encouraged to form a nurses' association in order to apply for membership and, thereby, contribute to elevating and maintaining the highest standards of nursing around the world as well as receive the benefits that naturally come from such powerful joint efforts. Membership in the ICN consists of national associations rather than of individual members. The council does, however, present citations of merit to outstanding individuals (Fig. 14–4).

Since the ICN was founded, it has held quadrennial congresses at which the nurses of the world meet to discuss professional problems (Fig. 14–5).

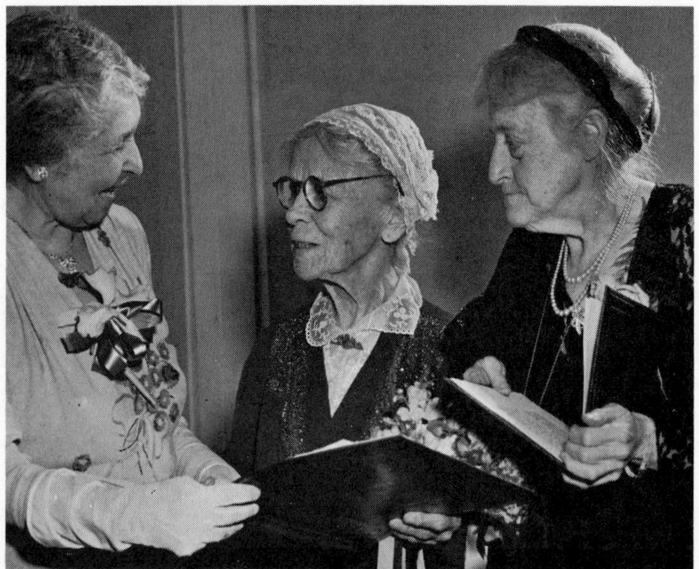

Figure 14–4. President Effie J. Taylor *(left)* presenting citations from the I.C.N. to Lavinia L. Dock *(center)* and Annie W. Goodrich, former ICN president, *(right)* on May 14, 1947. (Dolan collection.)

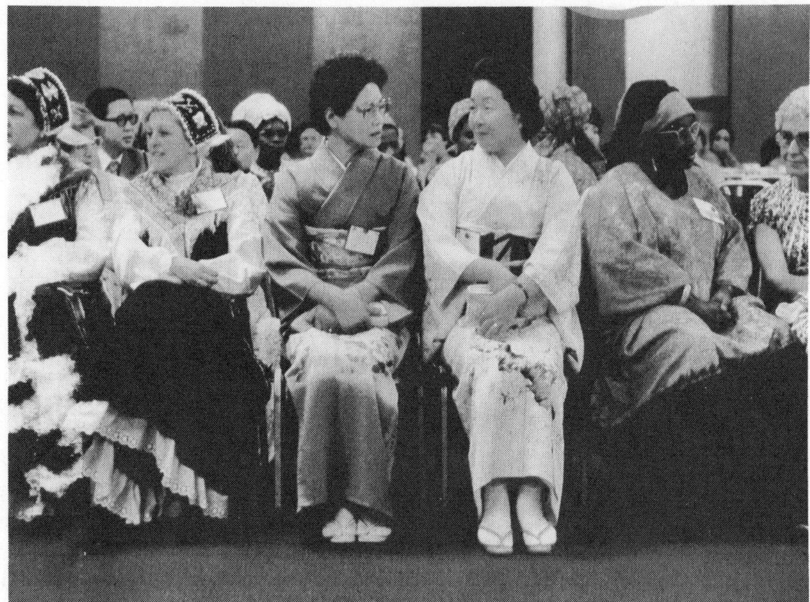

Figure 14–5. Nurses from 93 nations convene at ICN Congress in 1981. (Courtesy of *American Journal of Nursing*.)

ICN CONGRESSES

Year	*Place*	*Elected President*
1901	Buffalo, U.S.A.	Mrs. Bedford Fenwick, Great Britain
1904	Berlin, Germany	Miss Susan McGahey, Australia
1909	London, England	Sister Agnes Karll, Germany
1912	Cologne, Germany	Miss Annie W. Goodrich, U.S.A.
1915	San Francisco, U.S.A.	Mrs. Henry Tcherning, Denmark
1922	Copenhagen, Denmark	Baroness Mannerheim, Finland
1925	Helsinki, Finland	Miss Nina Gage, China
1927	Geneva, Switzerland	No election
1929	Montreal, Canada	Mlle. Chaptal, France
1933	Paris, France Brussels, Belgium	Dame Alicia Lloyd Still, Great Britain
1937	London, England	Miss Effie Taylor, U.S.A.
1947	Atlantic City, U.S.A.	Miss Gerda Hojer, Sweden
1949	Stockholm, Sweden	No election
1953	Petropolis, Brazil	Mlle. Marie Bihet, Belgium
1957	Rome, Italy	Miss Agnes Ohlson, U.S.A.
1961	Melbourne, Australia	Mlle. Alice Clamageran, France
1965	Frankfurt, Germany	Miss Alice Girard, Canada
1969	Montreal, Canada	Miss Margarethe Kruse, Denmark
1973	Mexico City, Mexico	Miss Dorothy Cornelius, U.S.A.
1977	Tokyo, Japan	Ms. Olive Anstey, Australia
1981	Los Angeles, U.S.A.	Ms. Eunice Muringo Kiereini, Kenya

NATIONAL ASSOCIATION OF COLORED GRADUATE NURSES

The National Association of Colored Graduate Nurses was organized in 1908 because of a need to break down discriminatory practices facing black nurses as well as to foster leadership in the membership. In 1951, after contributing many sound policies for the total profession of nursing as well as many leaders whose achievements have been exemplary (Fig. 14–6), the organiza-

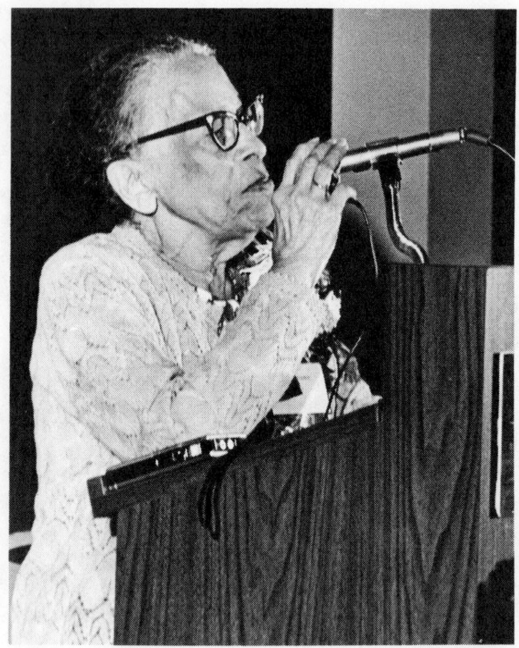

Figure 14–6. Mrs. Mabel K. Staupers, distinguished leader and author of *No Time for Prejudice,* presenting an address at the NACGN awards luncheon of the A.N.A. Commission on Human Rights in 1977. Mrs. Staupers, the last president of the N.A.C.G.N., has received many awards and honors for her great contributions to nursing and health care. (Courtesy of the American Nurses' Association.)

tion was dissolved by legal action of its members. At the Biennial Convention of the American Nurses' Association in Detroit in 1962, it was reported that integration had been achieved in every state so that qualified applicants may join their state nurses' association without discrimination due to race, creed or national background.

National League of Nursing Education

The National League of Nursing Education (NLNE) was founded in 1912 as a successor to the ASSTS. In 1932, the ANA and NLNE voted to make the NLNE the Department of Education of the ANA. Membership in the league was restricted to nurse educators. It was mandatory to hold membership in the ANA in order to become a member of NLNE. The two organizations did not conflict or duplicate functions.

The National Organization for Public Health Nursing

The *National Organization for Public Health Nursing* (NOPHN) was formed in 1912. Its official journal was called *Public Health Nursing.* The membership consisted of nurses actively engaged in community nursing as well as lay members interested in promoting the services of public health nurses. Nurses had to be members of the ANA in order to be members of the NOPHN. Each member received an enrollment number and a pin. This separate organization was needed because the role of the nurse in the community had become much different from that of the nurse in the hospital: the delivery of care differed; community nurses had a greater degree of independence; gave health teaching, carried out case-findings, made referrals and worked with consumer groups.

The Association of Collegiate Schools of Nursing

The *Association of Collegiate Schools of Nursing* was established in 1933 with the purpose of fostering nursing education on a professional and collegiate level, strengthening nursing school relationships with institutions of higher learning and encouraging research. This organization was a constituent member of the American Council on Education.

National League for Nursing

In 1952 the National League for Nursing (NLN) was formed by the fusion of the following organizations: National League of Nursing Education (founded 1912), National Organization for Public Health Nursing (1912), Association of Collegiate Schools of Nursing (1933), Joint Committee on Practical Nurses and Auxiliary Workers in Nursing Services (1945), Joint Committee on Careers in Nursing (1948), National Committee for the Improvement of Nurs-

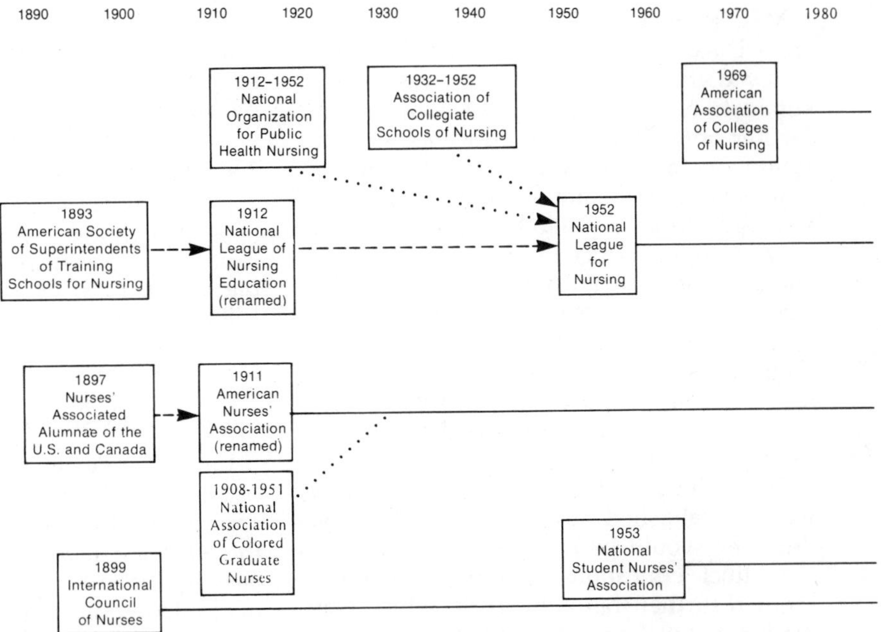

Figure 14–7. *The development of major nursing organizations in the United States.* Dashed line denotes developmental evolution of an organization. Dotted line denotes the merging of one organization into another.

ing Services (1949) and National Nursing Accrediting Service (1949).

State Nurses' Associations

In addressing the Associated Alumnae of Nurses in New York in 1900, Isabel Hampton Robb spoke of the steady and encouraging growth of the organization and the opportunities for achieving the goals of the nursing profession. She commented that it was time to involve and motivate nurses on a local level. She stated, "After deciding upon the formation of local associations we trust steps will be taken to formulate state associations, beginning in all probability with the State of New York." She discussed the need for nurses in every part of the country to work for legislation for registration.

> As many of us know, the question of registration for trained nurses has been long in our minds, but we were also aware that to advocate legislation for nurses eight or ten years ago would have been to "put the cart before the horse." At that time, no *esprit de corps* existed among the leaders in our schools. Nothing much in the way of systematic teaching was recognized; . . . there was no uniformity in curriculum and not even an attempt at a general education and ethical standard. Among the nurses there was no professional feeling . . . there was simply nothing organized or professional about us. Collectively we could neither qualify as a profession, a calling, or a trade.

Mrs. Robb continued her presentation by identifying what the essential ingredients would be for a profession versus a calling or a trade: "For to be a member of a profession implies more responsibility, more serious duties, a higher skill and work demanding a more thorough education than is required in many other vocations in life. But two things more are needful—organization and legislation." She believed that a calling implied a consecrated religious life and a trade involved manual labor. Through the years since her pronouncement, many nurses have fought against the educational requirements for membership in a profession and have spoken up for more "experience" to enhance the manual skills that for the first part of the century caused nurses to be considered domestics.[3]

[3]Robb, Isabel Hampton: *Educational Standards for Nurses.* Cleveland, E. C. Koeckert, 1907, pp. 173–177.

Mrs. Robb exhorted nurses to face the crucial issue of securing registration. She believed that New York State was ideally suited to achieve this project. One reason for her opinion was that educational institutions in the state were controlled by the University of the State of New York, which she said, "does not allow members of any profession to practice in the state until they show proper proofs that they have graduated from some recognized qualified school, and have also passed certain prescribed examinations in the studies taught in these schools. Only to those who satisfy these requirements is a license granted by the regents of the University."[4]

She opined that if similar requirements were established by graduate nurses, "nursing would be at once established on a distinct educational plane." She commented further that New York, which was the home "of the mother of training schools in this country," would be the fitting place to undertake such a monumental task as registration.

On April 17, 1901, the *New York State Nurses' Association* became the first state nurses' association in the country. This association has worked constantly through the years to secure statutory recognition of nursing as a legitimate profession. It had led the movements for:

1. recognition of the profession of nursing (1901–1903).
2. restriction of the use of the title "nurse" (1913–1920).
3. control of the practice of nursing (1933–1938).
4. delineation of the independent and distinct practice of nursing (1969–1972).[5]

The ANA is composed of 53 constituent state and territorial associations in 50 states, the District of Columbia, Guam and the Virgin Islands and over 900 district associations.

JOURNALS FOR NURSES

In the United States there was need for a professional magazine to establish communication among scattered groups of nurses. As early as 1896 Mrs. Robb suggested that the ANA should have its own official magazine.

As a history of the *American Journal of Nursing* recounts:

> In order to secure freedom of expression of opinion or criticism, or advocacy of plan or policy in nursing matters, it became evident that the journal must be something more than an adjunct. It must be independent, unhampered by fear, favor or prejudice in its expressions of truths, as seen and interpreted by nurses. To that end it must be owned, edited and controlled by nurses.[6]

In 1900 a stock company of nurses was organized for this purpose, and $2400 was contributed by hundreds of nurses to start the *American Journal of Nursing. Sophia Palmer*[7] of Rochester, N.Y., and *M.E.P. Davis,* of Philadelphia, both in active hospital work, made themselves personally and legally responsible for the venture. Miss Palmer became the editor and remained in that position until 1920.

On October 1, 1900, the first issue of the *American Journal of Nursing* was published. Since 1912 the magazine has been the property of the ANA and the official organ of this national nursing association. *Mary M. Roberts* was editor from 1920 to 1949; she retired after exerting remarkable influence on all fields of nursing. *Nell V. Beeby* was appointed editor of the journal in 1949. During her administration, the duties of this office broadened in scope to include two new publications, *Nursing Research* (1952) and *Nursing Outlook* (1953). As executive editor of the American Journal of Nursing Company as well as editor of the *American Journal of Nursing,* Miss Beeby carried out her duties with wisdom, and her death was a profound loss to the nursing profession.

[4]Robb, Isabel Hampton: *Educational Standards for Nurses.* Cleveland, E. C. Koeckert, 1907, p. 176.

[5]Driscoll, Veronica M.: *Legitimizing the Profession of Nursing: The Distinct Mission of the New York State Nurses' Association.* New York, New York State Nurses' Association, 1976.

[6]*The American Journal of Nursing and Its Company—A Chronicle, 1900–1975.* New York, American Journal of Nursing, 1975, p. 4.

[7]Miss Palmer began her training in 1876 under Linda Richards at Massachusetts General Hospital. She organized schools at St. Luke's, New Bedford, and at Garfield Memorial, Washington, D.C., and reorganized the school at Rochester City Hospital, N.Y. She helped to organize both national nursing associations, was president of the first nurses' examining board of New York, founded the *American Journal of Nursing* and was its editor for 20 years. She died in 1920.

Before the death of Miss Beeby in 1957, it had become apparent that the administration of the Journal Company was a heavy assignment. *Pearl McIver* served as executive director from 1957 to 1959, followed by *Lucy D. Germain* from 1959 to 1964; *Philip E. Day* was the publishing director from 1964 to 1981, and currently, Thelma M. Schorr is the president and publisher of the American Journal of Nursing Company.

The sudden death of *Jeanette White,* who replaced Miss Beeby, was another loss. *Edith Patton Lewis* assumed the *Journal's* editorial functions until December of 1959, when *Barbara G. Schutt* became editor. *Thelma M. Schorr* was the editor from 1971 to 1981. Figure 14–8 depicts the editorship of the *Journal* from 1900 to 1981. On August 1, 1981, *Mary Buswell Mallison* assumed the duties of editor of the American Journal of Nursing (Fig. 14–9).

In June 1982, *Nursing Outlook* underwent an organizational change and was converted to a bi-monthly publication. Columbia University School of Nursing is responsible for its editorship, but the magazine will be owned and published by the American Journal of Nursing Company.

The Trained Nurse and Hospital Review (later renamed *The Nursing World*) was established in 1888. It was the first nursing

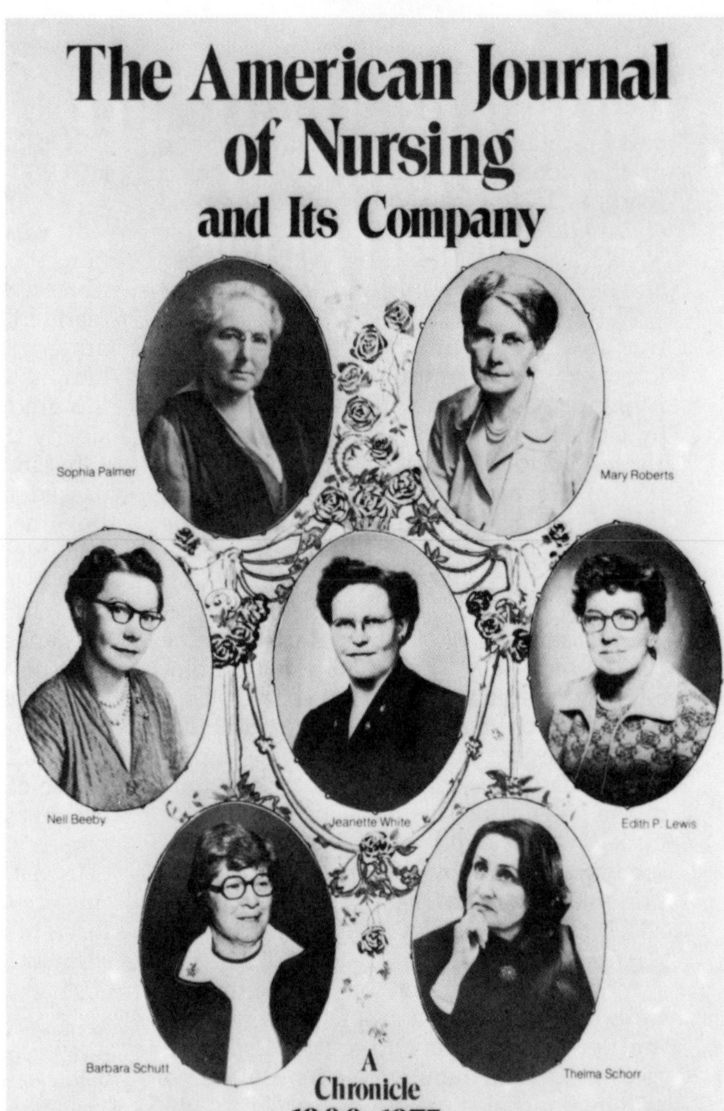

Figure 14–8. The editors of the *American Journal of Nursing* from 1900 to 1975. (Courtesy of the *American Journal of Nursing.*)

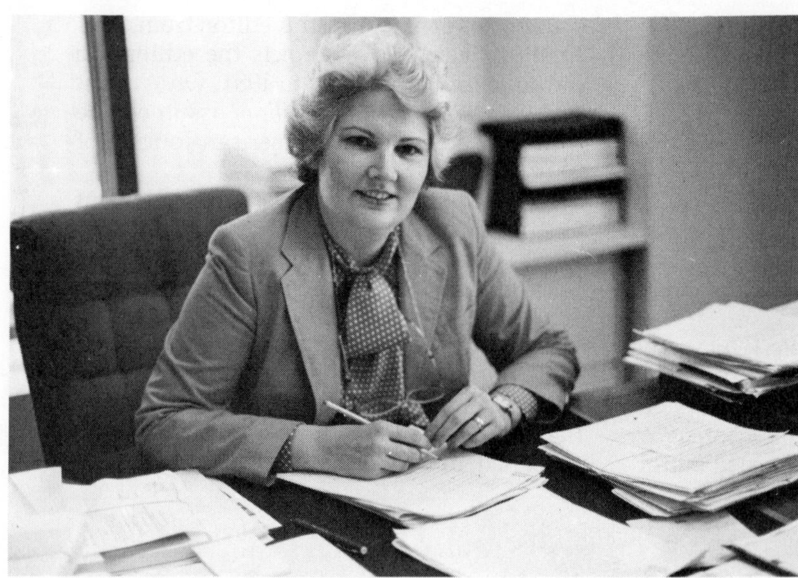

Figure 14–9. Mary B. Mallison, current editor of the *American Journal of Nursing*. (Courtesy of the *American Journal of Nursing*.)

and hospital journal of national circulation in this country and did valuable pioneer work. In 1889, it combined with the *Journal of Practical Nursing* and later it absorbed *The Nightingale, The Nurse, The Nursing World* and *The Nursing Record*.

The Canadian Nurse and Hospital Review was inaugurated in 1905 through the efforts of the Toronto General Hospital Alumnae Association. At first it was owned by a business firm, but in 1916 it was purchased by the Canadian National Association of Trained Nurses. Under its present title, *The Canadian Nurse*, the journal is the official organ of the Canadian Nurses' Association. Since 1959 an edition in French has been published, *L'Infirmière Canadienne*. *Ethel Incledon Johns* was the first full-time editor. Miss Johns had held many administrative positions in Canada, served as a field director for the Rockefeller Foundation in Europe and was director of studies of the committee for nursing organizations of the New York Hospital–Cornell Medical College Association. Miss Johns was succeeded as editor by *Margaret E. Kerr*. The present editor of *The Canadian Nurse* is *M. Anne Hanna*. *Claire L. Bigné* is editor of *L'Infirmière Canadienne*.

In the latter part of the twentieth century, there has been a proliferation of nursing journals pertinent to areas of specialization. By 1982 there were over a hundred nursing journals.

LEGISLATION FOR REGISTRATION OF NURSES

It was essential that nursing organizations protect the public from unqualified nurses. Legislation was provided that demanded the legal approval of schools of nursing, faculty preparation and curriculum, all of which were designed to prepare the graduate to fulfill professional responsibility (Fig. 14–10).

In 1891, the first registration bill was passed in Cape Colony, South Africa. By 1903 the states of North Carolina, New Jersey, New York and Virginia had passed laws establishing a legal system of registration. In Canada the first registration bill was enacted by the Province of Nova Scotia in 1910.

Eventually every state in the United States and every province in Canada passed registration laws. Other countries became aware of the need to control nursing practice by law and to register duly qualified nurses and took steps to do so.

In 1902, an editorial comment in the *American Journal of Nursing* presented a thought-provoking quotation from the *Philadelphia Medical Journal* of March 15, 1902:

> Trained nursing is a profession, not a trade, because it involves the intelligent application of certain general principles rather than mere manual dexterity acquired by constant repetition. . . . Trained nursing is now passing through a crisis

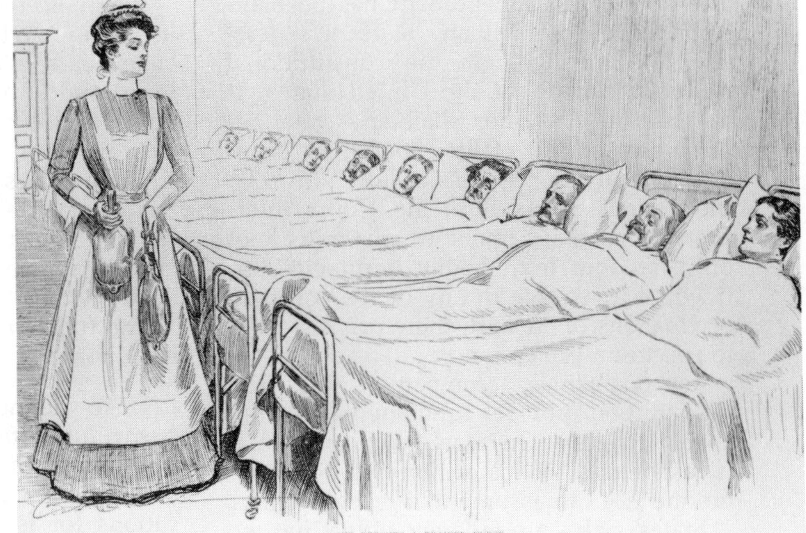

Figure 14–10. "She Becomes a Trained Nurse." In 1901 Charles Dana Gibson used his artistic skills to reflect on the value of legislation for registration of nurses. (Herrmann collection.)

such as affects all professions at some time, whatsoever they may be. The crisis is that for purposes of profit or from motives of economy various persons and institutions are taking advantage of the desire of various women to enter by easy routes a hitherto honorable calling, and thus causing a double injury: in providing a considerable number of unqualified persons with diplomas as trained nurses, and second in so increasing the supply of nurses that the profession—just as has happened to the medical profession—is being cheapened in the eyes of the public. . . . We have found it necessary to establish a State Medical Board, which imperfect as it is, has nevertheless served a most useful purpose. We have found it necessary to prescribe a minimum term of medical instruction, because men who could perhaps in a short time acquire enough information to pass the examination of the state board would not be sufficiently familiar with disease, as such, to render them qualified to practice medicine, and this also has proved good. The question now arises whether in view of the methods by which many so-called trained nurses are educated and let loose on an unguarded public, the state should not intervene, and at least limit an abuse *which is dangerous to the sick* and an injustice to women who have conscientiously prepared themselves for their chosen calling.[8]

Legal Basis for Nursing Practice

The legal basis for nursing is provided by the Constitution of the United States.

[8]"The State Control of Trained Nurses," *American Journal of Nursing*, p. 562, April 1902.

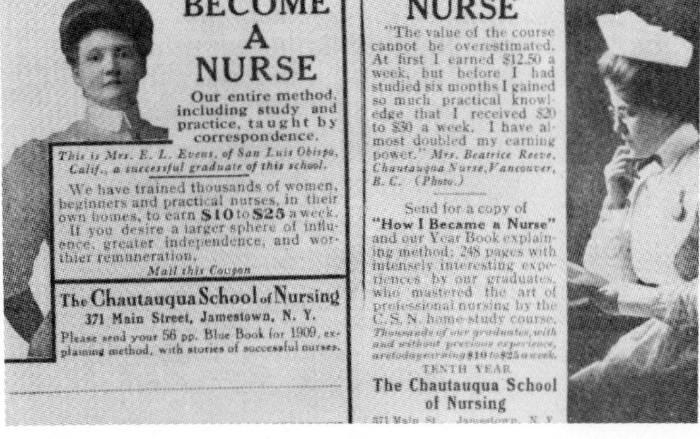

Figure 14–11. Advertisements for correspondence courses for "nurses." (Dolan collection.)

The Fourteenth Amendment has been interpreted to prohibit any state or federal law that infringes on the constitutional rights of citizens of the United States. It also states, ". . . nor shall any state deprive any person of life, liberty, or property without due process of law." In 1923, the United States Supreme Court interpreted this amendment to guarantee not only freedom from bodily harm but also freedom to engage in any of the common occupations of life and, therefore, the right to practice a profession.

Responsibilities accompany rights. The Constitution provides fundamental but not absolute rights. Therefore, each individual is responsible for his or her own acts, and no one else can assume that responsibility.

States' rights are inherent rights that the states did not surrender when becoming members of the Union under the Constitution of the United States. The legislature of a state is composed of elected members who vote on issues and pass statutes. These written laws establish regulations to protect the health and safety of the public. In addition each state has police powers that can be exercised to protect the health and safety of the public by preventing or constraining anyone from injuring the public.

Licensure was designed for the protection of the public. Among many groups that are licensed for the protection of the public are health care practitioners. Statutes define professional practice, set licensing requirements, impose penalties for infractions and establish administrative agencies known as state boards.

There is a difference between the passage of laws, which is under the purview of the legislature, and the implementation of laws, which is the responsibility of the state board. Only the state legislature is empowered to enact laws, and that authority cannot be delegated.

State Boards of Nurse Examiners

The implementation of enacted laws concerning nurses has been delegated to state boards of nursing, which are independent agencies within state governments that are charged with administering the law regulating the practice of nursing.

When licensing boards of nurse examiners were first formed, the members of the state board had to be selected for competency and knowledge because they had to help develop curricula, write examinations, and correct and grade these examinations. In many states the composition of the state board consisted solely of nurse educators, but in some states physicians were also included. Nurses were not members of the state boards of medical examiners.

The functions and responsibilities of the state board of nurse examiners were:

1. To define minimum standards and curriculum offerings for schools of nursing. These minimum standards included admission requirements for students and qualifications for faculty as well as approval of learning experiences.
2. To approve schools that met these established requirements or to deny approval.
3. To delineate qualifications to be met for eligibility to take the licensing examinations.
4. To administer the licensing examinations.
5. To grant or deny licensure.
6. To carry out disciplinary action by exercising the power to either reprimand a nurse or suspend or revoke a license. The decision would become effective after a professional hearing. This professional court was established so that persons would not be deprived of a livelihood "without due process of law."

The first nurse practice acts established permissive licensure, which allowed anyone to practice but forbade the nonlicensed or nonregistered nurse to use the title "registered nurse." The right to use that title was protected by law.

In a 1934 article on the essentials of a good nurse practice act, Elizabeth C. Burgess suggested the following:

> 1. That while the requirements for practice which are written into a law must be minimum, this minimum should be far above what we now accept and should be such that the person who becomes an R.N. should be a fully qualified person, safe to care for the sick.
> 2. That the time has passed when permissive acts meet needs. Nurse practice acts should compel all who make a nursing a profession, that is, who nurse for hire, to be licensed.
> 3. That in setting up provisions for much bet-

ter nursing education consideration must be given to two types of qualifications: (a) personal, which relates to health, education, and character; (b) the professional preparation.

And under this heading we are concerned with the length of the course, the facilities which can be provided, the organization of the faculty and its qualifications, with resources and the curriculum.

Provision must be made for the administration of the law, for examinations, for licences and registration, for fees, for reciprocity, and provision must be made for penalties.[9]

In answering the question of what should be the composition of the membership on a board of nurse examiners, she retorted that "if nurses are to control the practice of their profession, physicians should certainly not be members of the board of nurse examiners."

Miss Burgess felt the need for compulsory registration, and she stressed, "To me a great step forward would be taken if registration and licences were required of all professional nurses. I see no disadvantages to either the nurses or the public."[10] There were many problems inherent in interstate licensure. These problems were lessened with the formation of the *Bureau of State Boards of Nurse Examiners,* which was under the aegis of The American Nurses' Association until 1978. From 1950 until July 1982 every state used identical state board examinations, thus providing an important aspect of uniformity. The boards' tests originated from a test board pool conducted by the Department of Measurement and Guidance of the National League for Nursing. In 1951, the members attending the state board conference recommended and accepted the adoption of a national minimum passing score for state board examinations.

NURSING EDUCATION

When the first three schools of nursing that started in the United States sincerely attempted to pattern their independence in functioning after the Nightingale system, most members of the medical profession were vehemently opposed to the schools because the medical profession would lack the ability to *control* them. These early schools had contracted with hospitals for the provision of nursing services in exchange for educational services.

When expansion of hospital facilities occurred, a mushrooming in the development of schools of nursing resulted. It became apparent that the aims of the schools and those of the hospital were not in agreement. This conflict and the confusion resulting from the nursing schools' trying to serve two masters—nursing education and nursing service—resulted in the union of the two areas, and schools came under the purview of hospitals.

Because of the efforts of the stalwart, dedicated, courageous nursing leaders from the United States and Canada, many education reforms were initiated by the ASSTS.

In 1894, at the first annual convention of the ASSTS, the leaders stressed the importance of planning the entire educational program for the benefit of the student rather than for the convenience of the hospital nursing services.

In 1895, Mary Agnes Snively of Toronto presented a thought-provoking paper that emphasized the need for initiating uniformity of education for nursing by requiring a uniform matriculation examination for admission; specific prerequisite courses; a uniform length of the program in nursing education with a shortening of the workday and week; and an examination plan that would guarantee the possession of necessary theoretical background.

It is worthwhile to read Miss Snively's scholarly paper and note that she encouraged nurse leaders not to be frightened by "those who cry out in alarm against what they are pleased to call an attempt to educate nurses." She clearly delineated the need for a well-planned education for nurses.

At this same convention, Mrs. Isabel H. Robb, when pleading for a truly educational program, questioned the wisdom of the payment of an allowance to students. She referred to the practice of hospitals' paying each student 8 dollars a month for the first year and 12 dollars a month for the

---

[9]Burgess, Elizabeth C.: "A Good Nurse Practice ACT—What Are the Essentials?" *American Journal of Nursing,* p. 653, July 1934.

[10]Burgess, Elizabeth C.: "A Good Nurse Practice ACT—What Are the Essentials?" *American Journal of Nursing,* p. 655, July 1934.

second year. She noted, "We say in our circulars that 'this is in nowise intended as a salary but is allowed for uniforms, textbooks, and other expenses incidental to their training.' " Mrs. Robb then questioned whether this money was not intended as a remuneration for services rendered, and if not, why the amount was increased in the second year when in reality the cash expenses for the student were much greater in the first year. She proposed the establishment of a three-year program of an eight-hour day on a nonpayment plan. The pupils were to receive uniforms, board, room, laundry and a truly liberal education in exchange for the three years of service. She firmly believed that if schools were placed on a scholastic basis they would attract refined and intelligent students. Furthermore, if scholarships were provided, needy but highly competent women would receive an education. She commented, "I am not sure that nurses more than any others who are preparing to enter a scientific profession should expect to be self-supporting . . . and I do not believe that this arrangement would hinder any desirable additions to our numbers." Mrs. Robb believed that the money that had been given to students should be used to employ well-prepared head nurses.

Her constant gentle insistence that new ideas be tried prevailed against the illogical objections of those who were emotionally tied to the past and present.[11]

Adelaide Nutting presented an electrifying report at the 1896 convention entitled "A Statistical Report of Working Hours in Training Schools." This report revealed that work hours per day could total 15 hours per day, or 105 hours per week; in almost every school one lecture per week was given. Miss Nutting asked: "Now what are training schools? Are they charitable institutions? Is it a condition of employer and employee?" She answered her questions by emphatically stating that training schools were really educational institutions and that it was time that this fact was better appreciated. Miss Nutting continued:

> It should not be forgotten that the long hours of duty in wards may reduce pupils to a condition of servitude. It is not for the purpose of giving them more and better training that they are kept on duty so long, but rather that the amount of service rendered to the hospital may be increased and that the working force of the institution may for economy's sake be kept small. These long hours render it nearly impossible for a nurse to profit by the teaching for which her services are supposed to be given and with such long hours the teaching is merely offered as an advantage to attract applicants and is not deserving of any serious consideration.[12]

Sophia Palmer inveighed against using students to maintain service and lower the costs of operation of hospitals and schools. Her resolution to this effect read: "Be it resolved. That this Society condemns the practice of utilizing pupils in training as a means of revenue to the hospital or school."[13]

The resolution was adopted unanimously. In the Address of the President in 1897, Miss Nutting made a poignant plea:

> If we look into matters carefully, I think we shall find that in our profession we have still too low a standard of preliminary requirement, too short a course and too limited a curriculum, and that our examinations are somewhat superficial.
>
> Even if a woman possess many good qualities, without a basis of education and refinement we can never expect to obtain a training of the mind which will enable the nurse to observe, think and reason accurately.
>
> It may be natural that all hospitals should be wise to have their nursing provided for as cheaply as possible; but the time should be over in this country when training schools are maintained with this as their main object. . . . Our training schools should lessen in number, but improve in quality. Cities that are large enough, and have material enough to support two good training schools, should not maintain a dozen inferior ones . . . this subject [is] of gravest importance to us if we are working as we say we are, for a high standard and for the best interests of the profession generally.[14]

The necessity of establishing an adequate fee for service schedule and a salary scale that would be rewarding was presented by Diana Kimber in 1897.

---

[11]Dolan, Josephine A.: "Fusing the Past for Future Action." In *Three Score and Ten*, New York, National League for Nursing, 1963, p. 7.

[12]*Ibid.*, p. 8.

[13]*Third Annual Report*, American Society of Superintendents of Training Schools, 1896, p. 69.

[14]Nutting, M. Adelaide: Address of the President. *Fourth Annual Report*, American Society of Superintendents of Training Schools, 1897, pp. 8–9.

At the 1897 annual convention of the American Society of Superintendents of Training Schools, Lucy Walker, who was superintendent of nurses at the Pennsylvania Hospital Training School, gave a progress report about the acceptance by training schools of the lengthening of the program and the shortening of the workday. She reported, "Only one school [Johns Hopkins] has adopted it in connection with the extended course. The reason for this is . . . that the three years' course is of benefit to the hospital as well as to the nurse, whereas the eight hour day system benefits the nurse only."

In 1901, Dr. R. C. Cabot's article "Suggestions for the Improvement of Training Schools for Nurses" in *The Boston Medical and Surgical Journal* expressed dissatisfaction with the current system of training. In 1903, Dr. Francis Denny's report "The Need of an Institution for the Education of Nurses Independent of the Hospitals" in *The Boston Medical and Surgical Journal* stressed the benefits that might accrue if some educational institution would give instruction to the nurse before she entered the hospital. Dr. Denny encouraged nurses to be educated for a profession. He stated that "the nurse's diploma should come from this educational institution, rather than from the hospital. Its award should represent good work in the preliminary course, together with satisfactory service in a hospital in which there was a high standard of nursing."[15]

In the early part of this century the directors of nurses taught some of the classes, but the majority were given by medical practitioners and were called "doctor's lectures." The focus of the lectures was on hospital-based medical treatments rather than the role of the nurse in nursing intervention. Eventually textbooks for nurses were written by physicians, and later, nurses were asked to collaborate with them in their authorship. Two books were available, however, that stressed nursing care. One was written in 1910 by Emily A. M. Stoney, who had also written *Materia Medica for Nurses* and *Bacteriology and Surgical Technic for Nurses.* Miss Stoney, a graduate of the Training School for Nurses in Lawrence, Massachusetts, held the position of superintendent of the training school for nurses at Carney Hospital, Boston, and published *Practical Points in Nursing for Nurses in Private Practice.*[16] Recognizing a need for assisting all graduate nurses in keeping up-to-date and providing a sort of program of continuing education, she revised her book at frequent intervals. In the presentation of her data she indicated what nurses should observe and what response they should make. She stated that a physician had a myriad of ways of attacking a problem medically but the initial nursing response to a problem should follow a certain, sound, scientific plan of action. Stoney presented the scientific basis of nursing in a section entitled "Physiology and Descriptive Anatomy." She also included the nutritive aspects of patient care.

E. M. Clarke wrote a pocket-sized reference book entitled *The Nurses' "Enquire Within."*[17] In this book, published about the turn of the century, Clarke described briefly the symptoms of a condition or a disease entity and elaborated on the nurse's role. When indicated the nursing intervention was classified further into preventive or curative nursing care.

Isabel Hampton Robb noted, "Not so long ago neither medicine nor nursing were scientific in character. But the evolution of the one created a necessity for the other." In response to written and verbal assaults on the character of nursing, Mrs. Robb stated:

> To be sure there is the side to nursing so often spoken of as menial, but nothing dominated by the mind, and dignified by the way in which it is done can be derogatory; nor need the cultured and trained woman, when the emergency arises, shrink from unpleasant tasks. The spirit in which she does her work makes all the difference. Invested as she should be with the dignity of her profession and the cloak of love for suffering humanity, she can ennoble anything her hand may be called upon to do. . . .[18]

The trained nurse, then, is no longer to be regarded as a better trained, more useful, higher class servant, but as one who has knowledge

[15] Denny, Francis P.: "The need of an institution for the education of nurses independent of the hospitals." *Boston Medical and Surgical Journal,* June 18, 1903.

[16] Stoney, Emily A. M.: *Practical Points in Nursing for Nurses in Private Practice.* 4th ed. Philadelphia, W. B. Saunders Co., 1910.

[17] Clarke, E. M.: *The Nurses' "Enquire Within."* London, The Scientific Press.

[18] Robb, Isabel Hampton: *Nursing Ethics.* Cleveland, J. B. Savage, 1901, p. 35.

and is worthy of respect, consideration and due recompense. . . . She is also essentially an instructor; part of her duties have to do with the prevention of disease and sickness, as well as the relief of suffering humanity. In district nursing we are confronted with conditions which require the highest order of work, but the actual nursing of the patient is one of the least of the duties which the nurse is called upon to perform for the class of people with whom she meets. To this branch of our work no more appropriate name can be given than 'instructive nursing,' for educational in the best sense of the word it should be.[19]

In a period in history when nurses could not teach and answered questions with the familiar "I don't know, ask your doctor," Mrs. Robb attempted to encourage well-prepared nurses to expand their role:

These are some of the essentials in nursing by which it has come to be regarded as a profession, but there still remains much to be desired, much to work for, in order to add to its dignity and usefulness. As the standard of education and requirements become of a higher character and the training more efficient, the trained nurse will draw nearer to science and its demands and take a greater share as a social factor in solving the world's needs.[20]

The plight of the student of nursing was incorporated into one of the popular novels of the day, *K*, by Mary Roberts Rinehart. An editorial comment in the *American Journal of Nursing* castigated the author: "Writers of popular fiction have run riot in the field of nursing of late." While reading *McClure's Magazine* the editor was "attracted by the unusual title 'K' and found another story in which pupil nurses . . . appear. We understand that Mary Roberts Rinehart, the author, is a nurse, now the wife of a physician. We all know that literary license up to a certain point is permissible, but it seems almost unthinkable that a woman who assumed the ethical responsibilities of the nurse with her uniform would use her sisters in a way to, at once, cheapen the profession and rob it of its dignity."[21]

The editorial reflects the philosophy and thinking of some nurses in this period.

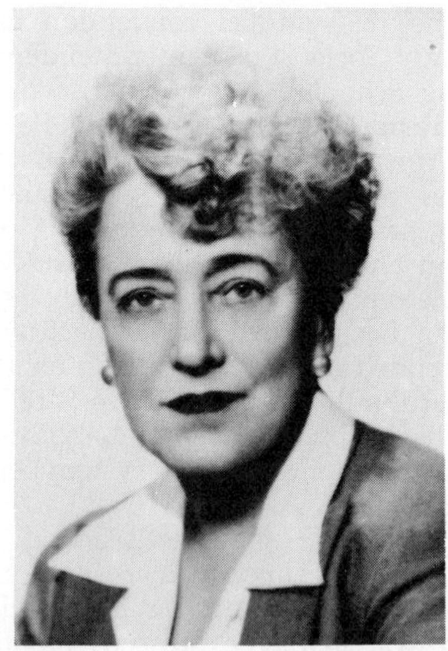

Figure 14–12. Mary Roberts Rinehart, nurse and famous novelist. (Courtesy of Frederick R. Rinehart.)

They were building their own concept of "professionalism" and resented any sign of criticism, especially from such a popular novelist as *Mary Roberts Rinehart,* who as a graduate nurse, described the plight and the "educational" program of the student and shared this information with the public (Fig. 14–12).

Continued Support for Upgrading Nursing Education

In the book *A Sound Economic Basis for Schools of Nursing,* Adelaide Nutting reported the need for a different pattern of education for nurses:

Heavy demands of the wards made it impossible for all students to attend their weekly lecture and it was always arranged that some students would choose to take very full notes and read them later to the assembled group of less fortunate. Lectures came under the category of privileges like 'hours off duty' to be granted 'hospital duties permitting.'[22]

It appeared that an occasional class was supplementary to the work experience or clinical practice. When there was a paucity

[19] *Ibid.*, p. 37.

[20] Robb, Isabel Hampton: *Nursing Ethics.* Cleveland, J. B. Savage, 1901, p. 37.

[21] "The Nurse in Fiction," *American Journal of Nursing, 15*:1075, 1915.

[22] Nutting, M. Adelaide: *A Sound Economic Basis for Schools of Nursing.* New York, G. P. Putnam's Sons, 1926, pp. 339–340.

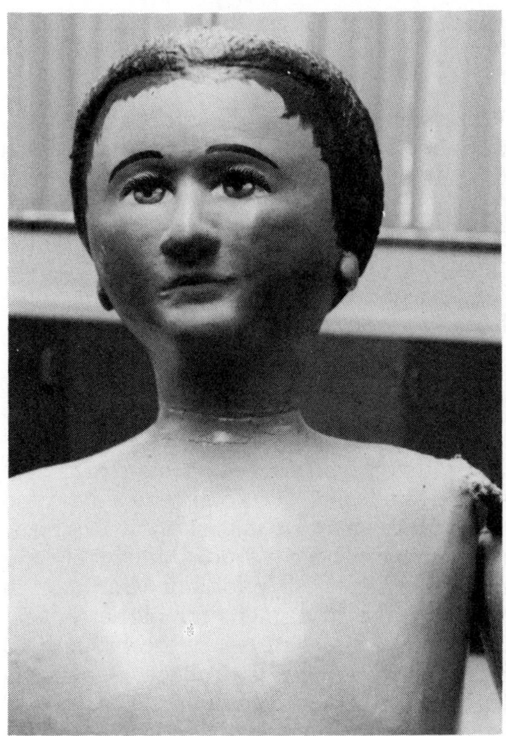

Figure 14–13. The original "Mrs. Chase" mannequin at Hartford Hospital. (Herrmann collection.)

of clinical experience, lengthening the time spent in the wards seemed a suitable solution even though it did not provide enrichment but rather "more of the same."

A scrutiny of progress in nursing education during its first 10 years reveals a change in terminology from "training" to "education," from "superintendent" to "director," from "probationer" or "probie" to "preliminary student," then to "preclinical student" and finally to "pre-professional student" and from "training school" to "school of nursing." The first preliminary courses varied from a few classes to a planned program lasting six months which included biological and social sciences and practical work on the mannequin frequently called *Mrs. Chase* (Fig. 14–13). The first adult Chase model doll was designed in 1911 by Mrs. Chase of Pawtucket, Rhode Island, at the request of Miss Lauder Sutherland, principal of the Hartford Hospital Training School.[23] It was Miss Sutherland's belief that students needed a practice room, later referred to as a laboratory, to increase their knowledge and technical skills (Fig. 14–14).

In 1903, arrangements were made with two technical schools—Drexel Institute in Philadelphia and Pratt Institute in Brooklyn—to offer a course of instruction covering one college year for students who wanted to enter a school of nursing. A student was to pay her own tuition and living expenses. This program was in sharp contrast to those in which students of nursing were paid a stipend to take a course in nursing in a hospital school. (The stipend was for the service that the student provided for the hospital.)

In 1915 at the Eighteenth Annual Convention of the American Nurses Associa-

[23]Herrmann, Eleanor K.: "Mrs. Chase: A Noble and Enduring Figure," *American Journal of Nursing*, Vol. 8, No. 1, p. 1836, October 1981.

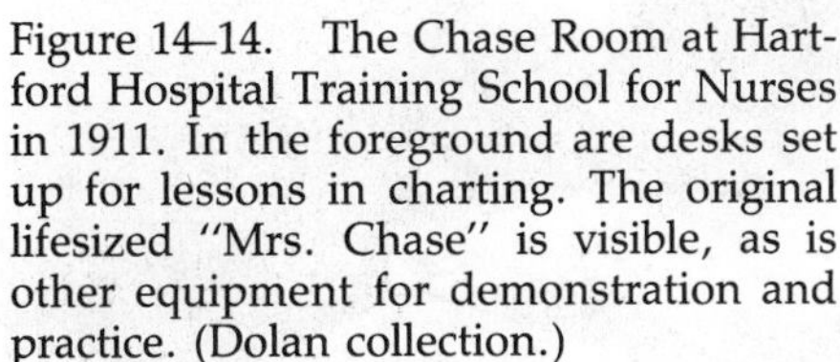

Figure 14–14. The Chase Room at Hartford Hospital Training School for Nurses in 1911. In the foreground are desks set up for lessons in charting. The original lifesized "Mrs. Chase" is visible, as is other equipment for demonstration and practice. (Dolan collection.)

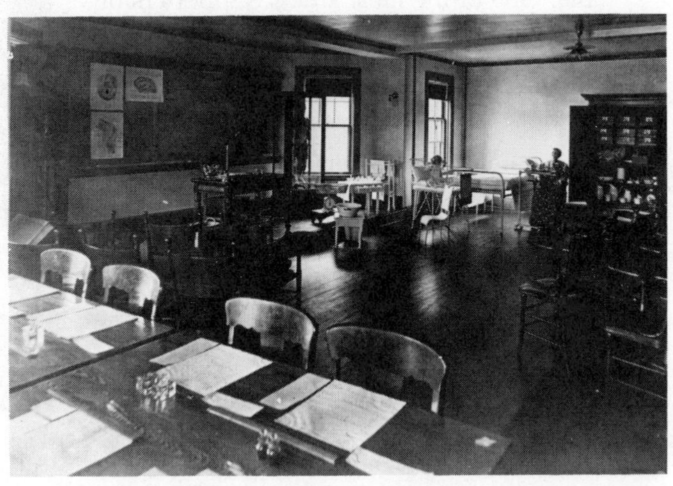

tion, Sara Parsons reflected with deep gratitude on the effect of the new American Red Cross Standards on Schools of Nursing.[24] She bemoaned the plight of the schools of nursing that "were so inaugurated that they proved not only a professional asset of great value but an economic advantage and they are still recognized as the cheapest possible way of getting the nursing work done in hospitals." For these reasons, she believed, there was an explosion in the numbers of schools of nursing. Sara Parsons mentioned the success of nursing in establishing state examinations and registration against the overwhelming opposition of hospitals. She expressed gratitude to Miss Jane Delano and the Red Cross Nursing Service for setting criteria for nurses desirous of joining the Red Cross. It was an honor to belong to the Red Cross Nursing Service, so pressure was exerted on schools to meet their new criteria for membership.

Nurses, both graduate and student, were beginning to rebel against the long hours of service, such as the 24-hour duty assignment. One nurse in 1915 wrote about the "awful indignities imposed upon both graduate and pupil special nurses in being asked to sleep on a cot in the same room with a patient." As late as 1933, some hospital bills identified nursing service charges.

In 1904, a number of lay leaders joined a medical leadership group in attempting to interest well-known universities in establishing schools of nursing as members of their academic family. At that time Harvard University was ready to undertake such a school if sufficient funds were available. One of the most ardent supporters of this project, *Alfred Worcester, M.D.*, decried the lack of nurse support for this project. He made a scathing evaluation of the problem:

> Even from the leaders of the nursing profession we have, with few exceptions, met only with condemnation. But our critics are not to blame. Their own education and training has been in hospitals only, and they fully believe that such education and training is all that is needed to fit women for highest usefulness in private nursing. Under this system, it is true, hospital nursing has been revolutionized, but nurses, alas, have been institutionalized.[25]

Worcester pleaded for a thorough education in "foundation sciences upon which the art of nursing depends, before they [the students] are given actual nursing service in the hospital wards." He also berated the "hospitals which own the training schools" as bearing the main responsibility "for shortcomings of modern nurses."

Nursing and University Affiliation

Another pioneering suggestion was presented by Isabel H. Robb; she advocated the establishment of state-supported schools of nursing. These schools, however, did not materialize. The efforts of Mrs. Robb in initiating the movement for higher education for graduate nurses were brought to fruition at Teachers' College, Columbia University. A one-year course in *hospital economics* was developed, and in 1907 *Adelaide Nutting* (Fig. 14–15) became the *first*

[24]Parsons, Sara E.: "The Effect of American Red Cross Standards on Training Schools, Nursing Organizations and the Nursing Profession," *American Journal of Nursing*, *15*:1008–1011, 1915.

[25]Worcester, Alfred, M.D.: *Nurses for Our Neighbors*. Boston, Houghton Mifflin Company, 1914, p. 70.

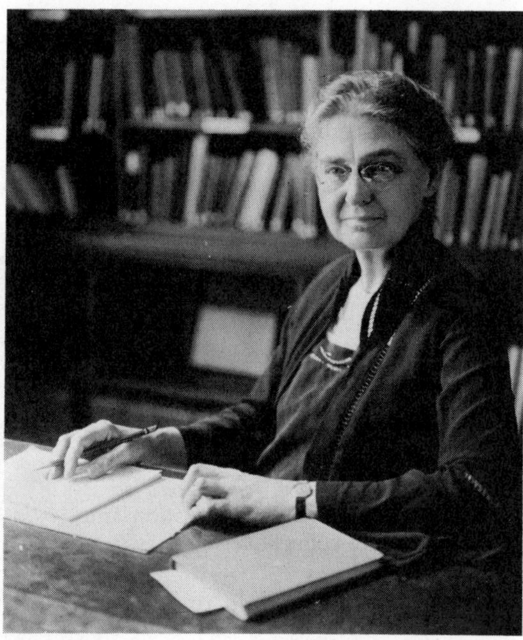

Figure 14–15. Mary Adelaide Nutting. (Dolan collection.)

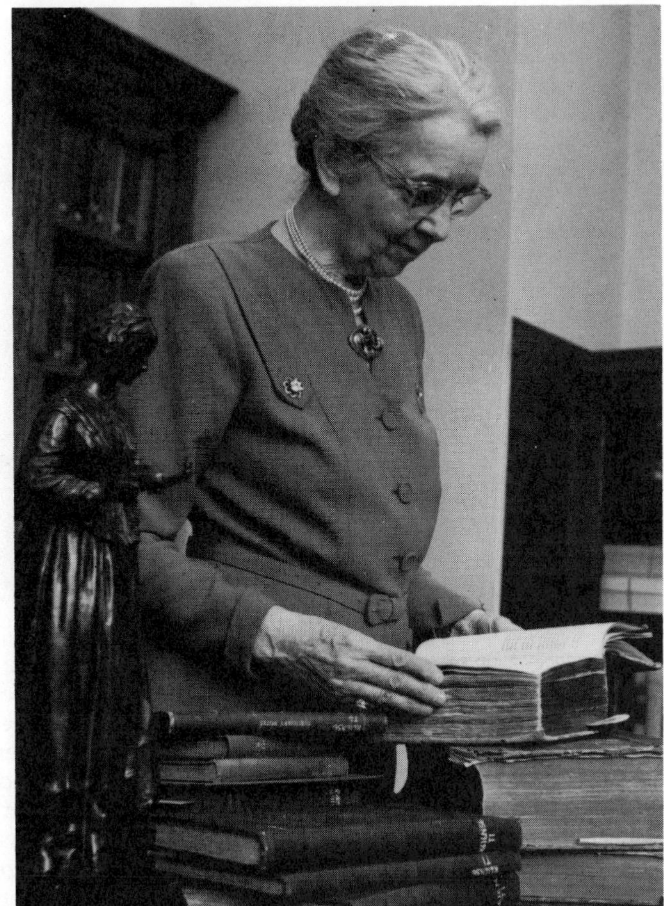

Figure 14–16. Isabel M. Stewart, esteemed nurse educator and renowned nurse historian. (Dolan collection.)

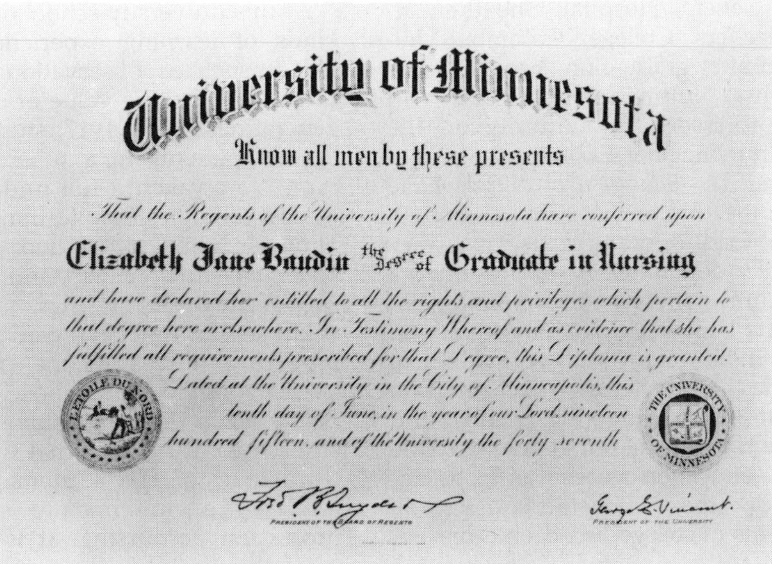

University of Minnesota

Know all men by these presents

That the Regents of the University of Minnesota have conferred upon

Elizabeth Jane Baudin the Degree of **Graduate in Nursing**

and have declared her entitled to all the rights and privileges which pertain to that degree here and elsewhere. In Testimony Whereof and as evidence that she has fulfilled all requirements prescribed for that Degree, this Diploma is granted.

Dated at the University in the City of Minneapolis, this tenth day of June, in the year of our Lord, nineteen hundred fifteen, and of the University the forty seventh

L'Etoile du Nord — The University of Minnesota

President of the Board of Regents — President of the University

Figure 14–17. University of Minnesota's "Degree of Graduate in Nursing" presented to Jane Baudin in 1915. (Courtesy of Mrs. Jane Baudin McKernan.)

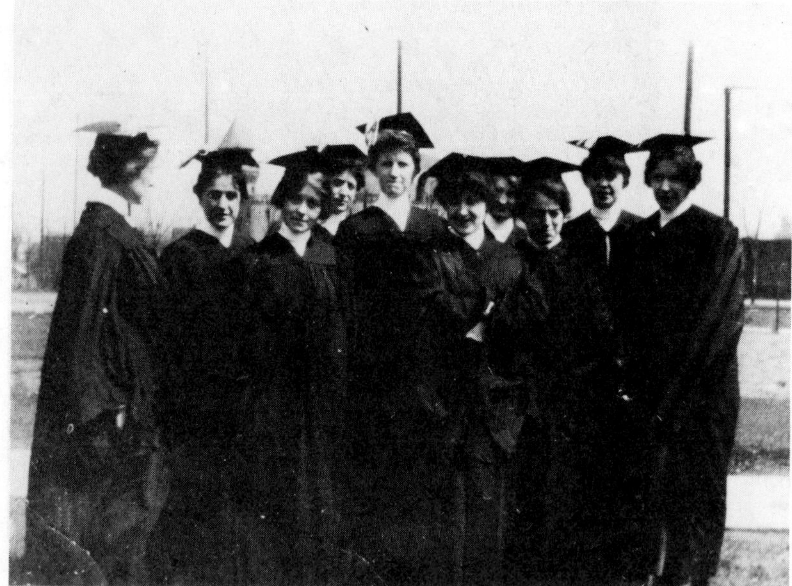

Figure 14–18. University of Minnesota School of Nursing's Class of 1915 participating in the commencement. (Courtesy of Mrs. Jane Baudin McKernan.)

professor of nursing in the world. Her advisory committee was a group of eminent nurses. Under her inspiration the school had a remarkable development and became a powerful influence in the nursing world.

When Miss Nutting retired in 1925, she was succeeded by *Isabel M. Stewart* (Fig. 14–16). Both these women were outstanding leaders in nursing education.

Miss Stewart, like Miss Nutting, was born in Canada and graduated from the Winnipeg General Hospital. She then attended Teachers' College, Columbia University and after graduation, became assistant to Miss Nutting and, in 1923, an associate professor. An authority on the history of nursing, her *Educational Status of Nursing* and *The Education of Nurses* have influenced the thinking of nursing leaders here and abroad for many years.

In 1909, *Dr. Richard O. Beard* presented a plan for a university school of nursing under the State University of Minnesota.[26] An academic environment was provided to nurture the first collegiate-type program for students of nursing (Figs. 14–17 and 14–18). The right of the nurse to receive the same good education as well as to be admitted under the same standards as all other students in college had been achieved. The social and cultural opportunities available to all university students were enjoyed by the students of nursing. The same science instructors who taught the medical students taught nursing students. In addition to the regular basic courses, such innovations as a course in invalid occupation were included to teach the importance of keeping convalescing patients pleasantly entertained. A manual was written at this time to assist nurses in their projects in diversional therapy.[27]

At this university school of nursing, new kinds of learning experiences were provided, such as observation in the dental clinics to learn the value of oral hygiene to general health. By 1917, students were caring for patients in a tuberculosis sanatorium "to awaken a full understanding" of the psychological implications of illness. As Thomas Mann recounted in *The Magic Mountain,* tuberculosis imposed a special way of life on its victims.

Lip service had been paid to the need for preparing nurses in the cultural setting used by other professions, but when Dr. Beard urged the establishment of a university school of nursing that would be an integral part of the academic program, he rendered a monumental service to the profession of nursing. It is interesting to

[26]Beard, Richard O.: "The University Education of the Nurse," *Teachers College Record,* 11:27–40, 1910.

[27]Tracy, Susan E.: *Studies in Invalid Occupation.* Boston, Whitcomb and Barrows, 1910.

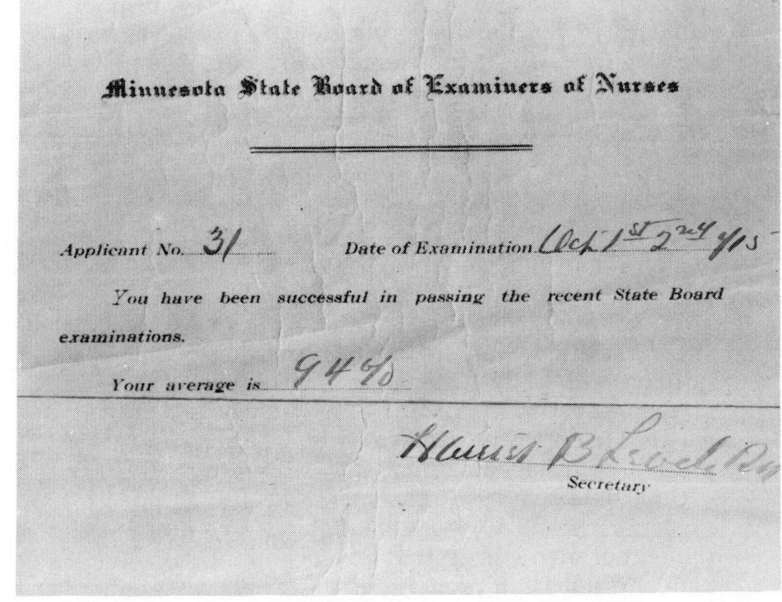

Minnesota State Board of Examiners of Nurses

Applicant No. 31 Date of Examination Oct 1st 2nd /15

You have been successful in passing the recent State Board examinations.

Your average is 94%

Harriet B Leach Rn
Secretary

Figure 14–19. The person taking the Minnesota State Board Examination for Nurses in 1915 took tests in many subjects but received only one final grade. (Courtesy of Mrs. Jane Baudin McKernan.)

note that nursing students in Minnesota took many examinations in their State Board series but only received one grade (Fig. 14–19).

As mentioned, Adelaide Nutting had been a catalyst in this university movement because she encouraged the separation of schools of nursing from hospital control and the provision of financial support for nurse education.[28] She hoped that the importance of the profession of nursing would be recognized by universities.

Two other champions of the cause of nursing were Drs. Washburn and Bur-

[28]Nutting, M. A.: *Educational Status of Nursing*. United States Bureau of Education, Bulletin No. 7, 1912.

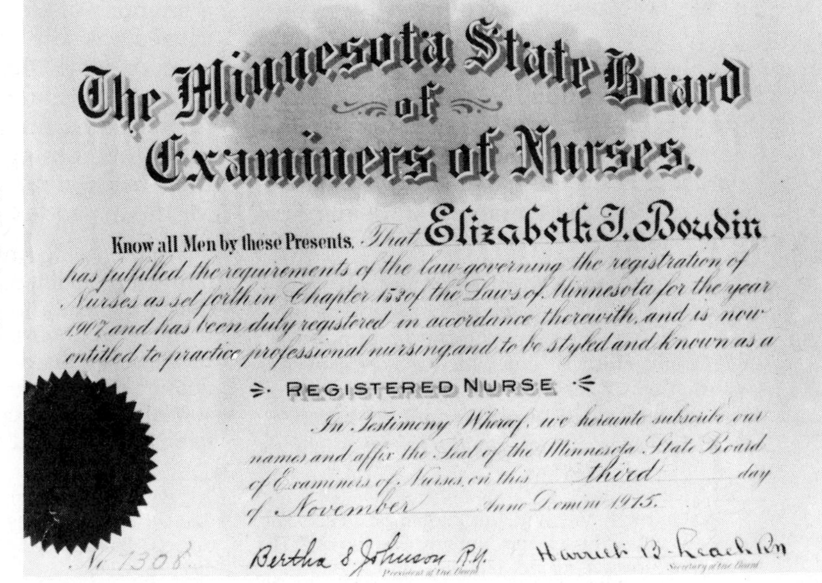

The Minnesota State Board of Examiners of Nurses.

Know all Men by these Presents, That Elizabeth J. Boudin has fulfilled the requirements of the law governing the registration of Nurses as set forth in Chapter 152 of the Laws of Minnesota for the year 1907 and has been duly registered in accordance therewith, and is now entitled to practice professional nursing, and to be styled and known as a

REGISTERED NURSE

In Testimony Whereof, we hereunto subscribe our names and affix the Seal of the Minnesota State Board of Examiners of Nurses, on this third day of November Anno Domini 1915.

No. 1308 Bertha S. Johnson R.N. President of the Board Harriet B. Leach Rn Secretary of the Board

Figure 14–20. Minnesota certificate of registration in 1915. Note the comment, "is now entitled to practice professional nursing." (Courtesy of Mrs. Jane Baudin McKernan.)

lingham,[29] who advocated raising the standard of the nursing profession by increasing the educational requirements for admission. They insisted that applicants' cultural values should be greatly considered.

In 1915, only 10 schools reported full-time paid instructors; in most schools the superintendent of nurses did most of the teaching, and physicians attempted to teach anatomy and other sciences by lecture. It was not until about 1920 that the "nursing arts" or "fundamentals of nursing" instructor existed, and for a long time her position and salary were lower than those of the "science" instructor—a nurse who was not necessarily prepared in biological, physical or behavioral sciences.

Until state board requirements came into existence, each director of nursing designed her own curriculum. Schools might plan and publish a program of classes and lectures, but there was no guarantee that it would actually be carried out.

One of the first publications of the NLNE, the successor of the ASSTS, was the *Standard Curriculum for Schools of Nursing*. The Education Committee of the NLNE worked on this publication from 1914 until it was published in 1917. The objective of the committee was to achieve uniformity in the programs of the schools of nursing and to assist in improvement of both course content and teaching methods.

Studies of Nursing Education

At the Proceedings of the Seventeenth Annual Convention of the ASSTS, Adelaide Nutting presented a report of the Committee on Education, which described a particularly dismal picture of the exhaustingly long hours of nursing students. She commented:

> [These] factors seem to be bound up in the relationship which the school bears to the hospital, a relationship of which the first and most far-reaching effect is that which makes it necessary for the school in order to do the work of the hospital to accept and admit in numbers candidates who do not qualify from the standpoint of age, general education, natural ability, and personal fitness for the difficult, responsible and important work of nursing.
>
> The Committee believes that the present policy of admitting such candidates into our schools for nurses will bring about a steady deterioration in the character of nursing in hospitals, homes, and in all fields of public and private work, and that this must be the inevitable outcome of a continued policy of lowering requirements for admission in order to secure numbers to maintain an unpaid service in the hospitals. The Committee feels that the necessity for admitting such candidates is due to a system which, though sanctioned by years of custom and tradition, is one which is entirely capable of alteration and modification. They believe that in view of this a close, careful and exhaustive study is now needed on the whole question of the education of the nurse, inclusive of the fields of professional work which she occupies.
>
> And the Committee further believes that such a study should be made by neither hospital authorities, physicians, or nurses, but by some scientific body able to bring an unprejudiced mind to the situation and to study it from the point of view of the public welfare.
>
> The Committee therefore recommends that this Society request the Carnegie Foundation for the Advancement of Teaching to make such a study.[30]

In speaking of the recommendation of the Committee on Education, Miss Nutting soberly reflected on the then-current problems as being the most serious faced by the nursing leaders. It was unbelievable that training schools were forced to take poorly educated people to meet the quantitative demands of hospitals, and this action caused, as she stated, "an unrest in our field of work that is pretty general." She commented that the lack of incentive found in the superintendents, teachers and students of nursing schools was because of their being unable to carry out their goals for the expanded role of nursing care.

> Women who enter the training school position, well qualified, full of ideals, ambition, enthusiasm, ready to give the very best that is in them, find themselves unable to go on with their work, discouraged and baffled, through nothing that they are responsible for, but through something that seems to be inherent in the situation and beyond their control.

---

[29]Washburn, F. A., and Burlingham, L. H.: "The Supply of Pupil Nurses and Nursing Standards." *The International Hospital Record*, January, 1913.

[30]*Proceedings of the Seventeenth Annual Convention of The American Society of Superintendents of Training Schools.* Baltimore, Maryland, J. H. Furst Company, 1911, p. 75.

Those who are striving to improve their training schools find themselves meeting actual conditions in the hospitals which make it extremely difficult and often impossible to carry out any reasonably satisfactory scheme of training and education. The very fact of ten hours a day duty in a school would block any good scheme of education ever suggested. A pupil who has been on duty ten hours cannot study, nor even listen intelligently.

We see hospital superintendents thinking that training schools are trying to pull away from hospitals, and we see training school superintendents struggling to be loyal to both hospital and training school and wondering how they can do well by both. In view of this unrest, and in view of the importance of the work of the nurse and the expansion of her field in the new demands that are being made upon her, we are wondering if it isn't time to make some serious study, scientifically, of this situation. Would it not be well to ask some scientific body—not hospitals, not medical people, not nurses, because we are all too deeply involved,—to make a study of the relation of the school to the hospital. Your committee therefore recommends that the Carnegie Foundation be asked to make such a study.[31]

Miss Annie W. Goodrich moved that the Carnegie Foundation be asked to make a comprehensive study of nursing and the education of nurses. The motion was approved by the membership. This study was to be undertaken by an objective person prepared in data gathering and data analysis, like Dr. Flexner. To insure that the study would present an accurate picture of nursing, the committee working with this individual was not to include anyone associated with the delivery of health care. Thus, nurses, physicians and hospital administrators, all of whom could be considered to have a vested interest in the matter, were to be excluded. Unfortunately, World War I intervened, and the plans for the study had to be tabled.

In 1912, nursing leaders discussed the need for liberal arts courses to be available to assist students in broadening the base for the development as professionals. An examination of the frustrations faced by able nursing leaders who tried to reform the curriculum by introducing or enhancing cultural pursuits was presented by Miss Parsons from the Massachusetts General Hospital Training School. She admitted that "the older schools must find themselves trying to crawl out from under the old system, where a new school starting may perhaps make its proper affiliations with a university."[32]

Need for Continuing Education

Edna L. Foley, like Florence Nightingale, was an ardent proponent of the need for constant upgrading of nursing education. She had graduated from Smith College before entering Hartford Hospital Training School and had received the great tribute from Smith College of an honorary Doctor of Science degree. At the 1912 convention of the Visiting Nurses Association of Chicago, Edna Foley as superintendent of the association urged the leaders of nursing to realize that expansion of knowledge and its implications for the nurse necessitated a program of continuing education as well as in-service education.

Each of the speakers at this convention begged that an experience in community nursing be provided for nursing students so that they would truly understand patient and family problems. Miss McKechnie regretted that "the graduate just out of the training school has the hospital point of view solely. She lacks the wider social view. I believe she will not get this point of view until she looks at her work from another side entirely; and besides a new point of view she must get a new feeling, a new attitude toward her work and toward society."[33]

Miss McKechnie also prodded nurses to use their observational and intellectual skills in making a nursing diagnosis and in promoting conservation of health. She cited as an example the family whose breadwinner is unwilling to work:

Such a case brings up the question of diagnosis and how that diagnosis shall be made. . . .

---

[31]*Proceedings of the Seventeenth Annual Convention of The American Society of Superintendents of Training Schools.* Baltimore, Maryland, J. H. Furst Company, 1911, p. 75.

[32]*Eighteenth Annual Report of American Society of Superintendents of Training Schools.* Baltimore, J. H. Furst, 1912, p. 37.

[33]*Eighteenth Annual Report of American Society of Superintendents of Training Schools.* Baltimore, J. H. Furst, 1912, p. 60.

Because of the more intimate relation which exists between the visiting nurse and the family, the nurse is able to get at the underlying causes of a man's idleness, and often to prove that his failure to support his family is due, not so much to fault in himself as to some physical defect or weakness. I believe it is becoming more and more obvious that in relief work, the knowledge of conditions gained by the visiting nurse, and her judgment of the case, must be taken into account in the making of every diagnosis, and in planning the treatment for every dependent family. The visiting nurse who believes that conservation of health and prevention of disease are the foundations upon which the wealth of the nation rests, is, while recognizing human frailties, to give friendly assistance and advice in obtaining employment, together with adequate aid.[34]

This story exemplifies the idea of helping people to help themselves. Miss McKechnie held that in order to provide the most complete plan of nursing care, the nurse must "keep up with all the wonderful developments of her time, and be gaining knowledge every day, every month, and every year as long as she is actively at work."[35]

The nurse educators recognized the need for nurses to have a broad educational and experiential base but reported the inability to provide these learning opportunities because of commitment to the hospitals with which they had become an integral part. The nurse educators discovered that when a community experience was permitted, patient care improved because "it is of very great benefit to the pupils in the consideration of their patients in the hospital. They appreciated their home situation"[36] and could provide a much more meaningful plan for nursing care.

Scientific management, a means of providing more time by using it more efficiently, was studied. The leaders of nursing were aware of the disastrous trap into which nurses were falling by assuming non-nursing tasks and leaving less time for nursing care activities. The need for nursing input in the design of buildings, equipment, new appliances and modern conveniences was discussed. Miss Giles asserted:

Scientific management can only be accomplished in a building erected on scientific lines, with the proper lighting, heating and ventilating plants, and with such arrangement of its apartments as shall best serve its purpose for the class of cases treated; the building being so constructed as to conserve the time, health, strength and nerve force of those who are engaged in this most interesting, absorbing and splendid work [of nursing].[37]

Miss Giles pleaded that the chance to aid in hospital design be given to nurses who know the *how* and *why* of hospital construction instead of persons whose social, political or financial prominence provided this opportunity. She quoted a case of a society woman who was a member of the board of trustees of a hospital and who, because of her abysmal ignorance of the workings of a hospital, entered the school of nursing and completed the course. Upon graduation, she asked to serve on the board again and was informed that "they feared her education and knowledge of hospital work would prejudice her in favor of the nursing staff. This young woman, when truly qualified . . . was deemed unworthy by those who had been her co-workers in the days of her real ignorance of hospital management."[38]

Miss Giles concluded by requesting that nurses realize that:

The structure should be an expression of its purpose; a hospital should stand for health, hygiene, strength, rest; a veritable refuge for those who seek its protection, cure, and care. . . .

As for equipment, it should be complete, and it is only complete when the institution can meet every demand made upon it. There should be everything necessary, in order that its staff of workers may use their skill and knowledge to the best advantage.[39]

In focusing on the paucity of properly prepared nurses, Miss Giles noted that it "is but false economy that the inadequate supply of nurses so often interferes with the education of the nurse, the welfare of the patient, and the reputation of the hospital."[40]

The Annual Reports of the ASSTS are replete with the comments of nurses who en-

[34] *Ibid.*, pp. 60–61.

[35] *Eighteenth Annual Report of American Society of Superintendents of Training Schools.* Baltimore, J. H. Furst, 1912, p. 62.

[36] *Ibid.*, p. 64.

[37] *Ibid.*, p. 104.

[38] *Eighteenth Annual Report of American Society of Superintendents of Training Schools.* Baltimore, J. H. Furst, 1912, p. 105.

[39] *Ibid.*, p. 106.

[40] *Ibid.*, p. 108.

couraged the consideration of ways of cutting costs for the hospital. The willingness with which some nurses took on non-nursing tasks is reflected in the report of savings to the hospital by such projects as making soap and ink.[41]

The famous scientific management specialist Frank Gilbreth was invited to address the leaders of nursing, and in 1912, he presented a paper on the application of scientific principles of management to the work of the nurse. He recommended that an analysis of nursing activities be conducted by an expert in time and motion study. Some nurses present believed that during the study greater speed would be required on their part in carrying out their activities. Mr. Gilbreth disabused them of this notion and emphasized the need for more labor-saving devices, for rest periods, for planning before performing and for assignment "to each worker of that work for which he is best suited" and said that it was waste of energy and lack of the right incentive that prevented the production of satisfying results in one's daily work.

Some of the recurrent issues that are observed in the annual reports of these very able educators include: the need for financial assistance for students; the importance of evaluative examinations for pre-admission as well as to measure achievement; the comparable value of theory and practice; the necessity of changing the status of the student of nursing from employee of the hospital to student; the disapproval of lowering nursing care standards by having inadequately prepared nurses employed by hospitals; the necessity for mandatory licensure in all states; the importance of making nursing a satisfying endeavor; the obligation of freeing nursing from hospital control; the desire for inclusion of programs of nursing within a university setting; and the significance of having a study of nursing and nursing education made by an impartial but knowledgeable group of national leaders free from paramedical or hospital manipulation.

Central schools were fairly common and successful in Europe. In them, preliminary nursing students from several schools received class instruction at one place, often at a university, under expert teachers. In this country such schools began (1900 to 1910) as affiliates of technical schools, colleges or other nursing schools.

Early in this century New York State established certain standards for accrediting its schools of nursing. Because most states had no registration laws and no boards of examiners at the time, it gradually became the custom for schools in other states to apply to New York for registration, thereby enabling them to prove that they were meeting the requirements of at least one group of nursing authorities.

THE ESTABLISHMENT OF MILITARY NURSING

At the close of the Spanish-American War, Dr. Anita McGee focussed her efforts on building the foundations for the Army Nurse Corps. It was through her efforts, with the support of the Nurses' Associated Alumnae (now the ANA), that the Army Reorganization Bill was written, which, when passed by Congress in 1901, established the *Army Nurse Corps* as a branch of the Army Medical Service. Nurses received letters of appointment and agreed to serve three years, but their functions and military status were not defined.

Dita H. Kinney, who was educated at Mills College in California and was a graduate of Massachusetts General Hospital, became Superintendent of the Corps (1901 to 1909). The second superintendent (1909–1912) was *Jane A. Delano,* a graduate of Bellevue, where she had been superintendent of nurses. Her leadership ability can be seen in her many accomplishments; she organized the *American Red Cross Nursing Service,* which included the surgeons general of the Army and Navy in its membership. She eventually resigned from the Army Nurse Corps to become the full-time director (without salary) of the Department of Nursing of the American Red Cross.

The major accomplishment of the Department of Nursing of the American Red Cross was the development of a system by which a group of member nurses could be relied upon to form a *reserve* both for military service and for emergency service with the American Red Cross. In order to join this reserve group, a nurse had to be a member of the ANA and the Army Nurse

[41]Dolan, Josephine A.: "Fusing The Past For Future Action." In *Three Score Years and Ten,* New York, National League for Nursing, 1963, p. 10.

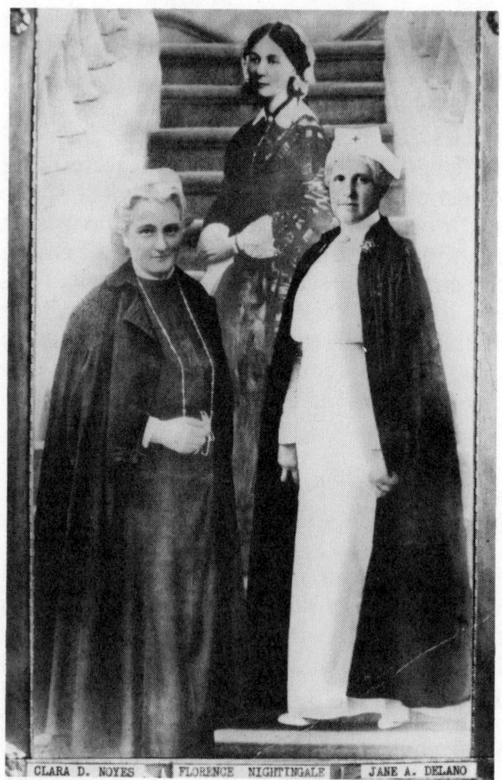

Figure 14–21. Two directors of the American Red Cross Nursing Service, Jane A. Delano, director from 1909 to 1919 *(right)* and Clara D. Noyes, director from 1919 to 1936 *(left)*. The inspirational force of Florence Nightingale is represented by her picture behind them. (Dolan collection.)

Corps as well as the American Red Cross Nursing Service. Members also had to be graduates of schools whose standards were well above those set by the state boards of nurse examiners.

Jane A. Delano directed the American Red Cross Nursing Service from 1909 to 1919. She was succeeded by Clara D. Noyes (Fig. 14–21), who left her position as director of nurses at Bellevue and Allied Hospitals in New York City. She was the current president of the NLNE. She served as its director from 1919 to 1936.

In May of 1908, the *Nurse Corps* of the *United States Navy* was established by act of Congress. *Esther Voorhees Hasson* was appointed first superintendent in August, and by October of that year the first 20 nurses had reported to the United States Naval Hospital, Washington D.C., for orientation and duty. The corps grew in number, and the members were assigned to naval hospitals.

In 1910, certain members of the Navy Nurse Corps were given assignments to serve outside the United States. By 1911, those nurses who were stationed at Guam had established a school of nursing for young native women in conjunction with the Navy's native hospital. The educational efforts of the members of the Navy Nurse Corps are also evident in other schools of nursing they organized, such as the one in Samoa.

WORLD WAR I

World War I was to create a huge demand for nurses, open up new fields of specialization, accelerate the educational processes that were already under way and awaken in the public a consciousness of the importance of good nursing.

For the first time in history, an adequate number of carefully selected nurses was available for military service. The vision and foresight of Jane Delano of the American Red Cross Nursing Service was responsible for this reservoir of nurses.

When war broke out in August 1914, no one thought that it would last more than a few months, but the American Red Cross immediately sent units of physicians and nurses to help in six countries of Europe. When the United States came into the war in 1917, the Red Cross Nursing Service became the reserve of the Army and Navy (Fig. 14–22).

At the request of the Queen of Bulgaria, *Helen Scott Hay,* of the Illinois Training School, Chicago, went overseas just before the war to establish a school of nursing. She remained as chief nurse of the American Red Cross in the Balkans and later in 1921 was chief nurse of the American Red Cross in Europe.

As the war went on and country after country was drawn into it, and millions of men became involved, the medical and nursing resources of the world were taxed to their utmost. Eventually, the personnel of civilian hospitals in every country were seriously depleted, and the sick civilians suffered from neglect.

The fighting was chiefly trench warfare, different from the modes used in previous

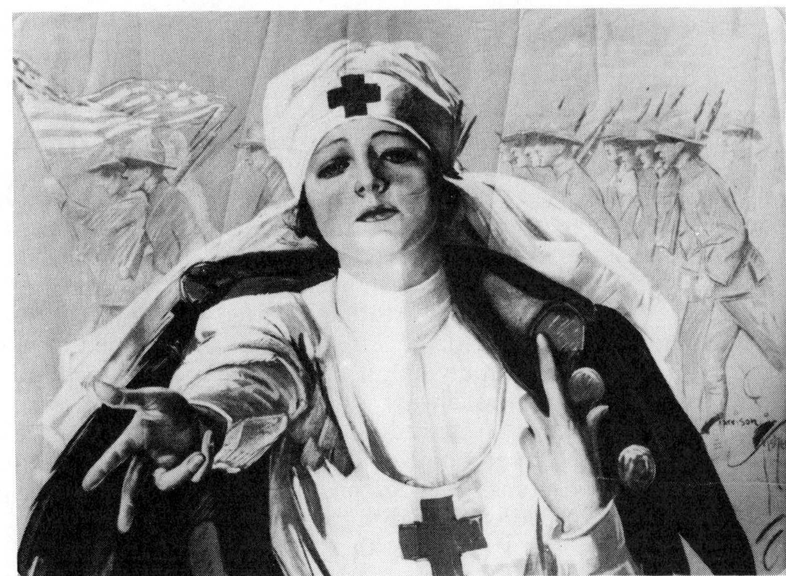

Figure 14–22. World War I recruitment poster by Harrison Fisher. (Herrmann collection.)

wars. The wounded went in a continuous stream from first aid station or field hospital to evacuation hospital (10 miles back), and within 24 hours to base hospitals, still farther away. There were no women nurses at the front, either in first aid stations or field hospitals. France, England and the United States each maintained separate hospitals; cooperation was always good. In addition to military hospitals, there were numerous auxiliary hospitals, often supported by private funds, in cities or distant villages, in the castles, chateaux or homes of the wealthy. In these hospitals the staff was composed of women, trained and untrained, and of men too old or unfit for the army, who often worked at no salary.

The *American Ambulance* at Paris, a private unit, included some famous surgeons and served throughout the war. From June 1915, Harvard University had a medical unit with the British in France, which remained there even after the war. Harvard's second unit arrived after America had entered the war.

Many other units such as the University of Minnesota–Mayo Clinic unit also responded to the call for assistance (Fig. 14–23). Two health catastrophes at this time stand out. The epidemic of typhus in Siberia in 1915, involving half a million civilians, was like a repetition of medieval days. The cause of typhus was discovered during the epidemic by Scottish and American doctors. A unit of American nurses served through that terrible time. In 1918, an epidemic of influenza became a pandemic as it reached France, the United States and other parts of the world. As their doctors and nurses dropped out with the infection, Army and civilian hospitals struggled with a dwindling staff until the

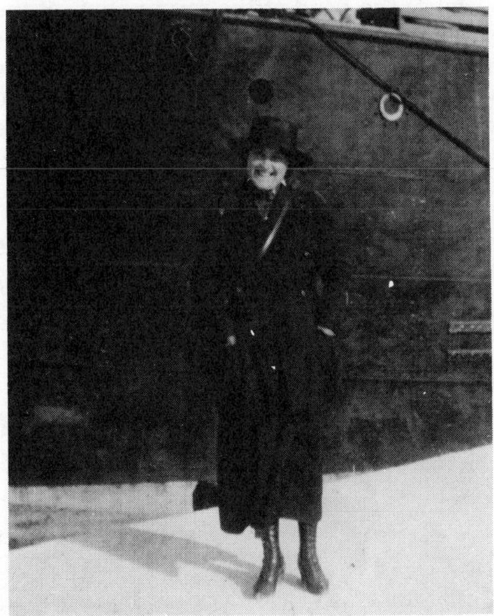

Figure 14–23. Elizabeth Jane Baudin of the University of Minnesota–Mayo Clinic Unit ready to board the steamer to be taken to her destination in the theater of operations of World War I. (Courtesy of Mrs. Jane Baudin McKernan.)

plight of both the servicemen and their families at home was pitiful.

Since trench warfare was the rule, most wounds were caused by shrapnel, a few by bombs and almost none by bullets. Wounds of the head and face were common. Poison gases were used for at least three years, and the men who survived them often never recovered from their effects. Mustard gas caused the greatest agony. The Carrel-Dakin method for treating infected wounds was developed.

Since so many supply ships were torpedoed and there was always doubt about supplies arriving, American doctors and nurses learned to economize. The value of well-prepared nurses was demonstrated as in the days of Florence Nightingale. Graduate nurses, accustomed as they were to emergencies and to group work, stepped into war conditions and adjusted themselves unhesitatingly to a new environment. Great problems were involved in providing sanitation for armies constantly on the move, dealing with communicable diseases, caring for severely damaged tissue and coping with the unusual results of "shell shock." In previous wars there had been well-defined battles that demanded collecting and caring for the wounded and burial of the dead at the termination of the battle. In this war, the so-called battles lasted for days, the dead were buried as best they could be or not at all, and the wounded were rescued under fire. There was always a stream of wounded, sometimes swelling, sometimes thinning, but never ceasing.

The members of the Navy Nurse Corps were utilized during World War I. The first Navy nurses assigned for transport duty reported aboard the U.S.S. George Washington, on which President Wilson sailed to France in 1918. The first Navy nurses to serve on board a hospital ship did so in 1920 aboard the U.S.S. Relief.

Although the nurses of World War I seemed to receive less public recognition in the United States than elsewhere, they had in their hearts the consciousness that they had done well and had the gratitude of the men. These nurses were honored in popular songs, such as "I Don't Want To Get Well" and "A Rose That Blooms in No Man's Land" (Fig. 14–24). The nurses felt great pride to have served in this historic war. "Never before had such a thing occurred, the sending across three thousand miles of danger-strewn seas of ten thousand soldier-women, to be part of a great expeditionary force." Praise came from General John Pershing in a letter addressed to the women of the American Expeditionary Forces:

> While the achievements of American Arms are still fresh in our memories, I desire to express my sincere appreciation of the work done by the women of the American Expeditionary Forces. The part played by women in winning the war has been an important one. Whether ministering to the sick or wounded, or engaged in the innumerable activities requiring your aid,

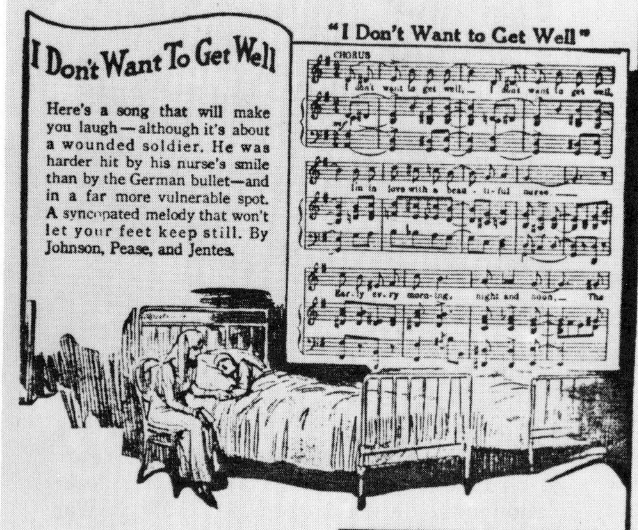
I Don't Want To Get Well
Here's a song that will make you laugh—although it's about a wounded soldier. He was harder hit by his nurse's smile than by the German bullet—and in a far more vulnerable spot. A syncopated melody that won't let your feet keep still. By Johnson, Pease, and Jentes.
"I Don't Want to Get Well"
CHORUS

Figure 14–24. Music as a form of tribute to the nurses of World War I. (Herrmann collection.)

the cheerfulness, loyalty and efficiency which have characterized your efforts deserve the highest praise. You have added new laurels to the already splendid record of American womanhood.

It is a privilege to testify that your glorious accomplishments in the war have given you a new place in the hearts of officers and men of the Army, and have earned for you the admiration of a grateful nation.

World War I made both military authorities and the public conscious of their dependence on nurses. An epidemic of pneumonia in 1917–1918 and the pandemic outbreak of influenza in 1918 emphasized the need for well-prepared nurses.

Army School of Nursing

In order to recruit many women who were motivated to study nursing, the *Army School of Nursing,* also known as the *Army Training School,* was organized in 1918 with *Annie W. Goodrich* as dean (Fig. 14–25). She was the originator of the plan for an Army school of nursing. Anna Jammé was her assistant. Established in 1918 as a war measure, the school was intended to be a permanent organization (Figs. 14–26 and 14–27). The course lasted for three years, and nine months' credit was given to college graduates. The work was centered in the Army hospitals, with affiliations in civilian hospitals. At the height of war enthusiasm, the applicants numbered in the thousands.

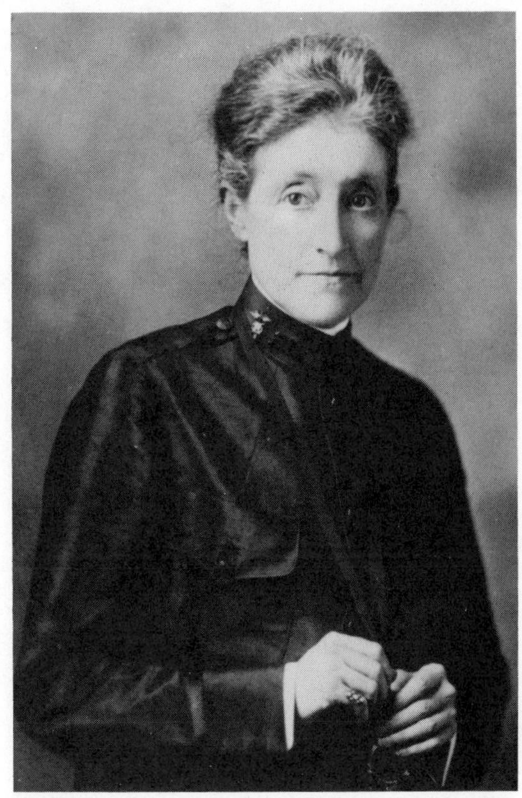

Figure 14–25. Annie W. Goodrich, dean of the Army School of Nursing. (Dolan collection.)

The first graduating class, in 1921, consisted of 500, with 400 graduating at the Walter Reed Hospital, Washington, D.C., and 100 at the Letterman Hospital, San Francisco (Fig. 14–28). It was unquestion-

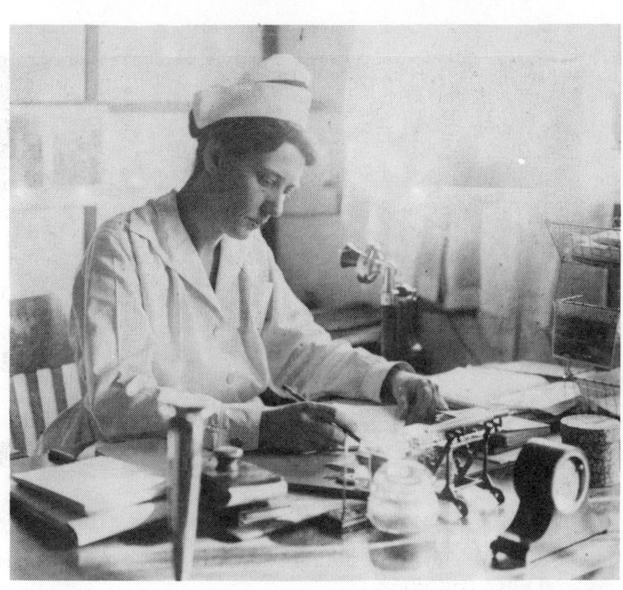

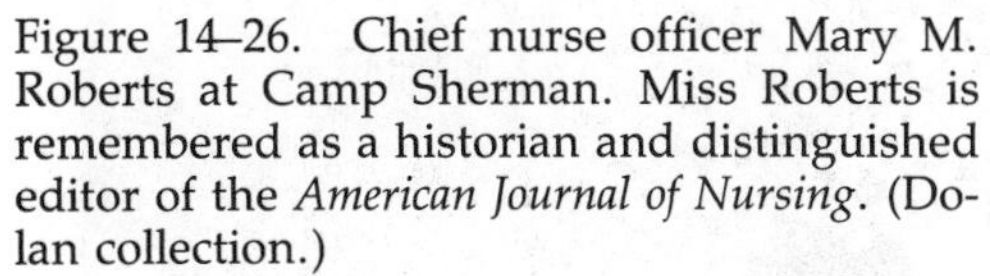

Figure 14–26. Chief nurse officer Mary M. Roberts at Camp Sherman. Miss Roberts is remembered as a historian and distinguished editor of the *American Journal of Nursing*. (Dolan collection.)

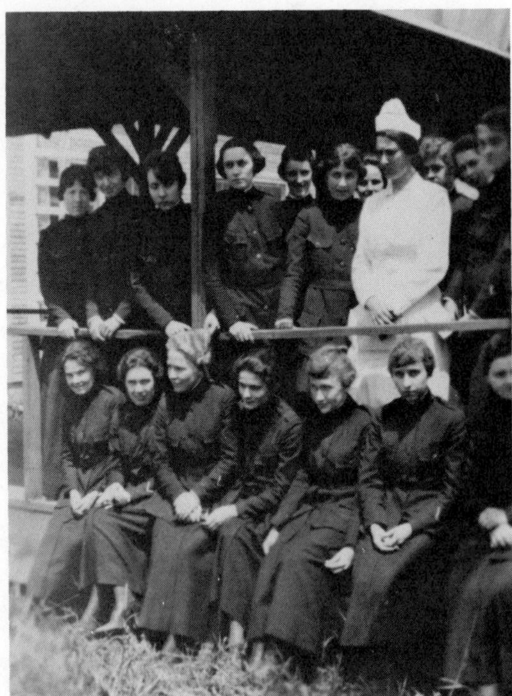

Figure 14–27. Army Training School students, called "Blue Birds," with the chief nurse officer, Mary M. Roberts, at Camp Sherman. (Dolan collection.)

ably the largest class of nurses ever graduated at one time. The school continued, but with smaller classes. It was discontinued in 1932 for economic reasons, and the last class graduated in 1933. This school was organized in an excellent fashion and set a superb example for all other schools to emulate.

Vassar Training Camp for Nurses

A tremendous spirit of patriotism and desire to cooperate with the war effort attracted a large number of college graduates to Vassar College for a preparatory course in nursing. The Vassar Training Camp for Nurses was established for the summer of 1918 by Vassar College. The idea for such a program came from Mrs. Minnie Comnock Blodgett, a Vassar alumna and member of the board of trustees. The plan was brought to fruition as a result of the efforts of Adelaide Nutting, chairman of the Committee on Nursing for the Council of National Defense, Isabel Stewart, chairman of the Curriculum Committee of NLNE, and Jane A. Delano, director of the Red Cross Department of Nursing. The program was financed by the American Red Cross, which voted funds "to establish and maintain a school of science applied to nursing at Vassar College during the summer of 1918"[42] that was open to college graduates only.

Graduates of the course chose a program and were admitted into selected nursing schools across the country. The accelerated

[42]Clappison, Gladys Bonner: *Vassar's Rainbow Division, 1918*. Iowa, Graphic Publishing Company, 1964, p. 2.

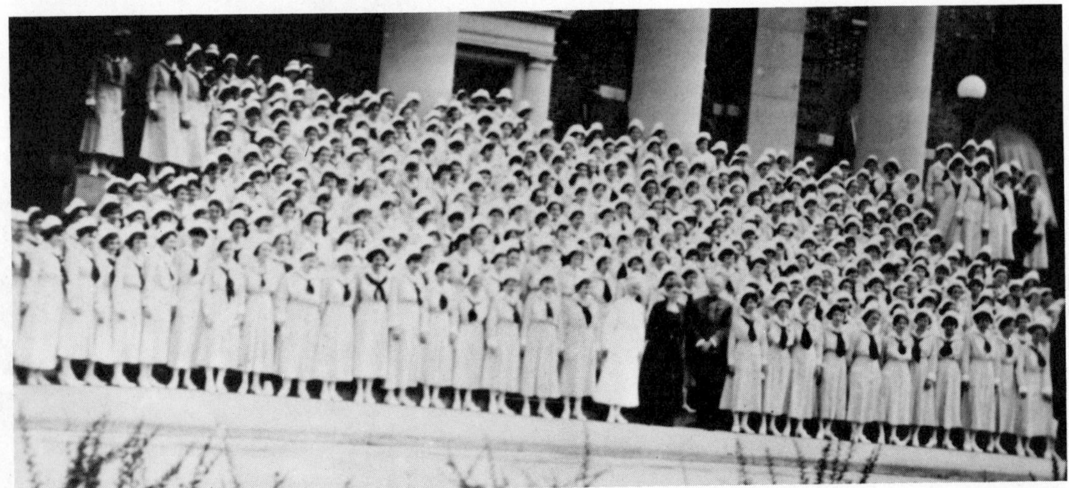

Figure 14–28. The graduating exercises of the Army Training School, with Annie W. Goodrich in attendance. (Dolan collection.)

program of nursing lasted two years and three months. The students wore the uniforms of the school with which they would be affiliated, and they thus came to be referred to as Vassar's Rainbow Division. A total of 435 students from 42 states representing 110 colleges participated in this exceptional program.

One of the members of this program, Katharine Densford Dreves (Fig. 14–29), has written her reminiscences of the experience, emphasizing the impact of the program.

> The camp brought college recognition to nursing; such a prestigious college as Vassar encouraged the effort to bring nursing out of its secluded hospital environment into higher education while conversely challenging colleges to accept responsibility for nurse preparation; it served to interest college women in nursing; the camp received the first large group of well-educated, versatile women, almost half of whom went on to complete the entire nursing course. In addition the camp enlisted national recognition of nursing by the public and of the need for public and private financial support of nursing.[43]

The teachers of the science courses and of nursing were some of the most illustrious in the world.[44] Many of the graduates became influential leaders of nursing. Katharine Densford Dreves became dean of the University of Minnesota School of Nursing, president of the ANA, and second vice-president of the ICN.

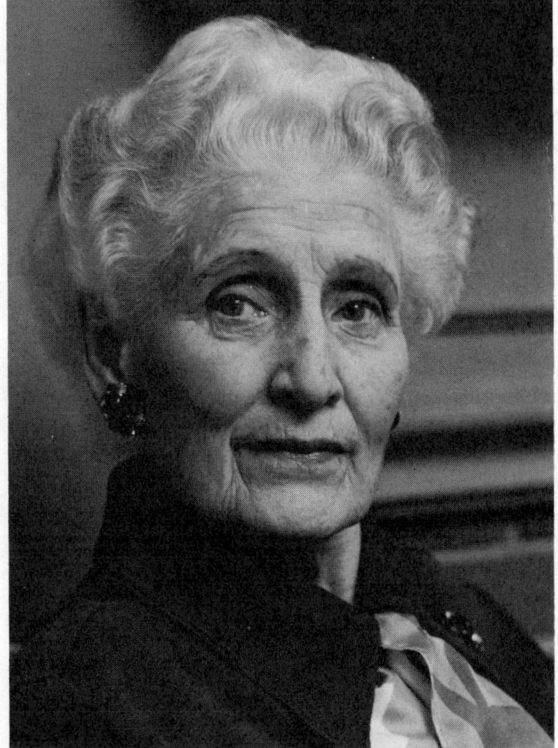

Figure 14–29. Katharine Densford Dreves, internationally famous leader of nursing. (Dolan collection.)

World War I—a Nurse Heroine

Edith Cavell was an English nurse who in 1909 founded a school of nursing in Brussels, Belgium. From the beginning of the war her hospital cared for both Allied and German soldiers without discrimination. She was arrested by the Germans on August 3, 1915, and was charged with helping Allied prisoners to escape. She did not deny the charge. Many governments exerted tremendous political pressure to save her life, but the German leaders refused, and she was shot October 12, 1915. It was recorded that "she died like a heroine."[45] The act stirred much public sentiment (Figs. 14–30 and 14–31). The courageous example of Edith Cavell in being unwilling to relinquish her role as a preserver of life for her patients even if it meant losing her own had a profound influence on the public and the nursing profession around the world.

The void that existed owing to the death of Edith Cavell bothered many people. The State of Massachusetts appointed and sponsored an "Edith Cavell Memorial Nurse from Massachusetts," whose services were intended to be a gift to the British nursing service for the duration of the war. Miss *Alice Fitzgerald* was chosen for this position. She was born in Florence, Italy, of American parents, both of whom were from Baltimore. She was educated in France, Switzerland and Germany and returned to

[43]Dreves, Katharine Densford: "Nurses in American History, Vassar Training Camp for Nurses," *American Journal of Nursing, 75*:2000–2002, 1975.

[44]Clappison, Gladys Bonner: *Vassar's Rainbow Division, 1918.* Iowa Graphic Publishing Company, 1964, pp. 331–339.

[45]Fitzgerald, Alice: *The Edith Cavell Nurse From Massachusetts.* Boston, W. A. Butterfield, 1917, p. 95.

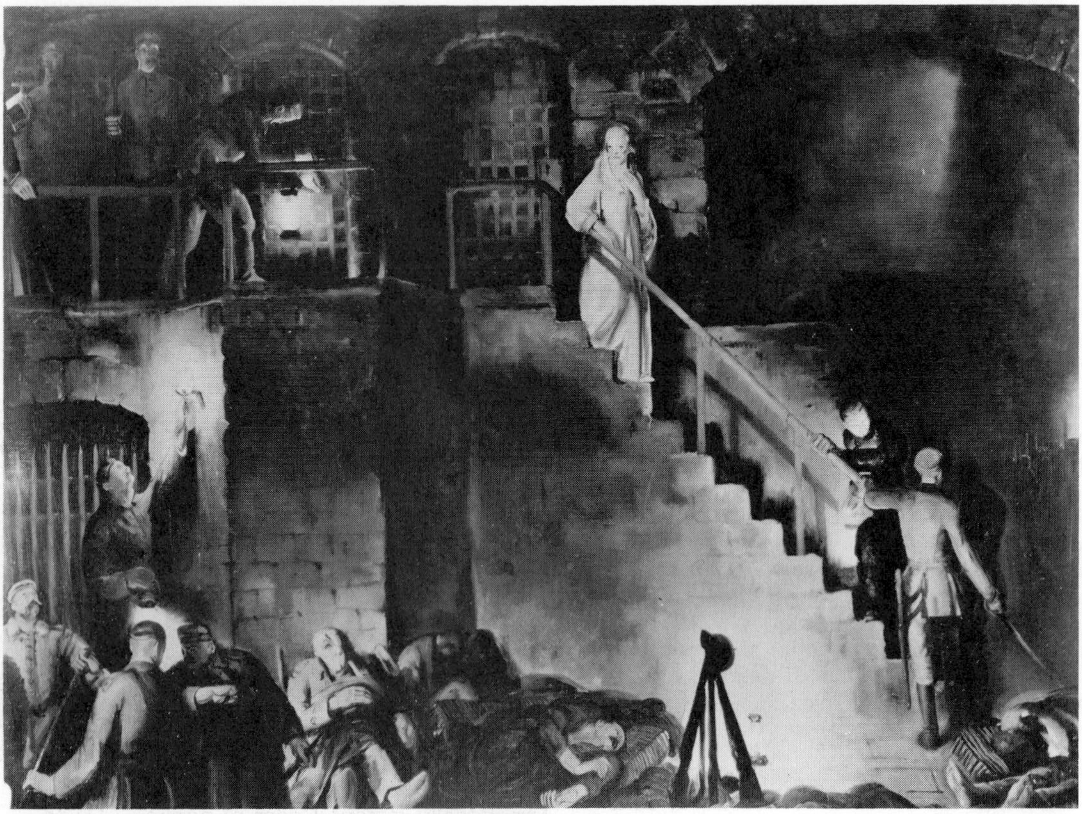

Figure 14–30. Edith Cavell directing the escape of soldiers from prison camp, by George W. Bellows. (Courtesy of Museum of Fine Arts, Springfield, Mass., James Philip Gray Collection.)

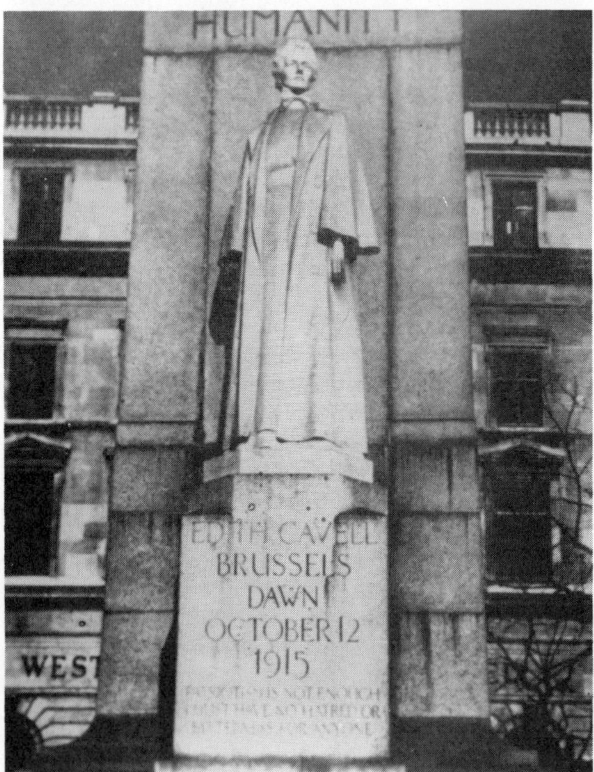

Figure 14–31. A monument honoring Edith Cavell, the international heroine, in London. (Dolan collection.)

the United States for her social debut in Baltimore. Miss Fitzgerald entered the school of nursing at Johns Hopkins from which she graduated in 1906. She held positions at Johns Hopkins and Bellevue Hospitals and then became director of nursing at a hospital in Wilkes Barre, Pennsylvania, and then at one in Indianapolis, Indiana. Her next assignment was as health director of Dana Hall, a finishing school in Wellesley, Massachusetts. It was from this post that she embarked on her historic assignment in 1916. She saw active service with the British in France for two years, and when the Americans entered the war, she joined the American Red Cross at their headquarters in Paris. Her duties were many and varied.

After the Armistice, Miss Fitzgerald became chief nurse for the American Red Cross for the whole of Europe and directed, supervised and inspected nursing and welfare work in these countries. In 1921, she organized the department of nursing of the recently created League of Red Cross Societies at Geneva. She helped in coordinating the relief efforts of the Red Cross and the Rockefeller Foundation.

After World War I

Because Canadian nurses had had officers' rank since 1906 and other countries gave their nurses a semi-official status, American nurses felt the need of rank. From the time of the Spanish-American War, prepared nurses endured lack of status because they had no real rank. This inhibited most nurses' freedom of action in implementing and executing the nursing regimen, curtailed their independence and placed them in a subservient role, a situation that often continued when they returned to the hospitals in the United States. In 1920, after the war was over, enough pressure was exerted so that "relative rank" as officers was granted to nurses.

Julia Stimson (1881–1948) graduated from Vassar before entering the New York Hospital School of Nursing. She succeeded Miss Goodrich as dean of the Army School of Nursing. Miss Stimson then held the position of superintendent of the Army Nurse Corps. She also shared the concern felt by the members of the nursing profession about the lack of rank for military nurses. When relative rank was awarded to nurses through the Army Reorganization Act of 1920, she became *Major Stimson.* She served later as president of the American Nurses' Association.

On November 11, 1918, the armistice was signed. Troops and medical units began to return home.

EVALUATION OF NURSING EDUCATION

After the war had terminated and the ghastly influenza pandemic had subsided, a hopeful, peaceful country could now assess its strengths as well as its weaknesses.

Many leaders in nursing had pleaded that educational programs for nurses be improved and located in a milieu that provided a sound, broad preparation for living as well as earning a living. Many leaders, utilizing data-collecting skills, eloquently presented facts that reflected a need for change. Miss Nutting's recommendation for a careful and exhaustive study of the education of the nurse "by some scientific body able to bring an unprejudiced mind to the situation and to study from the point of view of public welfare" was reconsidered.

The *Rockefeller Foundation* financed a survey of nursing education headed by *Dr. C. E. A. Winslow.* The findings and conclusions of this survey were published in February 1923 in a book called *Nursing and Nursing Education in the United States.* This remarkable report is frequently referred to as the *Goldmark Report,* after Josephine Goldmark (1877–1950), the member of this prestigious committee who recorded and compiled the data for the book (Fig. 14–32). The work should be read in its entirety, for many of its suggestions have not yet been appreciated or implemented.

The members of this committee were aware of many of the weaknesses in the educational preparation of nurse practitioners. It was evident that nursing education in 1922 was still on an apprenticeship basis—an earn-while-you-learn system—even though this type of preparation had been abandoned by other professions that demanded specialized education. It was apparent that nursing was still struggling with the problem of serving two masters; training schools were responsible for the care of the sick in the hospital and the ed-

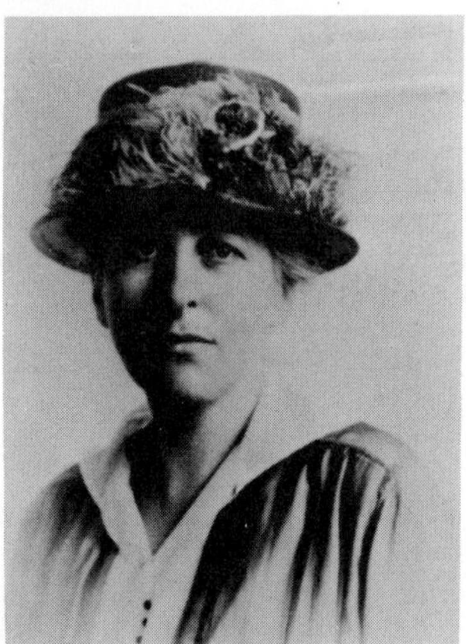

Figure 14–32. Josephine Goldmark (1877–1950). (Courtesy of Canady Library of Bryn Mawr College.)

ucation of the nurse. In stressful situations the first assumed the more important role while the second was neglected.

Many of the instructors were poorly prepared. In one hospital, the course in anatomy and physiology, which was of nine months' duration, was interrupted seven times by the entrance of a new class that studied the subject at whatever point it was being presented. The instructor explained "It makes no difference in anatomy, as one part is not dependent on another."[46]

The lack of well-prepared teachers was a problem, as was the quaint custom of admitting a student to replace every student who withdrew from the school. This custom occurred even in the "better" schools (Fig. 14–33). The following conclusions of the Goldmark Report are noteworthy:

Conclusion 1. That, since constructive health work and health teaching in families is best done by persons:

(a) capable of giving general health instruction, as distinguished from instruction in any one specialty; and

(b) capable of rendering bedside care at need;

the agent responsible for such constructive health work and health teaching in families should have completed the nurses' training. There will, of course, be need for the employment, in addition to the public health nurse, of other types of experts such as nutrition workers, social workers, occupational therapists, and the like.

That as soon as may be practicable all agencies, public or private, employing public health nurses, should require as a prerequisite for employment the basic hospital training, followed by a post-graduate course, including both class work and field work, in public health nursing.

Conclusion 2. That the career open to young women of high capacity, in public health nursing or in hospital supervision and nursing education, is one of the most attractive fields now open, in its promise of professional success and of rewarding public service; and that every effort should be made to attract such women into this field.

Conclusion 3. That for the care of persons suffering from serious and acute disease the safety of the patient, and the responsibility of the medical and nursing professions, demand the maintenance of the standards of educational attainment now generally accepted by the best sentiment of both professions and embodied in the legislation of the more progressive states; and that any attempt to lower these standards would be fraught with real danger to the public.

Conclusion 4. That steps should be taken through state legislation for the definition and licensure of a subsidiary grade of nursing service, the subsidiary type of worker to serve under practising physicians in the care of mild and chronic illness, and convalescence, and possibly to assist under the direction of the trained nurse in certain phases of hospital and visiting nursing.

Conclusion 5. That, while training schools for nurses have made remarkable progress, and while the best schools of today in many respects reach a high level of educational attainment, the average hospital training school is not organized on such a basis as to conform to the standards accepted in other educational fields; that the instruction in such schools is frequently casual and uncorrelated; that the educational needs and the health and strength of students are frequently sacrificed to practical hospital exigencies; that such shortcomings are primarily due to the lack of independent endowments for nursing education; that existing educational facilities are on the whole, in the majority of schools, inadequate for the preparation of the high grade of nurses required for the care of serious illness and . . . the fields of public health nursing and nursing education; and that one of the chief reasons for the lack of sufficient recruits, of a high type, to meet such needs lies precisely in the fact that the average hospital training school does not offer a sufficiently attractive avenue of entrance to this field.

Conclusion 6. That, with the necessary financial support and under a separate board or training school committee, organized primarily for educational purposes, it is possible, with

[46]Winslow, C. E. A., et al.: *Nursing and Nursing Education in the United States.* New York, The Macmillan Co., 1923, p. 224.

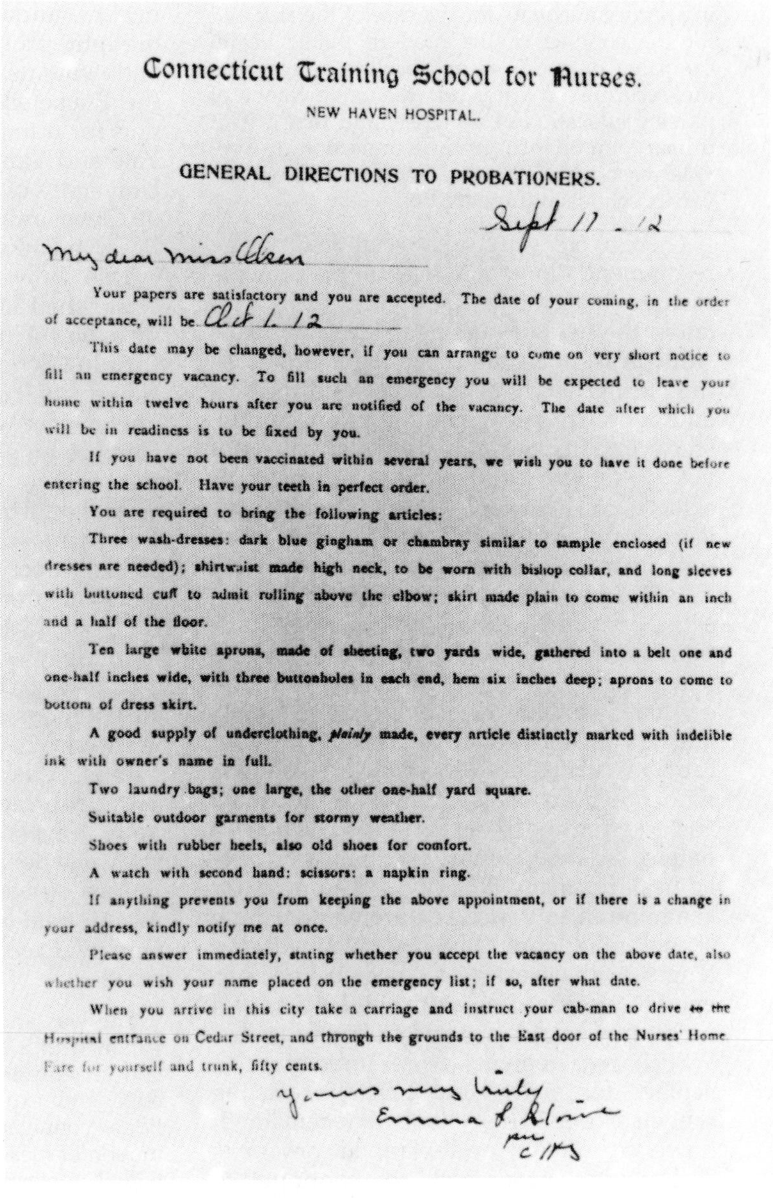

Connecticut Training School for Nurses.

NEW HAVEN HOSPITAL.

GENERAL DIRECTIONS TO PROBATIONERS.

Sept 17 . 12

My dear Miss Olsen

Your papers are satisfactory and you are accepted. The date of your coming, in the order of acceptance, will be Oct 1. 12

This date may be changed, however, if you can arrange to come on very short notice to fill an emergency vacancy. To fill such an emergency you will be expected to leave your home within twelve hours after you are notified of the vacancy. The date after which you will be in readiness is to be fixed by you.

If you have not been vaccinated within several years, we wish you to have it done before entering the school. Have your teeth in perfect order.

You are required to bring the following articles:

Three wash-dresses: dark blue gingham or chambray similar to sample enclosed (if new dresses are needed); shirtwaist made high neck, to be worn with bishop collar, and long sleeves with buttoned cuff to admit rolling above the elbow; skirt made plain to come within an inch and a half of the floor.

Ten large white aprons, made of sheeting, two yards wide, gathered into a belt one and one-half inches wide, with three buttonholes in each end, hem six inches deep; aprons to come to bottom of dress skirt.

A good supply of underclothing, *plainly* made, every article distinctly marked with indelible ink with owner's name in full.

Two laundry bags; one large, the other one-half yard square.

Suitable outdoor garments for stormy weather.

Shoes with rubber heels, also old shoes for comfort.

A watch with second hand: scissors: a napkin ring.

If anything prevents you from keeping the above appointment, or if there is a change in your address, kindly notify me at once.

Please answer immediately, stating whether you accept the vacancy on the above date, also whether you wish your name placed on the emergency list; if so, after what date.

When you arrive in this city take a carriage and instruct your cab-man to drive ~~to~~ the Hospital entrance on Cedar Street, and through the grounds to the East door of the Nurses' Home. Fare for yourself and trunk, fifty cents.

Yours very truly
Emma L. Stowe
per C.H.S.

Figure 14–33. Instructions to incoming student, Miss Beatrice Olsen, in 1912. (Courtesy Mrs. Beatrice Olsen Chesson.)

completion of a high school course or its equivalent as a prerequisite, to reduce the fundamental period of hospital training to 28 months, and at the same time, by eliminating unessential, non-educational routine, and adopting the principles laid down in Miss Goldmark's report, to organize the course along intensive and coordinated lines with such modifications as may be necessary for practical application; and that courses of this standard would be reasonably certain to attract students of high quality in increasing numbers.

Conclusion 7. Superintendents, supervisors, instructors, and public health nurses should in all cases receive special additional training beyond the basic nursing course.

Conclusion 8. That the development and strengthening of university schools of nursing of a high grade for the training of leaders is of fundamental importance in the furtherance of nursing education.

Conclusion 9. That when the licensure of a subsidiary grade of nursing service is provided for, the establishment of training courses in preparation for such service is highly desirable; that such courses should be conducted in special hospitals, in small unaffiliated general hospitals, or in separate sections of hospitals where nurses are also trained; and that the course should be of 8 or 9 months' duration; provided the standards of such schools be approved by the same educational board which governs nursing training schools.

Conclusion 10. That the development of nursing service adequate for the care of the sick and for the conduct of the modern public health campaign demands as an absolute prerequisite the securing of funds for the endowment of nursing education of all types; and that it is of primary importance, in this connection, to provide reasonably generous endowment for university schools of nursing.[47]

There were startling revelations, strong recommendations and slow improvements as the impact of this study gradually was felt in the field of nursing. This remarkable study was not shared with the public as the Flexner study of medicine and medical education had been. The significance of the study and its recommendations have not yet been fully understood, accepted or achieved. However, the earn-while-you-learn type of apprenticeship slowly died out; instructors began to be hired; poor schools closed; the amount of non-nursing service began to decline; the cost of educational programs started to increase; hospitals commenced hiring permanent staffs of graduate nurses, ward helpers and orderlies; and schools adopted acceptable educational curricula and initiated affiliations with other hospitals to provide adequate and well-rounded experiences. Unfortunately, lack of practical experience in public health nursing continued. The need for a minimum entrance requirement of high school graduation had to be faced; the length of the work week had to be shortened to include classes during the day; and night duty experience had to be reduced.

Such requirements were impossible to achieve for many, and half the existing schools closed. The schools that remained, however, offered well-planned programs and were encouraged to continue to improve.

DEVELOPMENT OF ENDOWED UNIVERSITY SCHOOLS OF NURSING

Two of the history-making results of the Rockefeller study were the establishment of endowed collegiate schools of nursing and the emphasis on the need for commitment to education and service in public health nursing. The Goldmark Report brought prompt response in the form of endowments. Through the generosity of the Rockefeller Foundation, financial support for nursing education was provided at Yale and Vanderbilt Universities and at the University of Toronto. Mrs. Frances Bolton of Cleveland provided support at Western Reserve University.

Yale University School of Nursing was established in 1923 on the fiftieth anniversary of the founding of the Connecticut Training School for Nurses, which the Yale University School of Nursing succeeded. The degree of Bachelor of Nursing was given to graduates from 1926 to 1936; then, the degree of Master of Nursing was awarded. The first dean was Annie W. Goodrich, who had been director of the Henry Street Settlement Nurse Service and assistant professor of nursing in Teachers' College, Columbia University. Her appointment was of historic significance because she accepted the deanship of the first autonomous nursing school within a university in the United States.

What this great lady exhibited to the president, administration and faculty at Yale University was described by University president Angell, who was president of Yale University when she joined his academic family. At the Twenty-Fifth Anniversary Exercises in 1949 (Fig. 14–34), he recalled:

> She was and is a woman of the finest cultivation with a broad and human outlook on life and an amazing sweep of professional knowledge and experience, deep and fiery convictions, courageous, indeed fearless in the promotion of measures she believes to be wise, and withal possessed of complete tolerance for persons and views at variance with her own convictions. In other words, being also highly imaginative and a fine administrator, she was the ideal choice as organizer and leader of the new school.

Being associated with a prestigious medical school, Dean Goodrich confronted criticism from the physicians of her "new experiment" of a curriculum that would produce a well-educated person capable of delivering "complete nursing care." President Angell relates that a good many physicians:

> had been schooled to regard the nurse as their purely personal property to be completely subservient to their every whim and ready instantly to execute any command, however unreasona-

[47]Winslow, C. E. A., et al.: *Nursing and Nursing Education in the United States.* New York, The Macmillan Company, 1923, p. 224.

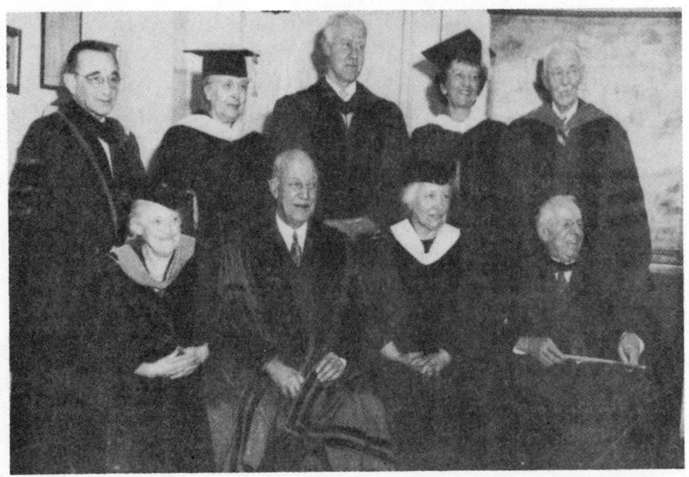

Figure 14–34. Speakers and guests of honor at the 25th anniversary celebration of the Yale School of Nursing. *Seated, left to right:* Dean Emeritus Annie W. Goodrich; President Charles Seymour of Yale University; Mrs. August Belmont; and James R. Angell, president emeritus. *Standing, left to right:* Dr. Milton C. Winternitz, professor of pathology; Dean Emeritus Effie J. Taylor; Dr. Alan Gregg of the Rockefeller Foundation; Dean Elizabeth S. Bixler; Dr. C.-E. A. Winslow, professor emeritus of public health at Yale University. (Dolan collection.)

ble. . . . Men of this kind were often fearful that nurses trained as the Yale School proposed to do would be overeducated, would be rebellious and indisposed to accept the dictatorial procedures of the physician or surgeon in charge.

He commented that the attitude of the medical group gradually changed.

The Yale curriculum was designed to give the student of nursing a sound scientific background upon which to build nursing skills in caring for "the whole patient." The teaching methods included the "patient nursing care method of assignment" on the patient units, "instead of the efficiency method," and the assigning of "nursing case papers" for class reports. Even the clinical practice laboratory provided the same focus. Contrast the case-oriented laboratory shown in Figure 14–35 with the task-oriented laboratory in Figure 14–14. Provision for educational leadership as well as a background in public health nursing was incorporated into the curriculum. Miss Goodrich encouraged the students to share with her and the faculty of nursing their critical evaluations of their clinical experience.

The teamwork needed between the medical and nursing professions in planning learning experiences for the nursing students served to clarify each as a separate and distinct discipline. It is recorded that "the mutual reliance upon intelligent co-operation, which characterizes a growing professional competence in both medical men and nurses, is doing away with the fears which in the past have prejudiced the cause of nursing education."

In recognition of the need for enrichment of learning, Dean Goodrich published a landmark article[48] that emphasized the benefits of the use of teaching films in increasing an understanding of nursing procedures.

[48]Goodrich, Annie W.: "Nursing Procedure Motion Picture," *American Journal of Nursing,* Vol. 32, 1932.

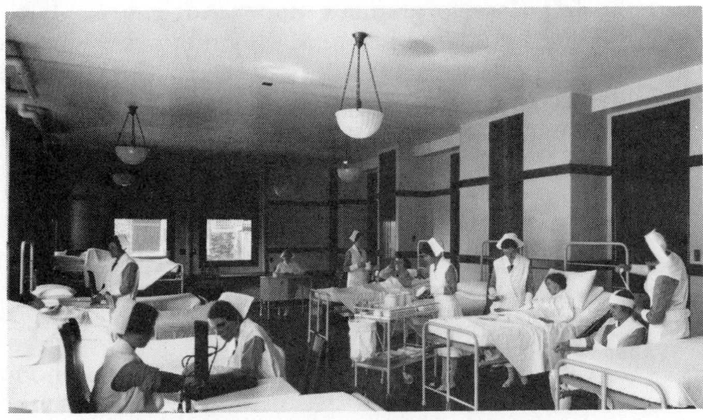

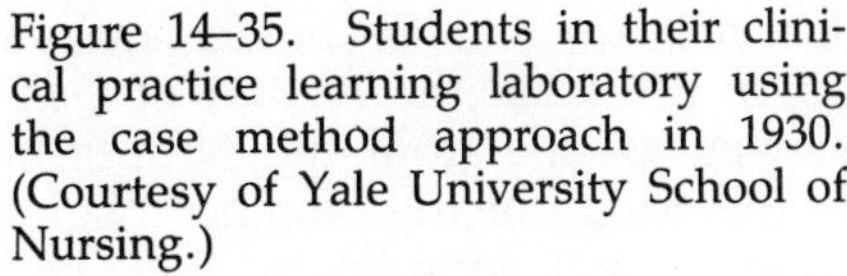

Figure 14–35. Students in their clinical practice learning laboratory using the case method approach in 1930. (Courtesy of Yale University School of Nursing.)

Annie W. Goodrich's leadership was sought by her colleagues nationally and internationally, for she was president of the ICN (1912–1915), the ANA (1916–1918) and the ACSN (1934–1936). For all of her contributions to her profession and the welfare of mankind, Dean Goodrich received many awards, among them the Medal of the National Institute of Social Science (1920); the Distinguished Service Medal of the United States (1923); the Medaille d'Honneur de l'Hygiène Publique (1928); the Silver Medal of the French Ministry of Social Welfare (1933); and the Bronze Medal of Belgium (1933). She also received such honorary degrees as Doctor of Science, Mount Holyoke College (1921); Master of Arts, Yale University (1923); and Doctor of Laws, Russell Sage College (1936). Her profession paid tribute by presenting her with the Walter Burns Saunders Medal and the Mary Adelaide Nutting Medal.

Annie W. Goodrich believed that collegiate nursing education was the preferred type of education for all nurses: "It is desirable that nursing education should find its place in the university, which is another way of saying that it belongs where all educational expressions have been increasingly placed, and for the reason that universal knowledge is here assembled and distributed in accordance with the needs of the students as future builders of the community."[49]

Miss Goodrich was succeeded as Dean of the Yale University School of Nursing by *Effie J. Taylor* (Fig. 14–36), who continued her high level of leadership. Dean Taylor was born in Hamilton, Ontario, Canada, and was educated at Hamilton Collegiate Institute and Wesleyan Ladies College before entering Johns Hopkins Hospital School of Nursing. Miss Taylor was a member of the last class to graduate under Adelaide Nutting's guidance before Miss Nutting assumed her role at Teachers' College, Columbia University. After functioning as a head nurse and then assistant superintendent at Johns Hopkins Hospital, Miss Taylor went on a study tour of existing psychiatric institutions. Upon her return she became first director of nursing services at the Henry Phipps Psychiatric Clinic, the first such university clinic in the United States. In 1926, as a member of the Yale faculty, she was reported by Dean Goodrich to be the "first and probably only professor in the world in psychiatric nursing." She served her profession as president of the NLNE (1933–1937) and as president of the ICN during the long and difficult years of World War II. The temporary office of the ICN was located in New Haven, Connecticut, during this crisis period.

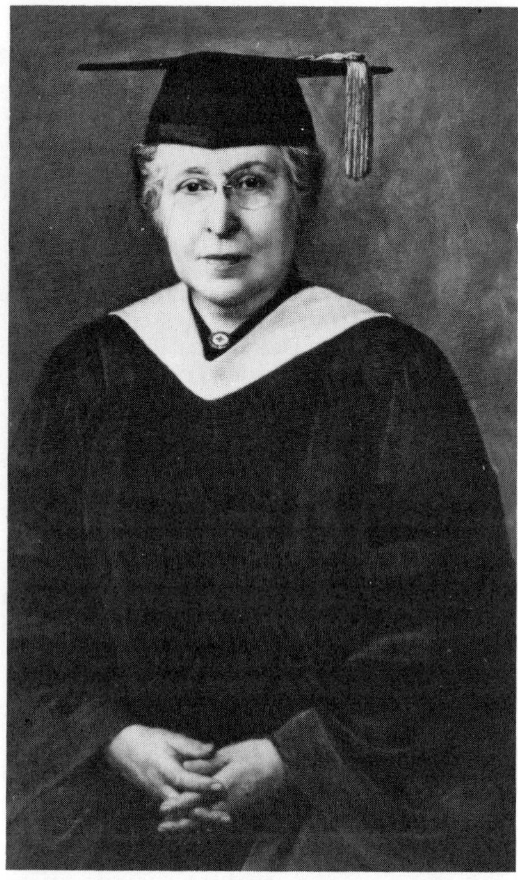

Figure 14–36. Dean Effie J. Taylor of Yale University School of Nursing. (Dolan collection.)

Many honors were bestowed on Dean Taylor in recognition of her achievements, including a badge of honor from the National Council of Nurses of Finland; a membership pin from the Nurses of Denmark as well as one from the Nurses of Norway; the Badge of the Florence Nightingale International Foundation; the Mary Adelaide Nutting Award; an honorary degree of Master of Arts from Yale; and an honorary degree of Doctor of Humane Letters (L.H.D.) from Keuka College. She

[49]Goodrich, Annie W.: "The School of Nursing and the Future," *Proceedings of the Thirty-eighth Annual Convention of the National League of Nursing Education*. New York, National Headquarters, 1932, p. 173.

was particularly proud of her pin from the American Red Cross and worked conscientiously in the activities of this organization.

At Western Reserve University, another leader with great vision also guided a significant pioneering venture in nursing education. *Mrs. Frances Payne Bolton* (1885–1977) devoted herself to public service and philanthropy. Her planning, encouragement and generosity were of great assistance to the nursing profession. She served in Congress for many years following the death of her husband, Congressman Chester C. Bolton. She was instrumental in the establishment of the Army School of Nursing in World War I and sponsored the bill creating the Cadet Nurse Corps in World War II. She financed the School of Nursing at Western Reserve that was named in her honor. She received many awards, including 16 honorary degrees. She became the first woman named as a Congressional delegate to the United Nations.

STUDY BY COMMITTEE ON THE GRADING OF NURSES

In 1925 the ANA sponsored the Committee on the Grading of Nurses, to undertake a five-year study of nursing and nurse education. The committee's members were lay men and women, physicians and nurses. Dr. May Ayres Burgess, an educator, psychologist and statistician, was the director, and Dr. Walter Darrach, a surgeon, was the chairman. Nurses themselves gave $115,000 to the project.

Participation in the first grading study was entirely voluntary. Of the 2,205 schools invited to participate, 1,458 accepted and sent back their reports. A 66 per cent return on so difficult a project was clear evidence of the widespread interest in this study.

Results of the data collection and analysis were returned to each participating school in a report that contained three sections: Section I—The Student Body; Section II—What Students Learn; and Section III—Who Controls the Schools.

In Section I, 59,612 students provided statements as to their education before entering the school. Sixty-five per cent were high school graduates, 26 per cent had completed some high school, seven per cent had had one or more years of college, 1 per cent had not gone beyond the eighth grade, and 1 per cent were college graduates.

In answer to the question on where the students had been on duty during the preceding 24 hours, 18 per cent of the 59,285 students reported having been on more than one hospital unit, 15 per cent in the diet kitchen (Fig. 14–37) and 10 per cent in the operating room.

Some of the replies caused considerable consternation in the minds of those who perused the reports. What educational experience was being provided for the 3,262 students in the record rooms? Were the 1,180 students in the drug rooms receiving educational experience (Figs. 14–38)? Were the 836 students in the main kitchens all learning dietetics? What were the learning experiences of the 677 students in the radiology departments and the 877 in the laboratories?

Of the additional students performing non-nursing tasks, 3,365 students were making surgical supplies, 505 reported that they had been on telephone switchboard duty; 552 had been assigned to the utility

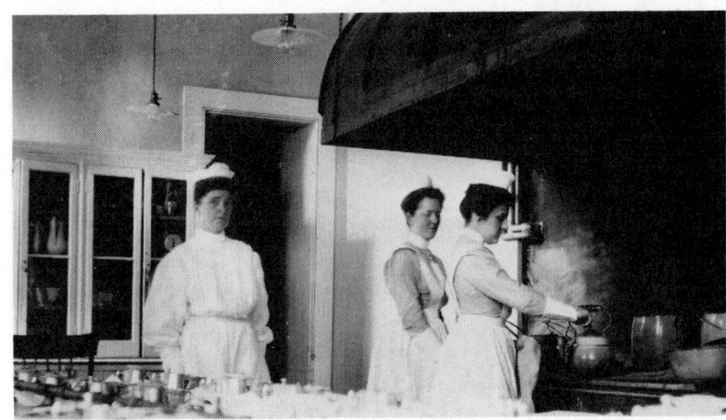

Figure 14–37. Students of nursing preparing meals in the diet kitchen. (Dolan collection.)

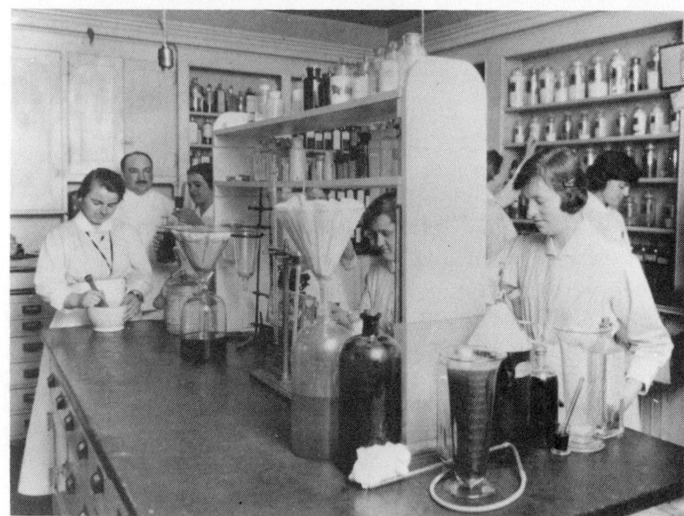

Figure 14–38. Students of nursing staffing the pharmacy and preparing solutions for hospital use. (Dolan collection.)

room; others reported "running the elevator," "painting furniture," "making curtains," "running errands," "mending gloves" and being engaged in other activities essential for the management of the hospital but of decidedly questionable educational value.

In Section III, in response to the question of who is responsible for the teaching in the schools, the fact that a preponderance of those teaching were physicians was documented. Of the 1,391 regular schools of nursing that responded, 42 per cent had no regular nurse instructor, 42 per cent had one nurse instructor, while 16 per cent had two or more.

Of the preparation for teaching of the nurse faculty, 42 per cent of the instructors had less than a high school diploma, 42 per cent were high school graduates, and 16 per cent had some college preparation. The need for continuing education to be better prepared for teaching and for keeping up to date was not recognized or accepted because the data collected showed that 85 per cent of those teaching had not received any

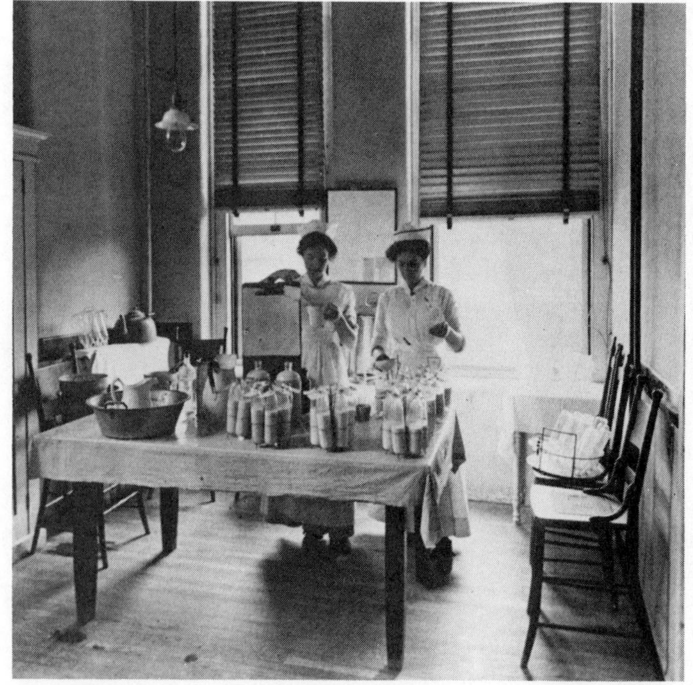

Figure 14–39. Students receiving experience in the formula room. (Dolan collection.)

TABLE 14–1. HOW FAST HAS NURSING GROWN? MEDICAL AND NURSING SCHOOLS AND GRADUATES, 1880–1926*

Year	Medical Schools	Nursing Schools	Medical Graduates	Nursing Graduates
1880	100	15	3,241	157
1890	133	35	4,454	471
1900	160	432	5,214	3,456
1910	131	1,129	4,440	8,140
1920	85	1,775	3,047	14,980
1926	79	2,155	3,962	17,522

*Practically all figures for nursing schools were taken from the various reports of the United States Bureau of Education; those for graduates of medical schools and colleges from the files of the Journal of the American Medical Association. (From Burgess, Dr. May Ayres: *Nurses, Patients and Pocketbooks,* 1928, p. 35.)

additional preparation after beginning to teach. This attitude on the part of the nursing staff encouraged a perpetuation of the status quo.

During the eight years of study, two reports were published. *Nurses, Patients and Pocketbooks* (1928) analyzed the supply and demand of nurses and emphasized the growth in schools. Table 14–1 contrasts the difference in numbers of schools of medicine and those of nursing. The actual number of schools of nursing was greater than that shown in the table because not all the schools were reported to the United States Bureau of Education. The effect of the Flexner study on schools of medicine was reflected in the decrease in the numbers and increase in the quality of programs of medical schools.

The other report, titled *Nursing Schools Today and Tomorrow* (1934), identified the large number of small schools that provided limited educational experience. The differences between adequate and inadequate schools was appalling.

In 1936, a significant pamphlet, *Essentials of a Good School of Nursing,* was published by the NLNE. It was revised in 1942.

The Committee on the Grading of Nurses believed that it was incumbent upon the committee to spell out succinctly what a professional nurse should know and be able to utilize in practice. They gave the following guidelines:

What Should a Professional Nurse Know and Be Able to Do?

1. All professional nurses, irrespective of the special field in which they have elected to practice, should be able to give [illegible] They should also have such [illegible] household arts as will enable [illegible] tively with the domestic emerg[illegible] of illness.

2. All professional nurses, irr[illegible] special field in which they have e[illegible] tice, should be able to observe an[illegible] interpret the physical manifestations of the patient's condition, and also the social and environmental factors which may hasten or delay his recovery.

3. All professional nurses should possess the special knowledge and skill which are required in dealing effectively with situations peculiar to certain common types of illness.

4. All professional nurses should be able to apply, in nursing situations, those principles of mental hygiene which make for a better understanding of the psychological factor in illness.

5. All professional nurses should be capable of taking part in the promotion of health and the prevention of disease.

6. All professional nurses should possess the essential knowledge and ability to teach measures to conserve health and to restore health.

7. All professional nurses should be able to cooperate effectively with the family, hospital personnel, and health and social agencies in the interest of patient and community.

8. Every nurse should be able, by means of the practice of her profession, to attain a measure of economic security and to provide for sickness and old age. It should be possible for her to conserve her physical resources, to seek mental stimulus by further study and experience, and to follow that way of life in which she finds those spiritual and cultural values which enrich and liberate human personality.[50]

Only a small fraction of those graduating from schools of nursing could meet these standards as presented in 1934.

Although there was a need for change and upgrading of schools of nursing, many schools were providing good programs as well as enriching them constantly. In the history of the Farrand Training School of Harper Hospital (Fig. 14–40) such progress was reported. The affiliation of this hospital school with an institution of higher learning was recounted thus:

A course, covering a forty-eight month period, is planned for young women who wish to take a combined college and nursing program leading to the Bachelor of Science Degree in Nursing from the College of the City of Detroit and the Diploma of Nursing from the Farrand

[50]Johns, Ethel, and Pfefferkorn, Blanche: *An Activity Analysis of Nursing.* Committee on the Grading of Nursing Schools. New York, 1934.

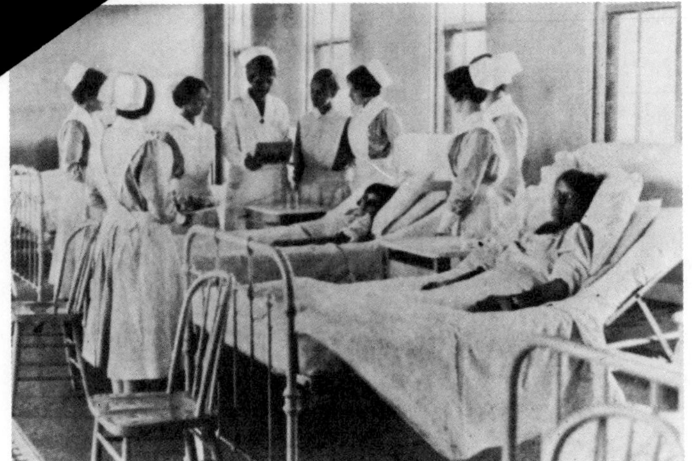

Figure 14–40. In the late 1920s at Farrand Training School, discussion of a nursing regimen was carried out on the clinical units and was referred to as a *nursing clinic*. (Dolan collection.)

Training School of Nursing connected with Harper Hospital.[51]

AN HONOR SOCIETY IN NURSING—SIGMA THETA TAU

During this traumatic period of building a solid foundation for programs in nursing education, some creative students were looking beyond the usual and aiming for scholastic recognition. They were determined to publicize their desires to foster high standards of professional nursing care and to encourage creative work that would stimulate research in nursing as well as promote the maximum development of each individual culturally, socially and professionally. To realize these goals of high scholastic endeavor an honor society in nursing was initiated in 1922 at Indiana University called *Sigma Theta Tau*.

In the early days of the century, the revelations of the studies of nursing as well as those of the Flexner Report in medicine were shocking to health care deliverers. Flexner recorded that the majority of medical students arrived at medical school without having completed high school. In contrast, the six founders of Sigma Theta Tau were high school graduates, and at least one had two years of college preparation prior to entrance into the University of Indiana Training School.

These students were encouraged to speak out for nurses and nursing, and to interpret, for the public, nursing and the advantages of university preparation for nursing practice. They were charged by the director of their school to be political activists for the betterment of society.

From 1922 to 1982, the chapters of this society have multiplied and the membership has increased. There are now 162 chapters of Sigma Theta Tau in colleges and universities across the country. The research accomplishments of members have been greatly publicized. It is of interest to note that the national honor society in medicine was established at the same university in 1916.

STUDIES ON NURSING IN CANADA

The leaders of nursing in Canada and the United States had worked closely and shared suggestions and developments, so their systems of nursing education and service paralleled each other.

Canadian educators and health professionals undertook a survey of nursing education at about the same time as their American counterparts but their approach and methods differed. The survey was sponsored jointly by the Canadian Nurses' Association and the Canadian Medical Association and was undertaken by Dr. George M. Weir, an educator and sociologist.[52]

The findings were similar to those of the

[51]Deans, Agnes G., and Austin, Anne L.: *The History of the Farrand Training School for Nurses.* Detroit, Michigan, Alumnae Association of the Farrand Training School, 1936, pp. 118–119.

[52]Weir, George M.: *Survey of Nursing Education in Canada.* Toronto, University of Toronto Press, 1932.

United States survey. The report stressed that the system of nurse education needed to be changed—to be removed from hospital control and brought into the general educational system in each province. The report exposed the weaknesses in education that rendered nursing service less complete. The processes of observation, analysis and reasoning had not been fostered. There was regret that problem solving, which affected patient care and the growth of the student, received little encouragement. Leaders of nursing studied this report with great appreciation.

RECOMMENDATIONS BY THE COMMITTEE ON THE COSTS OF MEDICAL CARE

During the course of these studies of nursing, another group was investigating not health care needs but the actual health care that Americans were receiving. The investigating committee consisted of 25 physicians, 15 lay people (including social scientists), two dentists, two nurses and one pharmacist: It was hardly a health-team approach to a crucial health problem. The two nurses who represented nursing were carefully chosen. One was Mary Roberts, whose knowledge of nursing was vast and whose position as editor of the *American Journal of Nursing* commanded respect; the other nurse was *Elizabeth Fox*, who was director of the Bureau of Public Health Nursing of the American Red Cross. She had a national reputation in nursing and had served as president of the National Organization of Public Health Nurses. She was described as "creative, dynamic and aggressive."

This committee conducted investigations to determine the adequacy of medical services in terms of quantity and quality, the distribution of costs and the economic status of the different professional groups supplying these services. Figure 14–41 graphically presents the financial plight of the largest group of health workers—nurses—that existed at that time.[53] This study indicated that there was an acute need for more and better service from all professional groups. The committee advocated the extension of group practice, including nursing practice, around such a distribution center as a hospital.

In the section on nursing, the report recommended that nursing education be thoroughly remodeled to provide "well-educated and well-qualified" registered nurses. Concomitantly, they suggested that "less well-trained but competent nursing aides or attendants be provided" and identified the need for *adequate* preparation for nurse-midwives. The committee stated:

> There should be a rearrangement of curricula and a revision of the fundamental purposes of many nursing schools, so that they will produce socially minded nurses with a preparation basic to all types of nursing service. The care of hospital patients is not, in and of itself, sufficient preparation for professional nursing. Nurses should be prepared not only for the practice of

[53]The Committee on the Costs of Medical Care: *Medical Care For The American People.* Chicago, University of Chicago Press, 1932, p. 15.

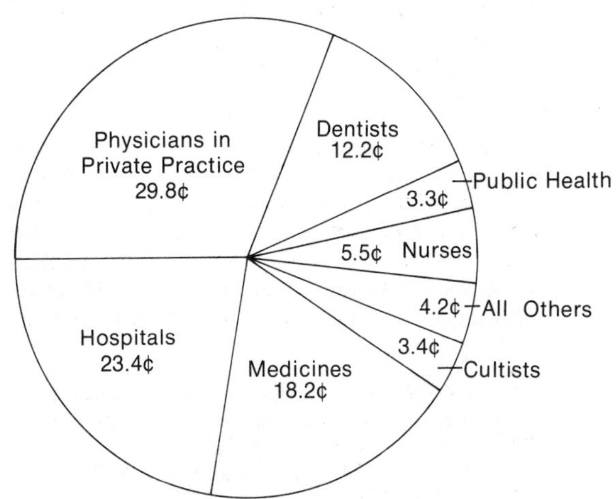

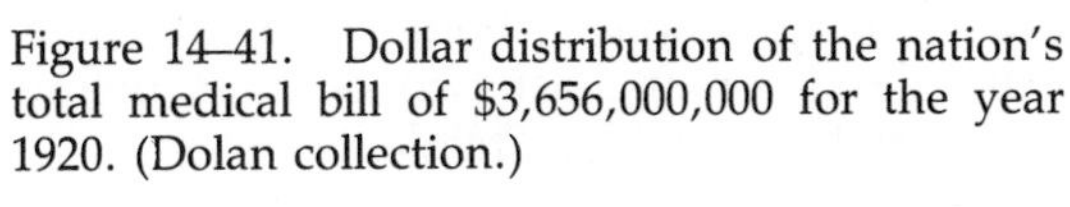
Figure 14–41. Dollar distribution of the nation's total medical bill of $3,656,000,000 for the year 1920. (Dolan collection.)

a profession but for life and its manifold home and community duties as well.[54]

The report exerted a remarkable influence on schools of nursing; the mere statement of unpleasant or discouraging facts stimulated action and brought marked improvement. Meanwhile nurse educators strove to provide faculty with guidelines.

NLNE PUBLICATIONS TO ENRICH CURRICULUM

In 1927, a revision of the NLNE's standard curriculum, entitled *Curriculum for Schools of Nursing,* was published. Because of misinterpretation, the word "standard" was deleted from the title. It was apparent that the Education Committee working on this revision was striving to incorporate recommendations from the Goldmark Report:

> It was definitely stipulated that the *elements* of public health nursing were to be considered as basic for *all* students regardless of the field of nursing they might plan to enter on graduation. More definite recognition was given to the care of the well child, to the health needs of the family and community and to the public health responsibilities of nurses. Psychology (including mental hygiene) was identified as an essential rather than a recommended subject, and communicable disease and psychiatric nursing were both more prominently featured in the clinical program.[55]

Nurse educators realized that there were stultifying aspects to the *Curriculum for Schools of Nursing,* which was used as a bible by faculty of schools of nursing. In order to create an educationally enriched program, a guide rather than a strict rule had to be devised. In 1937, a revision of the curriculum series was published which was retitled *A Curriculum Guide for Schools of Nursing.*

> It was specifically stated that the program outlined in the *Guide* was intended for students of *professional* calibre and qualifications, who were seriously preparing themselves for the practice of nursing as a *profession.* . . . A further assumption was that such schools would make every effort to adjust their programs to the resources and needs of a democractic society and to the advances of science especially in the fields of medicine and of education.[56]

The 1937 *Guide* contained a much broader and enriched presentation of scientific and nursing content. The application of social sciences to nursing received great attention. New approaches to the techniques of teaching and the role of clinical instructors were stressed. The work included the use of multimedia in teaching and learning. This project was intended to stimulate creativity in the development of essential curriculum content in order to keep pace with societal trends and scientific progress, but for many years some schools still adhered to the suggestions in this historic document. A further revision was unwarranted.

BALANCING NURSING SERVICE AND EDUCATION

More than 90 years ago Miss Florence Nightingale's foresight made her found her school of nursing as an *educational institution.* Among its outstanding features were that nurses were primarily students, being prepared for living as well as earning a living, heads of departments were chosen for their teaching and organizing ability, and the school was liberally endowed and thus in control of its own activities.

Though Miss Nightingale stated her principles clearly, they have been largely misunderstood. In consequence, many schools of nursing, from her time until now, have been organized with the purpose "of providing better nursing for the hospital." Even now these two different ends, nursing service and nursing education, are misunderstood. It is a well-recognized fact that there is *no other educational project in which students carry responsibility for the work* of an organization.

Economic pressure had been the chief cause of this confusion about the purpose of nursing schools, though the idea was discussed for at least two decades before any analysis of it was made.

Administrative Cost Analysis for Nursing Service and Nursing Education was a study made in 1940 under the sponsorship of the American Hospital Association and the Na-

[54]The Committee on the Costs of Medical Care: *Medical Care For The American People.* Chicago, University of Chicago Press, 1932, p. 142.

[55]Stewart, Isabel M.: *The Education of Nurses.* New York, The Macmillan Co., 1943, p. 223.

[56]*Ibid.*, p. 257.

tional League of Nursing Education. The study made sense of the chaos of ideas existing on the monetary value of student nurses' work. It worked out the number of hours' care given in each 24 hours to different types of patients, and the cost of housing, feeding and educating student nurses.

For more than half a century, directors of schools of nursing were perplexed by the problem of trying to educate their nurses and at the same time with the same personnel give care to patients in hospitals. As a rule, the two aims came into sharp conflict, and since the care of patients was of paramount importance, it was nursing education that assumed second place. For many years hospitals absorbed the nurse's whole time, including her social life; often her health was affected, and her personal life was given little consideration.

NURSING IN THE DEPRESSION

In the 1930s, the problems of the Great Depression caused a large oversupply of nurses, especially for private duty, which had become a luxury. The supply exceeded the demand, causing a lowering of income throughout all segments of nursing. Many nurses worked in hospitals for little more than room and board. In order to spread the work around, hospitals reduced service to an eight-hour day, which permitted three shifts. The economic security of nurses suffered a great setback.

Many people who needed health care could not afford it.[57] An important aspect of the federal government's recovery program was the passage of the Social Security Act, which introduced governmental involvement in health care.

[57]Fitzpatrick, M. Louise: "Nurses in American History; Nursing and the Great Depression," *American Journal of Nursing*, *75*:2188–2190, 1975.

Meanwhile within hospitals a *militaristic* image of the nurse was evolving. Military discipline pervaded the environment. There was an insistence on standing at attention when discussing patients with physicians or others of "higher rank" and holding doors open and entering elevators after others. It was stressed that one must not fraternize with "superiors," including interns.

The military influence extended even to the uniform a nurse wore. Stripes on one's cap reflected status. A probationer had no cap; after this period the "capping" ceremony occurred, and the first-year student wore a plain cap; the second year student donned a cap with one stripe; and the third-year student cap was adorned with two stripes. Dress review became part of the daily activities of the nurse, who had to stand for uniform inspection. Shoes had to be polished, the uniform had to be spotless, and the cap was not to be worn at a "sexy" angle.

The military influence was also apparent in the terms frequently used, such as "training" and "obeying orders" (other professionals had their services "requisitioned" but nurses "received orders"). Nurses were often not allowed to ask questions. Undesirable assignments such as scrubbing and cleaning were prevalent. Nurses were disciplined by losing late leaves and being curfewed. In many hospitals, they were forbidden to marry and were not allowed to show emotion in line of duty. The contrast between Nightingale School and schools in this country was startling.

THE HERITAGE OF NURSING

Conflicting Images in the Early Twentieth Century

No other profession could have had more staunchly loyal, politically enlightened, scholarly articulate and persistently undaunted leaders than those of the nursing profession who prevailed during this period.

The nurse leadership:

1. described the plight of and directions needed for nursing.

2. encouraged studies and surveys that provided accurate data to support their arguments.
3. were chagrined that the factual evidence, startling revelations and strong recommendations of the studies were not shared with the public.
4. fought to control and upgrade schools.
5. unified and strengthened nurses by forming nursing organizations and journals for communication.
6. encouraged nurse authors to write textbooks for nurses.
7. worked for establishment of a legal basis for protection of the public and the practice of qualified nurse practitioners.
8. welcomed university support for nursing education.
9. through the far-reaching efforts of community health nurses, worked with consumers and other health agencies to achieve remarkably sound health goals.

Conversely, certain nurses and vested interest groups ignored or challenged the incriminating data of the studies. These offenders included:

1. nurses who opposed change.
2. hospital administrators who ran institutions for profit at students' expense.
3. physicians who opposed "too much education" for nurses.

The public and some nurses and health workers viewed most nurses:

1. as classified "domestics" receiving "training" in a service agency.
2. as a source of cheap labor for nursing care and hospital housekeeping.
3. as "angels of mercy" because they worked so hard, for so little and for such long hours.
4. as essential to patient care because:
   a. patients went to hospitals for nursing care before the discovery of "miracle drugs" and modern surgical techniques. There was little "medical cure."
   b. patients with severe illnesses were nurtured back to health through the well-established knowledge and skills of nurses.
5. as developing a different scope of nursing practice because:
   a. new procedures and medications encouraged task-oriented assignments.
   b. nurses were encouraged to "take orders" and become physicians' assistants.
   c. nurses did not take the initiative in teaching patients or questioning medical practices and hospital routines.

Meanwhile a militaristic image of the nurse was evolving for both the student and the practicing nurse.

REFERENCE READINGS

Addams, Jane: *Forty Years at Hull House*. New York, The Macmillan Co., 1935.

American Journal of Nursing: *The Story of the Journal*. New York, American Journal of Nursing, 1950.

Boyd, Louie Croft: *State Registration for Nurses*. 2nd ed. Philadelphia, W. B. Saunders Co., 1915.

Breay, Margaret, and Fenwick, Ethel Gordon: *The History of the International Council of Nurses, 1899–1925*. Geneva, The International Council of Nurses, 1931.

Bridges, Daisy C.: *A History of the International Council of Nurses 1899–1964*. Philadelphia, J. B. Lippincott Co., 1967.

Burgess, May Ayres: *Nurses, Patients and Pocketbooks*. New York, National League of Nursing Education, 1928.

Burgess, May Ayres: *Nursing Schools Today and Tomorrow*. New York, National League of Nursing Education, 1934.

Committee on Nursing and Nursing Education in the United States: *Nursing and Nursing Education in the United States*. New York, The Macmillan Co., 1928.

Creighton, Helen: *Law Every Nurse Should Know*. 3rd ed. Philadelphia, W. B. Saunders Co., 1975.

Driscoll, Veronica M.: *Legitimizing the Profession of Nursing: The Distinct Mission of the New York State Nurses Association*. New York, New York State Nurses Association, 1976.

Faddis, Margene O.: *A School of Nursing Comes of Age*. Cleveland, The Alumni Association of The Frances Payne Bolton School of Nursing, 1973.

Fitzpatrick, M. Louise: *The National Organization for Public Health Nursing, 1912–1952: Development of a Practice Field*. New York, National League for Nursing, 1975.

Flanagan, Lyndia, Comp.: *One Strong Voice: The Story of the American Nurses' Association*. Kansas City, American Nurses' Association, 1976.

Gardner, Mary S.: *Public Health Nursing*. 3rd ed. New York, The Macmillan Co., 1936.

Gibbon, John Murray, and Matthewson, Mary S.: *Three Centuries of Canadian Nursing*. New York, The Macmillan Co., 1947.

Goodrich, Annie W.: *The Social and Ethical Significance of Nursing*. New York, The Macmillan Co., 1932.

Gray, James: *The University of Minnesota, 1851–1951*. Minneapolis, University of Minnesota Press, 1951.

Hermann, Eleanor K.: "Mrs. Chase: A Noble and Enduring Figure," *American Journal of Nursing, 8*(10):1836, 1981.

Johns, Ethel, and Pfefferkorn, Blanche: *An Activity Analysis of Nursing*. New York Committee on the Grading of Nursing Schools, 1934.

Lee, Eleanor: *History of the School of Nursing of the Presbyterian Hospital, New York, 1892–1942*. New York, G. P. Putnam's Sons, 1942.

Lesnik, Milton J., and Anderson, Bernice L.: *Legal Aspects of Nursing*. Philadelphia, J. B. Lippincott, 1947.

MacDonald, Lyn: *The Roses of No Man's Land*. London, Michael Joseph, 1980.

Marvin, Mary M.: "Research in Nursing—The Place of Research and Experimentation in Improving the Nursing Care of the Patient," *American Journal of Nursing*, 27:331, 1927.

Munson, H.: *The Story of the National League of Nursing Education*. Philadelphia, W. B. Saunders Co., 1934.

NACGN—Four Decades of Service. New York, The National Association of Colored Graduate Nurses, 1945.

Nursing Schools Today and Tomorrow. Final Report of the Committee on the Grading of Nursing Schools. New York, 1934.

National League of Nursing Education: *A Curriculum Guide for Schools of Nursing*. New York, National League of Nursing Education, 1937.

National League of Nursing Education: *Curriculum for Schools of Nursing*. New York, National League of Nursing Education, 1927.

National League of Nursing Education: *Essentials of a Good School of Nursing*. New York, National League of Nursing Education, 1936.

National League of Nursing Education: *Essentials of a Good School of Nursing*. Rev. ed., New York, National League of Nursing Education, 1942.

National League of Nursing Education: *Standard Curriculum for Schools of Nursing*. New York, National League of Nursing Education, 1917.

National Organization for Public Health Nursing: *Manual of Public Health Nursing*. Prepared by the NOPHN. New York, The Macmillan Co., 1926.

National Organization for Public Health Nursing: *The Public Health Nursing Curriculum Guide*. New York, National Organization for Public Health Nursing, 1942.

Nutting, M. Adelaide: *A Sound Economic Basis for Schools of Nursing*. New York, G. P. Putnam's Sons, 1926.

Rathbone, William: *The History and Progress of District Nursing*. New York, The Macmillan Co., 1890.

Roberts, Mary M.: *American Nursing*. New York, The Macmillan Co., 1954.

Stewart, Isabel M.: *The Education of Nurses*. New York, The Macmillan Co., 1943.

Thoms, Adah B.: *Pathfinders—A History of the Progress of Colored Graduate Nurses*. New York, Kay Printing House, 1929.

Wayland, Mary M.: *The Hospital Head Nurse*. New York, The Macmillan Co., 1938.

Winslow, C. E. A.: "The Role of the Visiting Nurse in the Campaign for Public Health," *American Journal of Nursing*, Vol. 11, 1911.

Zimmerman, Anne: "ANA—Its Record on Social Issues," *American Journal of Nursing*, 76:588–590, 1976.

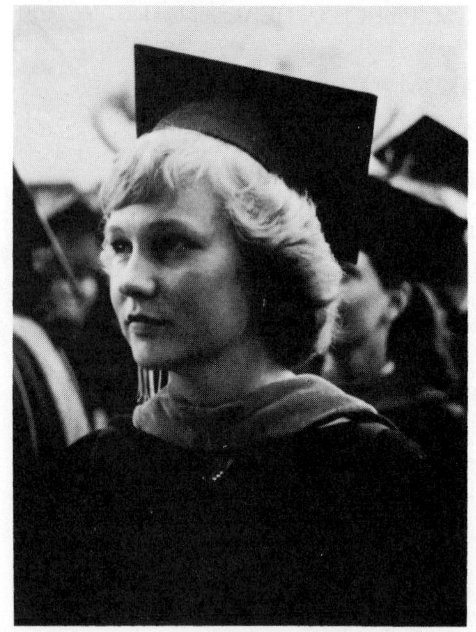

Nursing for the future. A 1982 graduate of the College of Nursing, Villanova University.

15 Nursing as a Continuing Social Force

THE GOVERNMENTAL INFLUENCE ON NURSING

NURSING AND WORLD WAR II

The Great Depression abated, but the catastrophic international conflict known as World War II loomed menacingly. This war was to have a dramatic impact on life for many years and a profound influence on nursing in the United States and other countries.

Early in 1941 the United States began drafting men by the thousands. As early as 1940 two American medical units went to Europe to help the Allies. Harvard University sent one to England, and an American-Scandinavian unit went to Poland. Many nurses responded to the government's appeal that they serve in the army camps established throughout the country.

Earlier, in the spring of 1940, our nursing leaders had comprehended the potential need for nursing service and had formed the *Nursing Council of National Defense,* composed of representatives from all the national nursing bodies: the American Nurses' Association (ANA), the National League of Nursing Education (NLNE), the National Organization for Public Health Nursing (NOPHN), the Red Cross Nursing Service, the federal nursing services, the Association of Collegiate Schools of Nursing and the National Association of Colored Graduate Nurses. Major Julia Stimson was chairman of this council. The council made plans to cooperate with similar councils in Canada and Central and South America. In 1942, this organization became the *National Nursing Council for War Service.* In order to increase the number of nurses for military service and at the same time to see that civilians were cared for, the council planned refresher courses for graduate nurses, pooled teaching staffs and made itself available for consultant service.

From 1940, a National Nurses' Committee on Procurement and Assignment, with branches in each state, considered and classified about 300,000 individual nurses as essential or nonessential to the war effort.

Wartime Nursing Education—The Cadet Nurse Corps

By means of the epoch-making Bolton Bill, the U.S. Congress appropriated $1,250,000 in 1941 and $3,500,000 in 1942 for nursing education. The bill was sponsored by Congresswoman Frances Payne Bolton (Fig. 15–1) from Ohio. This bill provided for refresher courses for graduate nurses, assistance to schools of nursing for construction of new facilities (nurses' homes, classrooms, laboratories) so that they might increase their enrollments, postgraduate courses, preparation for instructors and other personnel and training in midwifery and other specialties.

Never before had the government made such a financial commitment to nursing; still less had it concerned itself with the advancement of nursing. This bill was an important milestone in the history of American nursing.

In 1942, Mrs. Bolton sponsored a second bill in Congress, which created the *U.S. Cadet Nurse Corps*. This bill, which had been carefully planned by the *National Nursing Council for War Service*, aimed to increase the number of nurses in the country as rapidly as possible. In June 1943, the Bolton Act was passed by Congress, and the Corps became a fact. It was placed under the Division of Nurse Education of the U.S. Public Health Service. The Bolton Act created a system of government scholarships for qualified young women who wanted to be nurses (Fig. 15–2), the largest project for nursing education ever planned.

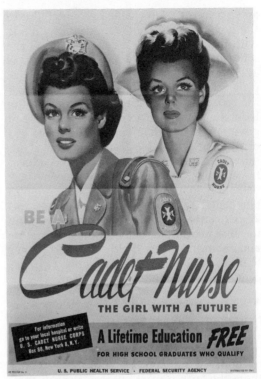

Figure 15–2. A recruitment poster emphasizing the wartime need and educational opportunities for those interested in nursing. (Dolan collection.)

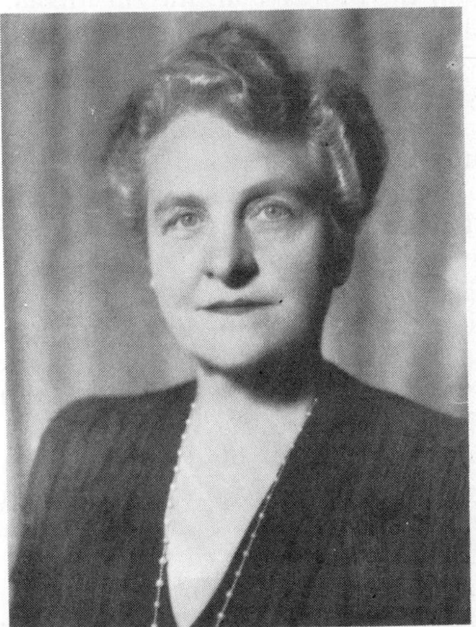

Figure 15–1. Hon. Frances Payne Bolton, sponsor in U.S. Congress of the bill that created the U.S. Cadet Nurse Corps. (Dolan collection.)

From 1943, about 95 per cent of all nursing students were enrolled in the Cadet Corps. Much publicity was given the Corps, and during its first year 65,000 students enrolled in it. The total number who joined the Corps was 179,000. The first two schools to enroll in the Corps were Freedman's Hospital School of Nursing and Providence Hospital School of Nursing.

Nurses on the staff of the U.S. Public Health Service and other nurse leaders recruited for this service provided assistance to the schools of nursing that participated in the Cadet Nurse Corps. With schools' acceptance of funds came accountability to the government. This responsibility, along with the freedom of students to attend the school of their choice now that money was available, acted as a catalyst to improve programs in nursing education. Through the reports that nursing schools sent to the federal government explaining their use of government funds, well-qualified leaders of nursing were able to obtain data about nursing education. In 1945, of the educational personnel in schools of nursing participating in the Corps' program, only 23 per cent had a baccalaureate degree, and 27 per cent were in the process of working for one. Four per cent of the instructors and administrators held degrees higher than the baccalaureate and only two per cent were working for such a degree.[1]

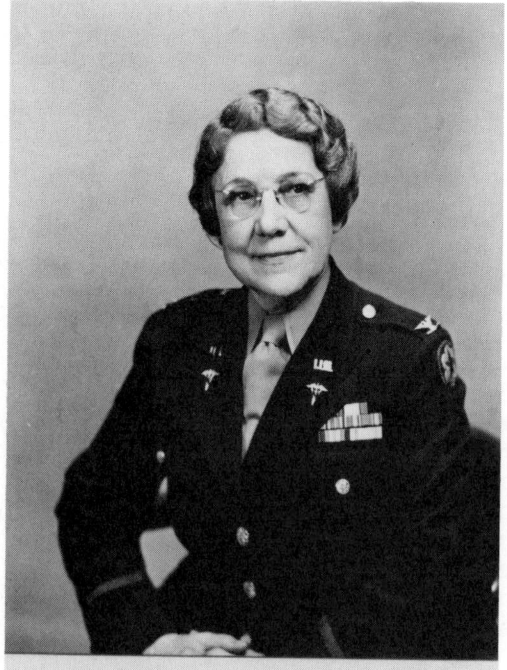

Figure 15–3. Colonel Florence A. Blanchfield, Chief, Army Nurse Corps (1943–1947). (Courtesy of the United States Army.)

Nurses in Military Services

"Relative" military rank had been granted to both Army and Navy nurses, giving them the authority of officers, though they were not commissioned. On June 22, 1944, President Roosevelt signed an executive order making the Corps an integral part of the Army, its personnel to receive the same pay and prerogatives as other officers. This order became effective on July 12, when the Corps numbered approximately 40,000 nurses. On April 16, 1947, the *Army-Navy Nurse Act* (Public Law 36) was enacted, which authorized permanent commissioned status for Army nurses. Florence A. Blanchfield became the first woman to be given a permanent commission in the regular Army as "Colonel" (Fig. 15–3).

The Army nurses were assigned to nine stations and 52 areas throughout the world; the Navy nurses, to a dozen hospital ships and more than 300 naval stations.

Some nurses did not go overseas but worked in the 80 Army hospitals in the United States. (There were about 600 Army hospitals abroad with 18,000 beds, 43 Navy hospitals and hospital ships with 10,000 berths.)

All through the war the work of nurses received special attention from the government and the public. Hundreds of significant decorations and citations were bestowed on them; 1619 nurses (approximately one out of every 40) were decorated with such medals as the Army Commendation ribbon, the Bronze Star, the Air Medal, the Distinguished Service Medal, the Silver Star and the Distinguished Flying Cross.

Regret was expressed by the government that no way was found, other than public commendation, to reward the no less heroic services of the instructors and thousands of personnel who remained on duty in civilian hospitals. Dr. Parran of the U.S. Public Health Service gave certificates "for meritorious service" to the instructors of more than a thousand schools who "prepared the largest classes of student nurses in history."

Nurses received high praise. "Those who know the record of the Army nurses since the days of the Crimea are not surprised that they proved themselves the equal of men under combat conditions."[2] "Their untiring service, their professional skill, and their unparalleled ability to sustain the morale of the wounded in their

[1] Brown, Esther Lucile: *Nursing For The Future*. New York, The Russell Sage Foundation, 1948, p. 49.

[2] Editorial, *New York Tribune*, 1943.

care will always reflect the highest credit to the Nurse Corps, U.S. Navy."[3]

Reintroduction of Men into Nursing

In World War II there were many well-qualified men nurses, who were not eligible to become commissioned officers of the Army Nurse Corps. This seems ironic in view of the fact that the first military nurses, in the Crusades, were male. On August 9, 1955, President Eisenhower remedied this situation by signing the Bolton Amendment to the Army-Navy Nurse Act of 1947. This amendment made it possible for qualified male nurses to become commissioned officers in the Army Nurse Corps Reserve.

For many years certain hospitals accepted men in their programs, though most gave the men a short course. The men were frequently not called "nurses," but "attendants."

In 1888, at Bellevue Hospital in New York, the Mills School was established with a two-year course for men; its graduates were called attendants, following the custom of the time. Bellevue had for a long time given a full course, so its male graduates were registered nurses. Frederick Jones, director of the school from 1921 to 1929, not only developed this school but also did much to promote the preparation of male nurses.

[3]Admiral William F. Halsey.

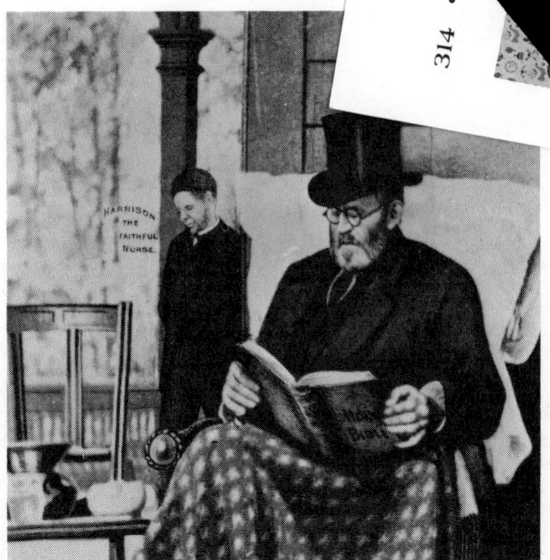

Figure 15–4. A famous gentleman, Ulysses S. Grant (1822–1885), American general and 18th President of the United States, being cared for during his last illness by Harrison, his nurse. (Dolan collection.)

Other early schools that trained male nurses were at Grace Hospital, Detroit, and Battle Creek Sanitarium, Battle Creek, Michigan; Boston City Hospital, Carney and St. Margaret's Hospital, Boston; St. Joseph's Hospital and the Pennsylvania Hospital in Philadelphia; and the Alexian Brothers hospitals in Chicago and St. Louis (Figs. 15–5 and 15–6).

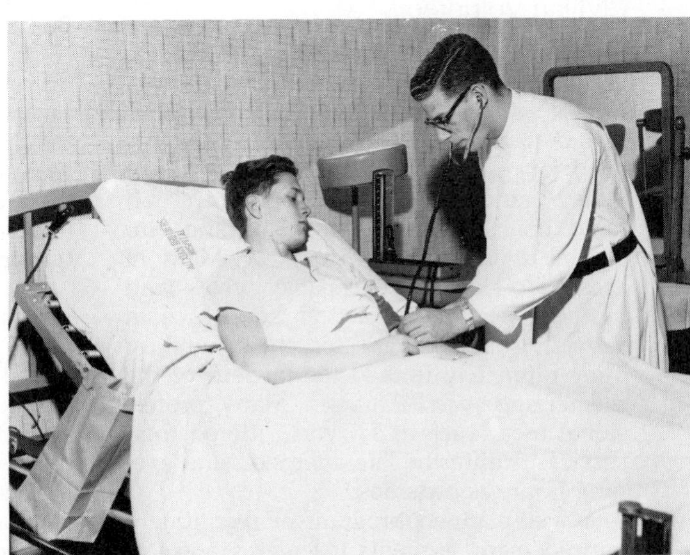

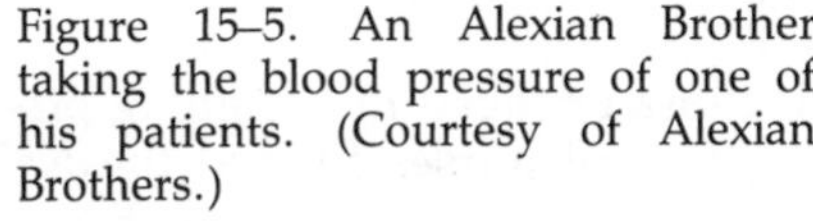

Figure 15–5. An Alexian Brother taking the blood pressure of one of his patients. (Courtesy of Alexian Brothers.)

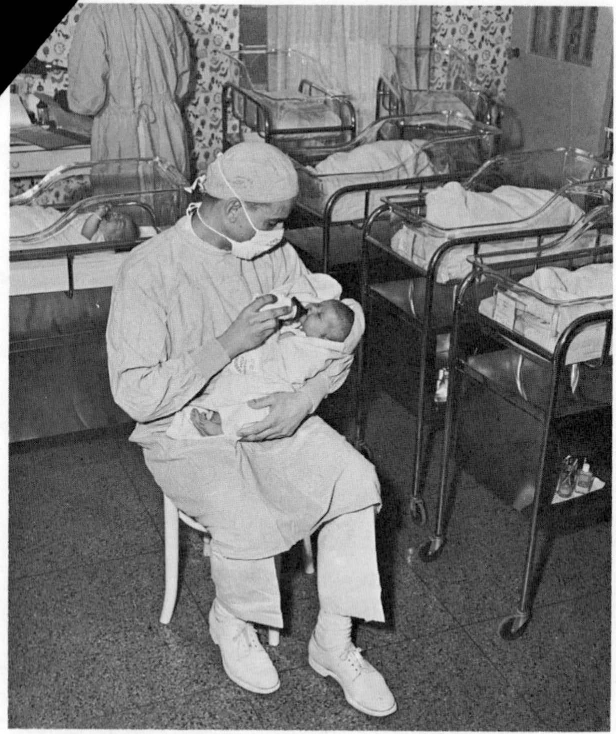

Figure 15–6. The nursery in Pennsylvania Hospital, Philadelphia. (Courtesy of Public Health Service, U.S. Department of Health, Education and Welfare.)

In 1943, there were four schools of nursing for men only: the Mills School in New York, the Pennsylvania Hospital School of Nursing for Men and the two Alexian Brothers' hospitals in Chicago and St. Louis. Now many more men are interested in nursing. Since 1948 the number of male students of nursing has increased dramatically.

Civilian Volunteers

The response to military needs for nursing care decreased the supply of registered nurses in civilian fields. Citizens volunteered to assist the hospitals in filling the need for nurse coverage. Great numbers of "Grey Ladies" and "Red Cross Aides" offered their services to hospitals and embarked upon a course in nursing. Many of these workers were capable wives and mothers who had practical experience in providing health care for their families. They ultimately formed the nucleus of the reemerging *practical nurses*. Many professional men, such as lawyers, offered their services during the late afternoon and evening hours as orderlies.

A well-planned program of recruitment enticed many students to enter schools of nursing. Patriotism and financial assistance were important lures.

Practical Nursing

Since 1880 there had been attempts at preparing practical nurses. In the early part of this century several excellent schools offered programs. Two of the pioneer schools were the Ballard School in New York and the Household Nursing Association in Boston.

One unwelcome development was the *correspondence school movement,* designed by businessmen for monetary gain, which offered correspondence courses in practical nursing (see Figure 14–10). It has been to the credit of many nurses that, in spite of tremendous opposition, these courses were terminated.

In 1941, those engaged in designing programs for practical nurses formed the *National Association for Practical Nurse Education*. This organization wanted most of the practical nursing programs to be part of the educational institutional structure. Vocational or technical schools often provided their services. These schools and their clinical practice opportunities have been approved by the State Board of Nurse Examiners in all states. Licensure for practical nurses (L.P.N.), or vocational nurses (L.V.N.) as they are called in several states, developed. By 1947, many states had passed statutes requiring licensure for practical nurses. The State Board Test Pool provided examinations for practical nurses. The Office of Education of the Federal Security Agency published a *Practical Nursing Curriculum* in 1950. In 1949, the *National Federation of Licensed Practical Nurses* (NFLPN) was formed "to foster high standards of practical nursing and to promote the welfare of the practical nurse to the end that the public will be served with the highest possible care."

In 1959, the National Association for Practical Nurse Education changed its name to the *National Association for Practical Nurse Education and Service* (NAPNES). The Council of Practical Nurse Programs of the National League for Nursing accredits these programs.

Having practical nurse representation on State Boards of Nurse Examiners has been a trend in many states.

MILITARY NURSE CORPS—AFTER WORLD WAR II

Later, during the Korean conflict and particularly during the Vietnam War, American military nurses provided valuable service to the nation. The development of the *Air Force Nurse Corps* on July 1, 1949, was an important event in military nursing. All three military nurse corps, those of the Army, the Navy and the Air Force, continue to support educational programs for nurses on active duty as well as for

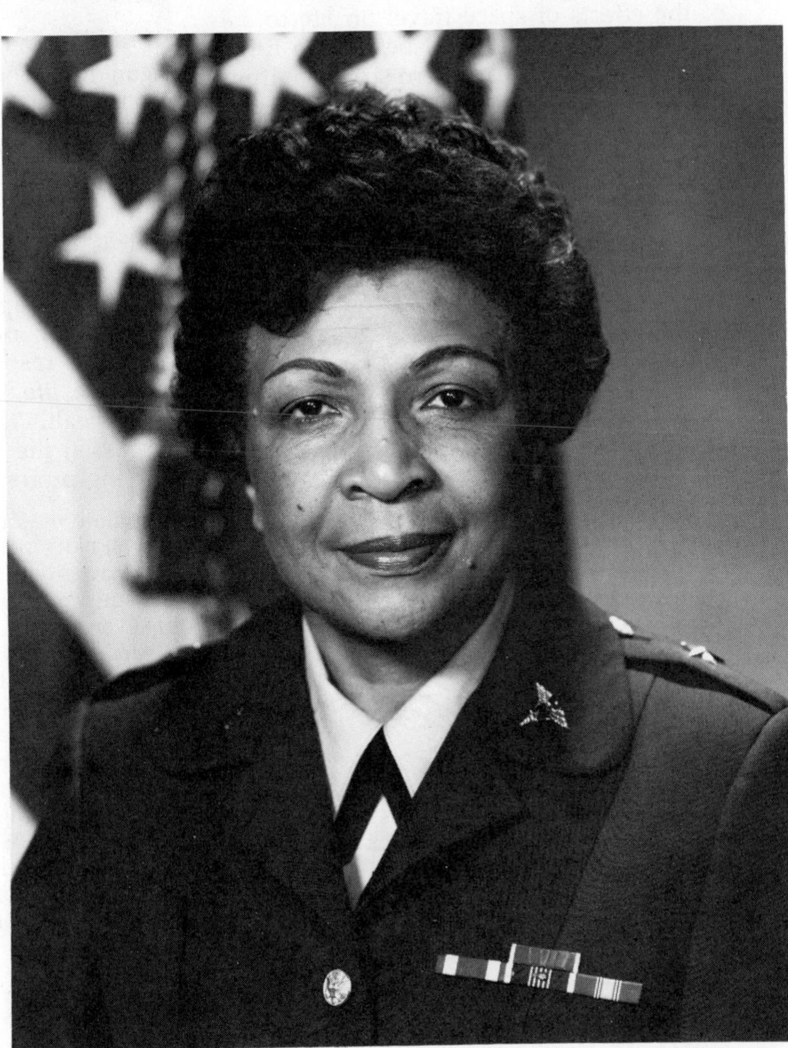

Figure 15–7. Brigadier General Hazle W. Johnson, Ph.D. (Courtesy of the United States Army. Photograph no. P–190481.)

nurses in reserve units. In addition, the Air Force and Army provide generous scholarship programs for nursing students. The Army Nurse Corps admits only those nurses who hold a baccalaureate degree in nursing. In 1979, Hazle W. Johnson, Ph.D., became the first black woman to attain the rank of Brigadier General and was appointed Chief Nurse of the Army Nurse Corps (Fig. 15–7).

Aerospace Nursing

Aerospace nursing is one of the newer specialties in nursing practice. Nurses receive educational experiences in order to assist people in adapting to a space environment. Nurses are assigned to the Air Force's *Bioastronautic Operational Support Unit* (BOSU). (Bioastronautics is the study of the effects of space travel on life to assure that the human will be able to function effectively in extraterrestrial environments.) *Major Pearl E. Tucker* became the first director of the BOSU nursing staff.

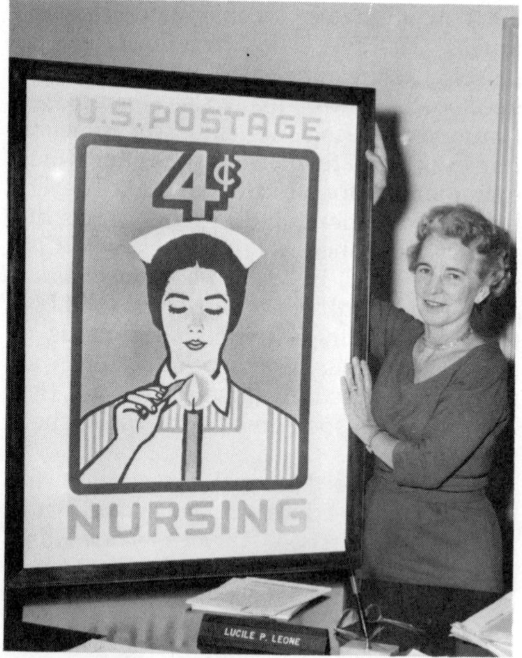

Figure 15–8. Lucile Petry Leone, Assistant Surgeon General of the United States Public Health Service, displaying the commemorative stamp. (Dolan collection.)

NURSES IN OTHER GOVERNMENT SERVICES

The Veterans' Administration, which represents the largest government-sponsored system of health care in the United States, employs the largest number of nurses. Nurses in the commissioned corps of the U.S. Public Health Service and other government programs and facilities, such as the clinical center of the National Institutes of Health, have made significant contributions to the advancement of clinical practice, research and technology in health care.

THE GOVERNMENT HONORS THE NURSING PROFESSION

In 1961, the United States government honored the nursing profession through the issuance of a commemorative stamp. The artist's depiction was representative of the public's image of the nurse at that time (Fig. 15–8). Many first-day covers, covers of stamps bearing marks showing that the stamps were mailed on the first day of their issuance, conveyed the message "science and a talent for mercy." One message, which appeared on a stamp honoring the nursing profession, stated, "The fundamental responsibility of the Nurse is to conserve life, alleviate suffering and promote health." President John F. Kennedy discussed the stamp in his message to the nursing profession:

> I salute the nursing profession of this Nation and all of its members who for more than a century have given strong leadership in translating scientific knowledge into better health for people everywhere.
>
> Modern nursing holds a high place in our system of health and medical care. We shall look to nursing even more as we move forward toward the development of better health services for all citizens in the years ahead.
>
> With the U.S. postage stamp to commemorate the nursing profession, the Government and the citizens of our country acknowledge with gratitude the advances you have already made, and we express our hopes and expectations for future progress in your own and the Nation's behalf.

Colonel Florence A. Blanchfield, Chief of the Army Nurse Corps, 1943–1947, became the first nurse or woman for whom a permanent army hospital was dedicated, when, in September 1982, the army community hospital in Fort Campbell, Kentucky, was named the Florence A. Blanchfield Army Community Hospital in her honor.

POSTWAR DEVELOPMENTS IN HEALTH CARE DELIVERY

In 1946, the *Hospital Survey and Construction Act,* also called the Hill-Burton Bill, was signed by President Harry S Truman. This bill provided a five-year federal grant-in-aid program to the states for the purpose of surveying health needs and planning and constructing necessary hospitals and health centers. The federal government paid one-third of the cost for the survey and construction; the individual states assumed the responsibility for the other two-thirds.

This act provided a challenging opportunity for nurses to be consulted and to make suggestions for the planning of work areas in which they would carry out their duties. Louise Waagen, chief of the Hospital Nursing Section, Division of Hospital Facilities of the United States Public Health Service stressed this challenge.[4]

The search for better methods of doing things, for labor-saving and step-saving devices and for the application of the principles of work simplification had long been undertaken in agriculture, industry and the home. Yet, although nursing assumed new functions, it still clung to old methods, and nurses frequently worked in antiquated work areas, walking miles and carrying heavy things.

The depletion in the ranks of nurse personnel during the war proved devastating to the civilian health care delivery system. The *case study method of patient care* was no longer feasible because of the acute shortages of nurses. A solution seemed to require a different assignment pattern using fewer well-prepared personnel. The *functional method of assignment* was designed for the task-oriented form of nursing that developed. This method of nursing resulted in fragmented care, which drew criticism from the recipients of the care and caused dissatisfaction among the providers. One nurse was assigned to give all the medications, another to take all the vital signs and a third to give all the treatments. Gone was the patient-centered approach; the family-centered approach was nonexistent. Critics decried the lack of "total patient care" or "comprehensive patient care." Clients queried, "Are hospitals made for people or vice versa?"

A change from this new unwelcome functional system to the more personalized approach was anticipated at the termination of the war. This stop-gap method continued, however, long after the war was over and the nursing staff had returned from service. The continuance of this unfortunate system was still blamed on the "shortage" of staff. Much discussion revolved around the perceived *qualitative shortage* in methods of health care delivery and providers of that care. The problems were compounded when staff of different educational backgrounds found they were assigned the same tasks.

In 1947, Mary Ella Chayer wrote a book entitled *Nursing in Modern Society,*[5] which made the members of the nursing profession aware of their current role and set the stage for another period of critical analysis of nursing and of nursing education. The foreword to this erudite work states that the book "constitutes a natural introduction . . . for it presents an enveloping concept of the true place of nursing today in the social background of which it is a part."

Miss Chayer stressed "A revolution is needed in nursing today. One is being experienced whether it is being recognized or not. Our time-honored methods of serving the public are no longer adequate. . . . Any institution that has permanence centers its activities around fundamental human needs."

Miss Chayer further indicated that as times changed and new knowledge was assembled, new techniques and skills in nursing would have to be developed. "What was good enough, or at least tolerated at

[4]Waagen, Louise: "The Hospital Survey and Construction Act," *American Journal of Nursing, 48*:361–363, 1948.

[5]Chayer, Mary Ella: *Nursing in Modern Society*. New York: G. P. Putnam's Sons, 1947.

one stage of development, is not good enough for another. The 'horse and buggy age' gives place to the 'atomic age,' with its new responsibilities and dangers."

Miss Chayer was prophetic in envisioning the revolution in nursing and health care delivery that was brewing, even though many of her contemporaries seemed not to be aware of it. There were to be marked changes in nursing education (basic, graduate and continuing); in the posture of the professional organization; in nursing service (roles and level of practice); in the total health care delivery system; in a delineation of the "nursing process"; and in licensure and definition of nursing practice.

NURSING EDUCATION

GENERAL STUDIES ON NURSING EDUCATION

The *National Nursing Council for War Service* was organized in 1942 as a coordinating council for the 14 national organizations concerned with nursing. This council's achievements were remarkable, and at the end of the war it continued as the *National Nursing Council* for the purpose of sponsoring three studies: a history of its own accomplishments, presented in *The History of the National Nursing Council* by Hope Newell; an economic survey of the nursing profession, compiled and distributed by the Bureau of Labor Statistics of the United States Department of Labor; and a study of nursing education. The National Nursing Council believed that the deficiencies in the quantity and quality of nursing service resulted from the prevailing system of nursing education.

The council obtained a financial grant from the Carnegie Foundation, and *Esther Lucile Brown,* Ph.D. (Fig. 15–9), director of the Department of Studies in the Professions at the Russell Sage Foundation, was appointed to carry out the study of nurse education. Because Dr. Brown had conducted studies and published findings on the role of education in the professions of social work, engineering, medicine and law and on how education for each could be molded to meet the needs of society, she was well prepared to conduct the survey.

The problem for this study of nurse education was the following: *How should a basic professional school of nursing be organized, administered, controlled and financed to prepare its graduates to meet community needs?*

It was essential to consider the function and place of the nurse in society before making recommendations for proper preparation. Three subordinate problems were identified:

1. What will be the probable nature of health services during the second half of the twentieth century and what nursing services will meet the needs of society most adequately?
2. What kind of education and training will prepare nurses most effectively to render these services?

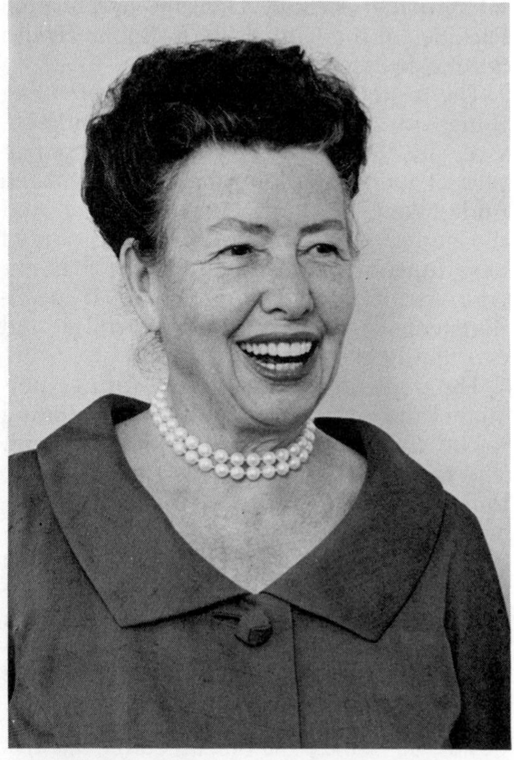

Figure 15–9. Esther Lucile Brown, Ph.D. (Dolan collection.)

3. How should this education be organized, controlled and financed?

Dr. Brown visited about 50 schools and held three regional conferences of nursing leaders in San Francisco, Chicago and Washington, D.C.[6] Her findings were interpreted and discussed, and in 1948, 28 recommendations were published in *Nursing for the Future.* These recommendations, briefly summarized, stressed the following needs:

—For nurses to study and analyze nursing functions.

—For nursing functions to be carried out by nursing-service teams.

—For clarification of the use of the term "professional," which should be used as the term is understood by educators.[7]

—For the university school of nursing to be autonomous, improve its programs, obtain a better-prepared faculty, seek the best available clinical facilities and have contracts with the clinical agency stating the privileges and obligations of both the degree-granting institution and the agency, including a statement concerning the use of the students' time exclusively for purposes of education.

—For positive steps to be taken by the nursing profession to create an atmosphere that attracts a carefully selected segment of the population.

—For provisions to be made within the university for distinguished hospital schools of nursing.

—For experimentation in shortening the course in hospital schools and at the same time making provisions for enriching their course of study. Dr. Brown stated, "A vast number of schools conducted by hospitals offer, in spite of improvements, apprenticeship training."

—To consider the use of psychiatric hospitals as agencies for affiliation in psychiatric nursing, rather than have these institutions conduct their own schools.

—To conduct a periodic examination of schools, to publish and distribute lists of accredited schools and to plan for periodic reexamination of schools.

—For the public to assume greater financial responsibility for nursing education.

—To provide a more substantial academic preparation for leadership in nursing education and in clinical nursing specialties.

—For improved programs in the educational preparation of the graduate nurse.

—For a study to plan for the distribution of schools on local and regional bases to serve the needs of the entire country.

—To improve in-service education and to achieve better interpersonal relationships within the hospital.

—For better interprofessional team relationships in more congenial hospital atmospheres.

—To increase the use of trained practical nurses, improve their educational preparation and enact sound legislation to safeguard their practice.

—For the greater use of men as nurses and for the employment of married nurses.

—For hospitals to assume a positive health function in the community and to have an increased awareness of the importance of the social and emotional factors involved in illness.

Many of the recommendations were not new. Florence Nightingale had discussed them, and other studies, such as the "Goldmark Report," had focused on them, but the problems remained and solutions still needed to be found.

This study, called the *Brown Report,* presented findings that pointed up the need for action if these long-range goals were to be secured. The importance of being aware of the needs of society in the second half of the twentieth century and preparing nurses to meet these needs were emphasized. The Brown Report quoted from the proceedings of a workshop organized by the National Nursing Council, which defined the future place of the professional nurse in nursing and in our society as a whole:

> It is the opinion of this group that in the latter half of the twentieth century, the professional nurse will be one who recognizes and understands the fundamental (health) needs of a person, sick or well, and who knows how these needs can best be met. She will possess a body of scientific nursing knowledge which is based upon and keeps pace with general scientific advancement, and she will be able to apply this knowledge in meeting the nursing needs of a person and a community. She must possess that kind of discriminative judgment which will enable her to recognize those activities which fall within the area of professional nursing and those activities which have been identified with

[6]An account of these conferences can be found in *A Thousand Think Together.* New York, National Nursing Council, 1948.

[7]"Careful consideration should be given to the fact that professional schools in most other fields have already come within degree-conferring institutions to such an extent that possession of a degree is fast becoming a criterion of a person's having received professional as contrasted with vocational training." (Brown, Esther L.: *Nursing for the Future.* New York, The Russell Sage Foundation, 1948, p. 77.)

the fields of other professional or nonprofessional groups.

She must be able to exert leadership in at least four different ways: (1) in making her unique contribution to the preventive and remedial aspects of illness; (2) in improving those nursing skills already in existence and developing new nursing skills; (3) in teaching and supervising other nurses and auxiliary workers; and (4) in cooperating with other professions in planning for positive health on community, state, national, and international levels.

In defining nursing itself, the Brown Report quoted Sister M. Olivia (Gowan) of the Catholic University of America:

> Nursing in its broadest sense may be defined as an art and a science which involves the whole patient—body, mind, and spirit; and promotes his spiritual, mental and physical health by teaching and by example; stresses health education and health preservation, as well as ministration to the sick; involves the care of the patient's environment—social and spiritual as well as physical; and gives health service to the family and community as well as to the individual.

The function of the professional nurse, and that of professional nursing, has been more than just carrying out treatments and assisting members of other professions. The nursing function should be that of *assisting patients.* Dr. Brown was impressed by the universal desire of nurses to nurse: "Nurses both want and like" to care for patients. She also noted that this desire was not satisfied because nurses were involved with non-nursing activities in archaic, energy-depleting hospital units.

With the publication of the Brown Report in 1948, the National Nursing Council, having achieved its last objective, was dissolved.

While the Brown Report was being made, the *Committee on the Function of Nursing,* appointed by the Division of Nursing Education of the Teachers College, Columbia University, was reviewing "a selected group of problems centering around the current and prospective shortages of nursing personnel."[8] The results of the discussion of this group were published in a book entitled *A Program for the Nursing Profession.* Eli Ginzberg was the chairman of the committee. Their proposals, which were summarized briefly at the end of the book were that:

a. The nursing function be subdivided among two groups of personnel—professional and practical nurses.

b. Relations be clarified and improved between the nurse and the other members of the medical and health team.

c. Suitable relations be developed among the various groups of nursing personnel who together comprise the nursing team.

d. The professional nurse complete a four-year course in a college- or university-affiliated school of nursing.

e. The practical nurse be graduated from a 9- to 12-month program in an approved school for practical nursing.

f. A goal of approximately 200,000 professional nurses for 1960 be established.

g. A goal of approximately 400,000 practical nurses for 1960 be established.

h. Conditions of pay and work in nursing be substantially improved and differentials in reward be instituted.

i. Research receive a heightened emphasis.

Reaction to both reports, but particularly the Brown Report, was violent, and much heated discussion was generated. Nevertheless, the enrichment of many programs commenced, the elimination of poor programs occurred and the accreditation process evolved into a more dynamic social and professional force.

The national nursing organizations formed a *Committee on Implementing the Brown Report,* with representatives from allied professional groups. The committee was eventually called the *National Committee for the Improvement of Nursing Services.* One of the important projects that this group sponsored was the *School Data Analysis:* By means of a questionnaire, a report of the practices in schools of nursing in 1949 was procured.

The schools cooperated wholeheartedly with the committee, and 97 per cent responded to the questionnaire. The data were analyzed, and the schools were classified against other participating schools, rather than against other criteria.[9] In November of 1949, the classification of schools appeared in the *American Journal of Nursing* under the heading "Interim Classification of Schools of Nursing Offering Basic Pro-

---

[8]The Committee on the Function of Nursing: *A Program for the Nursing Profession.* New York, The Macmillan Co., 1948, p. ix.

[9]Diploma and degree programs were graded separately.

grams." Nursing leaders and the *Journal* showed courage in publishing these data. They were subjected to great criticism by other members of the profession. The Interim Classification was published again in *Nursing Schools at the Mid-Century*,[10] together with a complete analysis of the data presented in an informative, graphic manner.

In 1949, the Russell Sage Foundation instituted an advisory service that was available to institutions of higher learning whose administration and faculty were interested in enriching their programs. Dr. Margaret Bridgman, former academic dean of Skidmore College, provided the service. The report of her activities, *Collegiate Education for Nursing*, was published in 1953.[11] This report served to stimulate improvement in baccalaureate programs for nurses. Concomitantly, the dichotomy between collegiate and diploma programs became more pronounced.

The nursing education programs of Canada have also faced scrutiny. For many years nursing leaders have voiced criticism of service-oriented programs for the preparation of nurses.

In the mid-1940's, Nettie D. Fidler, a member of the nursing faculty at the University of Toronto, was representative of those who continued to voice concerns of the nursing profession. In her 1944 report to the CNA general meeting, she identified three problem areas: the need for factual knowledge of the nursing requirements of the country; the probability that these would reveal the need for varied types of nursing services and of preparation for them; and the need for educational, i.e., financial, independence of nursing schools.[12]

In 1956, the Canadian Nurses' Association (CNA) inaugurated and financed a project to identify the strengths and weaknesses of the existing schools of nursing. A study of the value and feasibility of a national voluntary accreditation program for schools of nursing was carried out. This study became the *Pilot Project for the Evaluation of Schools of Nursing in Canada*, which was completed in 1960. Projects were undertaken to develop school improvement programs and to evaluate the quality of nursing service as well as to continue the move toward an accreditation program.

These large and expensive programs occupied the energies of the national association during the years 1960–1966, and the conclusions drawn from them form the philosophical and practical base from which the CNA now functions. Essentially, the CNA is committed to provide all reasonable help for effecting curriculum improvements in all schools of nursing. A consulting service is provided by national headquarters to work on request with provincial groups seeking to examine and improve educational processes.

Meanwhile, through provincial and national associations, nursing educators seek general acceptance, within and beyond the profession, of the principle that nurses should be prepared in educational institutions. Inseparable from this objective is the necessity of having educational programs developed and conducted primarily by educators and separated entirely from the requirement of providing service in exchange for training—an outmoded practice in conflict with modern concepts of education. Measurable evidence of progress towards this end was observed in 1966 when the Saskatchewan legislature made nursing education a responsibility of the province's education system.[13]

PREPARATION FOR THE DIFFERENT FUNCTIONS OF NURSING

A committee at Teachers College, Columbia University, was organized to focus on the problems and proposals confronting nursing and the need for differentiating between levels of preparation for functions of nursing. Professor R. Louise McManus proposed that there existed within the scope of nursing a differentiation of function.

The functions of nursing may be conceived as being of a spectrum range. Many functions involve the performance of skills and technics varying in difficulty and complexity and extending on a continuum, from the simplest performed by the mother and others, and easily

[10]National Committee for the Improvement of Nursing Services: *Nursing Schools at the Mid-Century*. New York: Osmond-Johnson, 1950.

[11]Bridgman, Margaret: *Collegiate Education for Nursing*. New York, Russell Sage Foundation, 1953.

[12]Canadian Nurses' Association: *The Leaf and the Lamp*. Ottawa, 1968, p. 5.

[13]Canadian Nurses' Association: *The Leaf and the Lamp*. Ottawa, 1968, p. 6.

picked up without training, to the most complex function demanding a very high degree of skills and expertness that can be developed only with considerable training. Many functions also demand judgment ranging from that based upon common knowledge to judgment that can be arrived at only by bringing to bear upon professional problems pertinent knowledge from an extensive reservoir of scientific information derived from many fields of study. The functions at one extreme of the range of the spectrum, those demanding a high degree of skill and judgment, must be the responsibility of nurses whose educational preparation has been of a professional type. Nurses who perform these functions can be assumed to need and to possess the breadth of scientific information with which to do reflective thinking and to have developed their higher intellectual powers and habits of reasoning, judging, and drawing inferences about nursing problems.[14]

A study on the differentiation of nursing functions was designed and carried to fruition by *Dr. Mildred Montag,* who published her findings in *The Education of Nursing Technicians.*[15] She used a simple diagram to present the concept of a continuum of nursing functions. (See figure at bottom of this page.) Dr. Montag differentiated the functions of nursing into the assisting, the technical and the professional functions. It was Dr. Montag's conviction that programs could be developed in appropriate agencies and educational institutions to prepare individuals to perform the various functions. Dr. Montag believed that the complex functions of nursing, requiring a high degree of skill, expertise and judgment, were acquired through the use of pertinent knowledge gained from intensive study. She described people who performed in this complex category as those who have obtained preparation of a professional type.[16]

This professional function was described as including:

1. The identification or diagnosis of the nursing problem and the recognition of its many interrelated aspects.
2. The decision upon a course of nursing action to be followed for the solution of the problem.
3. With the assistance of other members of the nursing and health team, both intraprofessional and interprofessional, the development of a satisfactory plan of nursing care, including therapeutic treatments for which the physician has delegated responsibility to the nurse.
4. The continued direction of the program of nursing toward its optimum accomplishment, and the performance of those aspects which demand the skill and judgment which she is best prepared to use.
5. The evaluation of the process and the results of nursing for the continuous improvement of the care of the patient and the practice of nursing.[17]

Dr. Montag believed that, at the other end of the spectrum, those performing the assisting function could be taught satisfactorily by on-the-job training in a service agency.

It was the middle section of the continuum, occupied by the technical nurse, to which she devoted her doctoral study. In their initial stages, the programs for technical nurses were experimental in nature. They were established under the aegis of a community or junior college, and an associate degree was granted. These associate degree programs were intended to be terminal.

The associate degree programs involved a curriculum of foundation courses in the

[14]Columbia University, Teachers College, Division of Nursing Education: *Regional Planning for Nursing and Nursing Education.* New York, The Macmillan Co., 1948, p. 54.

[15]Montag, Mildred: *The Education of Nursing Technicians.* New York, G. P. Putnam's Sons, 1951.

[16]Montag, Mildred: *The Education of Nursing Technicians.* New York, G. P. Putnam's Sons, 1951, p. 4.

[17]*Ibid.*, p. 55.

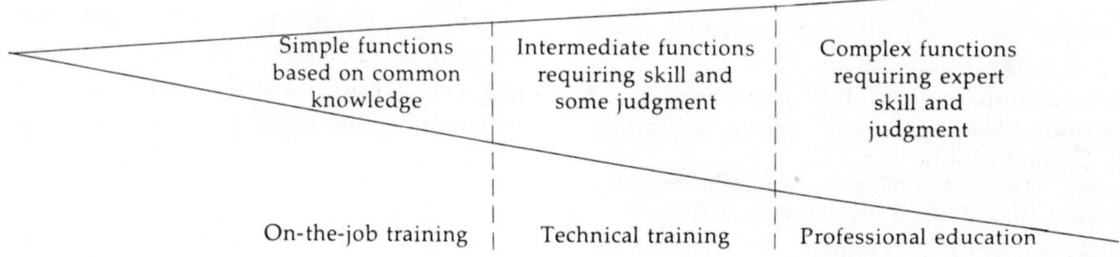

college setting and clinical courses and experiences in a hospital setting. The graduate of this program could assume the intermediate range of functions.

Following graduation, the avenue to licensure involved taking the same examinations as baccalaureate graduates and diploma school graduates. If these were passed the designation of registered nurse was obtained. These programs caused consternation, and many nurses and members of state boards of nurse examiners were not responsive to the request to permit associate degree programs to develop.

Montag proposed that the graduate of an associate degree nursing program function mainly by implementing the decisions of persons more expertly prepared and more experienced in nursing.

American Nurses Association's Study of Nursing Functions

A step forward was taken by the nursing profession when its members requested a study of all phases of nursing care. The ANA's House of Delegates approved this request at the 1950 convention, and endorsed the *ANA Program of Studies of Nursing Functions*. Thus was launched a five-year plan for research in nursing, which was financially supported by voluntary membership contributions. The earnest wish of all nurses seemed to be that nursing continue to be an important link in the chain of total health care.

In assuming its professional responsibility of undertaking research in nursing functions, the ANA had a threefold purpose:

1. To determine the functions and relationships of institutional nursing personnel of all types—professional nurses, practical nurses and auxiliary workers—in order to improve nursing care and to utilize nursing personnel most economically and effectively.
2. To determine what proportion of nursing time should be provided by each group in various situations.
3. To develop techniques for achieving the first two statements of purpose, which could be applied to all types of hospitals to obtain a national picture.

As a result of the ANA's interest, studies were made during a six-year period. Clara A. Hardin, associate executive secretary of the ANA, was appointed director of the Research and Statistics Unit, and at the 1956 ANA convention, the preliminary report *Nurses Invest in Patient Care* was released.

The ANA also stimulated a study of functions, standards and qualifications (F. S. & Q.)[18] for the practice of nursing, which was an invaluable guide for those who were planning curricula for future practitioners, those who were constructing job specifications and qualifications, those who were struggling to construct an acceptable definition for nursing, those who were trying to explain our profession to the general public and even those who were striving to defend an acceptable standard of conduct in nursing to lawyers and to courts.[19]

The ongoing change in functions continued to spawn studies, including a five-year project, which commenced in 1950 under the sponsorship of the ANA and the NLN. The results of this project were published in 1958 in *Twenty Thousand Nurses Tell Their Story*. It presented a sharp contrast to the 1930 *Activity Analysis of Nursing*.

In contemplating the study of the functions and standards of nursing care, people have scrutinized the area of nursing service. Many studies have been made and are still being carried out in this area. Notable among these has been an investigation of interpersonal relationships and their effect on patient recovery done by Leo Simmons at the New York Hospital.[20] Another point of interest was determining how many non-nursing tasks were being carried out by nurses. The Division of Nursing Resources of the U.S. Public Health Service conducted a study of this matter at the

---

[18]"American Nurses' Association statements of functions, standards and qualifications," *American Journal of Nursing*, 56:898, 1027, 1165, 1305, 1586, 1956.

[19]McIver, Pearl, and Anderson, Bernice: "Functions, Standards and Qualifications," *American Journal of Nursing*, 57:748–750, 1957.

[20]Simmons, Leo W.: *Studies in the Application of Social Science in Medicine and Nursing at New York Hospital—Cornell Medical Center*. New York, The Russell Sage Foundation, 1950.

Massachusetts General Hospital.[21] Another study in this type investigated the misuse of professional nursing personnel and made suggestions for using this personnel more effectively to achieve the greater satisfaction of nurses and patients. This project was carried out at Harper Hospital in Detroit,[22] and the feeling seemed to be that nursing should be given back to nurses. Also studied were the formations and uses of *nursing teams,* including the development of the philosophy of team work and its implementation.[23]

Self-Direction in Education—ANA

On May 4, 1960, at the forty-second convention of the ANA, held in Miami Beach, the delegates voted to accept from the Committee on Current and Long Term Goals a report that was to become the basis for continued discussion in the state associations. Included in this report was a section referred to as Goal Three, which stated:

> To insure that, within the next twenty to thirty years, the education basic to the professional practice of nursing for those who then enter the profession shall be secured in a program that provides the intellectual, technical and cultural components of both a professional and liberal education. Toward this end, the ANA shall promote the baccalaureate program so that in due course it becomes the basic educational foundation for professional nursing.

The ANA, the professional organization, was implementing its goals in becoming involved in self-analysis and self-direction, and for the first time, nurses were acting independently in making the decision to promote baccalaureate education.

Many states appointed committees to study the progress of nursing and nursing education.

The functions of the ANA Committee on Nursing Education were: to study and develop standards for nursing education and methods for their implementation; to evaluate scientific and educational developments as well as changes in health needs and practices; to determine implications for nursing education; and to encourage and stimulate research in all areas of nursing education.

ANA Position Paper of 1965. Acting to implement their goals, the Committee on Nursing Education prepared a position paper in 1965 that had as its major thesis: "Education for those who work in nursing should take place in institutions of learning within the general system of education." This paper was of tremendous historical significance because it was proposed and was approved by the membership of the ANA, meeting in biennial assembly in San Francisco in 1966.

Nursing practice has become exceedingly complex. The conditions of nursing are determined by the structure of society and its prevailing values. Professional nurses are required to master a complex, constantly enlarging body of knowledge and to make critical, independent judgments about patients and their care.

The essential components of professional nursing are those of care and cure. From the early Judeo-Christian base in nursing we know that the care aspect of nursing means more than "to take care of"; it means "caring for," "caring with" and "caring about" people in the broadest dimension. Caring is dealing with human beings under stress and, on occasion, over long periods. Other aspects of caring include comforting and supporting in times of anxiety, loneliness or helplessness, and listening, evaluating and intervening when necessary.

The cure aspect involves the promotion of health and healing. It requires assisting patients to understand their health problems and, through teaching, to cope with them. It includes carrying out a prescribed plan for care of the patient. The nurse, carrying out the cure aspect, shares the burden, with the community, of the responsibility for the health and welfare of all by participating in programs to prevent illness and maintain health. The curing function also encompasses the supervision and teaching of those who give any aspect of

---

[21] Olson, Appollinia F., and Tibbitts, Helen G.: *A Study of Head Nurse Functions in a General Hosital.* Public Health Monograph No. 3 (P.H.S. publication No. 107). Washington, D.C., United States Government Printing Office, 1951.

[22] Wright, Marion J.: *The Improvement of Patient Care.* New York, G. P. Putnam's Sons, 1954.

[23] Newcomb, Dorothy P.: *The Team Plan.* New York, G. P. Putnam's Sons, 1954.

nursing care, as well as participation in research or collaboration with those in other disciplines in research that results in more satisfying, scientific and better nursing care.

This rationale prompted the ANA Committee on Nursing Education to recommend that:

1. Minimum preparation for beginning professional nursing practice should be baccalaureate degree education in nursing.
2. Minimum preparation for beginning technical nursing practice should be associate degree education in nursing.
3. Education for assistants in the health service occupations should be short, intensive preservice programs in vocational education institutions rather than on-the-job training programs.

The technological advances in medicine that have stimulated impressive innovations in mechanical devices compel the profession to demand a scientific but humanistic nurse who can function in this environment and, in addition, provide compassionate personal care.

Colleges have been charged with designing programs to provide master clinical practitioners to assume faculty positions, with developing programs for continuing education and with encouraging research in nursing to expand the boundaries of nursing as an art and a science.

The ultimate aim of nursing education and nursing service is the improvement of nursing care. The primary aim of nursing education is to provide an environment in which the student of nursing can develop self-discipline, intellectual curiosity and the ability to think clearly and acquire knowledge necessary for practice. Nursing education will achieve its ultimate aim when recent advances in knowledge and findings from nursing research are incorporated into the program of nursing study.

The primary aim of nursing service should be to provide nursing care of the type needed and in the amount desired to those who require it. Nursing service achieves its ultimate aim when it provides a climate in which questions about practice can be raised and answers sought, in which nursing staffs continue to develop and learn and in which nurses work in collaboration with persons in other disciplines to provide improved services to clients.

These aims—educating nurses and providing clients with care—can be carried out only when nurses in education and in service recognize their interdependence and actively collaborate to achieve the ultimate aim of both—improved nursing care.

The ANA adopted structural changes as a result of the action of the House of Delegates in 1966. The *Nursing Practice Department,* created as a result of structural changes, devised plans to advance the clinical competence of practitioners of nursing. It encouraged recognition of professional achievement and research relative to the practice of nursing. Standards for nursing practice in various clinical areas and the process of certification of nurses were established.

In March of 1967 the newly established *Commission on Nursing Education* of the ANA identified four areas of need:

1. The need to delineate the "sphere of influence," responsibility and authority of nurses.
2. The need to identify inadequacies in the current system of education and health care.
3. The need to define the purpose and essential characteristics of education for nurse practitioners.
4. The need to identify functions for baccalaureate and associate degree graduates.

Open Curriculum in Nursing Education

In February 1970, the Board of Directors of the NLN approved the following statement:

> An open curriculum in nursing education is a system which takes into account the different purposes of the various types of programs but recognizes common areas of achievement. Such a system permits student mobility in the light of ability, changing career goals, and changing aspirations. It also requires clear delineation of the achievement expectations of nursing programs, from practical nursing through graduate education. It recognizes the possibility of mobility from other health related fields. It is an interrelated system of achievement in nursing educa-

tion with open doors rather than quantitative serial steps.[24]

The board of directors approved the following *Statement of Concern About Degree Programs for Nursing Students That Have No Major in Nursing* in October 1971:

> The National League for Nursing notes with concern the growth in the number of collegiate programs that have no major in nursing but are designed to appeal specifically to potential and enrolled nursing students and registered nurses. Publicity about these programs leads students to believe that they offer preparation for advanced positions in nursing or provide the base needed for further education in nursing when this is not the case.
>
> The programs in question lead to associate or baccalaureate degrees in such fields as applied science, biology, education, health science, occupational therapy, psychology, and sociology. Large blocks of credit are promised the student for nursing education obtained outside the college. The collegiate programs may provide the student with increased knowledge in the specified area of the major, but they do not offer additional preparation in nursing.[25]

Other suggestions for assisting individuals to obtain additional education have been proposed. According to the *career ladder* concept, for example, the student can progress from aide to practical nurse preparation to associate degree preparation to baccalaureate. The *external degree* concept enables an individual who possesses knowledge and ability equivalent to those of a person with a degree from an academic institution to take a battery of examinations, written and practical, and earn an undergraduate degree without attending a college or university.

Associate Degree Nursing Education

In the thirty years since their inception, associate degree programs have become the largest category of nursing programs in the United States. Unlike the original premise, which spawned their development, that the associate degree would complete the training for the graduate, the current view of the degree is as an entry point for professional nursing or the first step up an educational ladder. Many associate degree graduates continue their education and study for baccalaureate degrees in nursing following licensure as registered nurses.

Curriculum in Nursing Education

During the latter part of the twentieth century several distinctive developments occurred relative to curriculum development. One was the increased ability of nurse educators to design and implement professional education programs. Among the most significant developments were programs designed primarily to accommodate registered nurses who wished to study for a baccalaureate degree in nursing. In many ways, these programs were reminiscent of the early collegiate programs designed for registered nurses who had completed a diploma education. Some were exclusively upper division programs admitting only registered nurses, others were traditional baccalaureate programs, which offered credit by examination for the R.N. and another was the New York State Regents External Degree Program, considered controversial in the 1970s but generally accepted by the 1980s and accredited by the NLN in 1981.

Another important development in nursing curriculum design was the movement toward integration. This approach was a major departure from the former "medical" model. The new approach viewed nursing practice as a composite of knowledge and skills that are applied in a variety of practice settings for the care of individuals and members of groups and communities who are at varying levels of illness and wellness and who represent different ages and backgrounds. The integrated curriculum provided a conceptual approach to the study and teaching of nursing practice, with much attention given to systematic assessment, planning, implementation and evaluation of patient needs and nursing care. This approach was commonly referred to as the "nursing process." Attention to major concepts, such as the respon-

---

[24]National League for Nursing: *The Open Curriculum in Nursing Education*. New York, NLN, 1970.

[25]National League for Nursing: *A Statement of Concern About Degree Programs for Nursing Students That Have No Major in Nursing*. New York, NLN, 1971.

sibilities of nursing to those individuals requiring health maintenance, health restoration and health promotion and the use of conceptual frameworks and nursing diagnosis to organize educational exposure, characterized curriculum in professional nursing programs.

By the 1980s, there was once again realization that attention needed to be given to the preparation of administrators of nursing services and the education of teachers of nursing practice. It became increasingly apparent that a balance between the preparation of clinical specialists and role specialists needed to be monitored by the profession.

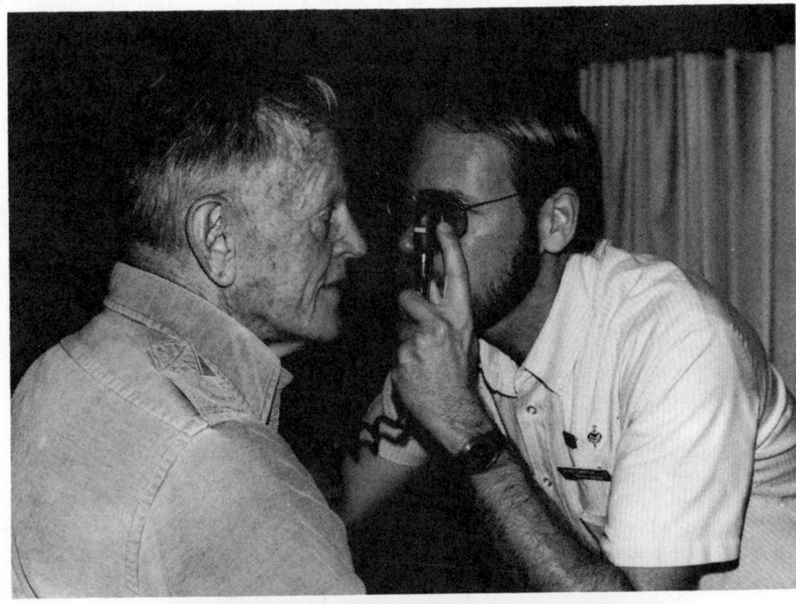

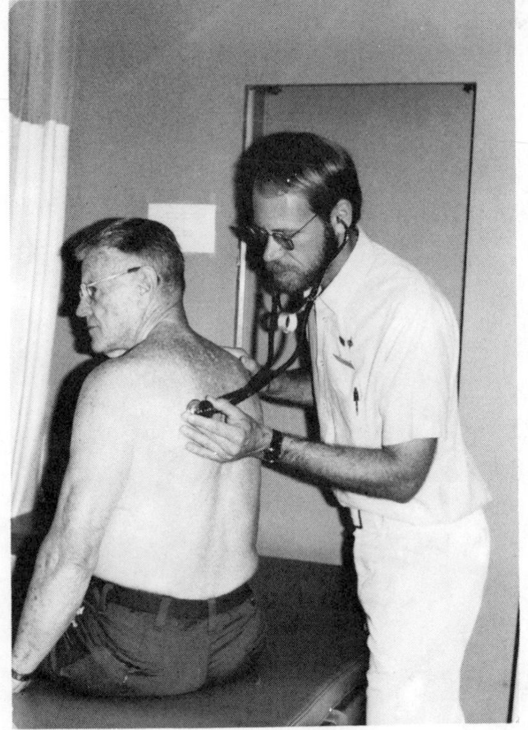

Figure 15–10. Master's degree–prepared clinical nurse specialist examining a patient. (Herrmann collection.) (Photographs by Ruth N. Knollmueller.)

Graduate Education in Nursing

In 1969, the ANA issued a *Statement on Graduate Education in Nursing:* "The major purpose of graduate study in nursing should be the preparation of nurse clinicians capable of improving nursing care through the advancement of nursing theory and science."

The assumptions that moved the membership of the ANA Commission on Nursing Education to prepare the preceding statement were the following:

> Graduate education is a more intensive and analytic extension of undergraduate education, enabling students to perceive and develop new relationships among the various factors and forces that affect nursing.
>
> There is now available an increasingly large body of nursing knowledge which appropriately and logically belongs in graduate education.
>
> Nursing must further develop and structure its body of knowledge, and add new knowledge that is relevant to both general and specialty practice.
>
> Corporate responsibility for the education of nurse clinicians capable of advancing nursing theory and science rests with institutions of higher learning.
>
> Nurses prepared at graduate levels can assume leadership in assessing the role of nursing in relation to changing concepts of health care, delineating action to bring about change, selecting that action most feasible at any given time, implementing decisions, and evaluating results in order to achieve quality nursing care.[26]

Master's degree programs have been increasing numerically and qualitatively. The proliferation of master's degree programs and the emphasis on the preparation of clinical specialists and nurse practitioners peaked in the late 1970s (Fig. 15–10). Such programs advanced the practice field, reinforced the autonomous role of nursing and established the primary care role of professional nurses. In 1982, there were 111 accredited master's degree programs.

Another development in the 1970s was the renewed interest in generic master's degree programs for basic nursing education and the development of the *first generic doctoral program in nursing* at the Frances Payne Bolton School of Nursing at Case Western Reserve University (Fig. 15–11). Nursing research and more sophisticated skills in physical and behavioral assessment as well as practice in establishing nursing diagnoses became integrated parts of the graduate program's curriculum. The inspiration for this Doctor of Nursing (N.D.) curriculum and degree came from a distinguished nurse leader, Dr. Rozella Schlotfeldt (Fig. 15–12). This three-year post–non-nursing baccalaureate program re-

[26]American Nurses' Association: *Statement on Graduate Education in Nursing*. New York, ANA, 1969, p. 2.

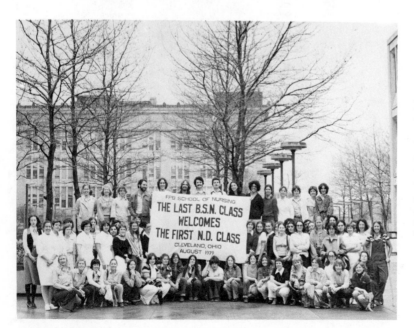

Figure 15–11. Nursing students of the last baccalaureate class at Frances Payne Bolton School of Nursing, Case Western University, Cleveland, Ohio, rally around the banner they sewed themselves proclaiming the beginning of the school's new doctor of nursing program. (Courtesy of Case Western Reserve University.)

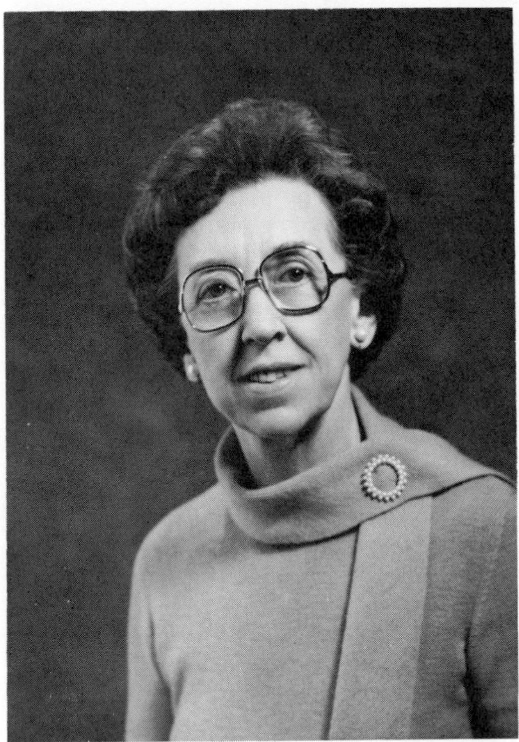

Figure 15–12. Rozella Schlotfeldt, Ph.D., a dynamic, innovative leader of nursing.

ceived not only the enthusiastic endorsement of the faculty of the nursing school but also that of the enrolled students.

The majority of schools of nursing now grant the Ph.D., with a growing number awarding the D.N.Sc., and a smaller number awarding the Ed.D. Many nurses choose to earn doctorates in allied and related fields.

CONTINUING EDUCATION

In the annals of nursing history many nurse leaders have emphasized the necessity of continuing one's education; notable among them were Florence Nightingale, Edna Foley and Mary Adelaide Nutting. Obviously, the concept of a planned program of learning experiences designed to broaden and enrich the scope of knowledge and skills after completion of the initial academic preparation is not a new one. Such programs can provide a vehicle for assuring continuing competence of nursing personnel in education and practice.

Continuing education programs have a specific focus; are short-term in length; are conducted in a variety of settings, such as colleges, universities, health agencies and professional organizations; are designed to meet the needs of professional people and are paid for by them; and provide evidence of participation through the awarding of *continuing education units* (CEUs). It has been proposed that the acquisition of CEUs be mandatory for relicensure.

Continuing education programs enable participants to improve or acquire new knowledge and skills; to change from one area of practice to another; and to assume greater responsibility for professional development and delivery of more improved service to the client and community.

Programs in continuing education differ markedly from those of *inservice education,* which are designed, paid for and conducted by the employing business or agency to meet the needs of its employees.

In addition to ongoing continuing education programs conducted by schools of nursing and health agencies, state nurses' associations and some national nursing organizations offer special conferences to meet the learning needs of nurses. Nursing Chataqua in Colorado and Nursing East in Pennsylvania are examples of two such regional programs.

ACCREDITATION— A STRENGTHENING PROCESS FOR NURSING EDUCATION

The National Nursing Accrediting Service (NNAS) was established in 1949. This organization represented the unification of accrediting services previously carried by the NOPHN, the NLNE, the Association of Collegiate Schools of Nursing, and the Council on Nursing Education of the Catholic Hospital Association. This accrediting service was responsible to a Joint Committee on Unification of Accrediting Activities, the membership of which represented the various nursing organizations, the American Medical Association, the American Hospital Association and the regional associations in higher education. This joint committee was in turn responsible to the joint board of directors of the six national nursing organizations.

When the reorganization of nursing organizations took place in 1952, because the new National League for Nursing (NLN) had been the descendant of the former American Society of Superintendents of Training Schools as well as the NLNE, it assumed the responsibility for all accrediting activities, even though it saw its function as that of "a community-oriented" association, rather than a professional organization for nursing.

The *Manual of Accrediting Educational Programs in Nursing* of the NNAS set forth the purposes of the accrediting service:

1. To stimulate progressive changes in nursing education that will improve nursing service and provide better health care.
2. To indicate, through published lists, institutions offering programs of nursing education worthy of public recognition.
3. To describe the characteristics of educational units offering programs of nursing education that are of superior quality.
4. To guide the prospective student in the selection of an educational unit offering programs in nursing.
5. To assist those responsible for schools and programs of nursing and state boards of nurse examiners in providing for better preparation of nurses.
6. To encourage, within each educational unit, self-evaluation and study of its own problems.
7. To encourage appropriate groups to engage in suitable experimentation and research in nursing and nursing service.[27]

Since its inception this group has carried on the important function of visiting, evaluating and accrediting schools of nursing. The accrediting service has also carried out a program of guidance for faculties of schools of nursing by conducting workshops and conferences. It publishes lists of accredited schools for the public, for prospective students of nursing and for guidance counselors in high schools.

Dr. Helen Nahm, who was director of the NLN accrediting service for seven years, wrote that this procedure of "accrediting programs in nursing can be looked upon as a last resort of nurse leaders to bring about improvements in nursing and nursing education"[28] inasmuch as the previous extensive studies, the publication of curriculum guides and the utilization of cost studies had failed to produce results. The famous "Grading Committee" studies of the NLN were inaugurated with the avowed intent of grading programs in nursing education and then sharing their standings with the public. In actuality the public was not made aware of the damaging data, although each school received a report indicating its standing in comparison with other schools.

The publishing of these lists of accredited schools and the sharing of these lists with guidance counsellors and the public proved a significant force for improving good schools, closing poor ones and, in general, upgrading nursing education.

Criteria published by the NLN in 1972 emphasize the progressive establishment in nursing of liberal and professional requirements, the development of nurses' leadership skills and ability to make decisions and exercise independent judgment and the necessity to stress the research process.

The accreditation process has become an important self-evaluation technique by which faculty record their evaluations, which are studied by a peer group, in furtherance of the concept of accountability to the profession, students, clients and the public.

LEGISLATION FOR FINANCING NURSING EDUCATION

Legislation, both state and federal, was enacted to encourage students to enter schools of nursing and to better prepare all nursing personnel—faculty members and nursing service staff members—in their particular areas of specialization. On the local level, many states have passed bills for scholarship aid for nurses.[29]

The most gratifying legislative accom-

[27]*Manual of Accrediting Educational Programs in Nursing*. New York, National Nursing Accrediting Service, 1949.

[28]Nahm, Helen: *What We Have Learned in the United States from More Than Thirty Years of Accreditation of Nursing Schools*. Unpublished manuscript, 1974.

[29]"Connecticut's scholarship aid program," *American Journal of Nursing*, 54:200–202, 1954.

plishment was the passage of the *Health Amendments Act* in 1956, which provided the opportunity for nurses to obtain advanced preparation for positions in administrations, supervision and teaching and in traineeships for public health personnel. It also provided for financial support for expansion and improvement of practical nurse programs under the direction of state vocational educational agencies.[30] This program has been quite successful in encouraging more academic preparation for nursing leadership.

With the passage of the *Nurse Training Act of 1964,* funds were made available for programs in nursing that either were fully accredited by the NLN or had reasonable assurance of receiving accreditation at an early date.

During the late 1970s and early 1980s, the amount of federal funding for nursing education declined sharply. Simultaneously, there was a decline in the number of students applying to nursing programs, due in part to the fact that there were fewer high school graduates as well as the expansion of opportunities for women in previously male-dominated occupations. A reordering of priorities for funding at the national level should place more emphasis on advanced preparation for nurses and continued stimulation of nursing research.

MAJOR REPORTS OF THE SECOND HALF OF THE TWENTIETH CENTURY

Many studies of nursing and nursing education were undertaken in the 1960s. (Nurses, as a group of workers, have been subjected to complete and constant scrutiny.) The National Commission for the Study of Nursing and Nursing Education was an independent group established by the ANA and the NLN. Its objective was to conduct a comprehensive study of nursing education in the United States. In 1963, the Surgeon General's Consultant Group on Nursing, in their document *Toward Quality in Nursing,* recommended an investigation of nursing education on a national level, with special emphasis on the responsibilities and skills needed for a high level of nursing care.[31]

In 1966, the Board of Directors of the American Nurses' Foundation voted a financial contribution to launch the study. Additional substantial sums of money were contributed by the Avalon and W. K. Kellogg foundations and an anonymous benefactor. The commission functioned as an autonomous group with W. Allen Wallis, president of the University of Rochester, as president. There were 12 people on the commission, three of whom were nurses. Jerome P. Lysaught was appointed director of the project and Charles H. Russell associate director.

In facing the magnitude of their assignment the commission determined that the following essential topics needed to be scrutinized: *the supply and demand for nurses, nursing roles and functions, the education of nurses* and *nursing careers.*

The final report with recommendations appeared in a book entitled *An Abstract for Action,* referred to as the *Lysaught Report.*[32] The commission held that change in nursing could be visualized in terms of four basic priorities.

A. Increased research into the practice of nursing and the education of nurses;
B. Improved educational systems and curricula based on the results of that research;
C. Clarification of roles and practice conjointly with other health professions to ensure the delivery of optimum care; and
D. Increased financial support for nurses and for nursing to ensure adequate career opportunities that will attract and retain the number of individuals required for quality health care in the coming years.[33]

In their acknowledgments the staff paid tribute to two historic documents—Abraham Flexner's *Medical Education in the United States and Canada* (1910) and Esther Lucile Brown's *Nursing For The Future* (1948).[34] It

[30] Jenney, Mary O., and Wehrwein, Annabel: "Federal traineeships—the first year," *American Journal of Nursing, 53*:1329–1332, 1953.

[31] U.S. Public Health Service: *Toward Quality in Nursing.* Report of the Surgeon General's Consultant Group on Nursing. Washington, D.C., U.S. Government Printing Office, 1963.

[32] Lysaught, Jerome P.: *An Abstract for Action.* New York, McGraw-Hill Book Co., 1970.

[33] *Ibid.,* p. 155.

[34] *Ibid.,* p. 98.

was reported that the decisions of Dr. Brown and this commission were remarkably similar. The important document of 1923 referred to as the *Goldmark Report (Nursing and Nursing Education in the United States)* received scant attention.

Scrutiny of Nursing Education

In focusing upon the dilemma of nursing education, the Lysaught report recognized the position taken by the ANA in 1965 that nursing education should take place in institutions of learning, but the study reported: "Many nurses, and even more physicians and [hospital] administrators feel that there is much to commend the hospital school approach."[35] The commission explained that societal trends, lack of qualified faculty, lack of qualified student applicants and the preference of students for programs that emphasized general education were instrumental in the reduction in the number of hospital-based schools of nursing. The stance of this commission in placing nursing education within institutions of higher education was stressed by the recommendation that:

> Each state have, or create, a master planning committee that will take nursing education under its purview, such committees to include representatives of nursing, education, other health professions, and the public, to recommend specific guidelines, means for implementation, and deadlines to ensure that nursing education is positioned in the mainstream of American educational patterns with its preparatory programs located in collegiate institutions.[36]

Another unusual recommendation was that "those hospital schools that are strong and vital, endowed with a qualified faculty, suitable educational facilities, and motivated for excellence be encouraged to seek and obtain regional accreditation and degree granting power."[37] It has not been the custom for service agencies that maintain educational programs to receive regional accreditation from general educational bodies nor to be empowered to award degrees.

It was recommended that all other hospital schools of nursing "move systematically and with dispatch to effect interinstitutional arrangements with collegiate institutions." Junior and senior collegiate institutions were encouraged to work cooperatively to develop programs with these hospital schools.

The commission also recommended that:

> The state master planning committees be charged with drawing up a plan for each state to determine the number and minimum size of institutions to receive institutional and individual student aid; [and that]
>
> Small programs be terminated or consolidated into larger programs in order to reduce the per unit costs of education and in order to make better allocation of qualified faculty.

Recommendations were made for the provision of financial assistance to nursing education, such as that:

> Nursing education institutions be encouraged and given federal and state awards and support grants proportional to the number of students enrolled, such moneys to be used to defray the expenses of operation and expansion, and to provide salary support for qualified faculty.
>
> Federal and state grants for building and construction of facilities be sharply increased to update and enlarge laboratory and classroom areas. There should, however, be an effort made at each institution having multiple preparatory programs to encourage and plan joint, cooperative use of buildings, laboratories, etc.
>
> Both state and regional committees explore the possibilities of sharing and increasing scarce faculty resources. A state, for example, might employ faculty through its university system to serve at several institutions for nursing education, while both state and regional associations could develop programs for the professional advancement of current and future faculty personnel.[38]

The commission studied the need for reexamination of accreditation of educational programs for nursing and recommended that a national committee of the

---

[35]*Ibid.*, p. 6.

[36]Lysaught, Jerome P.: *An Abstract for Action.* New York, McGraw-Hill Book Co., 1970, p. 107.

[37]*Ibid.*, p. 109.

[38]Lysaught, Jerome P.: *An Abstract for Action.* New York, McGraw-Hill Book Co., 1970, p. 112.

ANA and the NLN study and make recommendations for future accreditation.

In consideration of curricular needs, joint planning between the junior and senior collegiate levels was recommended to delineate "appropriate levels of general and specialized learning for the different types of educational institutions." It was stressed further that education is an open-ended process and that the opportunity to broaden one's education is a right of every individual.

In the area of graduate study and faculty development there should be adequate numbers of quality programs with permission withheld for the inauguration or expansion of weak ones. Graduate programs that prepare for positions in administration and education were seen to be of less value in society than those providing a clinical specialty.

The commission recommended that three specific types of preparation receive priority in the provision of financial assistance for graduate programs in nursing: programs for those individuals intending to teach nursing, those preparing for the master clinician role and those wishing to participate in the organization and delivery of nursing. The commission recommended that Congress continue to expand such programs as those established by the Health Manpower Act to:

> a. Provide educational loans to nurses pursuing graduate degrees with provision for part or whole forgiveness based on subsequent years of teaching;
> b. Provide postmaster and postdoctoral fellowships and traineeships for nursing faculty and master clinicians to permit added professional development and continuing reorientation to changing practice and developing health care delivery systems;
> c. Provide earmarked funds for faculty members of schools of nursing to enable them to obtain additional formal academic preparation equal to that required for regular appointment to faculty posts in collegiate institutions. These funds should have similar forgiveness features based on years of continuing service.[39]

The desire to seek innovative techniques to enhance learning effectiveness and efficiency resulted in the commission's recommendation that federal, state and private funds be made available to nursing institutions:

> a. In the form of small research grants or contracts to assess and evaluate the effectiveness of new media and technology for nursing education and to disseminate the results;
> b. In the form of grants and stipends to support short-term workshops to acquaint faculty members with new media and instructional materials;
> c. In the form of institutional grants or matching funds to permit the purchase and installation of media systems and the required technicians to maintain and operate them;
> d. In the form of demonstration grants to develop a limited number of centers so that faculty members may visit and have "actual" experience with these new media and materials.[40]

A true profession enlarges the body of knowledge it uses and improves its education and service through research. It was incumbent upon this commission to recommend that:

> Federal, state, and private funds be extended to support a limited number of institutions to establish or expand doctoral programs in nursing science. These programs should focus on developing research capabilities for the study of nursing practice and nursing education, and should undertake the specification and development of nursing theory and knowledge.
>
> The Federal Division of Nursing, the National Center for Health Services Research and Development, other governmental agencies, and private foundations provide research funds and contracts for basic and applied research into the nursing curriculum, articulation of educational systems, instructional practices, facilities design, etc., so that the most functional, effective, and economic approaches are taken in the education and development of future nurses.[41]

The commission recommended that the admission procedures be studied as well as placement tests and achievement tests to judge students' ease in retention and academic progression. The realm of academic counseling and opportunities for individual programs of instruction received scru-

[39]Lysaught, Jerome P.: *An Abstract for Action*. New York, McGraw-Hill Book Co., 1970, p. 118.

[40]*Ibid.*, p. 119.

[41]Lysaught, Jerome P.: *An Abstract for Action*. New York, McGraw-Hill Book Co., 1970, p. 120.

tiny. "Growing capacity to allow the student to learn at his own rate can mean acceleration for the talented as well as deceleration for the capable but less rapid learners."

The commission studied *continuing education* and even though the group recognized that the nurse is responsible for her own continual learning, the commission decided that provision for obtaining an enriched program of education is the obligation of the profession. Therefore the commission recommended that:

> The state master planning committee for nursing education identify one or more institutions to be responsible for regional coverage of continuing education programs for nurses within that area, and further that:
>
> a. Federal and state funds be utilized to plan and implement continuing education programs for nursing on either a statewide or broader basis (as suggested by the current interstate compacts for higher education); and
>
> b. In the face of changing health roles and functions, and the interdependence of the health professions, vigorous efforts be taken to have continuing education programs jointly planned and conducted by interdisciplinary teams.[42]

Attention was focused upon *in-service education* and the commission recommended that:

> Health care facilities, including hospitals, nursing homes, and other institutions, either individually or collectively through joint councils, provide professional training staffs to supervise and conduct in-service training and provide released time, facilities, and organizational support for the presentation of in-service nursing education as well as that for other occupations.[43]

In order to implement the various recommendations, the commission urged that:

> Federal, regional, state, and local governments adopt measures for the increased support of nursing research and education. Priority should be given to construction grants, institutional grants, advanced traineeships, and research grants and contracts. Further, we recommend that private funds and foundations support nursing research and educational innovations where such activities are not publicly aided. We believe that a useful guide for the beginnings of such a financial aid program would be in the amounts and distribution of funds authorized by Congress for fiscal 1970, with proportional increases from other public and private agencies.[44]

Nursing Careers

The commission examined nursing as a rewarding and satisfying career. It was acknowledged that there have been two traditional solutions to the problem of the shortage of nurses, namely constant campaigning to increase the number of students of nursing and increasing markedly the categories of helping personnel such as practical nurses, nurse aides, attendants and orderlies. The commission reiterated that "the profession must evaluate the current emphasis on quantity of nursing service to the near exclusion of quality considerations. The competency required of today's nurse practitioners makes it mandatory that prospective students be recruited through careful screening. Health personnel are not mere hands; and the growing complexity of care should serve to deemphasize our concern with numbers alone."

The commission perceived a lack of input from nurses in planning operations for health. "Until recently, the National Advisory Commission on Health Manpower had not a single nurse among its members, and only one nurse on any of its seven specialized panels." The American Hospital Association acquiesced to the request of nurse leadership, and nurses now have "a voice in all areas of its activities."

It is imperative that nurses assume an active role in the planning and action programs involving health care. Nurses must realize that changes in all aspects of care, such as new buildings, staffing patterns and treatments, have a direct influence on nurse activities. Nurses must have a voice in the determination of those things that affect nursing care. The commission recommended that "nurses be appointed to and hold membership in groups involved in health manpower planning at all governmental and regional levels."

Concern for the retention of qualified

[42] *Ibid.*, p. 122.
[43] *Ibid.*, p. 123.

[44] Lysaught, Jerome P.: *An Abstract for Action.* New York, McGraw-Hill Book Co., 1970, p. 124.

practitioners was expressed. The unhappiness and dissatisfaction of nurses was examined as were the many factors responsible for the loss of members from the profession. Career satisfaction seemed to be directly proportional to the ability to carry out the nursing care role. The impact of financial inequities between levels of nursing and between beginning and experienced practitioners was acknowledged. The commission noted that in order to retain capable nurse practitioners and to entice inactive but skilled nurses back into service, adequate financial reward and nursing care function incentive must be realized.

In order "to provide greater recognition for those who pursue a career in nursing service, and, just as importantly, improve the quality of care by retaining expert practitioners in their specialty," the commission recommended that "health management administrators and clinical directors of nursing service build on current improvements in starting salaries to create a strong reward system for remaining in clinical practice by developing schedules of substantially increasing salary levels for experienced nurses functioning in advanced capacities."

In appreciation of the view that "the present undifferentiated approach to clinical nursing skill should be revised," the commission recommended that:

> Personnel policies in all health care facilities should be so designed that they:
>
> a. Differentiate levels of responsibility in accord with the concepts of staff nurse, clinical nurse, and master clinician with appropriate intermediate grades. These levels should be designed according to the content of the position and the clinical proficiency required for competent performance;
>
> b. Provide for promotion granted on the basis of acquisition of the knowledge and demonstrated competence to perform in a given position.[45]

In order to ensure that nurses would be afforded "the opportunity to provide the highest quality of patient care," the commission believed that a "redirection of health care practices" must be effected that would relieve nurses of non-nursing activities and permit concentration on the nursing functions. To this end, it was recommended that:

> Health management administrators and clinical directors of nursing service establish conditions to promote optimum opportunity for excellence in nursing practice by providing such elements as sufficient staff to develop and execute a personal care plan for each individual, the opportunity to discharge appropriate nursing functions in client teaching, counseling, and rehabilitation, and the surveillance and evaluation of the nursing plan for care.[46]

The commission verified that "full excellence in the humane delivery of health care" will be achieved if and when *qualified personnel* are given the *time* to function as they desire and are prepared to do.

Well-prepared nurses will be retained or will return much more readily when programs in continuing education are utilized.

Provision for ongoing continuance of professional nurse membership revolves around the recruitment of students of nursing. The challenge of contemporary nursing should be publicized. A clear and correct interpretation should be presented. The need for the profession to disseminate accurate information to potential nursing students resulted in the recommendation that "state nurses' associations and state leagues for nursing undertake more effective dissemination of information to high school guidance counselors on the changing status of nursing, the opportunities for expanded clinical practice, the improving salary levels, and other career aspects of the profession."

The expansion of the scientific base of nursing with its new therapeutic treatments requires knowledgeable practitioners. The public must be assured of competency, and therefore licensure came under scrutiny. The commission recommended that all "states without mandatory licensure laws for registered nurses immediately adopt appropriate regulation to this effect."

In addition to initial licensure the commission considered the question of renewal of licensure to assure continued profes-

[45]Lysaught, Jerome P.: *An Abstract for Action.* New York, McGraw-Hill Book Co., 1970, p. 134.

[46]Lysaught, Jerome P.: *An Abstract for Action.* New York, McGraw-Hill Book Co., 1970, p. 135.

sional competency. Some states are considering requiring individuals to present documented evidence of participation in continuing education. The commission recommended that "all state licensure laws for nursing be revised to require periodic review of the individual's qualifications for practice as a condition for license renewal."

In order for nursing organizations to function effectively, to truly represent nursing, the commission recommended the following:

The national nursing organizations press forward in their current study of functions, structures, methods of representation, and interrelationships in order to determine:

a. Areas of overlap or duplication that could be eliminated;

b. Areas of need that are currently unmet; and

c. Areas or functions that could be transferred from one organization to another in light of changing systems and practice.[47]

The commission's plea for unified support by nurses is recognized in the recommendation that "individual nurses make a professional commitment to their organizations by joining and supporting one or more of them, at the same time ensuring that the organizations become more surely representative and more truly the designated spokesmen for nurses."

Implementation of the Lysaught Report

The emphasis of the Commission on Nursing Education turned from investigation to implementation. Although change had been noted after each of the preceding studies of nursing, the noticeable effects were not proportional to the input of significant data or to the pertinence of the suggestions for improvement. The commission felt a strong motivation to launch a plan to carry out their recommendations. It has been noted that energy and action can be generated after the publishing of the results of a study but eventually lethargy and inertia conquer. The members of this commission believed that "change is absolutely necessary to realize the potential contribution of nursing to the solution of our many health problems."

The implementation phase placed emphasis on the following:

1. The development and expansion of nursing practice together with a reexamination of role relationships among the health professions;
2. The repatterning of educational systems in nursing to meet current exigencies and provide a foundation for innovation; and
3. The emergence of an unambiguous profession that would, in fact, be a full partner in shaping health policy and in serving the needs of our people.[48]

Dr. Leroy E. Burney, former U.S. Public Health Service Surgeon General as well as president of the Milbank Memorial Fund, assumed the presidency of the commission. There were replacements in membership on this commission. Of the 20 members, five were nurses. Funds were supplied from the Kellogg Foundation with contributions from the NLN and ANA.

The continued efforts of the National Commission for the Study of Nursing and Nursing Education have been directed in three areas, that of joint practice, statewide planning and dissemination of information.

A tangible aspect of implementation was noted in the establishment of a National Joint Practice Commission in 1973. Their assignment was to discuss, study and make recommendations concerning the related roles of the nurse and physician in providing quality care. Approval for this was received from both the A.N.A. Board of Directors and the A.M.A. Board of Directors.

Although it made many pertinent recommendations, the Lysaught report has not been regarded as faultless. Perusal of primary historical documentation appeared to be nonexistent, resulting in many inaccuracies in historical viewpoint and content. Constructive criticism of the study has been published, and the weaknesses in basing changes on such an inexact foundation have been identified.[49]

[47]Lysaught, Jerome P.: An Abstract for Action. New York, McGraw-Hill Book Co., 1970, p. 144.

[48]Lysaught, Jerome: "From Abstract into Action," *Nursing Outlook, 20* (3):173, 1972.

[49]Christy, Theresa E., Poulin, Muriel A., and Hover, Julie: "An Appraisal of An Abstract for Action," *American Journal of Nursing, 71*:1574–1581, 1971.

In the content of the report many studies of nursing have been referred to as attesting "to the persistence of problems in the nursing profession" rather than to the persistence of those faced by the nursing profession.

RECENT STUDIES OF NURSING

During the 1970s and early 1980s several important studies were conducted that held great significance for nursing and nursing education.

Action in Affirmation: Toward an Unambiguous Profession of Nursing was a longitudinal follow-up on the recommendations of the National Commission for the Study of Nursing and Nursing Education. The investigation, financed by the Kellogg Foundation, examined changes in nursing role, careers and practice from 1973 to 1978 and progress in the implementation of the recommendations presented in Lysaught's *Abstract for Action*. The study concluded that considerable progress had been made on the proposals set forth in the original report. It also addressed the need for continuing attention to develop research to enlarge nursing's knowledge base to improve patient care, to advance collegiate education for nursing enrichment through clinical and research training and to develop systematic procedures for recognizing and certifying advanced clinical competence, with new patterns of compensation to reward expert practice.[50]

The Study of Credentialing in Nursing: A New Approach, undertaken by a study committee under the auspices of the ANA, was published in 1979. The study resulted from the resolution of the 1974 ANA House of Delegates "to examine the feasibility of accreditation of basic and graduate education." The committee attempted to assess the adequacy of credentialing mechanisms in nursing, including accreditation, certification and licensure. Among the recommendations of the study was a proposal that a national credentialing center be established to serve as a means of unifying and coordinating a comprehensive credentialing system for nursing.[51] Although the report met with much controversy, the 1982 ANA House of Delegates voted that such a center be established under the auspices of the ANA.

Another important study, which commenced in 1980, was that of the National Commission on Nursing. Its initial report and preliminary recommendations were published by the Hospital Research and Educational Trust in 1981. The commission, an independent group consisting of 30 individuals representing nursing and a wide range of other disciplines, was supported in its investigation by the American Hospital Association, Hospital Research and Educational Trust and American Hospital Supply Corporation. Although there were several specific charges given to the group, the primary reason for the commission's existence was to study the nursing shortage. The commission examined three major categories of relationships: those between nurses and other health care providers and agencies, those between the nursing profession and nursing education and nursing practice and those between nurses and the public. Five categories of issues provided a focus for the commission's work, including the status and image of nursing, the interface of education and practice, the effective management of resources, the relationships among nursing and others and the maturing of nursing as a profession.[52]

The preliminary report of the commission recommended the improvement of nurses' work environment and remuneration and the acceptance of baccalaureate education as a requisite for professional nursing practice. The impact and influence of the study's recommendations cannot yet be evaluated; however, they provide a blueprint for ongoing efforts that will greatly affect the profession in the coming decades.

A fourth study of importance commenced as a result of a Congressional mandate, in Section 113 of the Nurse Training

[50]Lysaught, Jerome P.: *Action in Affirmation: Toward an Unambiguous Profession of Nursing*. New York, McGraw-Hill Book Co., 1981, p. 191.

[51]*The Study of Credentialing in Nursing: A New Approach*. American Nurses' Association, 1979.

[52]National Commission on Nursing: *Initial Report and Preliminary Recommendations*. Chicago, The Hospital Research and Educational Trust, 1981.

TABLE 15–1. GROWTH OF SCHOOLS OF NURSING IN THE UNITED STATES—1873 TO 1973

Year	Number of Schools
1873	4
1888	22
1900	400
1910	1100
1920	3000
1923 Goldmark Report–"*Nursing and Nursing Education in the United States*"	
1930	1900
1940	1300
1948 Brown Report–"*Nursing For The Future*"	
1950	1190
1960	1137
1970	1355
1970 Lysaught Report–"*An Abstract For Action*"	
1973	1373

Act Amendments of 1979 (PL96-76), that a study in nursing and nursing education be conducted by the National Institute of Medicine. An interim report was issued in July 1981, with a final report expected in January 1983. The study grew out of the assertion made by the Carter administration that there was an adequate supply of nurses in the United States. The preliminary report focused on spiralling health care costs, maldistribution of nurses and health needs in rural areas. The reaction of organized nursing to the report, especially to the public assertions made regarding the self-serving nature of collegiate education as preparation for professional nursing practice, was extremely negative. The nursing profession views this report as a potential threat to professional advancement and awaits the final report and its

TABLE 15–3. PROGRAMS FOR REGISTERED NURSES AND LICENSED PRACTICAL NURSES—1970, 1975 AND 1980

Year	Total Basic R.N. Programs	Practical or Vocational
1970	1355	1253
1975	1375	1337
1980	1403	1319

recommendations while continuing to take serious issue with the Institute's six-month preliminary study.

Another landmark report called *Nursing—A Social Policy Statement* was developed by the ANA Congress for Nursing Practice and published by the ANA in 1980. The report defines the nature and scope of nursing practice and the criteria for specialists in nursing practice as well as their roles and functions. It discusses the importance of certification of specialties and the emerging categories of nursing diagnosis as foundations of the development of specialties in the future.

Marlene Kramer, Ph.D., did a study on the problems experienced by newly graduated nurses in making the transition from school to hospital and in becoming oriented to the administrative structure and function of hospital-based nursing. Her thought-provoking book, *Reality Shock,* contains her findings. In addition to other suggestions, she recommends that "preceptors" assist new graduates of nursing in making appropriate adjustments.

IMPACT OF STUDIES

Tables 15–1 to 15–3 reveal the discernible effects certain of these studies have had on nurses and nursing by illustrating trends in numbers and kinds of programs.

TABLE 15–2. SCHOOLS PREPARING STUDENTS FOR LICENSURE AS REGISTERED NURSES—1960–1980

Year	Total Number of Programs	Number and Type of Program		
		Diploma	*Associate Degree*	*Baccalaureate**
1960	1137	908	57	172
1965	1193	821	174	198
1970	1355	641	444	270
1975	1375	428	618	329
1980	1403	311	707	385*

*Includes three basic programs leading to a master's degree in nursing and one basic program leading to a doctorate.

PROGRESS OF NURSING ORGANIZATIONS

The effectiveness of the National Nursing Council for War Service, consisting of representatives of the six operative nursing organizations, pointed up the benefits of unity in action. At the termination of World War II, the need for a study to consider restructuring and unifying nursing groups to eliminate duplication as well as to strengthen the efforts of each was recognized. The group selected to conduct the study was the Raymond Rich Associates, which proposed that one or two organizations could be substituted for the six existing ones. This suggestion was accepted in 1950 when the proposal to have just two national organizations, the ANA and the NLN, was endorsed. The reorganization was completed in 1952, but the changes were not endorsed wholeheartedly or without expression of feelings of concern or disappointment. Many nurse leaders had wanted one organization.

At the biennial 1952 convention of the ANA, another milestone was reached when students of nursing voted to form a *National Student Nurse Association* under the sponsorship of the Coordinating Council of the ANA and the NLN. This association is composed of students enrolled in state-approved schools of professional nursing.

NATIONAL LEAGUE FOR NURSING

The National League for Nursing developed into a community organization to improve nursing, and thereby health services, through a coalition of community leaders, nurses, allied professionals, nursing service agencies and nursing schools. The NLN fosters community planning for nursing as a primary component of comprehensive health care, the development of nursing manpower and high standards of nursing service and education.

In May of 1967 at the biennial convention of this organization for nursing, a new structure was adopted. The new bylaws of the NLN, amended in 1967, were designed to provide a greater degree of flexibility in the structure of the organization. It was hoped that through this new form the national board of directors and the constituent leagues could achieve a closer working relationship to reinforce one another's goals and objectives.

Greater freedom was afforded the constituent leagues to determine boundaries. State boundaries could define the limits of a constituent league, or a section of a state or a union of several states might be chosen in order to provide the best milieu for the consideration of area needs.

The membership of the NLN consisted of individual members and agency members; the *Assembly of Constituent Leagues for Nursing* together with six regional assemblies that provided coordination of planning and action among the constituent leagues; and the councils of Associate Degree Programs, Baccalaureate and Higher Degree Programs, Diploma Programs, Practical Nursing Programs, Hospital and Related Institutional Nursing Services, Home Health Agencies and Community Health Services.

The League's Council of Hospital and Related Institutional Nursing Service has been active in providing continuing education workshops for agency as well as individual members.

In the early 1980s, the NLN underwent a major internal reorganization. Simultaneously, developments within the larger profession held great significance for the NLN. The National Council of State Boards of Nursing selected a commercial firm to develop the new professional licensing examination, thus removing that activity from the State Board Test Pool of the NLN. In the early 1980s, many issues concerning the process of NLN accreditation of nursing education programs surfaced. In 1981 the Council of Baccalaureate and Higher Degree Programs of the NLN voted to elect a board of review and members of the appeal panel. In addition, the council recommended that schools have more freedom in selecting accreditation site visitors.

In February 1982, the NLN issued a historic statement entitled "Nursing Roles—Scope and Preparation," which acknowledged the importance of the baccalaureate degree as an appropriate credential for professional nursing. This statement evoked tremendous reaction from NLN agency members. Diploma programs threatened to resign their memberships, and baccalaureate programs appaluded the courage of

NLN to finally take a stand on the issue of entry into practice. The 1983 biennial convention of the NLN in Philadelphia was viewed as a turning point in the history of the organization.

THE AMERICAN NURSES' ASSOCIATION

After the various reorganizations, the ANA's functions have been identified as follows:

To establish functions, standards, and qualifications for nursing practice.

To enunciate standards of nursing education and implement them through appropriate channels.

To establish a code of ethical conduct for practitioners.

To stimulate and promote research designed to enlarge the knowledge on which the practice of nursing is based.

To promote legislation and to speak for nurses in regard to legislative action.

To promote and protect the economic and general welfare of nurses.

To provide professional record service and assist states with counseling and placement activity.

To provide for the continued professional development of practitioners.

To represent nurses and serve as their spokesman with allied national and international organizations, government bodies and the public.

To serve as the official representative of the United States as a member of ICN.

To promote the general health and welfare of the public through all association programs, relationships and activities.

To promote relationships with the NSNA.

The structure of the ANA is designed to provide for these functions.

During recent years, the ANA has continued to represent the interests of the individual nurse. Through the state nurses' associations, economic and general welfare programs have expanded. Councils within the ANA, such as the *Council of Nurse Researchers*, have provided a forum for nurses who share common interests. In January 1973, the *American Academy of Nursing* was established to recognize nurses considered to have made major contributions to leadership and scholarship in the field.

At the ANA's 1982 convention, held in Washington, D.C., the House of Delegates voted a major by-law change that called for the restructuring of the ANA beginning in 1984. The new structure, termed the federation model, was developed through the combined efforts of the Washington State Nurses' Association and the New York State Nurses' Association. The reorganization specified that state nurses' associations be the central units of membership in the ANA and that the individual member belong to ANA through membership at the state level. The reorganization was viewed as a landmark in nursing history and an attempt to strengthen ANA while providing for flexibility and autonomy of state nurses' associations.

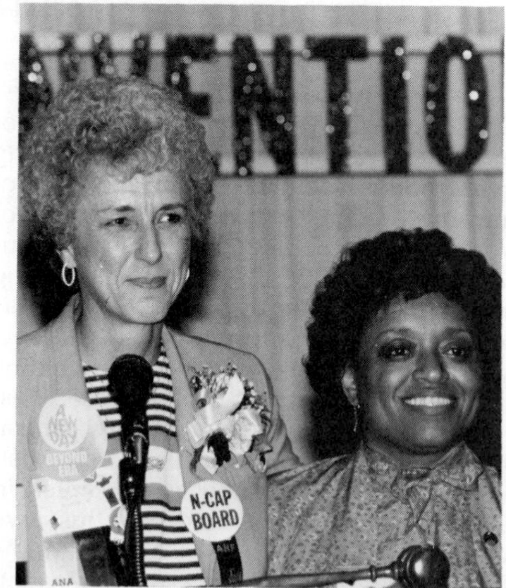

Figure 15–13. Eunice Cole, the newly elected president of the American Nurses' Association (*left*), with the outgoing president, Barbara Nichols (*right*), at the 1982 ANA convention. (Courtesy of the ANA.)

NATIONAL STUDENT NURSES' ASSOCIATION

The National Student Nurses' Association (NSNA) has expanded in size and influence since its inception in 1952. At its 25th convention in 1976 the following resolution on education for practice was adopted by the House of Delegates:

WHEREAS, education for the practice of nursing as registered nurses presently is through programs of two, three, four and five years in length and with differences in education content, and

WHEREAS, nurses graduating from these varying programs are being prepared for different types of practice, yet all are hired, for the most part, for similar beginning positions, and

WHEREAS, such variety in preparation for basic practice is confusing to the public, employers and nurses as well, and

WHEREAS, most of the health professions have a single route for basic practice at or above the baccalaureate; therefore be it

RESOLVED, that NSNA urge the gradual movement of all programs preparing for practice as registered nurses to the baccalaureate level, and be it

RESOLVED, that NSNA urge state boards of nursing, the American Nurses' Association, the National League for Nursing, the American Association of Colleges of Nursing and public groups to place a moratorium on the opening of *new* diploma and associate degree programs in nursing (in order to encourage more students to enter baccalaureate programs in nursing), and be it

RESOLVED, that NSNA work with other groups in nursing, the public and the legislators to increase the financial support for baccalaureate programs and that NSNA study educational philosophies of baccalaureate programs in order to strengthen such programs.

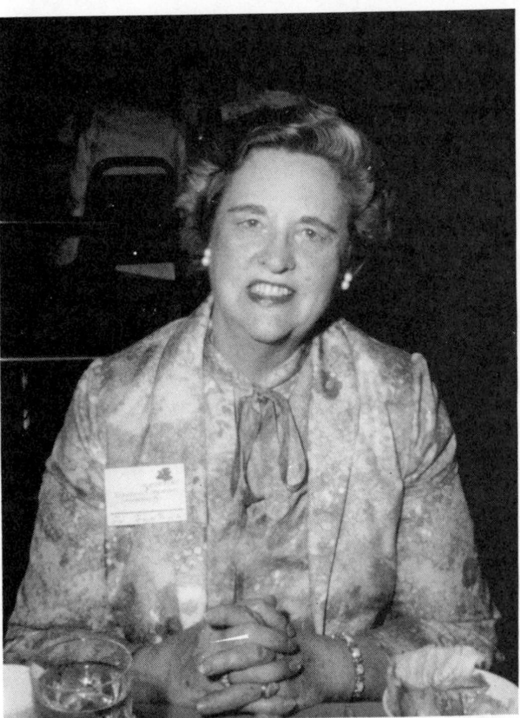

Figure 15–14. Dorothy A. Mereness, Ed.D., first president of the American Association of Colleges of Nursing.

THE AMERICAN ASSOCIATION OF COLLEGES OF NURSING

The American Association of Colleges of Nursing (AACN), founded in 1969 by approximately 40 deans of collegiate nursing programs, has become a significant force within nursing education. Through its legislative efforts, publications and continuing education offerings for deans, this association has advanced higher education for nurses and has influenced public policy concerning nursing and nursing education.

Through membership in the AACN, schools of nursing, represented by their respective deans, gain a forum for discussion of common concerns and become a political force for the promotion of higher educational programs in nursing.

POLITICAL ISSUES

One of the critical issues at stake for nursing in the last few years has been not just the economics of nursing but also the very precious opportunity to practice in a professional way. Barbara Schutt has pointed out that "practice issues are getting increasing attention at the bargaining table."[53] Dr. Schutt contacted all but three of the American Nurses' Association's 54 state and territorial constituents. She found that during the past decade there was a dramatic increase in the number of state nurses' associations that have negotiated nurses' contracts and that "numbers of contracts have increased five-fold to cover six times as many nurses."

The ANA has played a strategic role in this effort. The Economic and General Welfare Commission's chairman, Dr. Ada Jacox, has emphasized forcefully that the professional organization must help nurses to gain greater control over their practice. She said:

> Nurses have a great deal of knowledge about how to improve patient care. Many nurses are becoming less passive about what happens to patients and to nurses themselves in our con-

[53]Schutt, Barbara G.: "Collective Action for Professional Security," American Journal of Nursing, *73*:1946, 1973.

temporary health care system. . . . For a group of nurses to act collectively to improve care received by patients is professionalism in the truest sense.[54]

The control of nursing practice by nurses themselves has become one of the major issues facing the nursing profession. Maas and associates[55] have presented the thesis that "nurses claim their purpose is to deliver individualized health care . . . but most nurses lack the professional authority to control nursing care." This issue concerns one of the criteria of a profession, that of *autonomy.* Coupled with autonomy is *accountability* to the profession and to clients. The authors of this article condensed their beliefs into a diagram that emphasizes that professional nurse autonomy and authority are essential to client welfare (Fig. 15–15).

POLITICAL ACTION GROUPS

Nurses are becoming more involved in social and political action groups. Members of these groups are working with other nurses in learning how to communicate effectively with legislators and how to share the concerns of the nursing profession and to express the need for more effective health care with those responsible for legislation.

The ANA established an independent political action program in 1974 referred to as *Nurses for Political Action.* This group, which represents the legislative and political action arm of the ANA, is now called *N-CAP—Nurses' Coalition for Action in Politics.*

As a result of the efforts of this group, nurses have been encouraged to become social and political activists. They have noted that the role of the nurse has been broadened to include social activism and political expertise to achieve the rightful place of nursing in the health field; to share in federal health funding so that the delivery of nursing care will serve clients more effectively; and to reach legislative decision-makers as well as to develop policies and positions in health matters. Nursing must be included in a national health insurance plan so that nurses will be recognized as providers of health care and eligible for reimbursement for services.

Valeria Fleischhacker was the first director of N-CAP, and Helen Keller Bremberg is the current director.

[54]*Ibid.*, p. 1951.

[55]Maas, Meridean, Specht, Janet, and Jacox, Ada: "Nurse Autonomy—Reality Not Rhetoric," *American Journal of Nursing, 75*:2201, 1975.

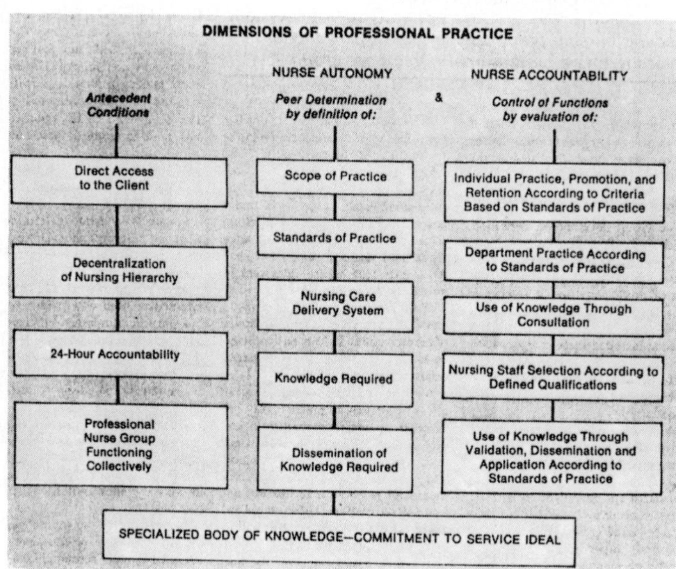

Figure 15–15. Chart of dimensions of professional practice. (From Maas and Jacox: *Guidelines for Nurse Autonomy–Patient Welfare.* New York, Appleton-Century-Crofts, 1977.)

NURSING FUNCTION AND PATIENT CARE

NURSING SERVICE PRACTICE MODALITIES

The staffing patterns of the twentieth century have tended to repeat themselves. Early in the century, when procedures were being developed to meet the demands of the new treatments, the *efficiency method* dominated the nursing scene. This method was suited to the task-oriented milieu into which nursing was permitting itself to drift.

The next pattern, the *case study method,* was designed and utilized by the new School of Nursing at Yale University. Dean Effie J. Taylor supported the merits of this system, which received great attention and was tried by many institutions for a number of years.

When Miss Taylor was asked to address the meeting of the American Hospital Association in 1926 on "Teaching Nursing by the Application of the Case Study Method," she announced that a more appropriate title for her address would be "Teaching Nursing Through a Study of the Patient as an Individual or as a Whole."[56] Dean Taylor informed the group that:

> The new psychology deals with man as an integrated organism and he cannot be interpreted through a study of his parts as entities separated from himself. His physical well-being is expressed through his behavior, which in turn is influenced and changed by environmental and mental attitudes. The human being is composite in nature and is made up of a group of systems which work in relation to each other, and a well man or woman is one whose system works in harmony toward a desired end which is the development of a healthy human being.

She shared with the group the idea that teaching nursing was just like teaching anything else in that one "sets objectives," which in turn "suggest the tools, the sequence and the way in which they will be used." The reason for lack of uniformity in nursing education and service, she believed, was that the leaders were not agreed on the objectives of nursing and "thus we are confusing the needs of the world, the community and the hospitals with nursing." She identified the rewards that would be gained if there was an agreement on objectives for nursing based on the needs of the client as a whole and if nurse leaders would discuss a plan of education for nursing that would prepare students to reach those objectives. She suggested that analysis might reveal that the confusion of nursing objectives was the outgrowth of a financial system in hospitals that did not provide adequately for nursing service. She reminded the hospital administrators that hospitals should exist primarily for patients.

In discussing what the case study method was and how it worked, she described it as involving the scientific method in "the collection, recording and classification of facts into series or sequences with the possibility of predicting future facts," and, therefore, according to Dean Taylor, the case study method of teaching nursing might well be termed a scientific method of work.

Dean Taylor reminded the association of the frustrations and disappointments experienced by both deliverers and receivers of the "efficiency method," which was task-oriented and which benefitted the hospital economically but in no other way. The efficiency method focused on the carrying out of procedures very much as the later "functional method" did.

In explaining the case study method, Dean Taylor showed clinical assignment sheets to demonstrate nurse coverage on the units at the School of Nursing at Yale University. In addition, she exhibited a student experience record that reflected the achievement of the objectives of the method and the benefits to clients of collaboration between nurses and physicians (Fig. 15–16).

When World War II created an acute shortage of nursing personnel, the old efficiency method reemerged in a less appealing form called the *functional method,* which was been described previously. This method was followed by the *team method,* which utilized differently prepared staff members and supposedly fit the assignment to the background of the provider of service.

The latest pattern resembles the case

[56]Taylor, Effie J.: "Teaching Nursing by the Application of the Case Study Method," *International Council of Nursing,* January 1927, pp. 1–16.

YALE UNIVERSITY · SCHOOL OF NURSING
STUDENT EXPERIENCE RECORD

Name: F. W. Class 1928

Date	Location	Time	Case No.	Patients Cared For	Medical Diagnosis	Observations of Symptoms and Signs Related to Medical Diagnosis	Family or Social Problems
[illegible]	I E	7-11 A.M.	1	Edward (16 yrs)	Tuberculosis of the left kidney with either a tuberculous lesion on the left side or a tuberculous nephritis. (X-ray shows a large kidney on the left side which would indicate that the lesion is on the left side.)	Blood clots and blood in urine. Frequent urination. Limited bladder capacity. Loss of weight. Puscells in urine Easy fatigue.	1. Teaching. *a)* Teaching patient hygienic laws, means of preventing spread of infection. *b)* Teaching step mo. precautions to prevent further occurrence of tuberculosis in family. (There is family history of tuberculosis). 2. Occupational therapy. Preparation of boy for future employment.
[illegible]	I E	7-11 A.M.	2	Gerald	Empyema — chronic, left. Jan. 20th. Operation. Resection of ribs. Plastic operation of skin.	Discharging wound. Cough. Profuse perspiration at night. Emaciation. Pain on abrupt motion. Weakness. Pain in neck and left shoulder. Inability to raise head, to move upper arm in horizontal position.	Patient has been living with relatives as own home is broken, so for years he has suffered an irregular hygienic routine. Education in hygiene is advisable. Long time hospital care is probable. Some interest must be devised for him in hospital, as he is impatient and active in mind.

PAGE 1.

YALE UNIVERSITY · SCHOOL OF NURSING
STUDENT EXPERIENCE RECORD

Name: F. W. Class 1928

Date	Case No.	Nursing Care, Treatments, Diets, Teaching Experience, Etc.	No. Times	Observations of Symptoms Related to Nursing Care, Treatments, Diets, Etc.	Job Analysis Student's Criticism of Work and Measurement of Achievement
[illegible]	1	A.M. care including complete bath. Forced fluids Teaching general laws of hygiene — importance of sleep, right kind of food, fresh air, importance of taking plenty of water, etc.	1	Boy is encouraged to sit up. Can do so easily and can help himself somewhat. Has little appetite owing to anaesthetic. Has pain in lower abdomen which is periodic and cramping	Student lacks ease and skill in handling patients, especially those who are post operative. Is not alert to foresee needs of patients nor to observe signs and symptoms. Is slow in movements — does not accomplish a thorough and finished piece of work in a limited time.
[illegible]	2	A.M. care including complete bath. Forced fluids. Patient on porch. Assistance with massage.	1, 1	Good appetite is evident. Patient is hopeful, and cooperates with doctors. He can move his upper arm more this week than last. Can now move it high in the vertical line.	During next week student must concentrate on the medical side of the problems, to thoroughly understand the medical sign and symptoms and those symptoms relating to nursing care which have been considerably neglected or confused so far.

PAGE 2.

Figure 15–16. Yale University student experience record of 1928, which reflects the concept of client-centered care. This record was both a learning and an evaluative tool. The medical assessment appears on page 1 of the card (*left*), and the nursing assessment appears on page 2 (*right*). This experience record differs from many student records of the time, which only reported what treatments had been used and whether tasks had been completed in the allotted time. (Dolan collection.)

study method and is called *primary nursing*. In this system the nurse is assigned to patients as their primary nurse for the length of their hospitalization. This method differs from the case study method in that the primary nurse has the responsibility for the *total* nursing care of the patient for 24 hours a day, seven days a week. This system provides the setting to utilize the nursing process. In the absence of the primary nurse, an associate nurse provides the care. Primary nursing has focussed on client welfare and family satisfaction rather than on meeting hospital demands by interchanging nursing personnel. It has provided a reclamation and an expansion of the traditional nursing functions of care and comfort. The consumers of the care (or significant others) are given the opportunity to play an active role in the decision making of the care process. Primary care provides a greater opportunity for physicians and nurses to collaborate for the good of their clients. Many clients and nurses have reported satisfaction with this system of nursing care.[57]

The delivery of nursing care has received input from the *telecommunications* field. Since 1973, hospitals have been utilizing computerized information systems, which serve to link departments and provide data of significance about the client (Figure 15–17). In addition to their administrative use for the hospital, these systems retrieve data, which assist in planning nursing care (Figure 15–18).

With this computer equipment it is possible to obtain clinical data to enhance the value of the *Problem-Oriented Medical Record* system; to search for information quickly; to encourage designing and storing personalized nursing care plans using nursing process standards and expected patient

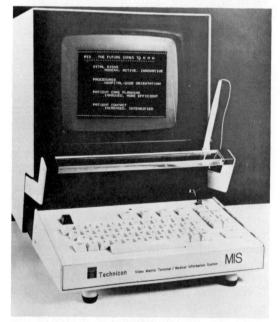

Figure 15–17. A data terminal ready to provide and record valuable patient information. (Courtesy of Methodist Medical Center, Omaha, Nebraska.)

[57]"Symposium on Primary Nursing," *The Nursing Clinics of North America*, 12:185–255, 1977.

```
4W-5566                NATIONAL INSTITUTES OF HEALTH CLINICAL CENTER
PAGE 001                                                     NURSING CARE PLAN
                           F 27 04W08A  INST/BR:N NI
ADM: 05/08/82                   JONES, JANE                  7:00 AM  6/25/82
==============================================================================
                                                 ASSOC NURSE:  PRESCOT, JOHN
PRIM NURSE:  SMITH, ANN
DX:  MULTIPLE SCLEROSIS...CARE CATEGORY IV...
REAL & POTENTIAL PROBLEMS:                                                ABS
5/9 DIFFICULTY WITH MOBILITY: R/T--PROGRESSION OF ILLNESS.
                                                 C/P:   D/L:
EXPECTED OUTCOMES                                                         ABS
   5/9   --NO PHYSICAL INJURY                    ODD    D/C
   5/9   --IDENTIFIES WANT TO PERF ACTIVITIES                             JJP
           INDEPENDENTLY                         ODD    D/C
NURSING ACTIONS                                                           ABS
   5/9   DISCUSS ABILITIES & LIMITATIONS W PT                             ABS
   5/9   DISCUSS ALTERNATE WAYS OF PERFORMING USUAL ACTIVITIES            JJP
   5/9   ENCOURAGE TO PARTICIPATE IN CARE TO MAXIMUM ABILITY              ABS
   5/9   ASSIST WITH ALL TRANSFERRING FROM BED TO W/C & COMMODE           JJP
   5/9   ENCOURAGE INDEPENDENCE
   5/19  HAVE SIDE RAILS UP AT ALL TIMES WHEN PT IS                       ABS
         RESTING IN BED & DURING SLEEPING HRS                             NJA
5/15 PAIN: R/T--MUSCLE SPASMS                    C/P:   D/L:
EXPECTED OUTCOMES
   6/9   --IDENTIFIES & USES SEVERAL TECHNIQUES TO                        JJP
         CONTROL PAIN                            QEPI   DOD               NJA
   6/19  --VERBALIZES SENSE OF CONTROL OVER      TUES   DOD
         DISCOMFORT
NURSING ACTIONS
         ASSESS TYPE, LOCATION, INTENSITY, &
```

This computer printout of a care plan at the NIH Clinical Centers includes current nursing diagnoses and prescribed actions, the schedule for charting on outcomes (C/P), and initials of the nurses.

Figure 15–18. A nursing care plan computer printout, which includes nursing diagnoses and prescribed actions. (Courtesy of National Institutes of Health Clinical Center.)

outcomes; and to provide a suitable vehicle for encouraging clinical research in general and nursing care research in particular. Edmunds states: "Such clinical research indicates the potential that computers have for facilitating retrospective and prospective, descriptive and experimental studies."[58]

NURSING PRACTICE—A NEW DEFINITION

Many states have been reexamining their definitions of the practice of nursing. New York State amended its practice act on February 9, 1972, and enacted the following definition:

> The practice of the profession of nursing as a registered professional nurse is defined as diagnosing and treating human responses to actual or potential health problems through such services as casefinding, health teaching, health counseling and provision of care supportive or restorative of life and well-being, and executing medical regimens prescribed by a licensed or otherwise legally authorized physician or dentist. A nursing regimen shall be consistent with and shall not vary from any existing medical regimen.

The definitions of terms used in the preceding are as follows:

> *"Diagnosing"* in the context of nursing practice means that identification of and discrimination between physical and psychosocial signs and symptoms essential to effective execution and management of the nursing regimen. Such diagnostic privilege is distinct from a medical diagnosis.
>
> *"Treating"* means selection and performance of those therapeutic measures essential to the effective execution and management of the nursing regimen, and execution of any prescribed medical regimen.
>
> *"Human Responses"* means those signs, symptoms and processes which denote the individual's interaction with an actual or potential health problem.

These new definitions in New York's practice act delineated the independent functions of nurses while adding a dependent one. As early as 1955, in their book *Nursing Practice and the Law,* Lesnik and Anderson described six independent activities and one dependent activity of the professional nurse:

> 1. Supervision of patients involving the whole management of care, requiring the application of principles based on the biological, physical, and social sciences.
> 2. Observation of symptoms and reactions including symptomatology of physical and mental conditions and need, requiring evaluation or the application of principles.
> 3. Adequate recording and reporting of facts including the evaluation of the whole care of the patient.

[58]Edmunds, Linda. "Computer-Assisted Nursing Care," *American Journal of Nursing, 82*:1076–1079, 1982.

4. Supervision of others, except the physician, in the care of patients.
5. Application and execution of nursing procedures and techniques.
6. Direction and education to secure physical and mental care.
7. Application and execution of legal orders of physicians concerning treatments and medications with an understanding of cause and effect thereof.

THE NURSING PROCESS

While working on a Western Council on Higher Education for Nursing project to define clinical content, Lucile Lewis became interested in defining the nursing process. She was convinced that the nursing process could characterize professional nursing and could assure its effectiveness in meeting the needs of clients. She believed that:

> The central focus of nursing is to help the person cope with his physiological, psychological and spiritual reactions to his health problems and maintain his integrity in these experiences. To be therapeutic, the nurse must contribute to the wholeness of man, to the interrelationships of the parts to the whole, to the person's here-and-now as well as to his future, to the health of all the parts so that the person may attain and maintain his highest potential.[59]

To implement the caring function, a systematic logical process was evolved, referred to as the nursing process. In a simplistic description this process consists of four steps:

1. Identifying the patient's needs—resulting in a nurse assessment or nursing diagnosis.
2. Planning solutions for these needs—devising plans referred to as a nursing care plan.
3. Implementing this plan of action.
4. Evaluating the results of the actions.

In the phase of *assessment*, there is a critical appraisal of all discernible factors (past, present and future) that actually or potentially affect the client's ability to cope with daily living. It has been stated that problems arise when needs cannot be met. This type of assessment lays the basis for individualized rather than routinized care.

In the second phase, the *planning* phase, the nurse works collaboratively with the client. Priorities are determined and a judgment is made as to who can best handle certain aspects of the plan. Goals are then set and a plan of action is designed to meet the goals—a nursing care plan.

After the plan is set and becomes operational, it is *implemented* by nursing intervention. Direct care involving physical care, emotional support or teaching, or indirect, supportive care may be given. This area is assigned to or referred to the person best prepared to care for the client.

In the *evaluation* phase, Florence Nightingale's advice to look at the effectiveness of nursing actions is followed. There is a deliberate consideration of the effectiveness of the nursing action—what made it successful or what factors led to lack of success? Evaluation is an ongoing process. *Reassessment* then follows.

Nursing is conceptualized as an analytical process in which knowledge from nursing, the biological, physical and social sciences and the humanities is used in the interaction with and response to a client who has a potential or actual health need. The nursing process is not a fragmented series of steps but a unified process.

STANDARDS OF NURSING PRACTICE

With the reorganization of the ANA in 1966, the concern of nurses to improve the nursing care of clients prompted the establishment of *Divisions on Practice:* Community Health Nursing Practice, Geriatric Nursing Practice, Maternal and Child Health Nursing Practice, Medical-Surgical Nursing Practice and Psychiatric and Mental Health Nursing Practice.

A priority item of the divisions was to identify and disseminate standards of nursing practice in each division. Therefore, in 1966, executive committees of the divisions appointed committees on standards to formulate guidelines and to commence the task of writing standards and concomitantly of devising ways to encourage their acceptance.

[59]Lewis, Lucile: "This I Believe About the Nursing Process—Key to Care," *Nursing Outlook, 68*:26–29, 1968.

By 1968, the *Congress for Nursing Practice* was constituted, with Ingeborg Mauksch, Ph.D., as chairperson. Among the functions of this body was the coordination of divisions that had been the responsibility of division chairpersons.

For the next several years, the committees worked conscientiously on producing the standards for practice. Sets of standards from each division were distributed at the ANA biennial convention in Detroit in 1972. The generic standards and those delineated by each of the specialty divisions were published in separate booklets in 1973 and 1974.[60] This significant basis for the evaluation of nursing performance has contributed to the aim of *accountability* for professional practice.

The ANA's next step involved serious consideration of ways of implementing these standards in practice. To this end the ANA Commission on Economic and General Welfare collaborated with the Congress for Nursing Practice. This resulted in the presentation of a resolution at the 1972 ANA convention entitled "Implementation of Standards of Nursing Practice Within the Employment Setting." A committee was convened with representatives from the Commission on Economic and General Welfare, each of the Divisions on Practice, the Commission on Nursing Education, the Commission on Nursing Service and the National Student Nurses' Association in addition to the Congress for Nursing Practice. The committee was charged by the congress to develop "guidelines for peer review, local joint practice, and nursing audit."

It has been expedient to have had the use of "nursing diagnosis" clarified by its inclusion in the ANA's *Standards for Nursing Practice*. The second standard states, "Nursing diagnoses are derived from health status data." This clarification of nursing diagnosis has marked significance for the practitioner of nursing and health colleagues and "in cases of alleged nursing malpractice."[61]

Peer Review

Peer review, as the name indicates, is the evaluation of nursing care by registered nurses using the accepted standards of nursing practice. The purposes of peer review are to appraise the quality and quantity of nursing care; to identify the strengths and weaknesses of such care; to provide evidence to be used as a basis for recommending new or changed policies and procedures to improve nursing care; and to identify those areas where patterns of practice demonstrate the need for more knowledge by the practitioners of nursing.

The peer review process includes two phases: (1) the appraisal of nursing care delivered by a group of nurses in a given setting (nursing professional standards review); and (2) the appraisal of nursing practiced by individual practitioners (nursing performance review). In 1973, the ANA developed guidelines for peer review committees with the suggestion that their implementation be given high priority.[62]

THE ANA CERTIFICATION PROGRAM

The ANA Certification Program was inaugurated to recognize expert practitioners—those nurses whose current practice demonstrates excellence. The use of the ANA's Standards of Nursing Practice has been one of the methods of evaluating excellence. Nurses must be currently engaged in clinical nursing practice to be eligible to apply for certification. Those who hold positions as administrators, consultants, educators and researchers may try for certification if they are also engaged in clinical practice.[63]

In 1950, an ANA committee proposed the establishment of means to recognize personal achievement and superior performance in nursing. In 1968, the Nursing

[60]American Nurses' Association: *Standards of Nursing Practice*. Kansas City, Missouri, American Nurses' Association, 1973.

[61]Bruce, Joan A., and Snyder, Marie E.: "The Right and Responsibility to Diagnose," *American Journal of Nursing*, *82*:646, 1982.

[62]American Nurses' Association: *Peer Review: Guidelines for Establishment of Committees*. Kansas City, Missouri, American Nurses' Association, 1973.

[63]American Nurses' Association: *Guidelines for Certification: Congress for Nursing Practice*. Kansas City, Missouri, American Nurses' Association, October 15, 1971.

Practice Department of the ANA defined certification as follows:

> Recognition of excellence in the practice of nursing is provided by the American Nurses' Association, the professional association for registered nurses, through the process of certification. The Association issues a formal statement attesting that the recipient has met special criteria for individual achievement and superior performance in a particular area of nursing practice.
>
> The objective of ANA certification is to improve nursing practice and to assure the public, employers, and members of allied professions that efforts are being made to recognize excellence in the practice of nursing. The process of certification affords direction for clinical content in educational programs. It also provides incentive for nurses to expand their knowledge and to make application of knowledge in their practice.[64]

ANA certification is based on assessment of knowledge through testing; demonstration of excellence in clinical practice through references, case studies and innovative projects; endorsement of colleagues through reference vouchers (peer endorsement); and evaluation of evidence.

The first certification examinations were administered in geriatric nursing in 1974 to 268 candidates and of that number 185 were successful. When the documentation was analyzed, 74 candidates were certified.

Certification is granted for a five-year period at the end of which practitioners may apply for recertification. Recertification assures continued competence in practice with periodic updating of knowledge and clinical expertise. Certification has been geared to one level of practitioner; however, future plans include certification of clinical specialty preparation at the master's degree level and above.

THE CODE FOR NURSES

An instrument to assist in the achievement of quality control has been the Code for Nurses which has been distributed by the ANA since 1950. The House of Delegates at the 37th Convention of ANA adopted this initial code in 1950, making the ANA the first national association to adopt such a code. In 1953 the International Code of Nursing Ethics, a revision of the ANA code, was adopted by the International Council of Nurses. In 1959 at the National Student Nurses' Association Convention, the Code for Professional Nurses, a third revision of the initial code, was accepted as a guide for student nurses. The Congress for Nursing Practice completed the fourth revision in 1976. This latest code places far less emphasis on nurse's dress and etiquette and far greater emphasis on the relationship between the nurse and client. *The Code for Nurses With Interpretive Statements* is directed toward present-day practice and emphasizes the role of the nurse as a client advocate. The first interpretive statement about self-determination of clients presents the nurse-client relationship as a cooperative endeavor with far greater emphasis on the accountability of the nurse to the client.

The editors of the *Encyclopedia of Bioethics* have applauded the ANA for its responsiveness to human needs: "The Code shows an awareness to social responsibility of nurses and does something about it." The code, with interpretive statements, appears in the four-volume interdisciplinary reference work being prepared by the Center for Bioethics, Kennedy Institute at Georgetown University.

The ANA provides a professional self-regulatory mechanism in this code.

> A code indicates a profession's acceptance of the responsibility and trust with which it has been invested by society. Upon entering the profession of nursing, each person inherits a measure of the responsibility and trust that has accrued to nursing over the years and the corresponding obligation to adhere to the profession's code of conduct and relationships for ethical practice.

The code reads as follows:

1. The nurse provides services with respect for human dignity and the uniqueness of the client unrestricted by considerations of social or economic status, personal attributes, or the nature of health problems.
2. The nurse safeguards the client's right to privacy by judiciously protecting information of a confidential nature.
3. The nurse acts to safeguard the client

---

[64]Nursing Practice Department, American Nurses' Association: *The Meaning of Certification*. Kansas City, Missouri, American Nurses' Association, September 1973, p. 1.

and the public when health care and safety are affected by the incompetent, unethical, or illegal practice of any person.

4. The nurse assumes responsibility and accountability for individual nursing judgments and actions.

5. The nurse maintains competence in nursing.

6. The nurse exercises informed judgment and uses individual competence and qualifications as criteria in seeking consultation, accepting responsibilities, and delegating nursing activities to others.

7. The nurse participates in activities that contribute to the ongoing development of the profession's body of knowledge.

8. The nurse participates in the profession's effort to implement and improve standards of nursing.

9. The nurse participates in the profession's efforts to establish and maintain conditions of employment conducive to high quality nursing care.

10. The nurse participates in the profession's effort to protect the public from misinformation and misrepresentation and to maintain the integrity of nursing.

11. The nurse collaborates with members of the health professions and other citizens in promoting community and national efforts to meet the health needs of the public.[65]

NURSING AND THE STUDY OF ETHICS

The study of ethics and its application to nursing practice and health care has been part of nursing education curricula since Florence Nightingale began influencing nursing education. In the early schools, a strong religious orientation frequently prevailed, and ethical considerations of practice were usually considered within the context of Christian values.

Following World War II, ethics in nursing education became integrated into courses in professional trends and issues in nursing. Except in church-related schools, the teaching of ethics usually revolved around a discussion of the ANA's Code for Nurses and was more secular in presentation.

Since the early 1970s, there has been a resurgence of interest in the inclusion of ethics and applied ethics in nursing education programs. The exploration of scientific knowledge, the expansion of technology and the advancement of medicine capable of extending life all contribute to the emergence of vital ethical issues confronting health care deliverers. Special courses in ethics designed to assist nursing students in analyzing ethical dilemmas, such as the beginning and end of human life, genetic engineering and other related topics, have been added to nursing programs. Required and elective courses in ethics are not uncommon in nursing programs today. In addition, fellowships for advanced study and research in health care ethics have been available to nurses through the Kennedy Institute at Georgetown University.

QUALITY ASSURANCE IN NURSING

Concern for accountability and cost effectiveness in the delivery of health care became a major issue in the 1970s. Nursing made great strides in developing systems that would assist nurses in determining the quality of their practice. Emphasis was placed on the importance of documenting the care given, which in turn would serve as objective evidence of the care provided. Two nurses, Maria Pnauff and Mabel Wandelt, pioneered this movement by developing systems that evaluated practice for the purpose of determining the quality of care rendered.

One of the major influences of the *accountability movement* was *consumerism*, a movement that has permeated every aspect of life today. Betz comments, "The simplest context in which to examine accountability is the paradigm of the exchange relationship between buyer and seller (either goods or services).[66] The health care delivery system has not been excluded in the obvious decline in public trust. Demands

[65]*Code For Nurses With Interpretive Statements*. Kansas City, Missouri, American Nurses' Association, 1976.

[66]Betz, Michael: "From Whence Accountability?" *Nursing and Health Care*, p. 482, November 1981.

for greater participation of consumers in the activities pertaining to health care providers have been documented.

PUBLIC ACCOUNTABILITY THROUGH LICENSURE

Ways to improve the quality of nursing care and the protection of practitioners delivering this care needed consideration. Many definitions of nursing practice in the state statutes were old and obsolete. These minimum standards for practice were too low and restrictive; did not identify an autonomous professional role; emphasized the dependent function and placed the nurse under the jurisdiction of another profession; were illness-oriented in focus; and did not reflect society's needs.

Changes in Licensure Laws

State licensure laws required one licensure examination, usually taken immediately upon graduation from a school of nursing, as the one and only check assuring minimal standards of professional practice. These licensure laws were enacted before the great increase in knowledge and technology and did not take into consideration that a licensed individual's knowledge could become outdated. Consumers of nursing care as well as professional team members should have the assurance that nurses are currently competent. To this end many states have been considering a continuing education requirement for relicensure of nurses.

Another area in the licensure process of nursing that has received consideration by consumer groups and has been changed in some states is the composition of the implementing boards carrying out the functions of the nurse practice acts. The consumer protection movement has affected the health fields in many areas. To assure that decisions are being made in the public interest, consumers have been demanding broader participation in policy making. Many have made important contributions to policy making in all areas of health care delivery and have sought improvements in the regulation of health manpower.

Another issue has been the centralization of licensing functions of health professionals in one licensing agency. One reason for this recommendation is the proliferation of "health workers" who are not protected by law. In 1973, the Massachusetts state legislature attempted a reorganization of the boards of examiners for the health professions, but was thwarted by the unanimous resolution of the membership asssembled at the NLN Convention in 1973 to eliminate the Massachusetts state board examination from the test pool if the state persisted in its reorganization plans.

Institutional licensure has been considered because of the large numbers of allied health workers. This change would remove the licensing authority from the current state boards of examiners and place it in the hands of the governing body of hospitals. Many groups of health professionals oppose this move for a variety of reasons. They fear that this change would lower the standards of health care while increasing the costs of hospital care. Many feel that accountability for health care would be redirected from the client to the hiring agency granting the licensure. It has been feared that the quality control of nursing by nurses could be weakened. Furthermore, those health workers practicing outside the hospital setting would not be covered, and it could be difficult to transfer from one institution to another.

One of the greatest threats to professional nursing today is sunset legislation affecting State Boards of Nurse Examiners. Sunset legislation is the passage of a bill in any state that mandates the dismantling of the State Boards of Nurse Examiners. Typically, the legislation provides for a review of a licensing board's efficiency and effectiveness. If the work of the board is judged inadequate or unsatisfactory, the board and its activities will cease to exist on the date specified in the legislation. If the board is judged necessary, new legislation must be introduced and passed, reestablishing the board or a similar mechanism.

The implications of sunset legislation are serious for nursing. Elimination of state boards of nursing leaves open to question the survival of individual licensure for nurses, and the status of the nursing profession without the boards of nursing performing the functions of regulating practice, determining disciplinary action for infractions of the nurse practice act and approving schools of nursing.

Such legislation has been passed, or is pending, in a large number of states. Cost containment in state government and fiscal accountability to taxpayers is frequently the rationale put forth as an explanation for the passage of such legislation. Political activity on the part of nurses concerning the issue of sunset legislation has become a focal point for many state nurses' associations and other interested groups.

Separate licensure was also under consideration. It would have provided for separate licensure for professional nurses and technical nurses as well as practical nurses who act as assistants. The objective of separate licensure was to make clear to the public and other professions the difference in nursing care and preparation for delivery of this care among the different groups. In 1977, at the New York State Nurses' Association convention, the membership approved introduction in the 1978 legislative session of a "1985 Proposal" (see definition of nursing practice on p. 345). The proposal would:

a. delete:
   1. the three definitions of terms included for clarification purposes only in 1972;
   2. all references to other disciplines, i.e., medicine and dentistry;
b. establish the baccalaureate degree in nursing as the educational requirement for licensure as a registered professional nurse;
c. establish the associate degree in nursing as the educational requirement for licensure as a registered associate nurse;
d. include grandfather provisions protecting the licenses of:
   1. those individuals licensed as registered professional nurses prior to the effective date of the legislation, authorizing these individuals to retain the title registered nurse.
   2. those individuals licensed as licensed practical nurses prior to the effective date of the legislation, authorizing these individuals to use the title registered associate nurse.

The NYSNA introduced a bill containing such a proposal into the legislature, but it was not passed.

The state board of nursing has remained the statutory body charged with the legal authority to regulate the practice of nursing in each state or territory of the United States. Beginning in the 1970s, the composition of state boards in some states expanded to include non-nurses as consumer members.

In 1978, at the ANA biennial convention in Hawaii, the ANA's formal ties with state boards were severed. The state boards had already established their own autonomous organization, the National Council of State Boards of Nursing. Based in Chicago, this voluntary association has no statutory power, although its member agencies (state boards) carry this power in their respective states. Each state board of nursing is represented by two delegates at council meetings, and policy adopted there is usually adopted by each state board, thus giving it the force of law.

In 1982, the National Council of State Boards of Nursing broke with tradition and implemented a new nurse licensing examination whose development it has initiated. Unlike the former examinations (the State Board Test Pool) developed under the auspices of NLN, the new examination was an integrated test instead of several separate tests in specific clinical specialties. It has one final score and was designed to better reflect the process orientation and integrated approaches of contemporary nursing curricula. Purchased through the National Council of State Boards but administered by each state board, the examination is called the NCLEX.

CHANGING NURSING ROLES

Various nursing roles evolved because of several aspects of health care, among them increased use of hospitals, a shortage of physicians (more specialists than general practitioners), greater consumer demand and poor utilization of nurses. Committees of nurses, physicians and hospitals decided that nurses could carry out certain medical functions (which they were already doing) although nurses are not protected by law when carrying out these functions.

In the 1960s, coronary care units were developing, and nurses were performing more medical functions. About the same time the American Academy of Pediatrics did a study that proved that most pediatricians' time was spent caring for well children when their efforts should be directed to caring for sick ones. The nurse as a pediatric associate emerged to provide care for the well child. In 1965, a program was designed for the preparation of the *pediatric nurse practitioner* (P.N.P.). In the same year a program was developed to prepare *physicians' assistants* (P.A.). In 1970, the American Medical Association, without consulting with the American Nurses' Association, proposed that nurses should be trained in the P.A. role. The ANA reacted violently to the proposal.

Numerous articles appeared contrasting the *extended* role (cure-oriented, physician extender) versus the *expanded* role (a broadening of the rightful care-oriented nursing role). In the extended role, authority is delegated by the physician who retains all decision-making power. Thus nursing is subordinate to another profession. In the expanded role, the nurse can utilize new approaches to meeting client needs based on enriched theoretical and clinical knowledge. This provides the opportunity for a collaboration between two professionals on a comparable level.

JOINT PRACTICE EFFORTS

In 1970, the Lysaught report recommended that in each state a joint practice commission be established. The *National Joint Practice Commission* was established in 1972 to make recommendations concerning the "congruent roles of the physician and the nurse in providing quality health care to the American people." The commission received financial support from the American Medical Association, the ANA and the W. K. Kellogg Foundation. Membership on the commission consisted of equal numbers of practicing nurses and physicians whose main interest was the public whom they served rather than the profession of which they were members. The goals identified by the commission were to examine the roles and functions of both professions and define new roles and relationships, to recommend changes in professional education to support new roles, to remove sources of professional differences and to assist in the development and support of state joint practice committees. A possible deterrent to the achievement of the goals was believed to be the lack of effective communication due to the position of nursing in the decision-making of the hospital organization. It was recognized that nursing had established its autonomy as a profession. In order for full collaboration between medicine and nursing to exist the commission recommended that nursing be given responsibility for the quality of nursing care it provides to patients and accountability for its ethical conduct and professional practices.

In 1977, the success of the work of the National Joint Practice Commission was rewarded by a W. K. Kellogg Foundation grant of $765,765. The project aimed to demonstrate in four hospitals of different size and type that collaborative practice between nurses and physicians in the hospital setting could be realized.

Each participating hospital introduced primary nursing, an integrated patient record system, nurse-physician joint evaluation of patient care and a nurse-physician joint practice committee and increased the involvement of nurses in clinical decision making.

The National Joint Practice Commission dissolved in 1980. A $147,244 W. K. Kellogg Foundation grant financed four conferences in 1982 to report on the findings of the four pilot projects:

> It was reported that the project proved successful at every hospital. A climate of trust and respect encouraged by collaboration allowed both nurses and physicians to function at their highest level of skills. . . . Communications improved; physicians began using nurses' notes; nursing care plans became an important tool for transmitting information. Nurses said they were finding greater satisfaction in their work. Physicians saw that patient care was better and supported use of the joint practice approach in other units.[67]

Many states have reported successful efforts of their State Nurses' Association–State Medical Association Joint Practice Committees in increasing collaboration between nurses and physicians.

One state joint practice committee reported to its respective state organizations that the trends in health care delivery

---

[67] "Kellogg to Fund Follow-Up Sessions on Joint Practice," *American Journal of Nursing, 81*:2134–2135, 1981.

seemed to perpetuate fragmentation of functions, creating a large variety of health care personnel with but a narrow range of skills. They recommended that when a new function is required, existing classes of occupations should be evaluated in order to ascertain whether the function of any could be redefined and expanded rather than inventing a new type of health worker.

In a guest editorial in the *American Nurse*, Luther Christman, Ph.D., described the need for nurses to design organizational structures that not only would encourage but also would permit the sharing of power. He states, "Nurses always have had *equity*—that is, a stake in the health care system, but they rarely have had *parity*, which is defined as equal . . . among groups."[68] Dr. Christman noted that the marked increase of prepared nurses at the graduate level has reduced the educational differences among health professional co-workers and has provided a cadre of well-qualified, scientifically prepared nurses to be partners in health care decision making. He remarked on the advantages of primary nursing care in providing client accountability.

NURSING THEORY AND NURSING RESEARCH

The first two criteria of a profession as identified by the Bixlers in their article on the professional status of nursing were:

> 1. A profession utilizes in its practice a well defined and well organized body of specialized knowledge which is on the intellectual level of higher learning.
> 2. A profession constantly enlarges the body of knowledge it uses and improves its technics of education and service by the use of the scientific method.[69]

The need for research in nursing has been recognized in articles in the *American Journal of Nursing* and by action of Boards of Directors of the ANA.

To establish a historical base for research in nursing one must inevitably turn to Florence Nightingale, who was a researcher of great skill. Her reforms in nursing were based on meticulous investigation; it has been recorded that "every set of plans was examined with infinite pains and treated in precise detail."

A portrait of Florence Nightingale as a statistician was brilliantly detailed in the Quarterly Publication of the American Statistical Association by the Assistant Statistician of the Metropolitan Life Insurance Company. He expressed admiration for her radical innovations in the nursing care of the sick; her unique accomplishments as reformer, administrator and nurse; and her work as a constructive compiler and interpreter of descriptive social statistics. "Her keen intellect, applied to . . . major projects . . . comprehended the utility of the statistical method as a means of developing a basis of established fact for social reform."

Miss Nightingale's study of available data on the death rate during the Crimean War convinced her that the greater number of deaths in hospitals need not have occurred. During the first seven months of the Crimean campaign, the mortality rate of 60 per cent occurred from disease alone, a rate that exceeded even that of the Great Plague in London and the death rate from cholera.

Her "Notes Affecting the Health Efficiency and Hospital Administration of the British Army" has been termed by statisticians a "treasury of authentic fact." She has been applauded as a pioneer in graphic illustration of statistics. Her diagrams were an innovation in the field of statistics. She used shaded or colored squares, circles and wedges to portray the deaths due to preventable causes in the hospitals during the Crimean War and the rate of mortality in the British Army.

Florence Nightingale used statistics to prevent the relocation of St. Thomas' Hospital to make way for a railway. She analyzed the origins of persons served by the hospital, tabulated the proportions of cases within certain radial distances and showed the probable effect on patients of the removal of the hospital to the several possible sites suggested. This method of fitting hospital accommodation to the needs of populations has been emphasized recently.

---

[68]Christman, Luther: "Shared Power: Mandate for Nursing Leadership," *The American Nurse*, November 15, 1977.

[69]Bixler, G. K., and Bixler, R. W.: "The Professional Status of Nursing," *American Journal of Nursing*, Vol. 45, 1945.

It represents a legitimate application of demographic principles to the study of the relief of human needs.

She was adept at influencing public opinion—distributing the data she compiled to influential people and the press.

Another of Florence Nightingale's projects resulted in "Notes on Hospitals," which revolutionized ideas of hospital construction. She highlighted the deplorable existence of hospital gangrene and hospital septicemia. Her efforts revealed the complete lack of scientific coordination in hospital administration.

Because of her recognized expertise as a statistician Miss Nightingale was elected to fellowship in the Royal Statistical Society (1858) and to honorary membership in the American Statistical Association (1874). She participated in designing the program of the Second Section of the International Statistical Congress in 1860. In 1861, she prepared a detailed paper on "Hospital Statistics and Hospital Plans" for the National Association for the Promotion of Social Science. In 1862, her model forms for hospitals to use to gather data and assess their strengths or shortcomings as healers were published in the *Journal of the Royal Statistical Society*. It was recorded that for her model forms to be utilized "demands . . . a more intelligent appreciation of and a finer enthusiasm for statistical facts" than was available in the hospital administration of that period.

Miss Nightingale outlined minimum requirements for a report form for the nature and result of surgical operations. This outline served as a nucleus for a paper read for her at the International Statistical Congress in 1863. She addressed a letter to the president of the International Statistical Congress that was read to the whole congress and adopted by it as a resolution. The resolution impressed upon governments the necessity for publishing more extensive and numerous abstracts of the statistical information in their possession. She was beseeching them to pool and share their knowledge for the benefit of mankind.

This research approach was, however, never transmitted as part of the Nightingale tradition. We now regretfully realize that a profession reshaped by nineteenth century research was then divorced from the discoveries for many decades, which perpetuated nursing's traditional way of thought. The development of inquiring minds was anathema in the "training school" system of our country—as was the fostering of the discipline and skills required for research. The development of the ability to think independently or to create new patterns of practice based on critical analysis and scientific inquiry was unthinkable in an era when students and nurses were forced to answer "I don't know, ask your doctor" when questioned by clients or their families. Nurses had learned never to ask "why" and as rarely as possible to ask "how." Truly the spirit of inquiry had been effectively checked.

It wasn't until after World War II that research was again utilized to assist in the solution of nursing problems. A vigorous attempt was made to encourage the habit of objective inquiry. The momentum generated by the plight of nurses stimulated an editorial in the December 1949 issue of the *American Journal of Nursing:*

> One of the most serious handicaps to effective research in nursing . . . has been our failure to make definite plans for scientific investigation. The nursing profession has made no concerted effort to promote, support, direct or evaluate research in nursing and there has been no central clearing house for exchange of information.
>
> There has been an appalling lack of research in the area most crucial for nursing—the nursing care of patients.

Ultimately the Board of Directors of ANA outlined a plan for studies of nursing functions. It was tragic to realize that in most of the proposals the researcher was to be a non-nurse. Nurses have been viewed with suspicion by other nurses when they became data gatherers in a research capacity.

Owing to the efforts of the Association of Collegiate Schools of Nursing, the journal *Nursing Research* was launched in 1952. In the first issue Helen L. Bunge's editorial described the dual purpose of the journal: "To inform members of the nursing profession and allied professions of the results of scientific studies in nursing, and to stimulate research in nursing."[70]

Numerous tributes have been paid to the leaders whose efforts stimulated the incep-

[70]Bunge, Helen L.: "A Cooperative Venture," *Nursing Research*, p. 5, June 1952.

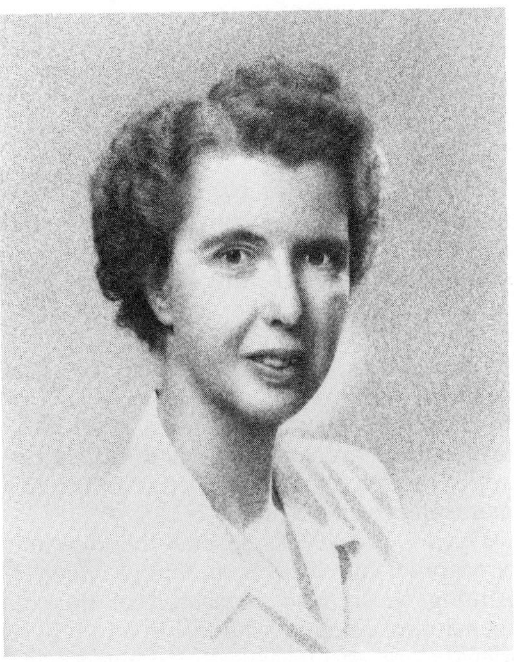

Figure 15–19. Helen Bunge, Ed.D., an outstanding nurse leader and strong advocate of nursing research. (Courtesy of the *American Journal of Nursing*.)

tion of this journal. Helen Bunge's leadership as chairman of the editorial board has been praised[71] and the summer 1962 issue, in its entirety, highlights the accomplishments of *Nursing Research.* There has been a continuity of skilled leadership in the editorial role, Dr. Lucille Notter having been editor from 1962 to 1973, and Dr. Elizabeth Carnegie from 1973 to 1978. Dr. Florence S. Downs is the current editor.

The American Nurses' Foundation, Inc. was established to encourage research studies. In 1955, the ANA gave $100,000 to this new organization to be used for studies of nursing functions.

A concerted effort began to be made by nurse leadership to encourage the formation of a body of knowledge—nursing science—while stimulating much-needed research studies in nursing care.

With more students and graduates using the nursing process, there should be heightened awareness of the urgent call for nursing practice research. There should emerge a greater appreciation of the need for evaluation and reassessment as an ongoing process and an increased facility in utilizing the scientific method and becoming involved in needed nursing research.

When findings from significant nursing research are implemented there should emerge innovative and client-satisfying patterns of care. A need for more interdependent research projects has been suggested as has been the allotment of more time and funds to allow faculty and master clinicians to participate in research.

Another aspect of research is in the area of historical research—bringing to light new knowledge and rediscovering what has previously been known as well as recording significant activities and thoughts of leaders through oral history.

In the past some leaders opined that nursing was based on intuition rather than on an accepted theory. There was agreement that patients were receiving routinized care that was too impersonal rather than individualized care. There was lack of planning and problem-solving in patient care; a series of unrelated procedures were being carried out. The question "Is this nursing?" constantly arose when activities

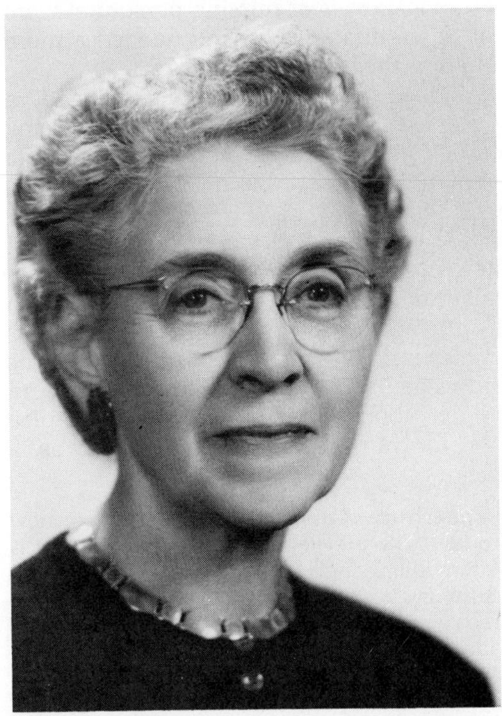

Figure 15–20. Anne L. Austin, a respected scholar and an outstanding researcher of nursing history. (Dolan collection.)

[71]Farrell, Marie: "Helen L. Bunge—An Idealist and a Realist," *Nursing Research, 11*:139, 1962.

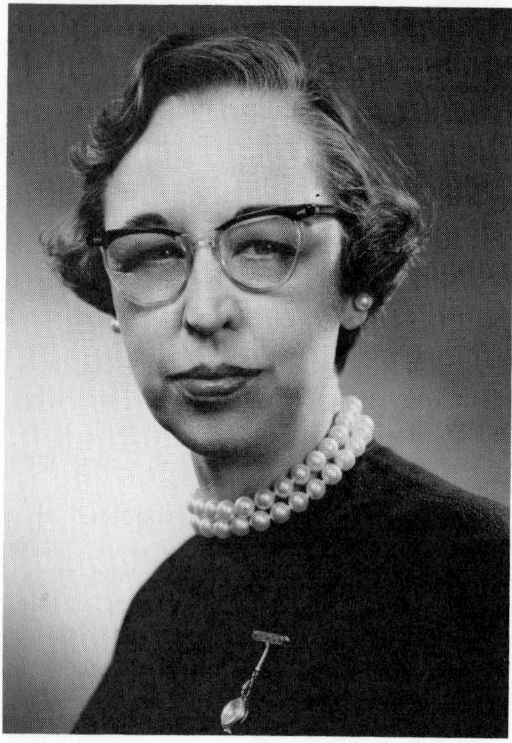

Figure 15–21. Martha E. Rogers, Sc.D. (Dolan collection.)

of various levels of nursing personnel were not differentiated. Nursing needed a more coherent theoretical structure.

As this need was being recognized, a conceptual framework of nursing was being studied, tested, taught and published by a scholarly leader of nursing, Martha E. Rogers, Sc.D (Fig. 15–21).[72] Dr. Rogers focussed on a timeless fact examined against the current framework of an incredibly sophisticated scientific setting: "The concern of nursing is with man in his entirety, his wholeness. Nursing's body of scientific knowledge seeks to describe, explain, and predict about human beings." Her plea was for nursing to be recognized as a *science:*

> The science of nursing is an emergent—a new product. The inevitability of its development is written in nursing's long commitment to human health and welfare. With today's rapid and unprecedented changes, new urgency has been added to the critical need for a body of scientific knowledge specific to nursing. Only as the science of nursing takes on form and substance can the art of nursing achieve new dimensions of artistry.
>
> The science of nursing aims to provide a body of abstract knowledge growing out of scientific research and logical analysis and capable of being translated into nursing practice.[73]

Dr. Rogers believed that the phenomenon of man was nursing's concern, and she has referred to nursing as a *humanistic science.* Her thought-provoking theory coupled with those of other leaders across the country set into motion a much needed set of designs for establishment of theoretical bases of nursing, thus requiring a change in curriculum patterns. Steps needed to be designed to prepare students of nursing to apply their scientific knowledge to the humanistic process of nursing.

During the 1970s, several theories and conceptual models of nursing emerged. Among those who pioneered in this dimension of nursing scholarship and whose ideas were enthusiastically received were Sister Callista Roy, Dorothea Orem, Betty Newman, Imogene King and Martha Rogers. Extensions of earlier definitions of nursing, such as that developed by *Virginia Henderson* (Fig. 15–22), attempted to provide a focus and system for viewing nursing and guiding nursing practice.

The essence of nursing has been constant through time—the caring about, caring with (involving the person), while caring for (genuine concern). This essence of nursing is what distinguishes nursing from other health professions. Historically nurses emerged in order to respond to actual or potential health problems. The increasing scientific base should cause an expansion of the concept of the nature of nursing, not a narrowing of it.

Virginia Henderson has defined nursing practice in the following way:

> The unique function of the nurse is to assist the individual (sick or well), in the performance of those activities contributing to health or its recovery (or to peaceful death) that he would perform unaided if he had the necessary strength, will, or knowledge. And to do this in such a way as to help him gain independence as rapidly as possible.[74]

---

[72]Rogers, Martha E.: *An Introduction to the Theoretical Basis of Nursing.* Philadelphia, F. A. Davis Co., 1970.

[73]Rogers, Martha E.: *An Introduction to the Theoretical Basis of Nursing.* Philadelphia, F. A. Davis Co., 1970, pp. 83, 86.

[74]Henderson, Virginia: *The Nature of Nursing.* New York, The Macmillan Co., 1966.

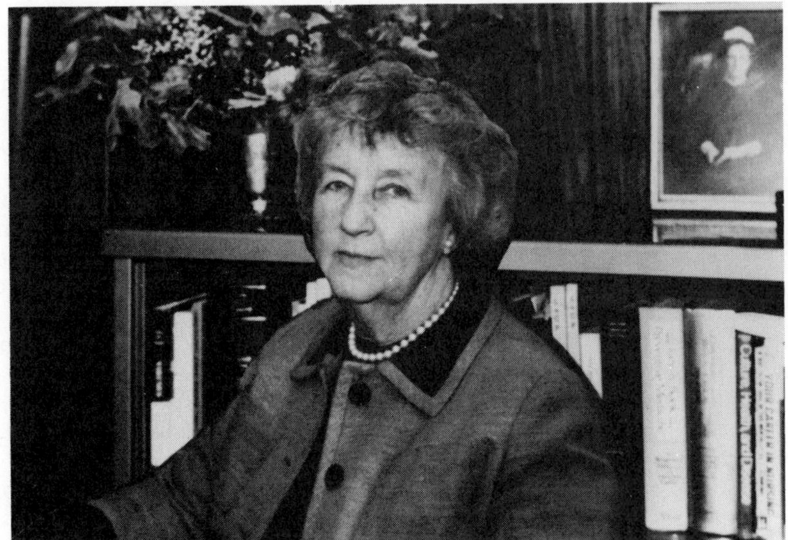

Figure 15–22. Virginia A. Henderson, internationally esteemed nurse and author, in front of a photograph of Annie W. Goodrich. (Courtesy of Ruth N. Knollmueller.)

THE HERITAGE OF NURSING

The Nurse as a Reemerging Social Force

Following the critical war years, there was a sense of enlightenment and of new opportunities for nurses in health care. New leadership appeared. The enrichment of education became channeled into effective practice and delivery of satisfying and acceptable nursing care for those we serve—the client, family and community.

1. Significant milestones in strengthening education for the delivery of care have been:
   a. a continuing succession of leaders with vision.
   b. a response to the impact of the documentation of the plight and needs of nursing through studies and surveys.
   c. participation in an accreditation process leading to self-analysis by nurse educators in regard to their programs and product.
   d. the publication of lists of accredited schools, producing social pressure for educational opportunities.
   e. financial support for nursing education (accountability accompanies acceptance of funds).
   f. self-analysis by and self-direction for the professional organization through the ANA Position Paper of 1965.
   g. the development of a theoretical basis for nursing—the science of nursing—and the emergence of "nursing" as an upper division college major without medical model bases.
   h. the delineation of steps in the nursing process.
   i. research findings of significance to nursing care.
   j. pressure for continuing education for nurses.
   k. the resolution by the NSNA for restructuring the preparation programs for professional nursing practice.

2. Significant aspects of the strengthening of quality control in the practice of nursing have been:

a. the change from the fragmented, depersonalized and dehumanizing task-oriented functional method to the individualized method of primary nursing with its round-the-clock client accountability.
b. the legal redefinition of nurse practice in nurse practice acts.
c. the revision of the Code for Nurses, which focuses on the accountability of the nurse as a client advocate.
d. the identification and dissemination by professional nurses of standards of nursing practice.
e. the evolution of peer review and professional standards review committees.
f. the recognition of the interest and demands of consumer groups in working with all professional groups—plus the value of their support in achieving nursing goals.
g. the emergence of certification and joint practice collaborative efforts.
h. membership of many nurses in political action groups to work for improvement of care; autonomy in professional activities; and promotion of protection of the public as well as the profession.

There has arisen the opportunity for a rebirth of the creative, independent, consumer-oriented role of the nurse in the health care system. A conceptualization of this role can be implemented in our current scientific society that encourages nursing to come back into its own because the health care system has always been ours even when our authority and accountability have been weak or invisible.

The professional ability to reassume this role demands cooperation and the development of nurse power. Society initially bestowed this role on nurses, but now nurses must fight to regain it by being prepared to act as advocates and deliverers of high-quality client care.

REFERENCE READINGS

The Study of Credentialing in Nursing: A New Approach. Vol. I. Kansas City, Mo., American Nurses' Association, 1979.

"ANA Votes Federation," *American Journal of Nursing, 82*:1246–1258, 1982.

Anderson, Bernice, E.: *Facilitation of the Interstate Movement of Nurses.* Philadelphia, J. B. Lippincott Co., 1950.

Armiger, Sister Bernadette: "Scholarship in Nursing," *Nursing Outlook,* 22:160–164, 1974.

Aydelotte, Myrtle K.: "Issues in Professional Nursing: The Need for Clinical Excellence," *Nursing Forum, 7*:72–86, 1968.

Brown, Amy F.: *Research in Nursing.* Philadelphia, W. B. Saunders Co., 1958.

Brown, Esther, Lucile: *Nursing For The Future.* New York, The Russell Sage Foundation, 1948.

Brown, Esther Lucile: *Nursing Reconsidered—A Study of Change: Part I—The Professional Role in Institutional Nursing.* Philadelphia, J. B. Lippincott Co., 1970.

Brown, Esther Lucile: *Nursing Reconsidered—A Study of Change: Part II—The Professional Role in Community Nursing.* Philadelphia, J. B. Lippincott, 1971.

Bruce, Joan A., and Snyder, Marie E.: "The Right and Responsibility to Diagnose," *American Journal of Nursing, 82*:645–646, 1982.

Carnegie, M. Elizabeth: *Historical Perspectives of Nursing Research.* Boston, Nursing Archive of Boston University, 1976.

Christy, Teresa: "Clinical Practice as a Function of Nursing Education: A Historical Analysis," *Nursing Outlook, 28*:493–497, 1980.

Committee on the Structure of National Nursing Organizations: *New Horizons in Nursing.* New York, The Macmillan Co., 1950.

Creighton, Helen: *Law Every Nurse Should Know*. Philadelphia, W. B. Saunders Co., 1975.
Edmunds, Linda: "Computer-Assisted Nursing Care," *American Journal of Nursing, 82*:1076–1079, 1982.
Fagan, Edna A.: "Diploma Schools Revisited," *Nursing Outlook, 22*:756–758, 1974.
Fagen, Claire, McClure, Margaret, and Schlotfeldt, Rozella: "Can We Bring Order out of the Chaos of Nursing Education?" *American Journal of Nursing, 76*:98–107, 1976.
Gelinas, Agnes: *Nursing and Nursing Education*. New York, Commonwealth Fund, 1946.
Gold, Harold, Jackson, Marjorie, Sachs, Barbara, and Van Meter, Margie: "Peer Review—A Working Experiment," *Nursing Outlook, 21*:634–636, 1973.
Gortner, Susan R.: "Scientific Accountability in Nursing," *Nursing Outlook, 22*:764–768, 1974.
Henderson, Virginia: *Nature of Nursing*. New York, Macmillan Co., 1966.
Infante, Mary Sue, Ed.: *Crisis Theory: A Framework for Nursing Practice*. Reston, Virginia, Reston Publishing Co., 1982.
Jacox, Ada K.: "Who Defines and Controls Nursing Practice?" *American Journal of Nursing, 69*:977–982, 1969.
Kramer, Marlene: *Reality Shock: Why Nurses Leave Nursing*. St. Louis, C.V. Mosby Co., 1974.
Lewis, Edith P.: *A Collection of Editorials From Nursing Outlook 1971–1980*. American Journal of Nursing Company, 1980.
Maas, Meridean, and Jacox, Ada: *Guidelines for Nurse Autonomy/Patient Welfare*. New York, Appleton-Century-Crofts, 1977.
Maas, Meridean, Specht, Janet, and Jacox, Ada: "Nurse Autonomy—Reality Not Rhetoric," *American Journal of Nursing, 75*:2201–2208, 1975.
Manthey, Marie: "Primary Nursing is Alive and Well in the Hospital," *American Journal of Nursing, 73*:83–87, 1973.
McGriff, Erline: "A Case for Mandatory Continuing Education in Nursing," *Nursing Outlook, 19*:726–730, 1971.
Montag, Mildred: *The Education of Nursing Technicians*. New York, G. P. Putnam's Sons, 1951.
Montag, Mildred: *Community College Education for Nursing*. New York, McGraw-Hill, 1959.
Mussallem, Helen K.: "The Changing Role of the Nurse," *American Journal of Nursing, 69*:514–517, 1969.
National Commission on Nursing: *Initial Report and Preliminary Recommendations*. Chicago, American Hospital Association and Hospital Research and Educational Trust, 1981.
Nuckolls, Katherine B.: "Who Decides What the Nurse Can Do?" *Nursing Outlook, 22*:626–631, 1974.
Parsons, Margaret, and Deloor, Ruth: "'. . . to care for him who shall have borne the battle . . .': The Veterans Administration Today," *Nursing and Health Care, 3*(3):126–131, 1982.
Phaneuf, Marie: *The Nursing Audit: Profile for Excellence*. New York, Appleton-Century-Crofts, 1972.
Quinn, Nancy K., and Somers, Anne R.: "The Patient's Bill of Rights: A Significant Aspect of the Consumer Revolution," *Nursing Outlook, 22*:240–244, 1974.
Rogers, Martha E.: *An Introduction to the Theoretical Basis of Nursing*. Philadelphia, F. A. Davis Co., 1970.
Rotkovich, Rachel: "The AD Nurse: A Nursing Service Perspective," *Nursing Outlook, 24*:234–236, 1976.
Safier, Gwendolyn: *Contemporary American Leaders in Nursing—An Oral History*. New York, McGraw-Hill, 1977.
Schlotfeldt, Rozella: "This I believe . . . Nursing is Health Care," *Nursing Outlook, 20*:245–246, 1972.
Schmalenberg, Claudia and Kramer, Marlene: *Coping with Reality Shock: Voices of Experience*. Wakefield, Massachusetts, Nursing Resources, 1979.
Schutt, Barbara G.: "Collective Action for Professional Security," *American Journal of Nursing, 73*:1946–1951, 1973.
Simmons, Leo W., and Henderson, Virginia: *Nursing Research*. New York: Appleton-Century-Crofts, 1964.
Smoyak, Shirley A.: "Is Practice Responding to Research?" *American Journal of Nursing, 76*:1146–1150, 1976.
Staupers, Mabel K.: *No Time For Prejudice*. New York, The Macmillan Co., 1961.
Taylor, Effie J.: "Teaching Nursing by the Application of the Case Study Method," *International Council of Nursing*, January 1927, p. 1–16.
Thibodeau, Janice A., and Hawkins, Joellen: *Primary Care: Nursing Management Across the Life Span*. Belmont, California, Wardsworth Health Sciences, 1983.
Thibodeau, Janice A.: *Nursing Models: Analysis and Evaluation*. Belmont, California, Wardsworth Health Sciences, 1983.
Walsh, Patricia L.: *Forever Sad the Heart*. New York, Avon Books, 1982.
Wandelt, Mabel A., and Ager, Joel: *Quality Patient Care Scale*. New York: Appleton-Century-Crofts, 1974.
Wandelt, Mabel, and Stewart, Doris Slater: *Slater Nursing Competencies Rating Scale*. New York, Appleton-Century-Crofts, 1975.

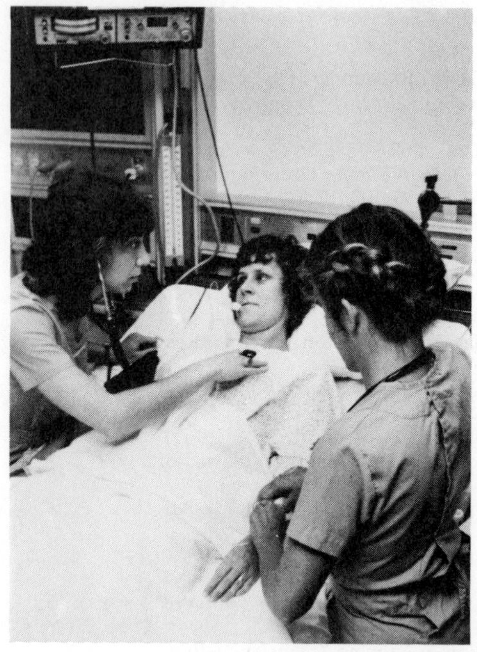

Blending the scientific, technical and humanistic skills of nursing for effective care in the late twentieth century. (Courtesy of the Framingham Union Hospital, Massachusetts.)

Perspectives on Nursing 16

NURSING—WHERE THE ACTION HAS BEEN IN THE TWENTIETH CENTURY

In reviewing the accomplishments of nursing we note that nursing has moved from a procedure-oriented approach to one that is oriented towards the individual, the family and the community. The location of the nurse's practice has been found within the fabric of life itself. The significant difference between nursing of past and present has been not *where* the nurse has practiced but the *quality* of the care that the nurse has provided.

Tremendous scientific discoveries along with the need for educational enrichment in order to comprehend them have become a fait accompli. It is not, however, the acquisition of a body of knowledge but its utilization in the delivery of nursing care that is rewarding to the provider and satisfying to the recipient of the care. During this century many complex threads of problems and progress have been woven into the fabric of client care and accountability.

NURSING IN ACUTE CARE SETTINGS

In the early years of this century, the patient and nurse were the main inhabitants of the hospital where "caring about," "caring with" and "caring for" were of paramount importance. The primary reason for admission of an acutely ill individual to a hospital was the need for nursing care. For the most part, the care consisted of continual skilled attention given to patients with a variety of illnesses that "had to run their course." Physicians' contributions were very modest and medical intervention had little impact. Although acutely ill individuals are still admitted to hospitals for nursing care, the practice of hospital nursing, like the practice of medicine, has changed dramatically.

The inception of antibiotics and technological equipment, the prolific increase in number and types of hospital personnel, the greater educational differential between health care providers and lastly the constraints of war service demands caused a weakening of the role of the nurse, whose efforts were absorbed in great measure by non-patient contact activities.

The most remarkable scientific advances have occurred since World War II with the steady progress made in the areas of medical science, technology and pharmacology. These advances, coupled with the development of highly specialized fields of medical practice, made it increasingly possible to successfully reverse many acute clinical conditions and to solve a host of other health problems, for people of all ages, that were previously incompatible with survival.

The changes also produced a hospital population with differing care needs, and gradually, general hospital wards were modified into specialized care units, which focused on the degree of illness of the patients rather than solely on the nature of their medical problems. Simultaneously, many hospitals began to concentrate on acute episodic illnesses that responded to short-term, high-technology treatment. Once clinical stability was achieved, patients were usually discharged from the hospital to recuperate elsewhere, thereby making the admission of other acutely ill patients possible. As a result, hospitals generally had a greater percentage of very sick patients than they had in the past, and the intensity of hospital nursing escalated accordingly.

To keep pace with this rapid evolution, nursing expanded its knowledge base, and as it grew in complexity, areas of specialization that broadly paralleled those of medicine were developed. Additionally, the activities of the professional nurses became pivotal to the coordination of all the nursing, medical and support services that patients received 24 hours a day, seven days a week.

During the 1950s and 1960s, many leaders strove to identify nursing problems and suggested that nurses realize their role and accept new solutions that were critical for client satisfaction as well as for strengthening delivery of nursing care. Consumers had criticized their "impersonal, fragmented care." By the mid-1960s, nurses had defined their roles even more clearly; titles such as Intensive Care Unit Nurses and Dialysis Nurses were common in hospitals. Implicit was the understanding that they were capable of exercising substantial independent judgment as the basis for timely and propitious nursing intervention rather than dependent on explicit instructions from physicians. At about the same time, master's degree–prepared clinical specialists also started to become part of the nursing force in acute care settings. They brought advanced clinical knowledge and expertise, understanding of research and evaluation processes and the ability to transform new research findings into clinical nursing practice. Their influence has increasingly elevated the quality of nursing care for acutely ill patients.

Currently, many acute care hospitals are expanding their specialized services even further. This is evident in the emergence of ultraspecialized areas, such as neurosurgical intensive care units, neonatal critical care units and coronary care units. With the growing complexity of medicine, new technologies and new responsibilities have entered the domain of acute care nursing. Many nurses are receiving special preparation in order to make their contributions in their unique areas of client care more effective. Nurses attend clinical conferences in nursing and receive reports of research findings in nursing care with great interest. That nurses are the basic component in the delivery of increasingly complex care is supported by the fact that 40 to 50 per cent of the total personnel budget in United States' hospitals is currently designated for nursing. Furthermore, acute care settings are seeing the appearance of more interdisciplinary health care teams of which nurses consistently continue to be influential members.[1] To appreciate the changes in the delivery of nursing care one must review the nursing service "assignment" patterns (see page 343).

NURSING IN THE COMMUNITY

The emphasis of the Goldmark Report on public health nursing focussed attention on the need for inclusion of community nursing as a learning experience for well-prepared nurses.

---

[1]National Commission on Nursing: *Initial Report and Preliminary Recommendations.* Chicago, American Hospital Association, Hospital and Educational Trust, 1981, pp. 12, 22.

At the close of the nineteenth century, sanitary inspectors in the United States visited schools and carried out a program of anticontagion service. Thousands of children were excluded from school because of pediculosis, ringworm, scabies, impetigo and trachoma.

Lillian D. Wald recognized the need for the well-prepared nurse to play a dynamic role in the detection of illness and to provide care for these persons and their families as well as to prevent disease and promote health.

Lillian Wald's first assignment as a graduate nurse was at the Juvenile Asylum in New York City, where she discovered the treatment of the children to be abysmally cruel. She enrolled at the Women's Medical College and, in her free time, conducted classes in home nursing for immigrants. The critical need for help for the poor and her strong interest in the role of the nurse caused her to realize that it was a strong, positive independent posture in nursing and not a medical role that she desired. She then terminated her medical education to concentrate on the now world-famous project of developing the "House" on Henry Street that became the Henry Street Visiting Nurse Service. This service, also known as the Henry Street Settlement, was established in 1893 and was the first nurses' settlement (Figs. 16–1 to 16–3).

As a result of Lillian Wald's motivation, lectures on public health nursing were inaugurated at Teachers' College, Columbia University, in 1899. In 1906, the Instructive District Nursing Association of Boston offered a postgraduate course in public health nursing. In 1910, Columbia University gave the first university course in public health nursing.

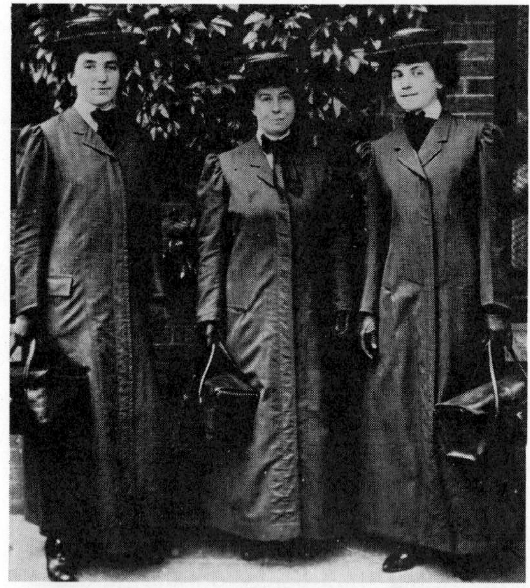

Figure 16–2. The official uniform adopted by the Henry Street Visiting Nurse Service in 1908. (Dolan collection.)

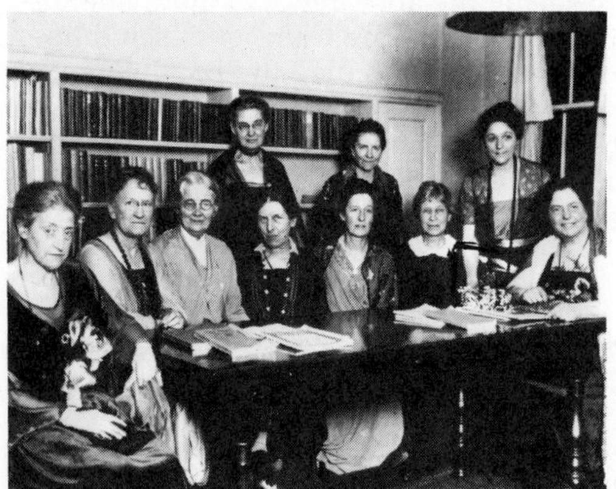

Figure 16–1. A group of nurse leaders at the opening of the Henry Street Visiting Nurse Service. *Left to right:* Annie W. Goodrich, Jane E. Hitchcock, Georgiana B. Judson, M. Adelaide Nutting, Henrietta Van Cleft, Rebecca Shatz, Mary Magonn Brown, Lavinia L. Dock, Elizabeth A. Frank and Lillian D. Wald. (Dolan collection.)

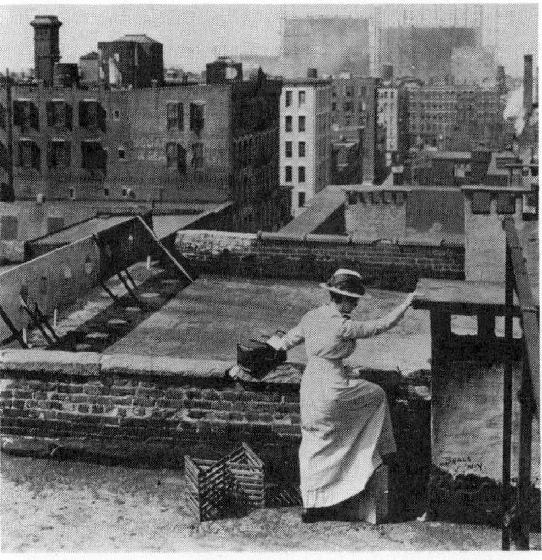

Figure 16–3. A nurse from the Henry Street Visiting Nurse Service takes a shortcut over the roofs of the tenements in New York's Lower East Side (ca. 1908). (Courtesy of Visiting Nurse Service of New York.)

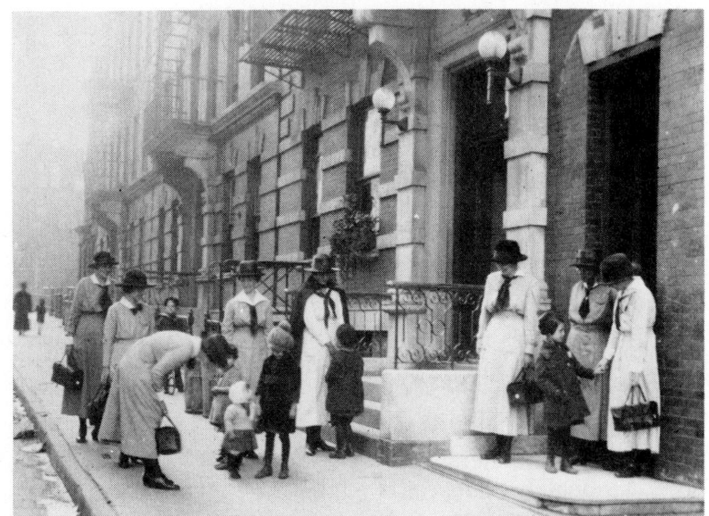

Figure 16–4. Community health nurses were soon accepted as missionaries of health. (Dolan collection.)

In 1900, the Board of Education of the City of New York established the first ungraded class for retarded children; in 1908, this act resulted in the creation of a separate department for special education for the mentally retarded.

Public health nursing began under voluntary philanthropic organizations that employed one or two nurses. The nurses' service demonstrated the value of public health nursing and attracted public attention and support, including that of local and state boards of health, which began to employ nurses (Fig. 16–4).

Today, nurses are making major contributions to health care in the community as visiting nurses, practitioners in ambulatory care settings and neighborhood health centers, health educators and promoters of health.

Rural Nursing

In 1912, Miss Wald prevailed upon Jacob Schiff to donate money to the Red Cross for the purpose of inaugurating a system of *rural nursing*. As a result of her efforts, the Rural Nursing Service, later called *Town and Country Nursing*, was established. The department's services reached vast neglected areas of the country.

The Nurse in Schools

In 1891 at the International Congress of Hygiene and Demography in England, Dr. Malcolm Morris proposed that a staff of specially educated nurses should visit the elementary schools regularly to examine the children. In 1892, *school nursing* was introduced into the school system in London. *Amy Hughes*, who had been superintendent of the Queen's Nurses, accepted the invitation to become the first school nurse. It was not until 1907 that an act was passed that provided for medical inspection of school children in England.

In her book, *Practical Hints on District Nursing*, Amy Hughes discussed the power of the movement of nurses in the community. "The power of keeping a home together, when the alternative is the workhouse, is a social question with far-reaching consequences. To shorten the breadwinner's illness . . . to save mothers of families from life-long effects of ignorance and neglect, to teach the proper management of infants and children, are gains to the community at large."[2] She further stated, "The true way to help the poor is to teach them to help themselves."

In 1902, Lillian Wald encouraged the use of nurses in the schools of New York. *Lina Rogers* (Fig. 16–5) was sent from the Henry Street Settlement to a school on a one-month trial basis. She visited four schools a day, spending about one hour in each school and making follow-up visits in the homes. Miss Rogers reported on the physical discomforts in some schools and on the

[2]Hughes, Amy: *Practical Hints on District Nursing*. London, The Scientific Press, pp. 2–3.

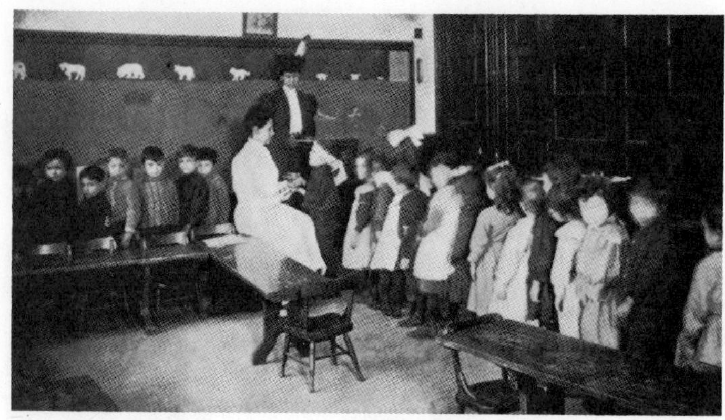

Figure 16–5. Miss Lina Rogers, the first school nurse, inspects school children. (Dolan collection.)

need for general improvement of the educational facilities as well as on the problems in the homes. This experiment was a successful one, and dispensaries were improvised with supplies furnished by the Board of Education. The nurses who were sent to assume the assignment of the school nurse felt the need for better education.

As early as 1903, New York City established the first municipally sponsored nursing service for children in schools, and Lina Rogers was employed by the Board of Health to direct this program. The area selected to be serviced by nurses encompassed four schools with 4500 pupils in the worst slums of the city. In this setting Miss Rogers carried out a program of communicable disease control. It has been recorded that she visited the poor in crowded, unhealthy tenements and instructed both parents and children in personal cleanliness and demonstrated simple treatments to improve health and prevent the spread of contagious diseases. Statistics reveal that as a result of this nurse leadership there was a marked reduction in the number of children absent from school. The identification of health needs and follow-through on the provision of necessary health facilities, as well as the utilization of the nurse as a health teacher, contributed to the success of the project and to the better health of the community. With the addition of many more nurses to the school system, treatment clinics were established in the schools, thus permitting students to receive care while attending school. School nurses visited newborn babies and mothers during the summer months, which had been the peak period for "cholera infantum," a disease that caused a high infant mortality rate. It has been estimated that 1200 more babies survived that first summer. These creative nurses recognized the importance of the application of their knowledge to health teaching. Pamphlets were written as another tool for dissemination of important health information.

In 1907, inspection for communicable diseases among school children was delegated to the school nurse, and school health programs were expanded.

Little Mother's Leagues (Fig. 16–6) were formed in the schools. Girls eight years old and over assumed the role of "little mother" and were taught how to care for their younger brothers and sisters. These leagues were received with enthusiasm and were a valuable asset to the health of the community.

In 1905, Miss Wald initiated school lunch programs. The Board of Education of New York City served the lunches, which were available to all children in the public school system. That same year Miss Wald recognized the need for a federal Children's Bureau; in 1912, this need was fulfilled when a federal agency was established to care specifically for children. Miss Wald was also instrumental in encouraging the organization of study halls, because she and her staff realized the inadequacy of most homes for study.

The nurse in a school setting has usually been employed by one of three agencies: a board of education, a local health department or a community nursing service. Certification requirements for nurses in a school system were enunciated without consultation with representatives of the nursing profession, so that a foundation in education rather than a good preparation in nursing has been required. It cannot be

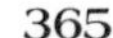

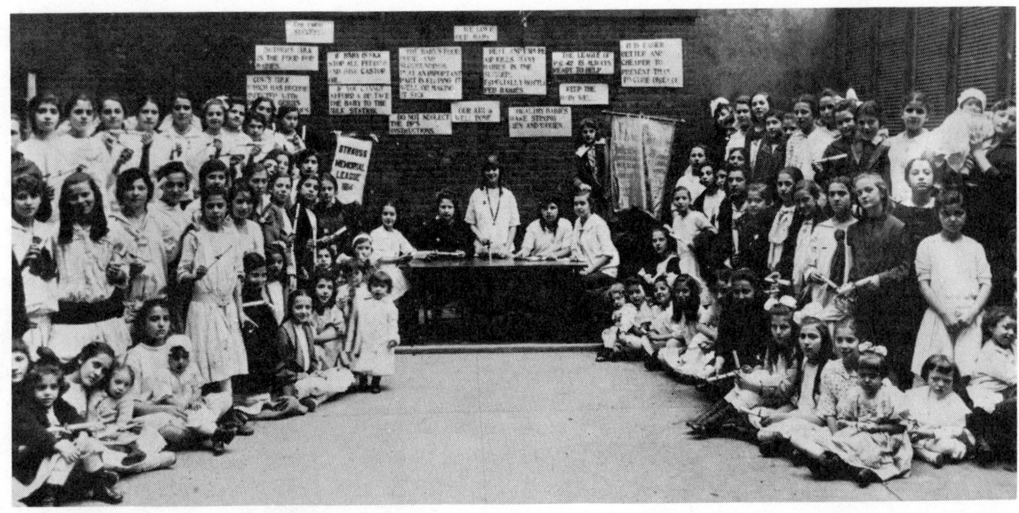

Figure 16–6. A positive and enthusiastic response to a call to participate in a Little Mother's League. (Courtesy of New York City Department of Health.)

denied that the educational requirements of certification broadened the background of school nurses.

In 1961, the American Nurses' Association (ANA) and, in 1962, the National League for Nursing (NLN) recommended that school nurses have a baccalaureate degree and field experience in school nursing at the undergraduate or graduate level. Elizabeth Stobo's efforts as director of a study by the NLN resulted in guidelines for the preparation of school nurses.[3]

In 1960, the California State Legislature passed the Fisher Bill, which lengthened the time required to prepare teachers from four years to five. This legislation called attention to the need for reevaluation of methods of preparation for the nurse in a school setting as well as for the classroom teacher.

The passage of this bill was followed by the publication of two significant documents, one by Anne Marks[4] on the delineation of guidelines for content of graduate programs in school nursing, and the other by Helen Florentine,[5] which discussed the

[3]Stobo, Elizabeth: *Findings of a Study Designed to Assist in the Development of Guidelines for the Preparation of Nurses for School Health Work*. New York, National League for Nursing, 1961.

[4]Marks, Anne P.: *School Nursing; Guidelines for Content of Graduate Programs of Study in the Specialty of School Nursing*. San Francisco, University of California School of Nursing, 1962.

[5]Florentine, Helen G.: *Preparation and the Role of Nurses in School Health Programs*. New York, National League for Nursing, 1962.

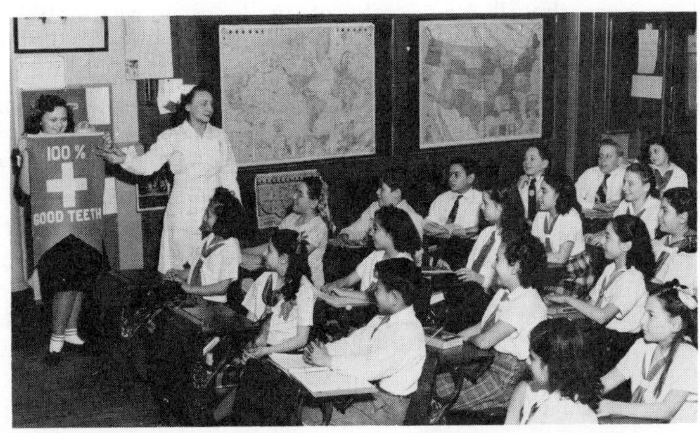

Figure 16–7. A school nurse in an officially recognized role of health teacher in the 1940s. The stereotypical image of the nurse role in "sick nursing" was perpetuated by the wearing of the uniform. (Dolan collection.)

preparation and role of the nurse in a program of school health.

San Francisco State College developed a supplementary program of 30 credits for graduate nurses who had earned a baccalaureate degree. Burtz described this program as well as the role for which the students were being prepared:

> The comprehensive role of the school nurse is one of an educator, which includes health counseling and guidance. She is the liaison between the school and the home. She works as a member of the health team in the school and . . . has special knowledge of . . . health problems. She interprets school problems to parents, and brings back to the teachers and principals the concerns of parents which affect the child's health.[6]

This program highlighted the need for nurses to have knowledge and understanding of the education process.

The University of Colorado developed a program to assist school nurses with baccalaureate degrees to become school nurse practitioners. The school nurse practitioner is expected to assess psychological, neurological and other problems that can affect the normal behavior of the child and his ability to learn. In addition to taking histories, doing physical examinations, giving immunizations and treating minor illnesses, the school nurse practitioner supervises tests to detect and evaluate evidence of problems of speech, sight, hearing, and posture and drug abuse.

Nursing's War Against Disease

Communicable diseases still continued to plague individuals, families and communities at the turn of the century. Attempts to prevent the spread of disease as well as return the ill to a state of wellness were noted. Nurses participated in the detection of communicable disease at the immigration centers (Fig. 16–8). Community nurses visited patients to assess their needs, and patients suffering from "consumption," or tuberculosis, called the white plague in the early part of this century, received special attention. These nurses distributed free milk and eggs to needy patients with tuberculosis. Because of their efforts, a tuberculosis pavilion was opened in Riverside Hospital and a tuberculosis dispensary was organized with nurses in charge. The need for instruction by a visiting nurse was essential for preventive as well as curative measures.

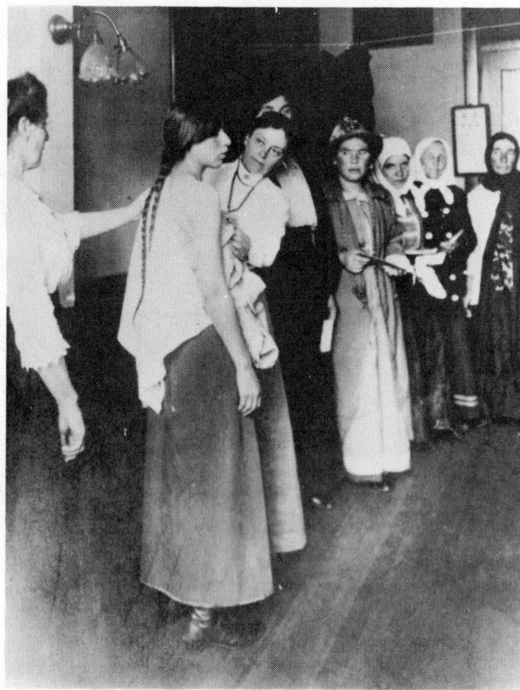

Figure 16–8. Nurse at immigrant detention center participating in a program of detection of communicable disease.

It was necessary to detect cases of tuberculosis in order to prevent the spread of the disease. Dr. William Osler was the motivating force behind a project to carry out plans to provide this service. In 1899, one of the women medical students at Johns Hopkins was selected to do follow-up work with dispensary patients in their homes. In 1900, through Dr. Osler's prompting, the *Laënnec Society of Baltimore* was founded, which disseminated information about the disease to the public. By 1903, the nurse replaced the medical student as dispenser of this information and gave complete home care, which included instruction for the patient and his family. In 1910, work with tuberculosis patients was absorbed by the City Boards of Health. By 1904, the National Association for the Study and Prevention of Tuberculosis had been organized. By 1907, the Boston Consumptives' Hospital had developed a tuberculosis vis-

[6]Burtz, Gudrun S.: "A Fifth Year for School Nurse Preparation," *Nursing Outlook, 17*:38–40, 1969.

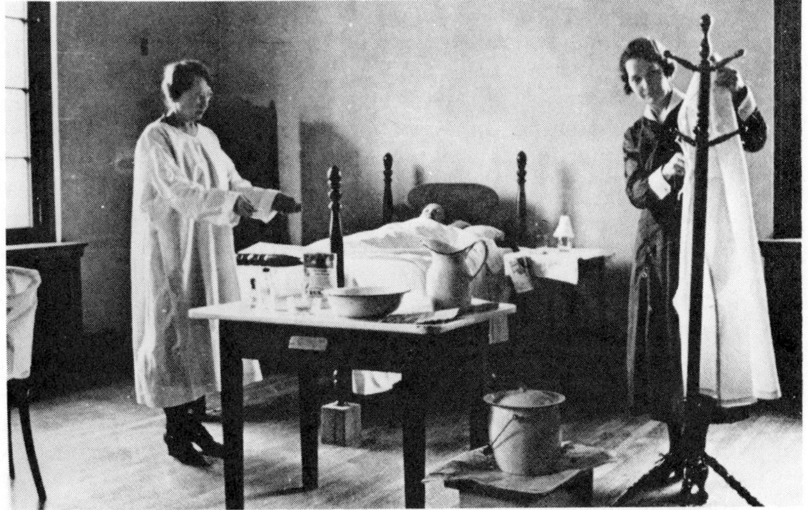

Figure 16–9. Pearl McIver and Sena Anderson demonstrate the home treatment of communicable disease referred to as the "isolation technique." (Dolan collection.)

iting nursing group within its Out-Patient Department, and by 1908, an affiliation had become effective between this nursing staff and the Boston School for Social Workers. In addition to "isolation hospitals" many general hospitals had special units for patients with communicable diseases. Hospital porches were used for patients with tuberculosis (Fig. 16–10).

Another specialized service within the overall coverage of nursing in the community was that of orthopedic nursing. Marguerite Wales, in her well-known book *The Public Health Nurse in Action,* estimated that in the 1930s there were "between 400,000 and 500,000 children under twenty-one years of age who were crippled by disease or conditions such as poliomyelitis, tuberculosis of bones and joints, birth injuries, injuries due to accidents, and congenital deformities."[7] *Jessie L. Stevenson,* consultant in orthopedic nursing for the National Organization for Public Health Nursing (NOPHN), stressed that nursing care of patients with orthopedic problems should be part of all nursing whether in the home or the hospital.

[7]Wales, Marguerite: *The Public Health Nurse in Action.* New York, The Macmillan Co., 1941, p. 252.

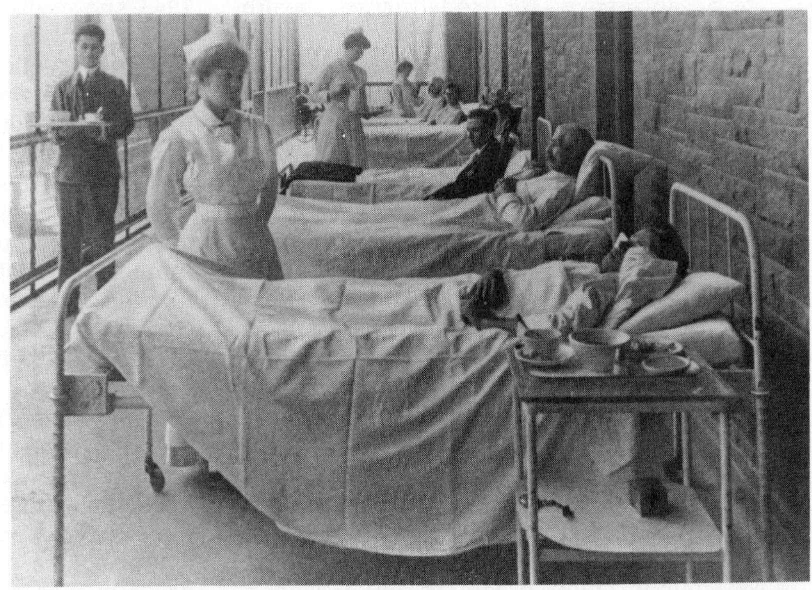

Figure 16–10. A porch in a general hospital where patients are convalescing from tuberculosis. (Dolan collection.)

The question of generalized nursing services versus specialized nursing services was studied in the 1920s by the American Red Cross. It was decided that specialized services isolate and concentrate on specific health entities while lacking the broader approach to the total physical, social, emotional and economic family problems taken by the generalized type of service.

Nursing and Life Insurance Projects

The history of the inception of community health nursing is replete with recorded evidence of the work of nurses in primary prevention. An example of this work was the affiliation of some community nurses with the *Metropolitan Life Insurance Company*. In 1909, this company launched a program that was to have a profound influence on the health of millions of people in the United States and Canada. The program's objective was the prolonging of life. The officers of the life insurance company made some assumptions that were stated in the form of ideals, purposes and beliefs. They believed that it would be possible:

1. to prevent unnecessary illness and premature death.
2. to carry out a campaign of education in primary prevention.
3. to encourage people to participate in community health projects.
4. to provide health messengers to carry out programs of education.
5. to strive for constructive health legislation.
6. to enlist the cooperative efforts of other health and welfare organizations in health promotion.
7. to use demonstrations coupled with printed materials as educational tools.

Lillian Wald offered the services of her community health nurses from Henry Street for this project. Thus began one of the most far-reaching and successful endeavors for the health of the American people. This project extended over nearly 44 years with 20 million policyholders receiving 100 million visits from nurses.

The value of public health nurses in primary prevention has been documented. They gave care to expectant and new mothers, brought health education into homes, set up storefront clinics, engaged in immunization programs and designed health teaching aids such as motion pictures, film strips, exhibits and pamphlets.

When the program was launched, in 1909, the life expectancy of the average American was 47 years. When the Metropolitan Life Insurance Agency terminated the Public Health Nursing Service in 1953, life expectancy had increased to 70 years.

Lillian Wald, like Florence Nightingale, had the ability to see beyond "what is" to "what could be."

In 1925, the *John Hancock Mutual Life Insurance Company* contracted for similar service. The value of health teaching and care in the conservation of life had been recognized.

Nursing and Social Issues

Miss Wald recognized that nursing leadership could penetrate any area where the health of people was in jeopardy. She became a member of the New York State Immigration Commission in 1909 and, upon making an inspection trip to two engineering projects, revealed the exploitation of immigrant workers and deplorable living and working conditions. As a result of her pleas, labor laws were better enforced and health and sanitary facilities were improved.

This kind of experience led Miss Wald to work for labor codes, which were enacted in 1910. That same year she was appointed to membership on the New York Joint Board of Sanitary Control. The board's first inspection revealed that two-thirds of the 1243 shops visited were defective in fire protection, sanitation or both. As a result of the inspection, standards were delineated that eliminated sweat-shops in tenements. Owing to Miss Wald's efforts as a member of the Factory Investigating Committee, fire drills became mandatory.

When illness invaded the home, a family of moderate means needed affordable nursing service to make the ill person comfortable and permit the family to continue their work. A solution to this problem appeared in 1909 in Brattleboro, Vermont, in the form of a program called *Household Nursing*. There were three types of workers in this program: graduate nurses, supervised nongraduate nurses, who performed household duties in addition to caring for the sick, and women who did housework in the homes of people with illness. This program was an early professional nurse, practical nurse and homemaker aid team plan.

In 1912, when the *National Organization for Public Health Nursing* (NOPHN) was instituted, Lillian Wald was elected the first president. Membership in this organization was conferred only upon nurses possessing specified professional qualifications. Agencies could possess corporate membership only if they employed nurses of whom a given percentage were eligible for membership. One of the chief aims of the NOPHN was to raise the educational standards for the practice of community nursing.

The U.S. Public Health Service openly proclaimed its dependence on the public health nurse. General Thomas Parran, when head of this service, said, "In this country more than any other, with the possible exception of Canada, there is almost complete recognition among public health officers and citizens alike of nursing as the spearhead of the whole public health movement. Dependence is placed upon it to advance new causes and to serve new needs."

The great foundations have aided materially in setting up public health programs and aiding public health work; they did not replace government projects, but supplemented them by providing services not undertaken by state and federal agencies. The *Rockefeller Foundation,* established in 1913, has as its stated goal: "To promote the well-being of mankind throughout the world."

When an epidemic of poliomyelitis struck New York City in 1916, the Henry Street Nursing Service gave meritorious service. At the termination of World War I when the Spanish influenza epidemic occurred in 1918, nurses again responded to the needs of the public. For example, in Lawrence, Massachusetts, the first case of influenza was reported on September 8, and the epidemic lasted until the latter part of October. The devastation was unbelievable. Pneumonia became a serious complication. At the outbreak of the epidemic, the armory was used as a temporary hospital, but later, an emergency open-air settlement was erected on the summit of Tower Hill overlooking the Merrimac River (Fig. 16–11). This settlement consisted of 100 tents furnished by military authorities,

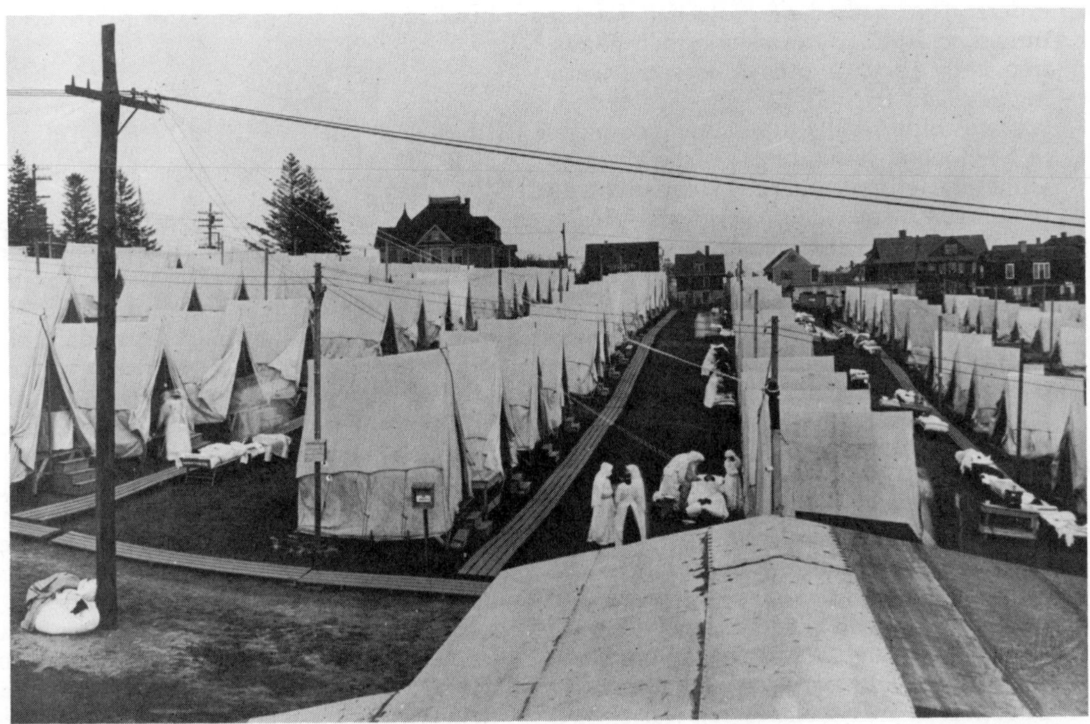

Figure 16–11. Tent City at Tower Hill (Emery Hill), the special hospital for victims of epidemic influenza in Lawrence, Massachusetts, on May 29, 1919. (Courtesy of American Red Cross.)

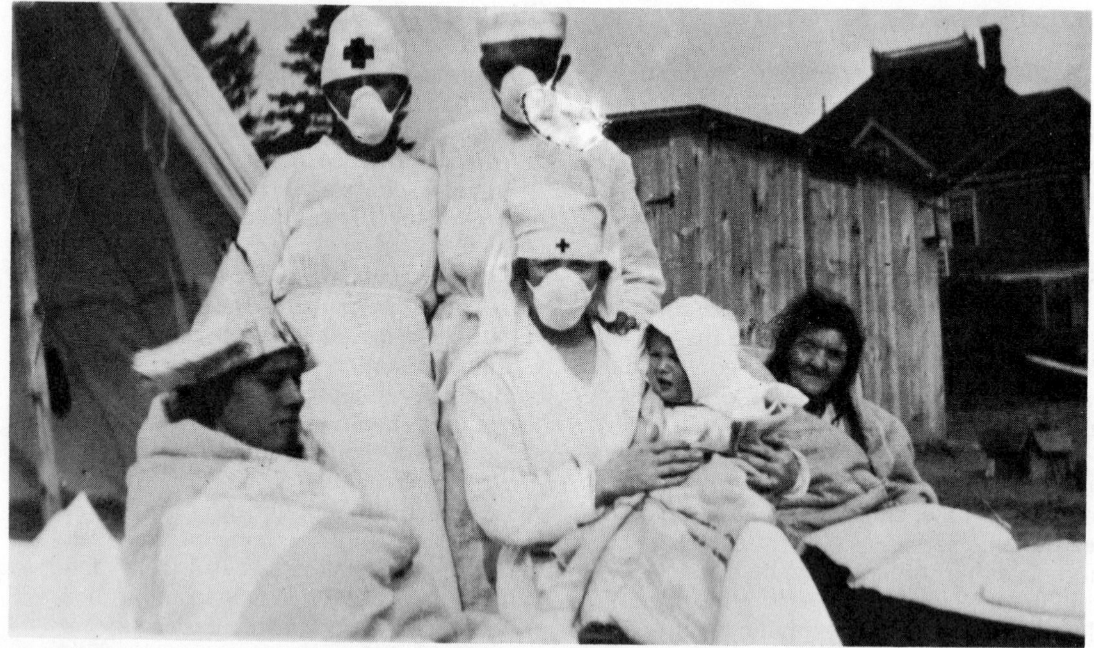

Figure 16–12. A closer view of Tent City shows the nurses and physicians wearing masks as a method of disease prevention. (Courtesy of Yvonne Charpentier, R. N.) (Dolan collection.)

each housing two patients. Many public health nurses were joined by volunteers, both lay people and members of religious orders. The method of protection for the nurses, in addition to washing their hands, frequently appears to have been the wearing of masks (Fig. 16–12).

It was reported that the surgeon general ordered wooden buildings to be erected on a hill for the treatment of the patients with pneumonia. The chairman of the Health Department in Lawrence received the orders at noon on a Sunday. By six o'clock, 40 carpenters started work erecting the building, which was 180 feet long and 15 feet wide, and by the following afternoon the building was ready for occupancy.

During this period in the city of Lawrence, 3155 cases of influenza were reported, with 215 deaths from influenza and 247 deaths from pneumonia. Before the "flu" pandemic terminated, 548,000 people in this country and 20 million worldwide had died of it.

Many leaders in the nursing field were staunch pacifists. Lavinia Dock worked ardently for world peace as did Annie W. Goodrich. In 1914, Lillian Wald was elected chairman of the American Union Against Militarism. Yet when the United States declared war, these nurse leaders made every effort to bind up the wounds of suffering humanity.

LEADERSHIP IN PUBLIC HEALTH NURSING

Mary Sewall Gardner (1871–1961) (Fig. 16–13) was one of the great leaders of nursing. She was born in Newton, Massachusetts, the daughter of Supreme Court Justice William Gardner and a direct descendant of a signer of the Declaration of Independence. Miss Gardner graduated from Miss Porter's School in Farmington, Connecticut, after traveling abroad for several years, and then entered Newport Hospital Training School for Nurses. She graduated from there in 1905 and founded the Providence Visiting Nurses' Association in Rhode Island, which she directed for 25 years.

Her book, *Public Health Nursing,* was published in 1916. It was the first and, for many years, the standard textbook in this field. Because her textbook was translated into French, Spanish, Japanese, Chinese

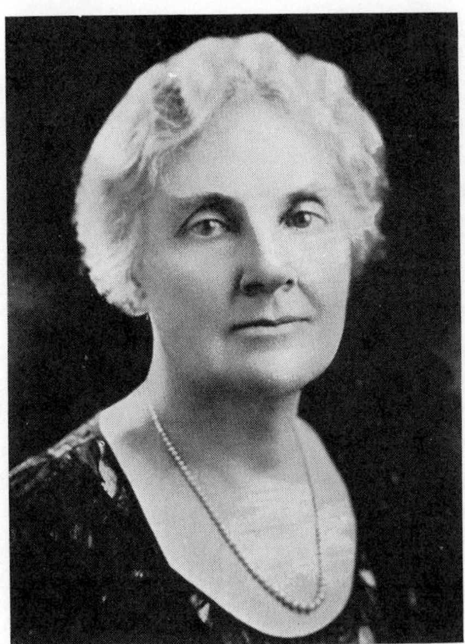

Figure 16–13. Mary Sewall Gardner. (Dolan collection.)

and Korean, she was recognized for many years as a national and international authority on public health nursing.

Miss Gardner assisted the Red Cross in Washington and Italy (with Edna Foley) and inspected Red Cross child welfare work in Europe. She served as the second president of the NOPHN and chairman of the public health nursing section of the International Council of Nurses (ICN). She wrote two novels of public health nursing, *So Build We* and *Katherine Kent*.

In 1918, Brown University awarded Miss Gardner an honorary Master of Arts degree because "she pioneered in making care of the sick an honored profession" and because she was "a gentlewoman whose writings and whose example have brought us healing of the body and inspiration of the spirit."

Dorothy Deming was born in New Haven, Connecticut, attended private schools and graduated from Vassar in 1914. She commenced work at Yale University Graduate School, where three generations of her family had preceded her. It was her intention to complete the requirements for a Ph.D. in American colonial history in 1918.

Dorothy Deming's doctoral research was published in monograph form by Yale University Press. These monographs became the historical highlights of the Connecticut Tercentenary Celebration in 1935. They have been regarded as significant historical documentation.

As a result of the emotional stress of her mother's death and the social and political pressures of the war effort, she engaged in volunteer work with the New Haven Visiting Nurses' Association. She was motivated to become a nurse and enrolled in Presbyterian Hospital in New York City. Dorothy Deming received a challenging senior year experience with the Henry Street Visiting Nurse Service. She joined the New Haven Visiting Nurses' Association after graduation but soon returned to Henry Street and commenced her meteoric rise in the field of public health nursing. Because of her writing skill, she became assistant editor and then editor of the magazine *Public Health Nursing*. Her next position of great influence was that of General Director of NOPHN. Dorothy Deming used her communication skills, her educational gifts and her sparkle and humor in creating the series of novels about nursing called the *Penny Marsh Series*, which were first printed in 1938 and were reprinted, through the eighteenth printing, until 1960. They were publicized as career novels.

Lavinia Lloyd Dock (Fig. 16–14) was another pioneer in public health nursing. She came from a cultured philanthropic family. She shared an interest in medicine with

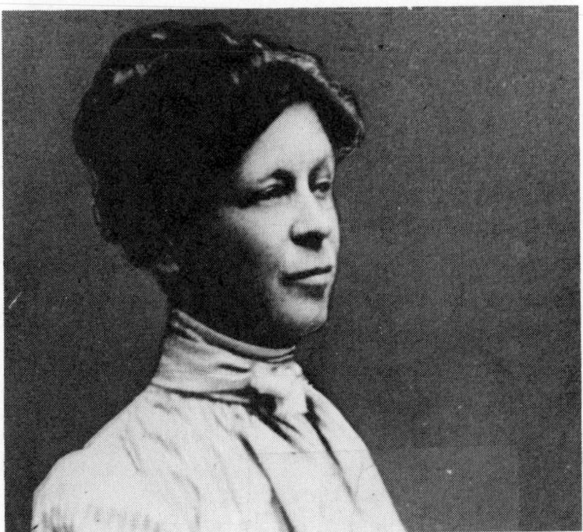

Figure 16–14. Lavinia L. Dock, a community health nurse, humanitarian, pacifist, world leader for nursing, and author and historian of renown. (Dolan collection.)

her brother, who became a professor of medicine in the schools of medicine at the University of Michigan and Washington University. Miss Dock entered Bellevue Training School for Nurses, from which she graduated in 1886. Her first assignment was with a pioneering effort called the United Workers of Norwich, Connecticut. This group wanted to try a three months' experiment whereby a trained nurse would take care of sickness in the community. Through Miss Dock's efforts the experiment was successful. She volunteered for service during a yellow fever epidemic, was one of the group of visiting nurses with the New York City Mission and finally became assistant to Isabel Hampton Robb at Johns Hopkins Hospital. After a brief experience as principal of the Illinois Training School for Nurses in Chicago, Miss Dock joined the Henry Street Settlement in New York City to work with Lillian Wald. Interest in her patients prompted Miss Dock to spend her free time studying languages.

It was Lavinia Dock's belief that a worldwide public health movement would emphasize prevention, thereby creating a need for a better-educated nurse than the typical bedside nurse of the time.

Miss Dock was the first secretary of the American Society of Superintendents of Training Schools for Nurses. In addition, she was the first secretary of the ICN. The nurses of the United States and the world profited by her wisdom and guidance as an officer of both organizations and a contributor of many articles to the early issues of the *American Journal of Nursing*. Her gift for writing is apparent in her early textbooks, *A Materia Medica for Nurses* and *Hygiene and Morality*, as well as in the magnificent four-volume *History of Nursing*, which she wrote in collaboration with M. Adelaide Nutting. This work remains a lasting memorial to two scholarly and gifted leaders of nursing.

Mary Beard was a member of the international health committee of the Rockefeller Foundation and was head of the American Red Cross Nursing Service. Ella Phillips Crandall, Edna Foley, Elizabeth G. Fox, Marguerite Wales, and Harriet Fulmer were also prominent in public health nursing early in this century.

As the century progressed, community health needs occasionally manifested unusual aspects. The 1930s brought poverty and unemployment to many. Low-cost housing was built on the Lower East Side owing to the vision and prodding of Miss Wald.

In addition to housing, the ancient system of almsgiving was reintroduced and agencies gave food to the "bread lines" of people. The *Works Progress Administration* (WPA) utilized the human resources of our country to assist in many welfare services.

A highly respected author, *Faith Baldwin*, wrote a popular book, *District Nurse*,[8] which she dedicated to "The V.N.A. and Welfare Nurses Everywhere." This book was widely read and served in its way to increase appreciation of the nurse in the community.

The Department of Philanthropic Information of the Central Hanover Bank and Trust Company issued a brochure entitled *The Public Health Nurse*. The purpose was to pay tribute to the unprecedented accomplishments of public health nurses and to broaden their financial base by encouraging "wise public giving" through a presentation of a "bird's-eye view of current activities and needs in that field." In urging financial support the bank officials quoted Dr. Howard W. Haggard:

> You who have done the work, and I who have watched as an interested spectator, do not need to have our emotions aroused. We have seen and we have heard. We know the stories of the tragedies averted and lives saved behind the bare records of those 29,000,000 visits last year. We have heard the sound of hoofbeats and creak of leather as a nurse on horseback rides alone at night over a rough mountain trail to a cabin, and there in the uncertain light of an oil lamp helps to bring a new life into the world. . . . The future of an American family has hung on her help and on her gift of the priceless knowledge of feeding, care, cleanliness, disease prevention.
>
> And again, in surroundings perhaps less picturesque, but none the less vital, we have heard the footsteps—often weary ones—of the nurse and the creak of the tenement stairs she mounts, and from above we have heard the cry of a fretting, feverish child to whom the nurse brings the soothing hand of comfort; and the sigh of a desperate mother to whom the nurse brings the clear, cold knowledge to solve those problems from which the tragedies of a home may come.

[8]Baldwin, Faith: *District Nurse*. Philadelphia, Blakiston Co., 1932.

You have heard those sounds for the millions of visits you have made; but there are a hundred million of our people who have not heard them. They have not seen, or felt, or known. Is it not then your duty to amplify these sounds so familiar to you until they reach the ears of every citizen, and reaching them, stir sentiment until a hundred million strong they join with their support to the work you carry out.[9]

Mary S. Gardner wrote of the important place the nurse held in the life of our country:

We see that she has had her effect on city and state legislation, and has influenced public opinion to effect non-legislative reform. We find her valued as a preventive agent and health instructor by municipalities and state bodies, and the usefulness of her statistics acknowledged by research workers.

. . . She is found in the juvenile courts and public playgrounds, in the department stores and big hotels, in the schools and factories, in the houses of small wage-earners and in the swarming tenements of the very poor. We find her in the big cities, the small towns, and to a limited extent in the rural districts and the lonely mountain regions. We find her dealing with tuberculosis, babies, mental cases, industrial workers, expectant mothers, and housing conditions.[10]

FAMILY NURSING

In the area of maternal and child health nursing, many changes have taken place since the beginning of the twentieth century. At the turn of the century nurses needed to know the hygiene of pregnancy; how to recognize approaching labor; how to help the physician and comfort the mother during labor; what supplies were necessary and how to prepare them; how to prepare the patient; when, why and how to examine; how to prevent septic infection; how to guard against hemorrhage; what symptoms precede eclampsia; what to do at a normal birth (with or without a physician); what to do at an instrumental delivery; how to prevent attacks of puer-

[9]Howard W. Haggard, M. D.: In *Public Health Nursing*, April, 1936.

[10]Gardner, Mary S.: *Public Health Nursing*. 3rd ed., New York, The Macmillan Co., 1936, pp. 39–40.

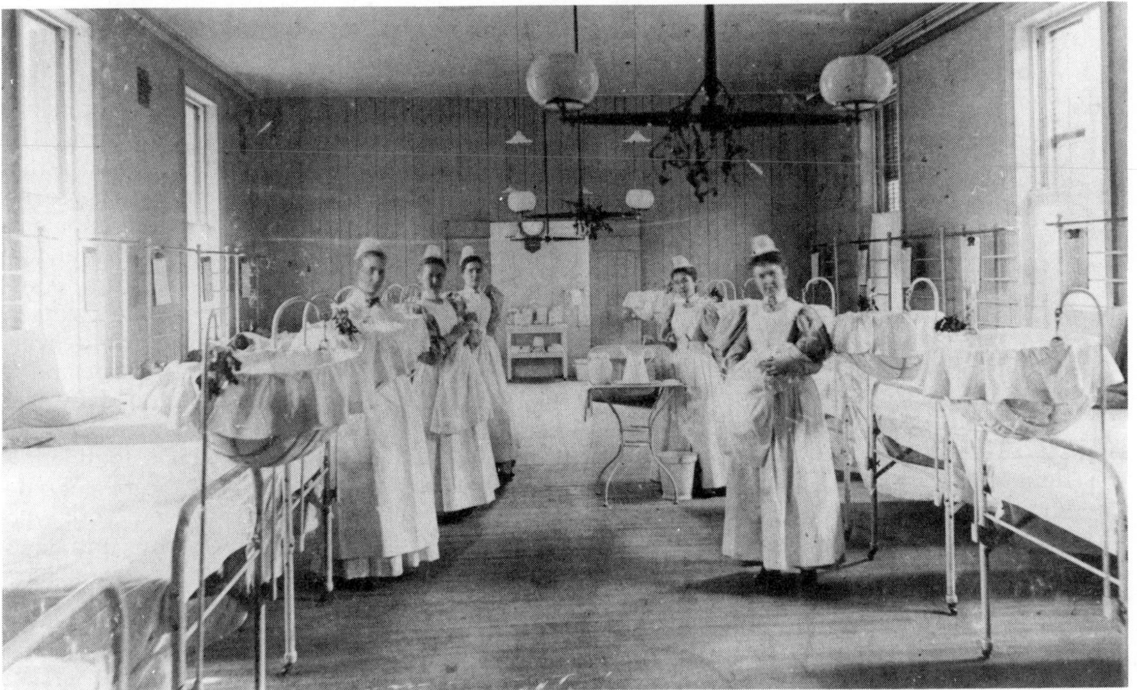

Figure 16–15. Babies "rooming-in" in bassinets at the foot of their mother's beds at the turn of the century. (Dolan collection.)

peral fever; how to provide the aftercare (with or without complications); and how to care for the new baby.[11]

Many nurses went into the homes of their clients and assisted at or even carried out the delivery of the newborn. These private duty nurses were engaged well in advance of the due date, and they stayed with the family for a certain length of time after the birth. It was a 24-hour duty assignment and having the baby was definitely a family affair. Many clients considered having the services of a nurse to be a status symbol.

In the 1920s a maternity center, the Maternity Center Association in New York City, was run by nurses. The nurses examined, taught, visited and helped the mother. They referred women to obstetricians and coordinated all other facilities.[12]

In the 1930s three phases of maternal care were recognized—prenatal, labor and delivery, and postnatal. The role of the nurse expanded. In addition she was the one who gave the pre-parent education.

The literature indicates that German and Russian obstetricians were reported to be using hypnosis to ease the pains of childbirth. In 1933, *Dr. Grantly Dick-Read* introduced a form of *natural childbirth*. Read believed that if a woman's fear and tension could be eradicated, the pain of childbirth would be eliminated or minimized. The women were taught the physical facts of childbirth and how to relax, exercise, concentrate and breathe properly. The nurse took an active role in the classes for prepared childbirth just as they do with the *Lamaze* method, introduced later.

Many women were anesthetized very heavily for the delivery process during the early decades of this century, and many hospital policies excluded fathers from the labor and delivery rooms.

By 1950, in many schools of nursing, a practice had been instituted whereby a student was assigned to a mother for whom she cared during labor and delivery. She helped with breathing exercises, gave back rubs and supported her patient emotionally. Many nurses and physicians realized that individual care was more important than a strict routine.[13]

In the 1950s, Grace–New Haven Hospital launched a pioneer experiment in which many mothers attended antepartal clinics during their entire pregnancy. The clinic provided classes given by obstetricians and obstetrical nurses, which included exercises and a tour of the obstetrical department. Everything was done to rid expectant mothers of their fears. Husbands were permitted to be with their wives in the labor and delivery room to provide emotional support and to assist in elimination of fear. After the delivery, the infant was placed in a plastic crib by the mother's bed. During the "rooming-in" period the mother and father became acquainted with and learned to care for their child (Fig. 16–16). Individualized care was given to mother and baby, and the family as a unit was emphasized.[14]

In Europe, *midwifery* has been considered an important specialty, with a two-year course commonly required. At one time in England nearly all state-registered nurses were registered midwives as well.

In the United States the subject had been neglected despite the fact that the maternal death rate was high and that a considerable number of untrained, ignorant midwives were practicing. The training of nurses in midwifery had been prevented by the attitude of the medical profession, which held that every woman should be aided in delivery by a physician. In actual fact, thousands of women live where no physician is available; other thousands employ incompetent midwives. In rural districts the need for the midwife-nurse is especially apparent. One million women annually in the United States have deliveries without the aid of a physician and a quarter of a million are attended by untrained people.

In 1911, Bellevue Hospital founded a *school of midwifery* to help care for the 40,000 mothers per year in New York who were assisted in delivery by untrained women. For many years there were nine

[11]Keith, Mary L.: "Preliminaries of Obstetric Nursing," *American Journal of Nursing*, 1:257, 1901.

[12]Stevens, Ann: "Maternity Center Work," *American Journal of Nursing*, 20:456–457, 1920.

[13]Corbin, Hazel: "Maternity Care Today and Tomorrow," *American Journal of Nursing*, *53*:201–204, 1953.

[14]Jensen, Faith E.: "Having a Baby is a Family Matter," *American Journal of Nursing*, *50*:674–675, 1950.

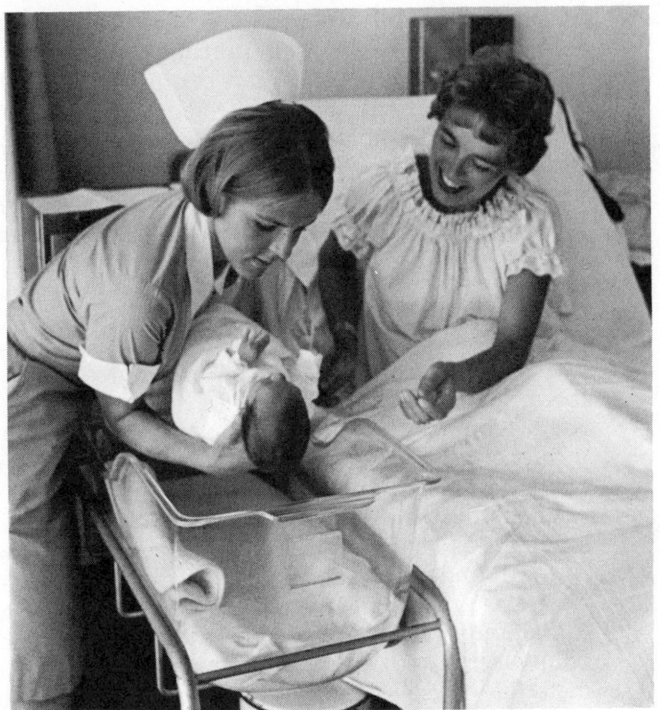

Figure 16–16. A student of nursing teaching a mother how to care for her newborn, who is "rooming-in" in the mother's hospital unit. (Courtesy of the University of Connecticut.)

centers offering courses and granting certificates in nurse-midwifery, such as the Maternity Center Association, which opened the first school for nurse-midwives in the United States, in cooperation with the Lobenstine Clinic, New York; Tuskegee Institute, Alabama; Mary Breckinridge's Frontier Nursing Service, Kentucky; and the Catholic Maternity Institute, Santa Fe, New Mexico.

Eventually, six schools offered certificates in nurse-midwifery in conjunction with a master's degree—Yale, Johns Hopkins, New York Medical College, Catholic University, Columbia University, and the University of Utah.

In 1925 the Catholic Maternity Institute was founded. Run by the Medical Mission Sisters, this organization now has centers in England, Holland and India. The sisters are fully trained physicians, pharmacists, nurses and technicians who do missionary work at home and abroad.

The first organized *midwifery service* in this country was the Frontier Nursing Service, founded by *Mary Breckinridge* (Fig. 16–17), a graduate of St. Luke's, New York, who had organized public health nursing in France. For many years, Mary Breckinridge used English-trained nurse-midwives since there were so few trained midwives in this country. Her nurses travelled on horseback to assist women in childbirth who lived in remote places; jeeps have now replaced the more traditional vehicle of travel. Mary Breckinridge's original plan

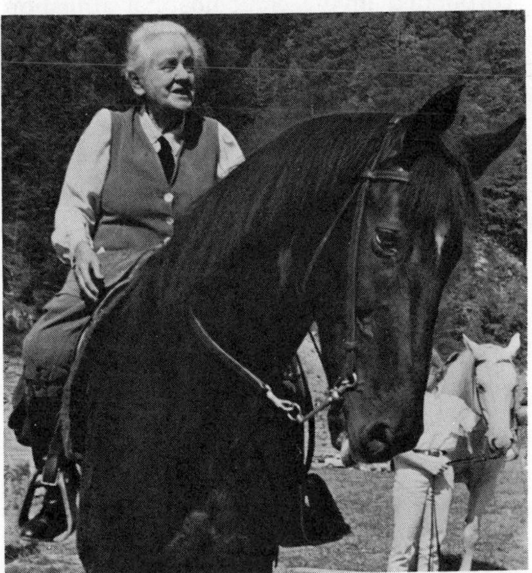

Figure 16–17. Mary Breckinridge at age 82 on her horse "Doc." (Courtesy of *Courier-Journal* and *Louisville Times*.)

of family-centered care prompted the need for her nurses to be well prepared, and each of her nursing staff had certification as a nurse-midwife. She implemented her philosophy of helping people to help themselves by including the people in the community in the planning of the programs of the Frontier Nursing Service. Mary Breckinridge's goal, to provide a program of good health care for all persons in an area of severe social and economic deprivation, has been realized.

Gertrude Isaacs, who was the first nurse to earn a *Doctor of Nursing Science* degree, has been in charge of the Family Nurse educational program of the Frontier Nursing Service.[15]

Vanderbilt University School of Nursing inaugurated an eight-week field experience at the Frontier Nursing Service as part of their master's program in Family Nursing.

Maternity care is again using nurse-midwifery services. Dorothea Lang, who directs the Nurse-Midwifery Program of the New York City Department of Health, described the current role and function of the nurse-midwife as those of a specialist who combines two disciplines—nursing and midwifery.[16] The maternity program in New York City provided services in the community health centers of the Department of Health, which then affiliated with nearby hospitals. The nurse-midwife has been incorporated in the clinic-hospital affiliation program and "acts as a liaison between the clinic and hospital teams and may serve as an 'ombudsman' for patients."[17] The care of the newborn is an essential aspect of the service. Dorothea Lang described the interdisciplinary and interdependency functions of the nurse-midwife:

> The Certified Nurse-Midwife assumes many of the functions of the physician as they relate to the medically uncomplicated patient. However, she does not assume the ultimate responsibility, which continues to rest with the medical staff. Neither does she assume the responsibility of the nursing care of the patient, which falls within the realm of nursing, but rather she extends and supplements some of the nursing services so that patients may benefit more fully from the existing maternity, newborn, and interconceptional care programs.[18]

Referrals play an important role in the functions of the nurse-midwife, who refers her patient for continuity of care to a public health nurse, nutritionist, social worker or dentist, if needed, and to an affiliating hospital if specialized services are required.

Changes have been noted in the 1970s in family structure, parenting patterns and the scope and delivery of maternity care. The involvement of the recipients of nursing services in the planning and execution of their care has been described by Sharon S. Rising.[19] The consumer-oriented nurse-midwifery service at the University of Minnesota has received a warm response from clients.

Midwifery is probably the oldest clinical specialty in nursing that has its focus on a healthy process. Its roots are deeply imbedded in biblical records as well as oral

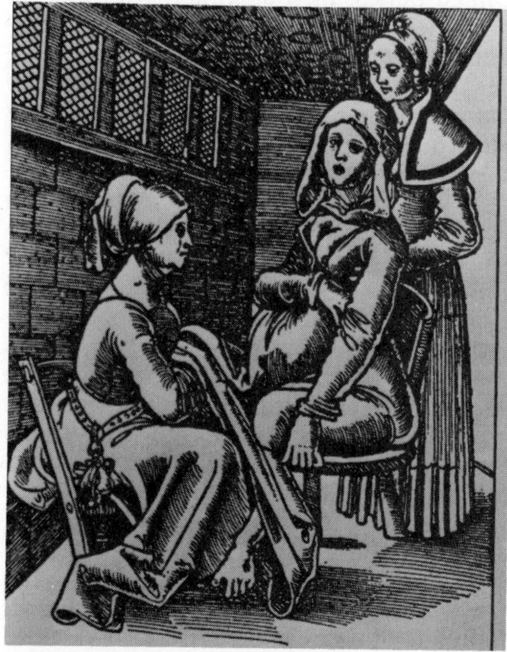

Figure 16–18. A medieval woodcut of a midwife delivering a woman seated on an obstetrical stool. (Dolan collection.)

[15]Schutt, Barbara G.: "Frontier's Family Nurses," *American Journal of Nursing,* 72:903–909, 1972.

[16]Lang, Dorothea: "Providing Maternity Care Through a Nurse Midwifery Service Program," *The Nursing Clinics of North America,* Philadelphia, W. B. Saunders Co., 4:509–520, 1969.

[17]*Ibid.*, p. 516.

[18]*Ibid.*, p. 512.

[19]Rising, Sharon Schindler: "A Consumer-Oriented Nurse-Midwivery Service," *Nursing Clinics of North America,* 10:251–262, 1975.

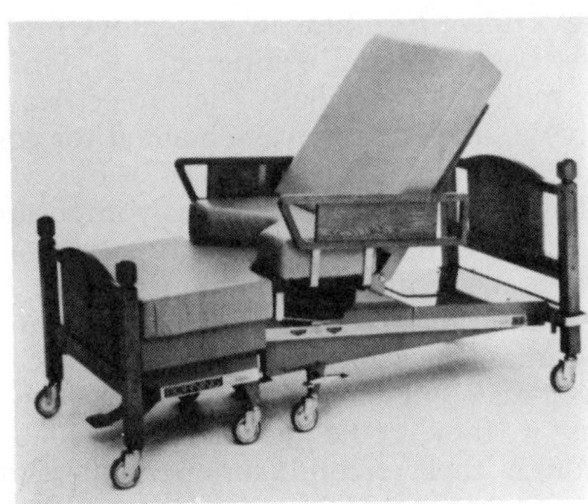

Figure 16–19. Modern childbearing bed adjusts to make either a birthing chair or a delivery table for management of complications. The bed eliminates patient transfers because it is used during labor, delivery, recovery and the post-natal stay. (Compare this 1980 bed with the adjustable 1880 bed on page 209.) (Courtesy of Yale-New Haven Hospital.)

tradition and writings of ancient cultures. One of the reemerging aspects of natural childbirth has been the reintroduction of the sitting position of delivery on "obstetrical chairs" (Figs. 16–18 and 16–19). Today, nurse-midwives are playing an ever significant role in family-centered health care. In some states, third-party insurance reimbursement for midwifery services has been obtained. In addition, birthing centers, such as the service developed by Ruth Lubic at the Maternity Center Association in New York City, are being established in hospitals and free-standing maternity centers. Concern for women's health has stimulated a growing number of nurses to specialize in this area of practice. Certification is obtained from the *American College of Nurse Midwives*.

NURSING CARE OF CHILDREN

In 1865, an unusual charity known as *St. John's Guild* was founded by Reverend Alvak Wiswall. It carried out an extensive program among the poor in the crowded areas of New York City. The plans included a volunteer visitor for every block of tenement houses so that in times of great destitution or sickness every family could be visited and cared for. In 1874, the guild established a floating hospital (Fig. 16–20) so that mothers could take their sick children from their "dens" to the cool breezes of the river to breathe fresh air. The members of the guild could not refuse the pleas of elderly people to be given this healthful opportunity.

Another interesting and important nursing contribution to child care took place when the *Boston Floating Hospital* (Fig. 16–21) began in 1894. The hospital started its tour of duty as a rented excursion boat which was towed around Boston Harbor, to give indigent mothers and their sick babies relief from the summer heat. From its inception it provided substantial education of infant feeding and disease in children,

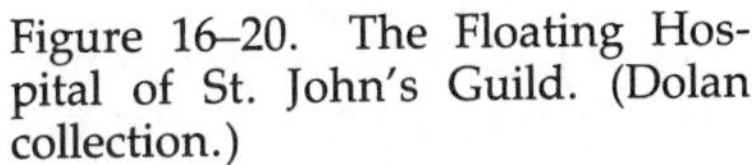

Figure 16–20. The Floating Hospital of St. John's Guild. (Dolan collection.)

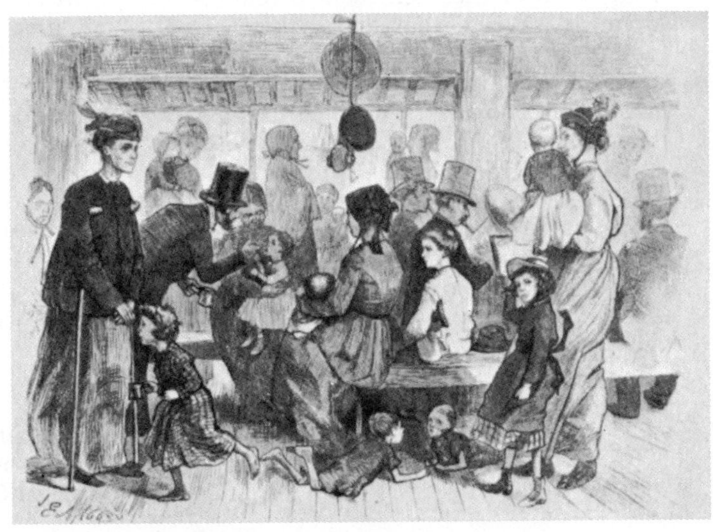

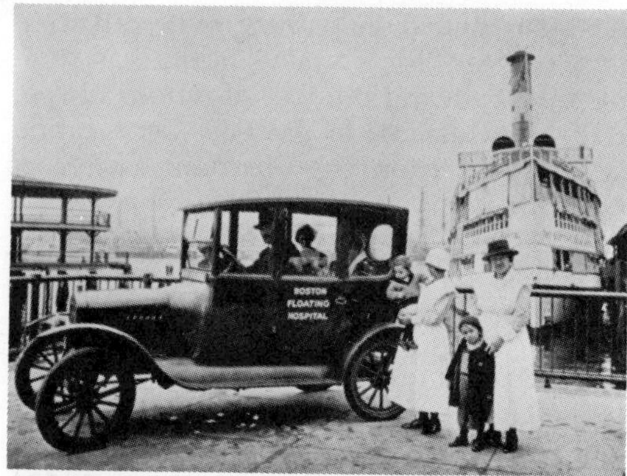

Figure 16–21. Returning children to their homes from a day's health care on the Boston Floating Hospital. (Dolan collection.)

especially infectious summer diarrhea and dysentery.

The story of the Boston Floating Hospital is interesting. In the 1890s when humanitarianism was reflected in the organization of philanthropic enterprises, certain writers had served as catalysts for the development of such enterprises. *Edward Everett Hale* (1822–1909), for example, in two of his books, *Ten Times One Is Ten* and *In His Name,* stimulated the formation of several groups dedicated to helping the destitute, the sick, the aged and the malnourished. It is reported that on a hot summer night in 1893, the Reverend Rufus Toby, a close friend of Mr. Hale, was returning home from an exhausting day in Boston. He noted the large numbers of mothers who were carrying infants across the South Boston Bridge trying to escape the heat and congestion of their tenement dwellings. It occurred to him that an excursion boat might provide this escape. Money was obtained for five trips through the efforts of many influential persons such as Edward Everett Hale.[20]

The first trip took place on July 25, 1894, when the rented barge *Clifford* was towed away from Pickett's Wharf in East Boston. In order to obtain passage aboard this boat, a mother had to acquire an admission ticket from a physician for herself and her sick child. The *Clifford,* which was used ordinarily for Sunday excursions and moonlight cruises, underwent a transformation: The cruise furniture was removed and cots, bassinets and equipment for sterilizing milk were installed. The project was a success, and money was obtained for continued service.

This project was tremendously important in coping with the care and treatment of infants with infectious summer diarrhea, frequently referred to as cholera infantum. The infant mortality rate from this disease was exceedingly high. Parents believed that if they could keep children alive through their second summer, the children's chances of survival increased remarkably.

The need for a staff of physicians and nurses to diagnose and treat the various pediatric disorders was of paramount importance. In 1897, the Boston Floating Hospital became incorporated and very sick infants began to be kept on board as in-patients. With this action, the hospital provided care for sick infants, a learning experience for students of nursing and medicine and an opportunity for research in the problems of the sick child.

In 1900, among the assigned duties of the nurses of the Boston Floating Hospital was to provide instruction for mothers on care of well children, including preparation of formulas, in addition to care and treatment of sick ones. *The nurses of this hospital participated in many research projects.* The first recorded research involved the observation and treatment of diarrhea. It attracted the notice of Dr. Simon Flexner of the University of Pennsylvania, who came on board to observe this research.

In 1921, a law was passed in Boston that required pasteurization of milk, and a downward trend was noted in the incidence of summer diarrhea. This development focused attention on infant nutrition. Human milk banks were instituted, and research commenced on the chemistry of milk and suitability of formulas.

One morning in June 1927, after the Boston Floating Hospital had been refurbished for another season, a fire destroyed the entire structure, including records. This institution had served a vital need at a time of urgency, so it was decided to build a permanent children's hospital, which joined with Tufts Medical School and the Boston Dispensary to become the New England Medical Center.

---

[20]Beaven, Paul: "A History of the Boston Floating Hospital," *Pediatrics,* Vol. 19, No. 4, 1957.

Only in the last 100 years have we had children's hospitals and separate departments for the care of children in general hospitals (Fig. 16–22). Many a child with a childhood affliction was cared for at home. Emphasis was on the disease rather than the child.

In 1908, *Sister Amy* (Fig. 16–23) of the Sisters of St. Margaret presented a program of specialization in nursing care for sick children at the Fourteenth Annual Meeting of the American Society of Superintendents of Training Schools. In carrying out the program, a study of the normal growth and development of the child was proffered.

In reviewing the development of nursing in child care, Blake stated:

> Recognition of the need for special instruction of nurses in the care of children roughly parallels the development of separate units for the care of children which appeared first in foundling homes, then in the children's hospitals and finally in the pediatric units within general hospitals. Associated with some of the earliest children's hospitals—those in Philadelphia, Denver, Boston and New York—schools were established which were devoted to the training of nurses in the care of sick children. But it was not until departments of pediatrics were firmly established in medical schools that pediatrics became a compulsory part of the undergraduate nursing school curriculum. University graduate study of pediatric nursing did not appear until the fourth decade of this century. Supplementary courses for registered nurses were given in many children's hospitals, but the development of university programs of study leading to specialization in the field are of comparatively recent origin.[21]

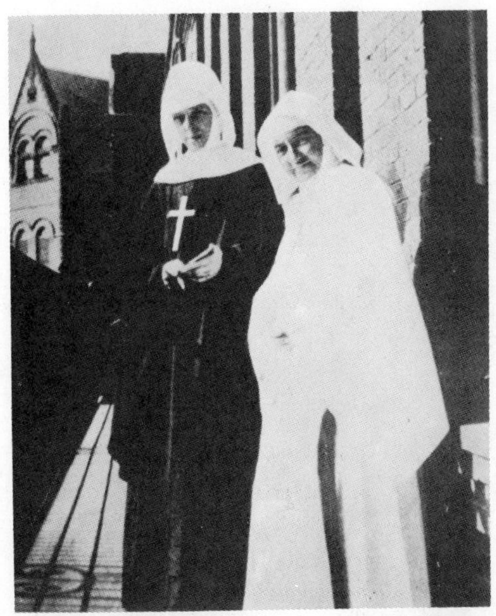

Figure 16–23. Sister Amy and Sister Lucilla of the Episcopal Sisters of St. Margaret, who first directed and staffed the Children's Hospital in Boston. (Dolan collection.)

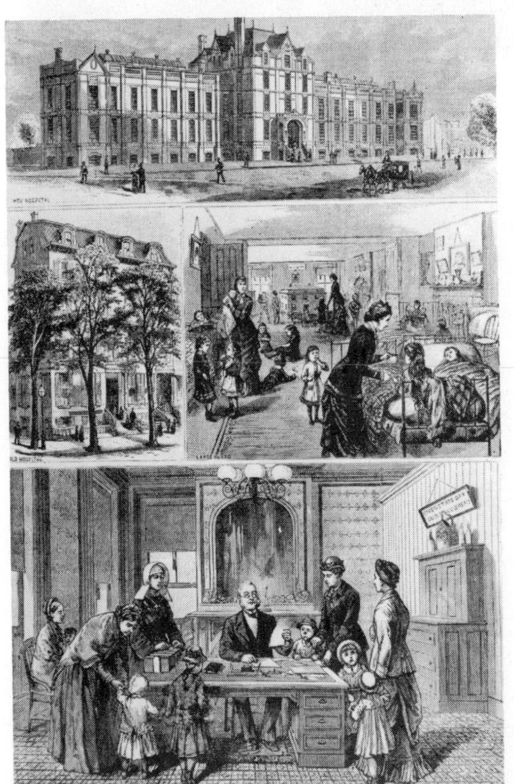

Figure 16–22. Beginnings of Children's Hospital in Boston as seen in 1881: *(top to bottom)* the Huntington Avenue Hospital; the Rutland Street Hospital; a ward in the Rutland Street Hospital; the outpatient department on Washington Street. (Courtesy of Children's Hospital, Boston.)

The well-prepared nurse in a child care setting joins with many other specialists, such as child psychologists, psychiatrists and nutritionists, in providing health care and identifying new knowledge. The nurse not only gives nursing care but acts as a "liaison between children, doctors, parents and other professional and ancillary workers who are involved in the provision of care"[22] (Fig. 16–24).

[21]Blake, Florence G., and Wright, F. Howell: *Essentials of Pediatric Nursing*. 7th ed. Philadelphia, J. B. Lippincott, 1963, p. 2.

[22]*Ibid.*, p. 3.

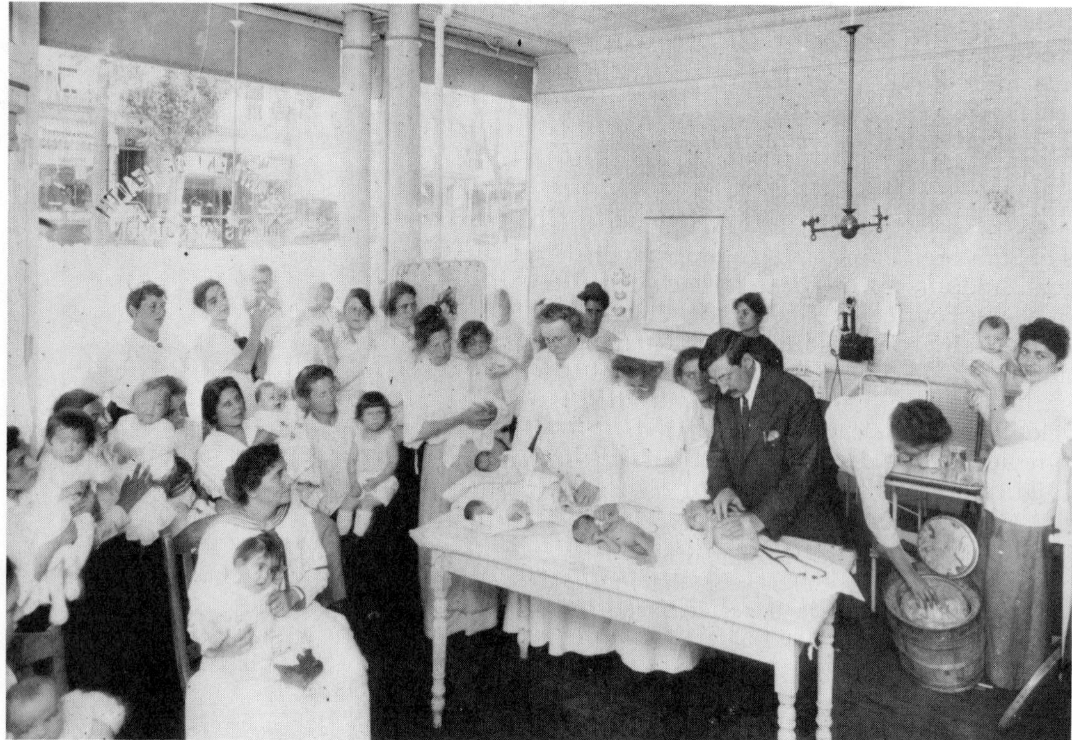

Figure 16–24. A storefront clinic at the turn of the century where two nurses and a physician conduct physical assessments. (Dolan collection.)

At the beginning of the twentieth century, the causes of many diseases, most of them communicable, were unknown. Illnesses were prolonged and serious, were a medical challenge, and often necessitated skilled nursing care at home. Parents fought against members of their families' being sent to general hospitals or isolation hospitals for care (Figs. 16–26 and 16–27). The frightening aspects of the isolation procedures coupled with limited visiting hours and the general discouragement of mem bers of the family visiting the ill member produced serious emotional stress. In a period when antibiotics were nonexistent, the time-consuming aspects of isolation techniques minimized the consideration of the child's need for emotional support from his family and the need of companionship and toys.

The discovery of antibiotics, the advances in medical knowledge, including those in nutrition and psychology, plus a marked change in all aspects of health care delivery and hospitalization have produced demands for a new role for nursing practice. At the present time, many programs

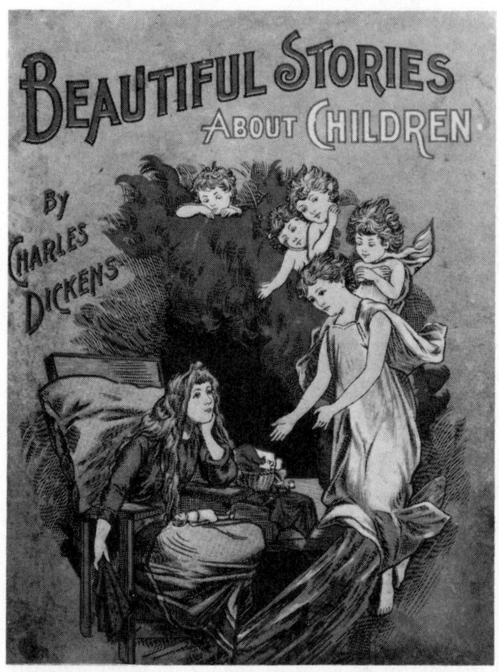

Figure 16–25. A cover from a book of stories by Charles Dickens. The book offered emotional support for children with long-term illnesses and prepared them for a life after death. (Dolan collection.)

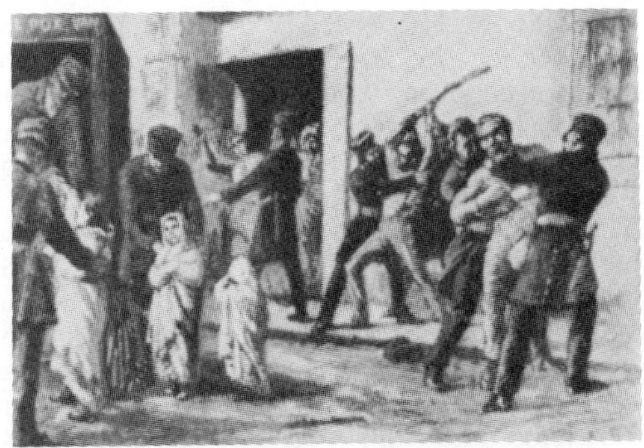

Figure 16–26. During an outbreak of smallpox in Montreal in 1885, fathers fought police officers while children were herded into a van that took them to a pest house. (Dolan collection.)

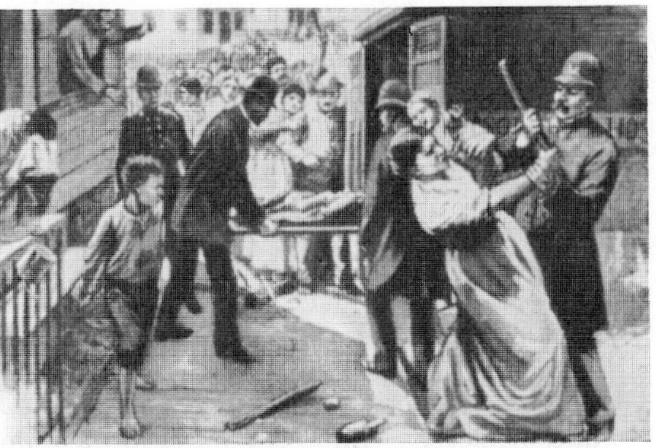

Figure 16–27. Families resisting police in Milwaukee in 1886 during a typhoid epidemic. Patients were brought to the isolation hospital. (Dolan collection.)

and resources are available to assist in the provision of child care (Fig. 16–28). Even the hospital setting has returned to a family-centered form of care but with the enriched dimension of the application of behavioral, biological and health science principles. Provision for permitting mothers or members of the family to "room-in" has been available for some time. In addition there has been a trend toward the lengthening of visiting hours.

In a "Symposium on Family-Centered Care in a Pediatric Setting,"[23] the benefits of the delivery of care in a milieu which is geared to a more healthful life for the child and his family are presented as are the role of the nurse and the components of nursing in such a family-centered setting. Coping with the problem of death and dying for a child and the family; assisting the adolescent's quest for self-identity in family-centered care; and finding ways of introducing programs for staff development to encourage implementation of family-centered nursing care between the hospital and home are important in providing the most satisfying and therapeutically sound child care.

Yet not all children receive this kind of

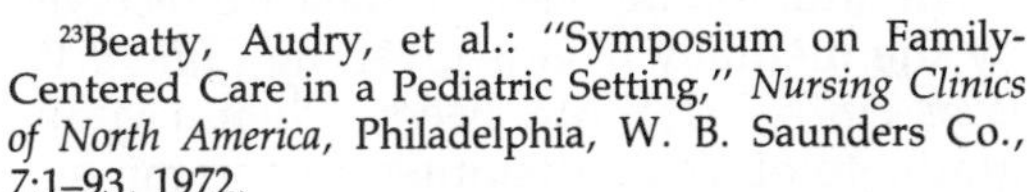

[23]Beatty, Audry, et al.: "Symposium on Family-Centered Care in a Pediatric Setting," *Nursing Clinics of North America*, Philadelphia, W. B. Saunders Co., 7:1–93, 1972.

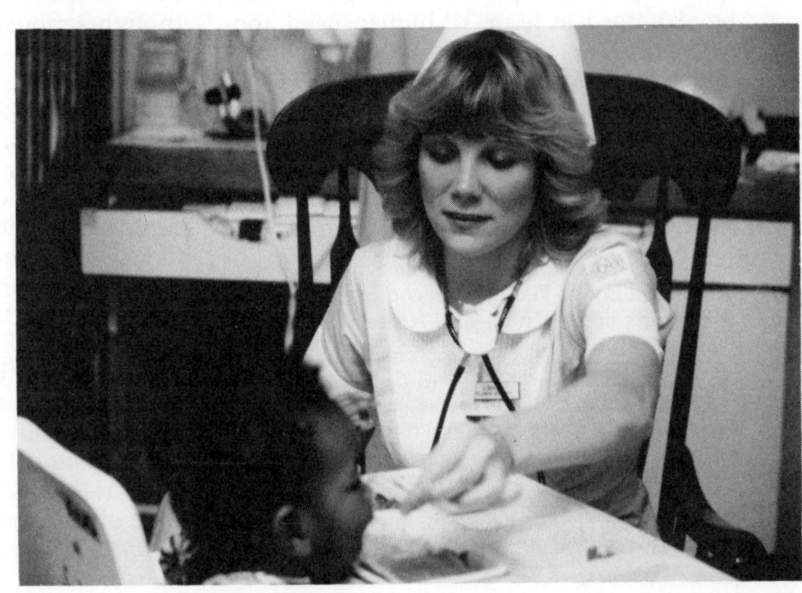

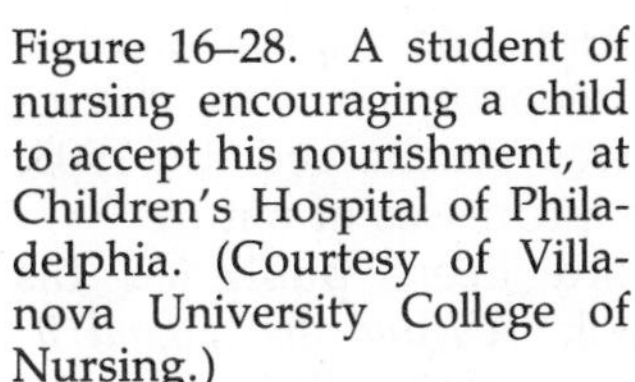

Figure 16–28. A student of nursing encouraging a child to accept his nourishment, at Children's Hospital of Philadelphia. (Courtesy of Villanova University College of Nursing.)

satisfaction because they do not receive the benefits of a program in good health care. A tragic plight that afflicts many children is the "battered child" syndrome. In 1961, Lester Anderson wrote his famous work "Slaughter of the Innocents," which described vividly the brutal treatment of some children.

Joan Hopkins has urged the nursing profession to "assume its role in the tremendous responsibility of case-finding, prevention and treatment of the abused and neglected child. No other profession has the opportunity to spend as much meaningful time with these patients and their families as does the nurse."[24] The members of the health professions are protected by law in many states from liability for reporting suspected cases of child abuse and neglect, and nurses are being called upon to testify. On a more positive note, nurses have been conducting classes that focus on the concept of "mothering the mother so she can mother the child."

Many infants and children need and receive very special and complicated health care. Many of the clinical settings, technical procedures and nursing skills were presented in a "Symposium on Care of the Infant and Young Child."[25]

In an article entitled "The Pediatric Nurse Practitioner," by Andrews and Yankaver, appearing in the March, 1971, issue of the *American Journal of Nursing*, the role of the pediatric nurse practitioner was discussed. The writers stated that "the effects of current shortages in pediatric manpower can be expressed in terms of human need and suffering. The pediatric nurse practitioner appears to offer an acceptable, practical, and workable contribution toward alleviating the manpower shortage."

A joint statement was issued by the ANA and the American Academy of Pediatrics:

> The American Nurses' Association and American Academy of Pediatrics recognize collaborative efforts are essential to increase the quality, availability and accessibility of child health care in the U.S.A. In order to meet the health care needs of children, it is essential that the skills inherent in the nursing and medical professions be utilized more efficiently in the delivery of child health care.
>
> Innovative methods are needed to utilize these professional skills more fully. One such innovative approach is the development of the Pediatric Nurse Associate program. This program will enable nurses, both in practice and reentering practice, to update and expand their knowledge and skills. It is essential that physicians become more aware of the skills and abilities of the nursing profession and that such skills be expanded in the area of ambulatory child health to enable both the nurse and the physician to devote their efforts in the delivery of child health care to the areas of their respective professional expertise.

ROLE OF THE PSYCHIATRIC–MENTAL HEALTH NURSE

The changes that took place in the role of the nurse, the inception of hospitals devoted exclusively to the care of the mentally ill, and the beginnings of the disciplines of psychiatry and psychology as fields of endeavor all played significant roles in the development of psychiatric and mental health nursing.

An illuminating view of the care received by the mentally ill was given by *Clifford W. Beers* (1876–1945). Mr. Beers, when a young graduate of Yale, attempted to commit suicide by jumping from the fourth story window of his home. He was rescued, and though seriously injured, he was alive. He was incarcerated for three years in various institutions for the mentally ill. His treatment vacillated between indifference and cruelty. At one period, he was kept in a straitjacket for 21 consecutive days and nights. He became firmly determined to devote his energies to the improvement of the care of the mentally ill. His chance came after he was discharged in 1903, cured only by the processes of nature.

In 1908, Clifford Beers published his epoch-making book, *A Mind that Found Itself*. This book was a frank, disarming picture of his illness, the way he was treated and the unbelievable sufferings to which he was subjected. In 1908 in his native state of Connecticut he founded a *Society of Mental Hygiene*, whose purposes were "to

---

[24]Hopkins, Joan: "The Nurse and the Abused Child," *Nursing Clinics of North America*, Philadelphia, W. B. Saunders Co., 5:597, 1970.

[25]Rothrock, E. Cleves, et al.: "Symposium on Care of the Infant and Young Child," *Nursing Clinics of North America*, Philadelphia, W. B. Saunders Co., 5:373–448, 1970.

work for the conservation of mental health, to help prevent nervous and mental disorders and mental defects and to help raise the standards of care for those suffering from any of these disorders." In 1909, through Beers' efforts, a *National Committee of Mental Hygiene* was established with essentially the same purposes. In 1930 in Washington, D.C., the representatives of 53 nations joined in establishing the *International Committee for Mental Hygiene.* Clifford Beers and his accomplishments exemplify how a client who is dissatisfied with the delivery of care can propose and obtain a much more enriched form of care.

The prevention, early detection and acceptance of prompt psychiatric care has now been advocated. The public has developed a greater acceptance of mental illness as an illness of the body rather than as a mysterious affliction of which one should be ashamed.

When Nicholas Brown died in 1841, he left a bequest of $30,000 for a retreat for the insane; thus, in 1844, the Rhode Island legislature issued a charter for the building of a "Rhode Island Asylum for the Insane," also called Butler Hospital. This hospital became one of the foremost institutions of its kind in the United States; it continued to treat the mentally ill until its closing in 1955. Because of public pressure, a new board of directors and a successful financial campaign, the institution was reopened in 1957 as the Butler Health Center, serving various health and welfare agencies. In its modern approach to the problems of the mentally ill, Butler Health Center is still carrying on the great tradition it established almost a century and a half ago.

In recent times psychiatric hospitals have been replaced in many areas by community mental health centers. A better understanding of emotional problems, psychiatric disorders, medications and treatments by better-prepared psychiatrists, clinical psychologists and professional nurses has contributed to the progress made in this area of health care.

In the early part of the century the position of the nurse treating mental illness was not very high because many nurses had a very meager background in basic principles of psychology and psychiatry and their tasks became merely custodial. This emphasis on custodial care reflected the philosophy and policies of the institutions for the mentally ill. Physical restraints produced an intolerable condition for both patients and attendants. The resulting increased agitation, injury to skin surfaces and inability to eat produced pathetically unhappy patients. Methods of forced feedings increased the discomfort, and the resultant "cerebral congestion" was supposedly relieved by cold wet therapy followed by the administration of sedatives.

The first school to give nurses psychiatric preparation was established at McLean Hospital in Waverly, Massachusetts, in 1882. Gradually there was a growing appreciation of the therapeutic role of the psychiatric nurse. Santos related:

> Paralleling the growth of psychiatric thought, psychiatric nursing by 1900 had become an organized discipline with its own body of knowledge and techniques, and with its emphasis on the nursing of the whole person. Nevertheless, it was suffused with the static custodial concepts of the psychiatric treatment of the time that it served.[26]

An important contribution to the history of the evolution of the nurse has been published under the leadership of Esta Carini, Ph.D., former chief of nurses of the Department of Mental Health of the State of Connecticut.[27] The book describes the changing scene for both the patients and nursing personnel in three state hospitals in one state. It reflects the nurse's evolution from custodian to psychiatric aide; from apprentice nurse to student of nursing; and from keeper to psychiatric nurse. An increasing awareness of the extent of mental illness as a national health problem focussed attention on the magnitude of the emotional needs of all people and the obligation of all health workers to understand human behavior. The National Mental Health Act of 1946 provided funds for the improvement of mental health and upgrading of the treatment of the mentally ill

[26]Santos, Elvin, and Stainbrook, Edward: "A History of Psychiatric Nursing in the Nineteenth Century," *Journal of the History of Medicine and Allied Sciences*, Winter 1949, p. 59.

[27]Carini, Esta, Douglas, Dorothy, Heck, Lois, and Pearson, Marguerite: *The Mentally Ill in Connecticut: Changing Patterns of Care and the Evolution of Psychiatric Nursing—1636–1972*. Hartford, State of Connecticut, 1974.

through research and the education of professional personnel. Schmahl wrote:

> After years of struggling to retain the integrity of nursing . . . nursing leaders suddenly found support for their efforts from a new development in the medical field—the recognition of the contributions that psychiatry could make to the care of all patients.[28]

The integration of psychiatry with medical treatment enhanced the role of the psychiatric nurse. Nursing contributions were also recognized as a result of the increased use of somatic treatments, such as insulin shock, electroshock, sleep therapy and psychosurgery.

The psychiatric nurse has become a member of a professional team in a therapeutic community. Her therapeutic role has been described as to "support and encourage the patient in his participation in the total treatment by acting as a clarifier and interpreter when the patient encounters difficulty, [to] collaborate with the physician in therapy, and most importantly, to serve as the transmitter of the therapeutic culture to the patient."[29]

Nurse educators began to encourage all students of nursing to receive preparation in this field because patients of all ages in homes and in general hospitals as well as in psychiatric institutions needed psychiatrically oriented nursing care. Attempts were made, with financial support from the government, to integrate psychiatric principles into the curriculum of professional schools of nursing. Many collegiate schools responded to this challenge, and a five-year study was made at the Skidmore College Department of Nursing "to investigate and demonstrate the ways in which the various resources at the department's command could be utilized to foster the student's awareness of psychiatric concepts and techniques and to help her apply them in the nursing care of all patients." The report of this study by Jane Schmahl was entitled *Experiment in Change; An Interdisciplinary Approach to the Integration of Psychiatric Content in Baccalaureate Nursing Education.*

The psychiatric nurse aims to create an environment in which the patient can develop new behavior patterns and work out his own problems. Mental illness is overcome by a growth process, so experiences promoting the growth process are encouraged, and interpersonal relationships provide the learning experiences necessary for growth.[30]

In 1963, federal legislation authorized funding for community mental health centers. Provision for *preventive* services was an essential part of this legislation.

The nurse with psychiatric–mental health preparation functions in more than psychiatric and general hospitals. This specialist works in halfway houses, community health clinics and community mental health centers and encourages community involvement in these programs. The skills of such a person are used to help combat particular mental health problems such as drug addiction, suicide, child abuse, juvenile delinquency, alcoholism and many other emotional disturbances.

Many modalities of treatment have been used in patient care, among them recreational therapy, art therapy, music therapy, occupational and recreational therapy and dance therapy. Marion Chace at St. Elizabeth's Hospital in Washington was one of the first dance therapists to report her use of the dance as therapy, including its use in nonverbal communication.

The task of demonstrating competence as a psychotherapist "on the same level and with the same type of patient" as her co-workers—psychiatric social case workers, clinical psychologists and psychiatrists—still confronts the psychiatric nurse.[31] The nurse who is responsive to community and individual mental health needs must become involved in social change.

NURSING IN OCCUPATIONAL HEALTH

It is difficult to trace the actual beginnings of the field of *industrial nursing* be-

[28]Schmahl, Janet: *Experiment in Change; An Interdisciplinary Approach to the Integration of Psychiatric Content in Baccalaureate Nursing Education*. New York, The Macmillan Co., 1966, p. 12.

[29]Kalkman, Marion, and Davis, Anne: *New Dimensions in Mental Health—Psychiatric Nursing*. New York, McGraw-Hill Book Co., 1974.

[30]Gregg, Dorothy: "The Psychiatric Nurse's Role." In *Psychiatric Nursing*. Dubuque, Iowa, William C. Brown Co., 1966, p. 178.

[31]Stokes, Gertrude: "Extending the Role of the Psychiatric-Mental Health Nurse in Community Mental Health," *The Nursing Clinics of North America*, Philadelphia, W. B. Saunders Co., 5:639, 1970.

cause many individual firms had for years employed a single nurse. A few employers established hospitals for injured employees. The Manufacturing Company of Lowell, Massachusetts, had such a hospital in 1859. The next hospital was probably a log cabin in Lead, South Dakota, which was built in 1877 for people with mining injuries. In 1881, the Colorado Fuel and Iron Company of Pueblo established an industrial hospital, which was staffed by male nurses. Even the Union Pacific Railroad established a hospital in 1893. In 1895, the Proctor Marble Company in Vermont become the first industrial plant to employ a nurse to visit and give nursing care to sick employees. Her name was *Ada Stewart* (Mrs. Markoff). In 1897, another early project, the Employees' Benefit Association of John Wanamaker's department store in Philadelphia, was established.

The idea of "industrial nursing" has been supplanted by a broader concept—that of the nurse in the field of occupational health. The nurse in this field has been employed in factories, department stores, telephone companies and many other enterprises.

Employee health care has been largely a twentieth-century development, and until about 1920, there was little general interest in it. Even now some employers do not realize that half-sick workers do not produce as much as they could, that absence from illness cuts into profits and that it pays to care for the health of employees. Insurance companies first called attention to these facts, and when workmen's compensation laws were enacted employers began to recognize the value of health care. The National Safety Council has done much in the prevention of accidents and occupational hazards and illnesses.

In 1917, Boston University became probably the first college in the United States to give a course in industrial nursing. Simmons College established such a course in 1919 (for college graduates), discontinued it, and began it again in 1942. The University of Minnesota, Wayne University, Detroit University and Columbia University gave similar courses.

The nurse in occupational health not only needs to know basic nursing and prevention of disease but also needs to be well versed in industrial hazards, safety rules, labor laws (including legal limitations and liability), plant hygiene, community hygiene and whatever health programs are being undertaken. The nurse may be consultant to state hygiene departments in the U.S. Public Health Service.

In 1942, the *American Association of Industrial Nurses* was formed. In 1944, the ANA created a section for industrial nurses.

The leadership in occupational health nursing has been recognized. As a faculty member in the Graduate School of Public Health at Yale and later as chief of the Occupational Health Nursing Section of the U.S. Public Health Service, *Mary Louise Brown* contributed much through her guidance and her literary efforts to the development of occupational health nursing and the improvement of the role of the nurse in such a program.

Many others have given direction and leadership in this field. A contribution of significance was Marjorie Keller's four-year study that resulted in the identification of occupational health content for the professional nursing curriculum.[32] In a "Symposium on Occupational Health Nursing,"[33] key issues were identified and proposals for their solution were presented.

An important milestone occurred when the *Occupational Safety and Health Act* was signed by President Richard M. Nixon on December 29, 1970. This act, which became effective in July 1971, had implications for nurses as employees and health professionals. The purpose of this act was:

> To assure safe and healthful working conditions for working men and women; by authorizing enforcement of the standards developed under the Act; by assisting and encouraging the States in their efforts to assure safe and healthful working conditions; by providing for research, information, education and training in the field of occupational safety and health; and for other purposes.

The current need for the occupational health nurse to be a well-educated generalist with special preparation in occupational health has been stressed.

---

[32]Keller, Marjorie J., in association with May, W. T.: *Occupational Health Content in Baccalaureate Nursing Education*. Cincinnati, U.S. Department of Health, Education, and Welfare, Environmental Control Administration, 1970.

[33]Keller, Marjorie J., et al.: "Symposium on Occupational Health Nursing," *The Nursing Clinics of North America*, Philadelphia, W. B. Saunders Co., 7:95–182, 1972.

Maureen Cushing, a nurse and practicing attorney, has addressed the issue of occupational nurses' legal responsibilities when applying their physical assessment skills in the area of duty.[34]

NURSING CARE OF THE ELDERLY

Dr. Howard Rusk has said: "We have added years to life, now add life to the years." Life has been lengthened in the twentieth century, and we have greater numbers of older citizens owing to many factors, among them the control of communicable diseases, lowered infant mortality, improved child care, increased nutritional information and better-balanced diets.

The addition of the spark that can enrich and enliven the extension of life has been the responsibility of the nurse. Gerontological nursing is a relatively new field in the modern health care system; in fact, geriatrics was not established as a medical specialty until almost 1940. Yet historically and culturally, the elderly have received reverential treatment; nursing care of the elderly was developed as a special field of endeavor by St. Helena, the Dowager-Empress of the Roman Empire.

In the early part of this century the elderly who were also poor were sent to a "poorhouse" or "almshouse," where what nursing care was available was limited to the infirmary. Caroline Barlett Crane vividly described the pathetic conditions in 1907.[35] She stated, "And of all that motley assemblage of human beings who were once carelessly consigned to oblivion in the county poorhouse, presently none will be left except—the aged and infirm. . . . Homeless, friendless poor old men and women: these are—and will become more and more—the great body of our almshouse population." Crane explained that the insane were removed to asylums and the children to special hospitals based on their needs but the aged were left to deteriorate in these bleak, cheerless surroundings.

The despair and rejection felt by the elderly when they had to leave family, friends and possessions were depicted in the poignant ballad by Will Carleton, "Over the Hill to the Poorhouse." A striking similarity can be noted between the feelings of an elderly woman of the late nineteenth century and those of many older people who today face admission to convalescent homes.

It was gradually recognized that nursing of the elderly requires special skills, a sense of humor, modification of the patient's diet and provision for regular exercise in fresh air. Recreational therapy began to receive emphasis.[36]

The term geriatrics was first used in 1909 in a New York medical journal article written by Dr. Nascher, who, in 1914, wrote the first American textbook on geriatrics. The first university course in the problems of the aged was offered in 1933 by the University of Minnesota in a Human Development program. A group of physicians formed the American Geriatric Society in 1942 to promote the organized study of medical problems of older people, and in 1945, physicians, biologists and psychologists organized the American Gerontological Society to sponsor research on the problems of aging.

The first textbook devoted to understanding the nursing contribution to the care of the aged was written by Kathleen Newton.[37]

In 1970 a definition of geriatric nursing was enunciated as follows:

> Geriatric nursing is concerned with the assessment of nursing needs of older people, planning and implementing nursing care to meet these needs, and evaluating the effectiveness of such care to achieve and maintain a level of wellness consistent with the limitations imposed by the aging process.[38]

The geriatric nurse must be sensitive to the special problems of the elderly, appreciating their basic desire to be accepted as

[34]Cushing, Maureen, R.N., J.D.: "An Occupational Nurse's Liability," *American Journal of Nursing, 81*:2207, 1981.

[35]Crane, Caroline Barlett: "Almshouse Nursing: The Human Need; The Professional Opportunity," *American Journal of Nursing, 7*:874–877, 1907.

[36]Breeze, Jessie: "The Care of the Aged," *American Journal of Nursing, 9*:826–828, 1909.

[37]Newton, Kathleen: *Geriatric Nursing*. St. Louis, C. V. Mosby Co., 1950.

[38]"Standards for Geriatric Nursing Practice," *American Journal of Nursing, 70*:1894, 1970.

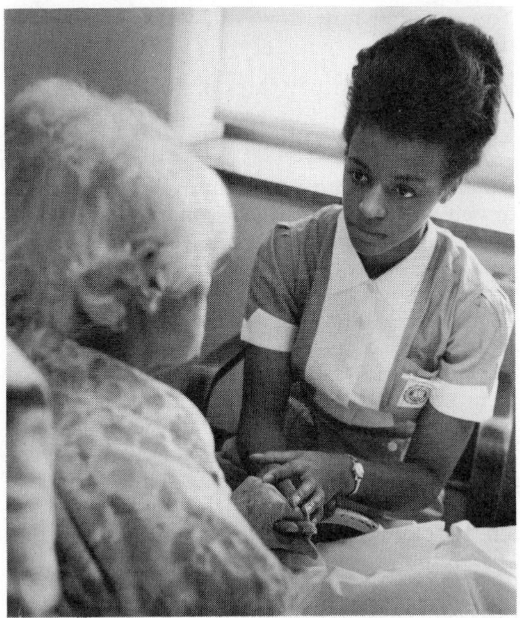

Figure 16–29. A student of nursing listens with compassion to her patient, who squeezes her hand appreciatively. (Courtesy of University of Connecticut.)

useful, contributing members of society (Fig. 16–29). In carrying out this definition, the nurse is challenged to use her skills and ability to preserve the proper functioning of the mind and body as long as possible.

In 1968, the ANA developed the first standards for the practice of geriatric nursing.

The *Andrus Foundation* of the National Retired Teachers' Association–American Association of Retired Persons (NRTA-AARP) has distributed grant monies in the hundreds of thousands of dollars to universities whose research projects in the field of aging have been approved. This group's constant encouragement provides a stimulus for support of research in gerontological nursing.

Nurses' commitment to "enriching the quality of life" prompted a meeting in Cleveland, Ohio, of nurses in gerontological practice to prepare a positive statement on gerontological nursing that would be distributed to every delegate to the 1981 White House Conference on Aging. The meeting was chaired by Chief Public Health Service Nurse Officer Faye Abdellah. The ANA's Division on Gerontological Nursing Practice, the Cleveland Clinic and the Upjohn Health Care Services were the sponsoring groups. Four fundamental needs were delineated to reinforce the nursing role: to change reimbursement policies; to prepare nurses to care for older adults; to design creative concepts of wellness and to encourage nursing research that addresses the health issues of older adults.

Another positive step was taken when the *ANA Task Force on Aging* distributed a statement entitled *Gerontological Nursing: The Positive Difference in Health Care for Older Adults* to White House staff members, technical committees and National Health and Social Service Groups involved in the conference.

The challenge for the well-prepared nurse in meeting the needs of the elderly remains one of infinite and compassionate concern.

Institutions whose philosophy of patient care coincide with these standards have achieved the comfort, satisfaction and praise of patients and families. "The nurse, in caring for the geriatric patient can be the enabler who, on the strength of her beliefs, provides the impetus for drive in the patient, the motivation for self-realization."[39]

Remotivation therapy, which encourages group interaction to help patients toward reality, was tried. After several sessions it was concluded that "a positive change in the mood tone of older patients occurred when new, younger, and concerned people took them out of their rooms and involved them in group interaction. . . . If nursing is to be more than meeting patients' physical needs, it is necessary to increase our understanding of older peoples' need for psycho-social stimulation."[40]

Many elderly people remain in their homes, and their nursing care may be provided by community nurses from visiting nurses associations (Fig. 16–30). Beyond giving actual nursing care, the nurse can act as a resource person: She can assist in obtaining additional funds and in finding suitable housing for her patients; in persuading the elderly to join Senior Citizen or Golden Age groups; in encouraging obtaining the spiritual advisor who is needed;

[39]Dupuis, P. H.: "Old is Beautiful," *Nursing Outlook, 18*:26, 1970.

[40]Moody, L., et al.: "Moving the Past into the Present," *American Journal of Nursing, 70*:2356, 1970.

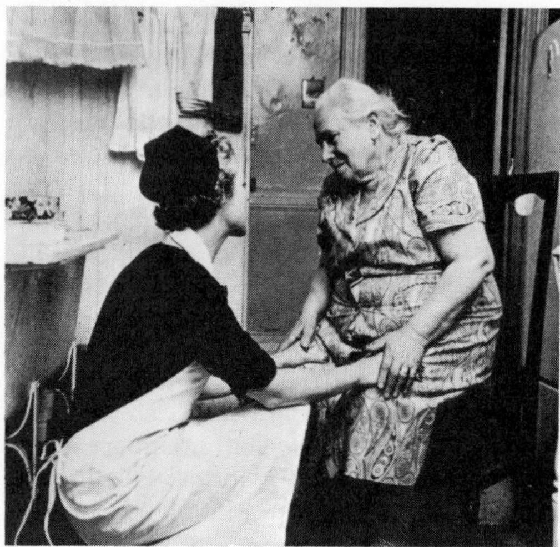

Figure 16–30. A community health nurse listens attentively to her patient's tale of distress. (Dolan collection.)

in contracting with the Meals-on-Wheels project, and in many other ways.

The elderly remain one of the most underprivileged groups in our society, particularly those in some extended care facilities that are reminiscent of the facilities described previously by Crane in 1907.

In expanding the area of specialty for the delivery of care to the elderly, the broader term "gerontological nursing" is now used. The current Standards for Nursing Practice reflect a concern with caring for both well and ill elderly persons. Certification in the area of gerontological nursing practice has become a reality.

NURSING CARE OF THE DYING

Throughout the ages people have needed a special kind of assistance when they faced death. Henry Fielding in *Amelia* observed: "It hath often been said . . . that it is not death, but dying that is terrible."

Florence Nightingale pleaded for nurses to use special skills in meeting the needs of dying persons when she wrote:

> But the long chronic case, who knows too well himself, and who has been told by his physician that he will never enter active life again, who feels that every month he has to give up something he could do the month before . . . oh, spare such sufferers your chattering hopes. You do not know how you worry and weary them.

Almost a century later a student of nursing who was dying wrote a poignant plea to nurses when she said:

> I am a student nurse. I am dying. I write this to you who are, and will become, nurses in the hope that by my sharing my feelings with you, you may someday be better able to help those who share my experience.
>
> I'm out of the hospital now—perhaps for a month, for six months, perhaps for a year . . . but no one likes to talk about such things. In fact, no one likes to talk about much at all. Nursing must be advancing, but I wish it would hurry. We're taught not to be overly cheery now, to omit the "Everything's fine" routine, and we have done pretty well. But now one is left in a lonely silent void. With the protective "Fine, fine" gone, the staff is left with only their own vulnerability and fear. The dying patient is not yet seen as a person and thus cannot be communicated with as such. He is a symbol of what every human fears and what we each know, at least academically, that we too must someday face. What did they say in psychiatric nursing about meeting pathology with pathology to the detriment of both patient and nurse? And there was a lot about knowing one's own feelings before you could help another with his. How true.
>
> But for me, fear is today and dying is now. You slip in and out of my room, give me medications and check my blood pressure. Is it because I am a student nurse, myself, or just a human being, that I sense your fright? And your fear enhances mine. Why are you afraid? I am the one who is dying!
>
> I know, you feel insecure, don't know what to say, don't know what to do. But please believe me, if you care, you can't go wrong. Just admit that you care. That is really for what we search. We may ask for whys and wherefores, but we don't really expect answers. Don't run away . . . wait . . . all I want to know is that there will be someone to hold my hand when I need it. I am afraid. Death may get to be a routine to you, but it is new to me. You may not see me as unique, but I've never died before. To me, once is pretty unique!
>
> You whisper about my youth, but when one is dying, is he really so young anymore? I have lots I wish we could talk about. It really would not take much more of your time because you are in here quite a bit anyway.
>
> If only we could be honest, both admit our fears, touch one another. If you really care, would you lose so much of your valuable professionalism if you even cried with me? Just

person to person? Then, it might not be so hard to die . . . in a hospital . . . with friends close by.[41]

Rose Hawthorne Lathrop (1851–1926), the brilliant and beautiful daughter of Nathaniel Hawthorne, has been credited with carrying on a most successful campaign in the interests of patients suffering with cancer. In the early 1890s, she visited her seamstress, who was dying of cancer on New York's Welfare Island. She was appalled by the poor care the victims of cancer received, at their anguish, which was not relieved by any kind of emotional support, and at the absence of human love throughout their days of illness and especially at their time of death. It became apparent that patients afflicted with incurable cancer were not wanted in hospitals and, in many instances, were not permitted to remain in their own homes.

Rose Hawthorne Lathrop determined to be of assistance to the poor victims of this serious malady, which was not then understood. She received three months' training in simple nursing techniques and in the care of cancer victims. Her next step was to rent a tenement in the slum sections where she could be closer to those patients who needed her.

In 1898, an artist friend of Rose's named *Alice Huber* joined her in her work. Large quarters were needed to provide accommodations to make it easier to give nursing care when it was needed. They purchased a three-story brick building at 426 Cherry Street in New York City and over the door they placed the words: "St. Rose's Free Home for Incurable Cancer," and the quotation: "I was sick and ye visited Me." Both Rose and Alice had become members of the Third Order of St. Dominic.

Gradually, the demand for more nurses became evident, and Rose Hawthorne Lathrop became the foundress of the order of sisters called *Servants of Relief for Incurable Cancer,* now called Hawthorne Dominicans. The membership of her religious family grew, as did the hospitals that they built and the quality of care rendered to many more patients. Of her work Rose once wrote:

> I am trying to serve the poor as a servant. I wish to serve the cancerous poor because they are avoided more than any other class of sufferers; and I wish to go to them as a poor creature myself, though able to help them through gifts from friends and relatives and public kindness. It is by humility and sacrifice alone that we feel the holy spirit of pity.

In *St. Christopher's Hospice* in Sydenham near London, a woman directs a most remarkable program. Dame Cicely Saunders, M.D., (Fig. 16–31), nurse, medical social worker and now a physician, is the moti-

[41]"Death in the First Person," *American Journal of Nursing,* Vol. 70, 1970.

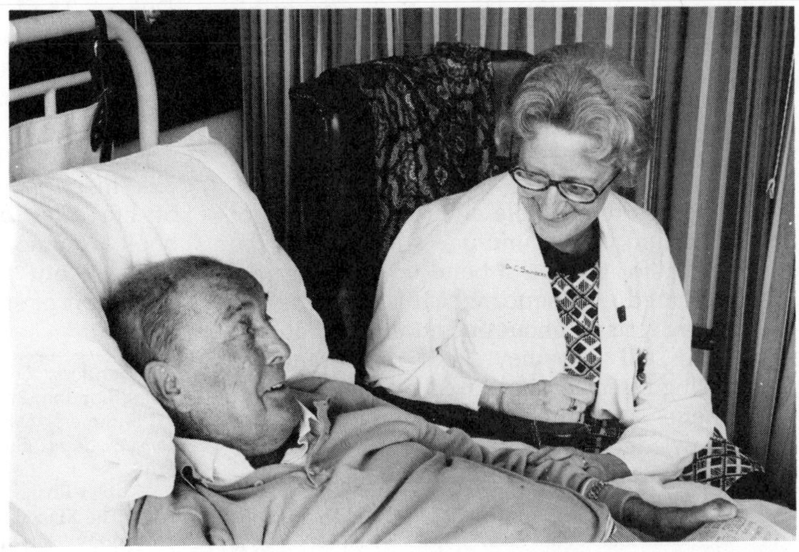

Figure 16–31. Dame Cicely Saunders, D.B.E., F.R.C.P., Medical Director, St. Christopher's Hospice. (Photograph by Derek Bayes.) (Dolan collection.)

vating force behind the project as well as its director.[42]

Dr. Saunders received preparation for nursing at the Nightingale School, St. Thomas' Hospital, during World War II and received an honors certificate. She then earned a degree in philosophy, politics and economics at Oxford and a diploma in public administration. She assumed a position as hospital almoner at St. Thomas', where she became vitally interested in patients with terminal illness. She then "read medicine at St. Thomas', becoming a physician." A three-year fellowship in the Department of Pharmacology at St. Mary's Medical School permitted her to carry out research on analgesics and other drugs used in the treatment of patients with terminal illness.

It was Dr. Saunders' dream that a milieu could be created in which a person who was dying could be cared for in a very special way. Dr. Saunders planned such a project, and her hope and dreams were described in a March 1965 *American Journal of Nursing* article, "The Last Stages of Life." Her dreams were brought to fruition and serve as a model for what can be achieved when people really believe in an ideal.

An extension of St. Christopher's Hospice is the outpatient plan to assist a patient to attain his desire of dying at home among family if possible. During this period, service is provided to the patient and his family, and readmission to the Hospice is readily accomplished whenever it is needed. A relative knows that even in his own home he isn't carrying the fear and worry alone, for the staff continues their concerned care to those within the Hospice or those within their own homes, giving total care—social, psychological and spiritual.

In this remarkable enterprise, a sense of community and mutual support can be seen, "for there is a bond in suffering and in shared experience which is expressed in caring for and about one another." Patients have said that they "find reassurance in feeling cared for and loved by the staff. . . . There is comfort and strength in the knowledge that whatever your weakness or uncertainty of faith, those about you believe in the meaningfulness of life and in the essential value of each person."

The rejuvenation of the *hospice movement* has been a boon to society. In this century we have progressed from "homes for incurables" with all they denote to hospices where expertise in terminal care is practiced.

Dr. Saunders has shared very generously her philosophy and experiences in the hope that greater numbers of terminally ill patients will receive better care.[43] Her staff exemplify her philosophy of care in their nursing practice. A manual supplied by the hospice reflects their views:

> It is not easy to convey the tremendous challenge and sense of achievement in working with people who are soon to die except by being exposed to and involved in the situation, but the role of the nurse is clear and unique.
>
> She has to refute the saying 'What cannot be cured must be endured' and is in a very privileged position in the caring team all of whom will be there as a 15th century folk saying has suggested, 'to cure sometimes' and 'to relieve often,' for she will be there 'to comfort always.' "[44]

Florence Wald, former dean of the School of Nursing at Yale University, directed "A Nurse's Study of the Care for Dying Patients," a project that has resulted in the establishment of a hospice in Connecticut similar to St. Christopher's.

A psychiatrist, Elisabeth Kubler-Ross, has written a thought-provoking and informative book entitled *On Death and Dying*.[45] The book focusses on the meaning of death to those who are dying and the five stages that a dying patient experiences before death occurs. It has been viewed as a discourse on the art of human dialogue.

A bestseller that provides documented case histories reveals that there is evidence of life after death.[46] The author of this book, Raymond Moody, M.D., has been carrying out an investigation of the phenomenon of survival after bodily death. Its

[42]"Christmas at St. Christopher's," *American Journal of Nursing*, *71*:2325–2330, 1971.

[43]Saunders, Cecily: "Care of the Dying," *Nursing Times*, London, 2nd Ed., 1976 (Special supplement).

[44]Summers, Dorothy H., and Young, Joan M.: *To Comfort Always*. Sydenham, St. Christopher's Hospice, p. 18.

[45]Kubler-Ross, Elisabeth: *On Death and Dying*. New York, The Macmillan Co., 1969.

[46]Moody, Raymond A.: *Life After Life*. Georgia, Mockingbird Books, 1975.

relevance to nurses who are caring for clients and families facing death is apparent.

NURSING PRACTICE—LEADERSHIP IN ACTION

Many courageous individuals have taken a nontraditional approach to the delivery of nursing care. Several of these people who have dared to try something different in the hope of better care for a greater number of people will be considered.

Innovators in Nursing Care

President Franklin Roosevelt brought the problem of infantile paralysis to national attention. There was increased interest in and funding for research for the prevention and treatment of this crippling disease.

Sister Elizabeth Kenny of Australia (Fig. 16–32) was known as a teacher of special forms of treatment for infantile paralysis. She is an example of a nurse who, in making a nursing diagnosis, made an important contribution to the care of many patients. An independent practitioner, she assessed the needs and plight of the patients who developed polio. In contrast to medical methods, her plan of nursing intervention involved the use of heat followed by passive and, later, active exercises. Strong nurturing skills emphasized the "caring with" aspect of nursing care. Her plan of care was based on scientific principles and careful consideration of the comfort of her patient. The heat treatments that she devised have been used for the relief of many patients and are known as the *Kenny treatments*. She accepted the challenge to aid victims of infantile paralysis, not by purposeful design but in response to a need that she alone could fulfill. She achieved remarkably successful results in contrast to the crippling effects of traditional medical treatment. The success of her nursing intervention was received at first with great hostility by many members of the medical profession. Eventually a Sister Kenny Institute was incorporated into health facilities in Minneapolis, Minnesota. A new and expanded Kenny Institute was opened on June 21, 1976.

Lydia Hall was the inspirational mover behind the philosophy and work of the *Loeb Center for Nursing and Rehabilitation* at Montefiore Hospital, which opened in 1963 (Fig. 16–33). At the dedication ceremonies on November 29, 1962, *Lucile Petry Leone*, Chief Nurse Officer, U.S. Public Health Service, commented, "This is forefront thinking of our century; this is innovation, experimentation, courageous embodiment in a living institution of a realistic dream of services for people." She concluded her speech by praising this institution, which exemplifies "dedication to restoration of each patient's fullest creative capacity—pa-

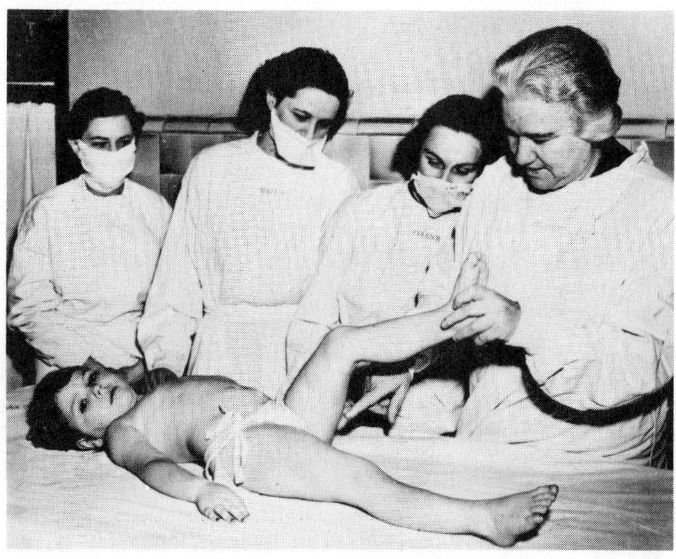

Figure 16–32. Sister Elizabeth Kenny demonstrating to other nurses the importance of muscle reeducation. (Courtesy of the *Minneapolis Star*.)

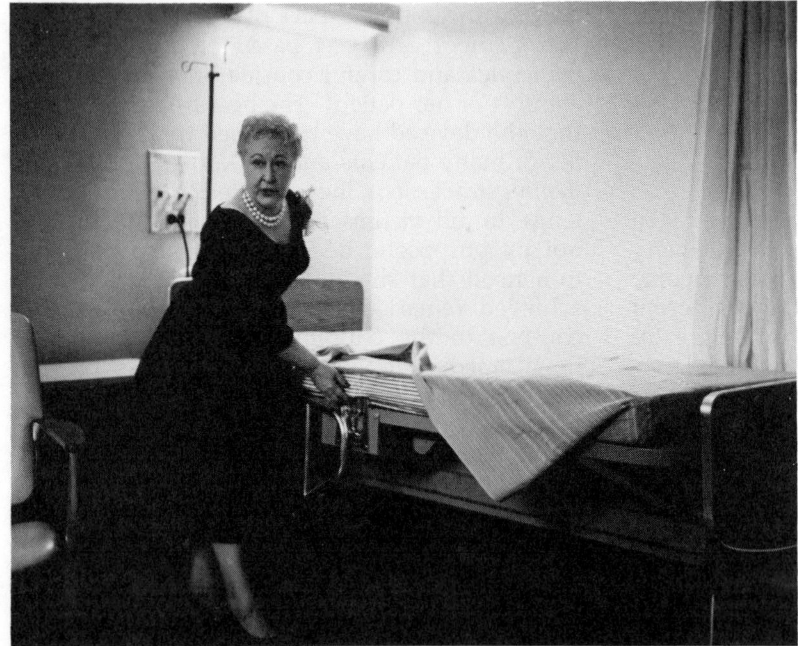

Figure 16–33. Mrs. Lydia Hall demonstrates the operation of a modern mechanized bed at the dedication ceremonies of the Loeb Center for Nursing and Rehabilitation in 1962. (Courtesy of Loeb Center for Nursing of Montefiore Hospital.)

tient by patient—through therapeutic nursing." The Loeb Center provides professional nursing service in an institutional setting that bridges the gap between the general hospital and the home. At Loeb, only professional nurses provide the nursing care. In the delivery of care, this nursing center is comparable to an extension of a community nursing service in an institutional setting. Mrs. Hall stated, "The nurse is the chief therapeutic agent and the final effector in providing interrelated patient care. Medicine and allied fields offer ancillary therapy." She also said: "At Loeb, the presumption is that, as he needs less medical care, he needs not only more nursing care, but more *professional* nursing care and teaching."

The patient, his family and the nurse analyze and solve those problems that must be tackled in order to achieve maximal health for the patient. The design of the building carries out Lydia Hall's philosophy of caring. The building contains the most modern equipment and allows for the most handicapped person to be comfortable and enjoy attractive surroundings. The design reflects the message of the staff: "We are with you in your efforts to gain health."[47] The distinguished director of the center, Lydia Hall, had a capable assistant who shared her dreams and goals and assisted in carrying them to fruition. *Genrose Alfano* (Fig. 16–34) succeeded her leader and has continued the direction of this famous center with great skill.

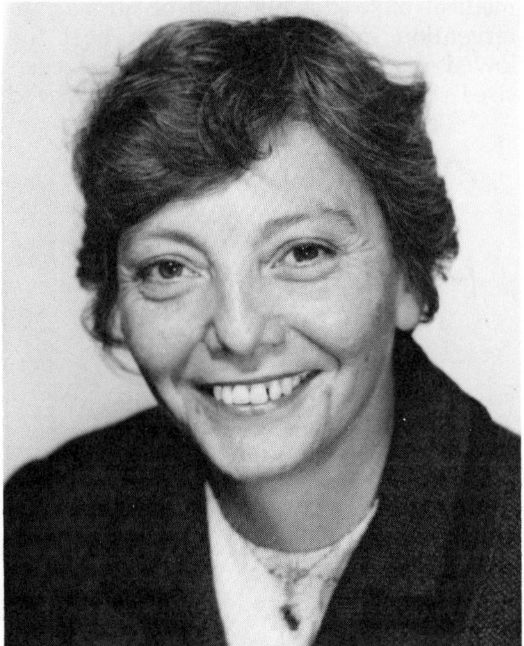

Figure 16–34. Gentrose J. Alfano, current director of Loeb Center for Nursing and Rehabilitation.

[47]Hall, Lydia E.: "A Center for Nursing," *Nursing Outlook*, Vol. 11, 1963.

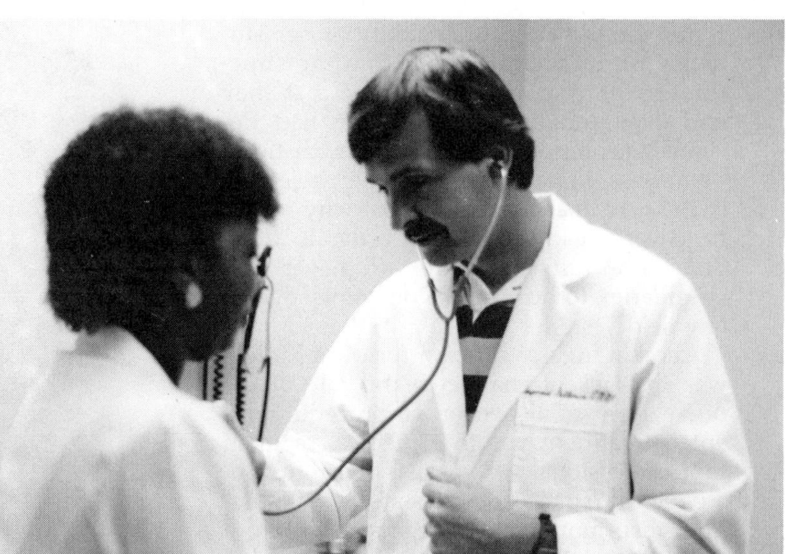

Figure 16–35. Raymond Fellows, M.S., Advanced Registered Nurse Practitioner, Certified Nurse Midwife, and officer of the United States Public Health Service, practices in Indiantown, Florida. He has been accorded hospital privileges at the Martin Memorial Hospital in Stuart, Florida. (Dolan collection.)

NURSES IN PRIMARY CARE

University programs have increased the numbers of well-qualified clinical specialists in order to enhance the delivery of nursing care. Many of these nurses have been attracted to the areas of *primary care.* In this area, the health care deliverer, who usually is the first member of the health care delivery system with whom the client has contact, retains primary responsibility for and provides for continuity in the care of the client throughout hospitalization or treatment. Primary care encourages the holistic approach.

In 1977, the role of the nurse in primary care was delineated in the film *Portrait of a Nurse.* This film describes the activities of *Jean Steele,* a nurse who takes full responsibility for a patient and responds to his health needs. This care includes client's participation. When the services of other health care providers are indicated, the client is referred to a physician, social worker, nutritionist or other person. The client returns to the nurse for continuance of care.

Some nurses in primary care participate in private practice, and some share private practice with a physician. Many states are providing *clinical privileges* for non-hospital-based nurses (Fig. 16–35).

M. Lucille Kinlein (Fig. 16–36), in hanging her shingle outside her office in May of 1971, identified herself as an *independent generalist nurse.* In addition to her independent practice, Miss Kinlein was a member of the faculty of Georgetown University School of Nursing.

Many frustrations and "irreconcilables,"

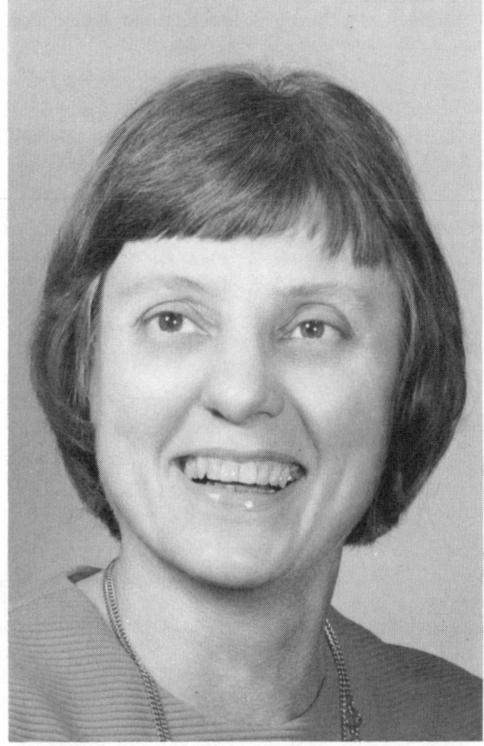

Figure 16–36. M. Lucille Kinlein, independent generalist nurse. (Dolan collection.)

a prime one being the inability of her students to practice nursing within the structure of the scientific framework that they had been taught and that they had designed, prompted her to break with tradition. Miss Kinlein described her objection to the perennial questions about why nurses need certain knowledge in order to function as a nurse: "There are never any boundaries to acquisition of knowledge in any field."[48]

Another area of concern for Miss Kinlein was the lack of change in the role of the nurse from a dispenser of procedure-oriented treatment within a medical regimen to a professional who assists the return of a patient to an acceptable state of wellness. The insurmountable pressures within a hospital structure frequently prevented the giving of the kind of nursing care that was needed. Only at great physical and emotional cost could the nurse give the kind of care that the patient needed. The nurse's lack of authority versus her responsibility prompted the decision that responsibility for *nursing* should require "control over what I did to achieve any nursing goals."

Another leader, *Dr. Dolores Krieger*, who is a professor of nursing at New York University, has focused her attention and skills on utilizing in practice the theory of *therapeutic touch* (Fig. 16–37). Certain aspects of this therapy have been recognized historically, and under her scientific and humanistic guidance, its significance in healing has been rediscovered.

Another remarkable personage is *Mother Teresa*, a Yugoslavian who gave up a comfortable teaching position in favor of ministering to the needs of lepers, cripples, dying derelicts, abandoned children and starving adults in troubled, underprivileged Calcutta (Fig. 16–38). Mother Teresa and the members of the nursing order she founded, the *Order of the Missionaries of Charity*, which was recognized as an order in 1960, are highly respected and loved. There are no religious barriers to the people for whom they care, as many patients are Moslem or Hindu in addition to Christian. The sisters wear a blue-edged white

[48]Kinlein, M. Lucille: "Independent Nurse Practitioner," *Nursing Outlook*, 20:22–24, 1972.

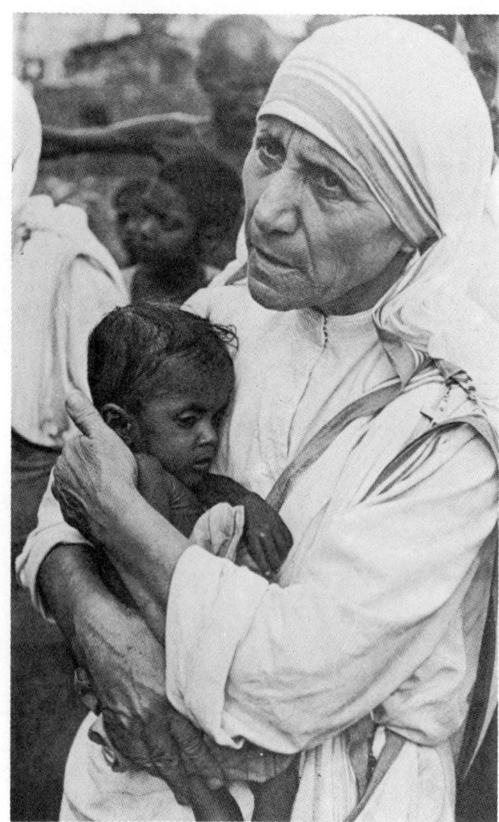

Figure 16–38. Mother Teresa shows loving concern for one of her precious patients. (Dolan collection.)

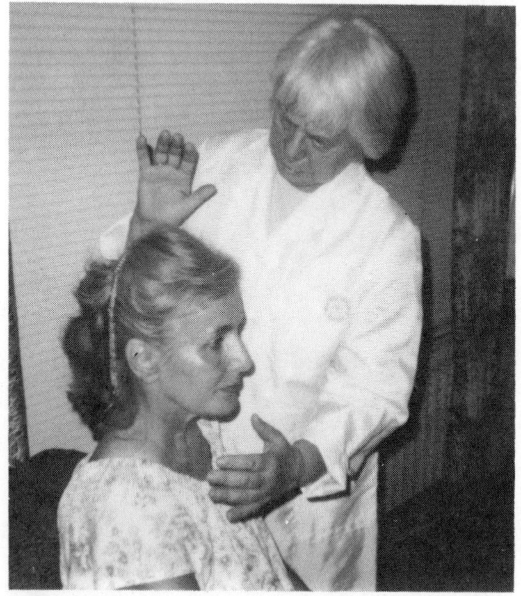

Figure 16–37. Dolores Krieger, Ph.D., treating her client with "therapeutic touch."

sari, modeled on the saris of the poor Indian women. They tend the poor in the streets, in their homes and in the hospices, which they have opened to care for children, the destitute, the dying and the lepers. The plight of the poor in India is reflected in the names given to the hospices: "Home for Dying Destitutes," and "Home for Sick, Crippled and Unwanted Children." Half of the patients have tuberculosis complicated by malnutrition. Life for these sisters is obviously precious, and its destruction by abortion or euthanasia is unacceptable to them.

Mother Teresa says to everyone, "Come do something for God," and she has hundreds of volunteers a day to assist her. Her community has expanded numerically and now has branches in Rome, Australia, Latin America and Holland. Mother Teresa was awarded the *Nobel Peace Prize* in 1980.

These leaders have reflected in action what Rozella Schlotfeldt has emphasized: "Nursing is health care." It is her contention that the "goal of nursing as a field of professional endeavor is to help people attain, retain and regain health. . . . Nurses must take primary responsibility for health care." She has summarized her charge to leaders of nursing:

> They must help students search for and find means to motivate persons to utilize their own resources to seek health—and these include teaching, counseling, stimulating, inquiring, and inspiring. Nurses must identify and explicate nursing therapies and teach their students to become proficient in sustaining, supporting, comforting, and helping persons during periods of infirmity, deprivation, disfigurement, changes in life style, crises, and periods of development and decline. Through compensating for an individual's inadequacies and adjusting his environmental circumstances, nurses must promote his motivation to seek health and his use of his own resources to attain, retain, or regain optimal health and function. Nursing, succinctly stated, is health care.[49]

RECOGNITION OF LEADERSHIP

Many nurses have been honored for their contributions to the health and welfare of others. One such person was *Lillian D. Wald*. It is gratifying to note and interesting to ponder the recognition she has received. As early as 1912, Mount Holyoke College awarded her the degree of Doctor of Laws, with the citation: "Lillian D. Wald, friend of those who need friends, originator of far-reaching municipal and national movements for the care of the sick and the poor and little children, a citizen of whom our greatest American city may be proud, we confer upon you the degree of Doctor of Laws and admit you to all its rights and privileges."

In 1913, Lillian Wald was awarded the medal of the National Institute of Social Sciences for "distinguished services rendered to humanity." In 1923, the Rotary Club of New York bestowed their first service medal "in recognition of her lifelong service to the world as sociologist, organizer and publicist." Miss Wald was referred to as a "student of the needs of the poor, organizer of agencies for better health, friend of the nurse, guardian and champion of the cause of childhood, and loving servant of needy humanity."

In 1926, *Better Times* magazine, a journal of sociology, presented her with a medal for distinguished social services because of her efforts to make public health nursing become "a vast city-wide, extra-mural hospital, the records of which constitute a valuable contribution to scientific knowledge."

In 1930, Smith College awarded her an honorary degree of Doctor of Laws with the citation: "Lillian D. Wald, founder and head of the Henry Street Settlement, organizer of district nursing, originator of the work of the School Nurse and of the Federal Children's Bureau, active supporter of all enlightened effort for the welfare of the community, internationally known as an indomitable fighter for justice, mercy and freedom."

Even in the United States Congressional Record of 1934, Lillian Wald received commendation: "Her vision and courage have been largely responsible for the legislation resulting in minimum wage, workmen's compensation, the protection of women and children in factories, and the abolition of child labor."

In 1937 Mayor La Guardia presented her with the Certificate for Distinguished Service to the City of New York with the com-

[49]Schlotfeldt, Rozella M.: "This I Believe—Nursing is Health Care," *Nursing Outlook, 20*:245–246, 1972.

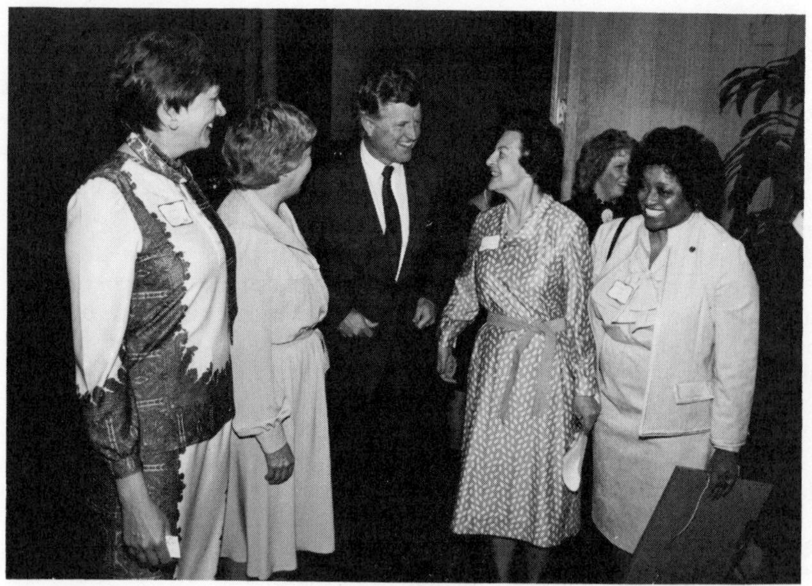

Figure 16–39. At the festivities of Nurse Recognition Day, nursing leaders took the opportunity to honor lawmakers who had been supportive of nursing. *Left to right:* Judith A. Yates, Executive Director of the American Nurses' Association, Billye J. Brown, President of the American Association of Colleges of Nursing, Senator Edward M. Kennedy, Elsa L. Brown, President of the National League for Nursing and Barbara Nichols, President of the American Nurses' Association. (Courtesy of National League for Nursing.)

ment: "I would not have wanted to assume the responsibilities of my office in 1933 if Lillian Wald had not pioneered in 1893."

On September 12, 1971, Lillian D. Wald received the highest tribute among a distinguished list of awards when she joined other outstanding Americans in the *Hall of Fame for Great Americans*. Her bust and tablet stand in the Colonnade at New York University. This accolade to a great person, a great leader and a great nurse can be shared by a profession of which she was proud.

A tribute to all nurses was celebrated on May 6, 1982, when President Ronald Reagan proclaimed that day to be *National Nurse Recognition Day*. In turn, the presidents of three national nursing organizations, the American Association of Colleges of Nursing, the ANA and the NLN, utilized the festivities in Washington to honor lawmakers who have been strong supporters of nursing in national legislative affairs (Fig. 16–39). The lawmakers honored were Senator Edward M. Kennedy, Massachusetts; Senator Lowell P. Weicker, Jr., Connecticut; Congresswoman Barbara A. Mikulski, Maryland; Congressman Carl D. Pursell, Michigan; and Congressman Henry A. Waxman, California.

In reviewing our historical heritage, we find that individual nurses have been applauded by having statues erected in their honor, by receiving professional recognition, military decorations, government awards, honorary doctoral degrees, and appointments or elections to high government positions and by having streets and mountains named for them. The profession as well as individuals have been honored through such acts as the issuance of commemorative postage stamps, the making of official proclamations and the designing of stained-glass windows and special chapels in their honor, as in Westminster Abbey.

The poet *Robert Frost* recorded his gratitude to his private duty nurse days before his death on January 29, 1963, in Peter Bent Brigham Hospital by writing his last poem in her honor. The first six lines were directed solely to her and the last four are from his "Dust of Snow."

> I met you on a cloudy
> dark day and when you
> smiled and spoke my
> room was filled with
> sunshine.
>
> The way you smiled at me
> Has given my heart a
> change of mood
> and saved some part
> of a day I had rued.

Nursing indeed possesses a rich historical heritage.

THE HERITAGE OF NURSING

The Image of the Profession of Nursing as a Social Force Must Be Maintained to Secure the Confidence and Support of the Public

1. The concern of the profession of nursing for the quality of its service constitutes the basis of its responsibility to the public and to its own profession.
   a. A profession must control its practice in order to guarantee the quality of its service.
   b. Accepted standards of practice must be implemented to assure that this guarantee is being met. The Standards of Nursing Practice, which were designed by nurses, encompass:
      (1) the collection of data about the health status of the client that is systematic and continuous (accessible, communicated and recorded).
      (2) nursing diagnoses derived from health status data.
      (3) nursing care plans based on goals derived from nursing diagnoses, including priorities and prescribed nursing approaches to achieve these goals.
      (4) nursing intervention that assists the client in achieving his maximum health potential.
      (5) evaluation of achievement of goals determined jointly by the client and nurse.
      (6) reassessment, reordering of priorities, new goal setting and revision of the plan of nursing care on the basis of this evaluation.
   c. Both the scope and theoretical basis of the nursing practice itself are changed as research findings warrant.
2. Nurses have received appreciation from clients and have been recognized publicly for notable achievements in nursing.
3. Nurses have endured in the face of obstacles and opposition.
4. Today the image of the professional nurse should reflect the reclamation of our lost role:
   a. To utilize in practice the scientific and humanistic basis of nursing, including efforts in health maintenance and use of nurturing skills, so completely that the artistic aspect of nursing reemerges.
   b. To regain freedom of action to design creative and innovative approaches for the delivery of nursing care.
   c. To contribute to better health care through independent/interdependent role collaboration.

Historically, nurses developed their role in antiquity and defined it in the last half of the twentieth century. There is a challenge now to build on this rich inheritance from professionally gifted ancestors, who were courageous, creative, competent, concerned and compassionate people.

Florence Nightingale's statement: "No system can endure that does not march . . . to stand still is to go backward" admonishes nurses to build on past achievements while using analytical skills creatively to develop new bodies of knowledge for the delivery of health care.

REFERENCE READINGS

Aiken, Linda: *Nursing in the 1980's: Crises, Opportunities, Challenges*. Philadelphia, J. B. Lippincott Co., 1982.

Amacher, Nancy Jean: "Touch is a Way of Caring," *American Journal of Nursing, 73*:852–854, 1973.

Barnett, Kathryn: "A Theoretical Construct of the Concepts of Touch As They Relate to Nursing," *Nursing Research, 31*:102–110, 1972.

Bowar-Ferres, Susan: "Loeb Center and Its Philosophy of Nursing," *American Journal of Nursing, 75*:810–815, 1975.

Brainard, Annie M.: *The Evolution of Public Health Nursing*. Philadelphia, W. B. Saunders Company, 1922.

Breckinridge, Mary: *Wide Neighborhood*. New York, Harper and Brothers, 1952.

Chayer, Mary Ella: *School Nursing*. New York, G. P. Putnam's Sons, 1937.

Christman, Luther: "Moral Dilemmas for Practitioners in a Changing Society," *Journal of Nursing Administration*, 1973.

Churchill, Fleetwood: *On the Theory and Practice of Midwifery*. Philadelphia, Blanchard and Lea, 1851.

Cohn, Victor: *Sister Kenny—the Woman Who Challenged the Doctors*. Minneapolis, University of Minnesota Press, 1975.

Curtin, Leah L.: "Human Values in Nursing," *Journal of the New York State Nurses' Association, 8*(4):31–40, 1977.

de Chardin, Pierre Teilhard: *The Phenomenon of Man*. New York, Harper and Brothers, 1959.

DeMaio, Dorothy: "The Born-Again Nurse," *Nursing Outlook, 27*:272–273, 1979.

Dubos, Rene: *So Human an Animal*. New York, Charles Scribner's Sons, 1968.

Duffs, R. L.: *Lillian Wald, Neighbor and Crusader*. New York, The Macmillan Co., 1938.

Forty-fifth Annual Report and Log 1915–1963 of the Maternity Center Association. New York, Maternity Center Association, 1964.

Gardner, Mary S.: *Public Health Nursing*. 3rd ed., New York, The Macmillan Co., 1936.

Gilbert, Ruth: *The Public Health Nurse and Her Patient*. New York, The Commonwealth Fund, 1940.

Goostray, Stella: *Fifty Years, A History of the School of Nursing. The Children's Hospital, Boston*. Boston, Alumnae Association of the Children's Hospital School of Nursing, 1940.

Hassenplug, Lulu W.: "Unified Action—Nursing's Ticket to Viability and Visibility in the 1980's," *The Journal of the New York State Nurses' Association, 8*(4):7–18, 1977.

Horn, Beverly M.: "Cultural Components and Postpartal Care," *Nursing and Health Care*, 2:516–517, 1981.

Jacox, Ada: "Address to the Next Generation," *Nursing Outlook, 26*:38–41, 1978.

Kinlein, M. Lucille: "The Self-Care Concept," *American Journal of Nursing, 77*:598–601, 1977.

Krieger, Dolores: "Therapeutic Touch: The Imprimatur of Nursing," *American Journal of Nursing, 75*:784–787, 1975.

Leahy, Kathleen, and Cobb, M. Marguerite: *Fundamentals of Public Health Nursing*. New York, McGraw-Hill Book Co., 1966.

Lubic, Ruth Watson: "Comprehensive Maternity Care as an Ambulatory Service—Maternity Center Association's Birth Alternative," *Journal of the New York State Nurses' Association, 8*(4):19–24, 1977.

McGrath, Bethel J.: *Nursing in Commerce and Industry*. New York, The Commonwealth Fund, 1946.

Morrissey, A. B.: *Rehabilitation Nursing*. New York, G. P. Putnam's Sons, 1951.

Mussallem, Helen K.: "The Changing Role of the Nurse," *American Journal of Nursing, 69*:514–517, 1969.

Oda, Dorothy S.: "A Viewpoint on School Nursing," *American Journal of Nursing, 81*:1677–1678, 1981.

Poole, Ernest: *Nurses on Horseback*. New York, The Macmillan Co., 1933.

Reid, Joseph, and Phillips, Maxine: "Child Welfare Since 1912," *Children Today, 0*:13–18, 1972.

Riehl, Joan P., and Roy, Sister Callista: *Conceptual Models for Nursing Practice*. New York, Appleton-Century-Crofts, 1974.

Robinson, Thelma: "School Nurse Practitioners on the Job," *American Journal of Nursing, 81*:1674–1676, 1981.

Russell, William Logie: *The New York Hospital—A History of the Psychiatric Service, 1771–1936*. New York, Columbia University Press, 1945.

Saunders, Dame Cicely, Summers, Dorothy H., and Teller, Neville: *Hospice: The Living Idea*. Philadelphia, W. B. Saunders Company, 1981.

Sheahan, Sister Dorothy: "Scanning the Seventies," *Nursing Outlook, 26*:33–37, 1978.

Smith, Shirley P., Jepson, Virginia, and Perloff, Evelyn: "Attitudes of Nursing Care Providers Toward Elderly Patients," *Nursing aad Health Care, 3*:93–98, 1982.

Stewart, Isabel M., and Austin, Anne L.: *A History of Nursing*. New York, G. P. Putnam's Sons, 1962.

Struthers, Lina Rogers: *The School Nurse*. New York, G. P. Putnam's Sons, 1917.
Styles, Margretta M.: "Dialogue Across the Decades," *Nursing Outlook, 26*:28–32, 1978.
Tinkham, Catherine, and Voorhees, Eleanor: *Community Health Nursing—Evolution and Process*. New York, Appleton-Century-Crofts, 1972.
Wald, Lillian D.: *The House on Henry Street*. New York, Henry Holt and Company, 1915.
Wales, Marguerite: *The Public Health Nurse in Action*. New York, The Macmillan Co., 1969.
Waters, Ysabella: *Visiting Nursing in the United States*. New York, Charities Publication Committee, 1909.

INDEX

Page numbers in *italics* indicate illustrations. Page numbers followed by t indicate tables.